Human Communication Disorders

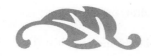

Human Communication Disorders

An Introduction

Eighth Edition

Noma B. Anderson

University of Tennessee Health Science Center, Memphis

George H. Shames

University of Pittsburgh, Emeritus

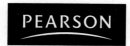

Boston   Columbus   Indianapolis   New York   San Francisco   Upper Saddle River
Amsterdam   Cape Town   Dubai   London   Madrid   Milan   Munich   Paris   Montreal   Toronto
Delhi   Mexico City   São Paulo   Sydney   Hong Kong   Seoul   Singapore   Taipei   Tokyo

Vice President and Editor in Chief: Jeffery W. Johnston

Executive Editor and Publisher: Stephen D. Dragin

Editorial Assistant: Jamie Bushell

Vice President, Director of Marketing: Margaret Waples

Senior Marketing Manager: Christopher D. Barry

Senior Managing Editor: Pamela D. Bennett

Senior Project Manager: Linda Hillis Bayma

Senior Operations Supervisor: Matthew Ottenweller

Senior Art Director: Diane Lorenzo

Cover Designer: Jason Moore

Cover Art: SuperStock

Full-Service Project Management: Chitra Ganesan/PreMediaGlobal

Composition: PreMediaGlobal

Printer/Binder: Courier Kendallville, Inc.

Cover Printer: Lehigh Phoenix Color/Hagerstown

Text Font: Minion

Credits and acknowledgments borrowed from other sources and reproduced, with permission, in this textbook appear on appropriate page within text.

Every effort has been made to provide accurate and current Internet information in this book. However, the Internet and information posted on it are constantly changing, so it is inevitable that some of the Internet addresses listed in this textbook will change.

Chapter Opener Photo Credits: Katelyn Metzger/Merrill, p. 1; Barbara Schwartz/Merrill, p. 16; istockphoto.com, pp. 54, 110, 164, 305, 380, 469; Comstock Images/Thinkstock Royalty Free, p. 84; Laura Bolesta/Merrill, p. 132; National Institutes of Health, p. 202; George Dodson/PH College, p. 238; Studi-Oh Medical Art/PH College, p. 272; Creatas/Thinkstock Royalty Free, pp. 331, 361; Scott Cunningham/Merrill, p. 406; Tom Wilcox/Merrill, p. 440; Bob Daemmrich/Bob Daemmrich Photography, Inc., p. 501.

Library of Congress Cataloging-in-Publication Data

Human communication disorders : an introduction / [edited by] Noma B. Anderson, George H. Shames.—8th ed.

    p. cm.

    ISBN-13: 978-0-13-706133-4

    ISBN-10: 0-13-706133-1

  1. Communicative disorders.   I. Shames, George H.   II. Anderson, Noma B.   III. Title.

RC423.H847 2011

362.196'855—dc22

2010019210

10 9 8 7 6 5 4 3 2 1

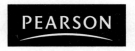

www.pearsonhighered.com

ISBN-13: 978-0-13-706133-4

ISBN-10:   0-13-706133-1

Contents

PART TWO

Disorders of Speech

CHAPTER SIX

Articulatory and Phonological Disorders
Richard G. Schwartz and Klara Marton   132

CHAPTER SEVEN

Stuttering and Other Disorders of Fluency
Peter R. Ramig and Ryan Pollard   164

PART THREE

Disorders of Language

CHAPTER ELEVEN

Developmental Language Impairment During the Preschool Years

Catherine K. Bacon and M. Jeanne Wilcox   305

CHAPTER TWELVE

Language Disabilities in School-Age Children and Youth

Barbara Culatta and Elisabeth Wiig   331

CHAPTER THIRTEEN

From Emergent Literacy to Literacy: Development and Disorders

CHAPTER FOURTEEN

Aphasia and Related Acquired Language Disorders

CHAPTER FIFTEEN

Augmentative and Alternative Communication

Kathleen A. Kangas and Lyle L. Lloyd   406

PART FOUR

Disorders of Swallowing

CHAPTER SIXTEEN

Swallowing: Process and Disorders

Barbara C. Sonies   440

Preface

The purpose of the eighth edition of *Human Communication Disorders: An Introduction* is to lead you into an exploration of the discipline of human communication and communication disorders and the professions of audiology, speech-language pathology, and speech, language, and hearing sciences. As editors, we continue to be proud that your guides for this exploratory journey are the authors who have contributed to *Human Communication Disorders: An Introduction*, each a leading authority in his or her area of practice and research. As you begin your journey to become an audiologist, a speech-language pathologist, or a speech, language, hearing scientist, *Human Communication Disorders: An Introduction* will guide you into the extraordinary breadth of the discipline.

New to This Edition

The eighth edition has focused on making the style and content of the chapters more student friendly, while continuing to impart up-to-date research and evidence-based clinical practice information.

- The language of the chapters is more student friendly.
- The definition and discussion of evidence-based practice have been expanded to include client expectations and decision making, in addition to existing research findings and clinician experience.
- The authors discuss the most relevant current research that has been published.
- Websites of interest have been updated.
- Cultural and linguistic diversity is infused throughout the chapters.
- Evidence-based practice discussions have increased in the clinically oriented chapters.

About This Book

In many ways, audiology, speech-language pathology, and speech, language, and hearing sciences are unique. These are relatively young professions that are continually evolving. This evolution comes from advances in research and in evidence-based practice occurring both within the discipline and in other disciplines such as psychology, neuroanatomy, neurophysiology, education, genetics, linguistics, engineering, medical research, ethics, and human growth and development. The significant influences of these other disciplines make human communication sciences and disorders unique by being a truly interdisciplinary subject. As you read this text, in pursuit of greater understanding about the discipline, you will realize the influences of these related disciplines.

Another unique quality of human communication sciences and disorders is that audiology, speech-language pathology, and speech, language, and hearing sciences are rewarding professions. Tremendous pride is felt by those who conduct the research and provide the clinical service that improve the quality of life for those who are faced with communication problems. Our professions are also unique because they cover the entire human life span. Additionally, professionals in this discipline have the opportunity to explore an interesting diversity of options. Over the course of one's professional life, one can work in many different settings, with individuals with different types of communication disorders, and with individuals of differing ages. These settings include public and private schools, day-care centers, rehabilitation centers, hospitals, nursing homes, hospices, colleges and universities, private practice, and patients' homes. This eighth edition of *Human Communication Disorders: An Introduction* presents these unique qualities of the professions. We have tried to blend the various parts of our professions into a cohesive picture of a complex discipline.

This text is for the beginner who may be a communication sciences and disorders student or a student curious about the discipline, but very well may be a special educator, a classroom teacher, a school principal, a hospital administrator, a rehabilitation professional, or a parent. As the editors, we have sustained the depth of scholarship of the contributors that has characterized the previous seven editions and have maintained the overall introductory level of the text. We hope the textbook will also help readers become informed citizens, whatever their profession.

Within this eighth edition of *Human Communication Disorders: An Introduction*, the first chapter introduces the concept that these professions are based on service. In the first chapter, various *wh-* questions are addressed: Who is served? What services are provided? Where are services provided? When are services provided? How are services provided? And even: Why serve? This last question involves discussion of evidence-based practice, an intersection of research and clinical practice and patient values and beliefs.

Organization of This Text

Three features are presented throughout the chapters in this eighth edition: cultural and linguistic diversity, evidence-based practice, and case studies. This edition is divided into five major parts. Following the introductory chapter, Part I covers normal aspects of human communication and provides information about theoretical and scientific principles that underlie the communication process. Parts 2 through 5 cover the disorder categories. Part 2 presents disorders of speech, Part 3 discusses disorders of language, Part 4 explores disorders of swallowing, and Part 5 analyzes disorders of hearing. Each chapter places the disorders in perspective, discusses basic theories of causation, introduces identifying characteristics, and presents an overview of procedures for evaluation and treatment. Although we have divided the disorders of human communication into these disorder categories (i.e., speech, language, swallowing, hearing), such a presentation loses the very real perspective that there are seldom distinct separations among communication disorders. Speech disorders can have co-occurring involvement of disabled language, hearing disorders can affect speech and language development, and very often, individuals present with more than one disorder category.

Each chapter begins with personal perspectives of the authors in which they discuss how and why they became interested in pursuing a career in communication disorders. Our thinking is that it may be enlightening, as you begin your study of this discipline, to learn how leading authorities made decisions similar to those that you are presently making. The chapters also present concrete, real-life case studies to help you better understand some of the human, social, and emotional aspects of the content of the chapter. Additionally, most chapters provide study questions for your review as well as a list of related readings.

Human communication and its disorders are part of the overall human experience. Each of us exists as a uniquely synthesized unit. The momentary focus by *Human Communication Disorders: An Introduction* on separate aspects of communication in separate chapters reflects our own attempt to analyze a complex process in order to try to understand it. But when we communicate, the body and mind respond together as a unit; it is this synthesis that we are concerned with in this text.

It is also recognized that this mind-body synthesis functions in a multicultural environment. Each of the various cultures represented in our communities brings a unique history and a set of values, mores, and beliefs, as well as linguistic variations that could influence how we deal with specific communication issues and problems. Perceptions and evaluations of the definition of "normal" versus "abnormal" communication may vary from culture to culture, as may the means of addressing communication disorders. Therefore, diagnosis and treatment need to be influenced by the cultural background of the individual. The contributing authors include discussions of cultural and linguistic diversity in their chapters.

Acknowledgments

Throughout the publication history of *Human Communication Disorders: An Introduction*, the authors of the chapters have all been recognized experts. We are delighted that so many of these authors have continued with us. We want to welcome the new author and coauthors who have contributed to the eighth edition: Shawna M. Dell, Ann W. Kummer, Klara Marton, Ryan Pollard, and Bari Hoffman Ruddy. We would also like to thank the following reviewers of this edition for their time and input: Anthony DeFeo, University of Arizona; Diane Ferrand, University of Nebraska, Lincoln; Jo Shackelford, Western Kentucky University; and Helen Sharp, Western Michigan University.

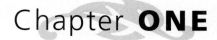

Chapter ONE

Introduction

*Human Communication Disorders:
A Philosophy and Practice of Science
in Service*

Noma B. Anderson
University of Tennessee Health Science Center, Memphis

Shelly Chabon
Portland State University

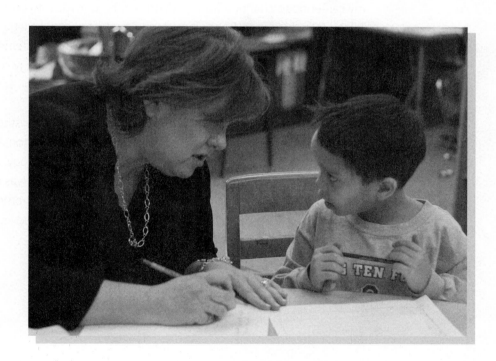

personal PERSPECTIVE

NOMA ANDERSON

Helen Keller was a national hero in the 1950s, when I grew up. There were lots of media stories about her, and quite often Ms. Keller would be interviewed. There she would be, on my black-and-white television, communicating—this extraordinary individual who was both blind and deaf. Long before the play and movie *The Miracle Worker,* I knew I was looking at a miracle. Beside her, facilitating her communication, was her teacher, Annie Sullivan. Of course, I admired and was awed by Helen Keller. However, I was intrigued by her teacher. How did she teach this extraordinary person to do such an extraordinary thing as to communicate? The teacher must be as exceptional as the student. From watching Helen Keller on television on numerous occasions, I wanted to be an Annie Sullivan. I recall being delighted when I learned the teacher's name—Sullivan. I was young when I became inspired by Annie Sullivan and Helen Keller. In fact, for years I had forgotten my impressions about this dynamic teacher–student dyad.

As I matriculated through elementary school, and junior high, and senior high, my career goals changed from pediatrician, to journalist, to clinical psychologist. Taking Introduction to Psychology during my first year in college was depressing for me because the spark I had anticipated didn't happen. I remembered my early interest and thought I would try a speech-language pathology course. I found the spark! It was 1967 when I became a speech correction major at the University of North Carolina at Greensboro.

I completed my undergraduate education at Hampton Institute, where I gained tremendous educational experiences and support. At Hampton, I was exposed to a broad foundation in speech-language pathology and audiology; I was exposed to the growing corpus of information of sociolinguistics; and I was encouraged by the department chair, Robert Screen, to earn my doctorate and return to Hampton to teach. What a vision statement for a young 21-year-old—become a faculty member in speech-language pathology at my alma mater. I did!

personal PERSPECTIVE

SHELLY CHABON

I literally stumbled upon the profession of speech-language pathology. While running to a sophomore English literature class, I tripped over some CSD brochures that had been tossed into the middle of the hallway. Although not a student of Freudian theory, I decided that this was no mere accident. I arranged to observe a few therapy sessions in the university clinic. I knew very little about the field at that time other than it was where I belonged. So it seems this day marked me for life. I had fallen for speech-language pathology in a big way.

Through this profession I have met many lifelong friends (including my husband and the coauthor of this chapter); learned, relearned, and unlearned a great deal; and grown wiser because of the lessons taught to me by my students and by the children with communication disorders and their families that I have been fortunate enough to serve. Recently, I came across my well-worn copies of the very same brochure that precipitated my interest in Communication Sciences and Disorders. Thirty years later I can honestly say that I have never regretted that serendipitous fall that led me down this rewarding career path.

We can fix without serving. And we can help without serving. And we can serve without fixing or helping. . . . fixing and helping may often be the work of the ego, and service the work of the soul.

Rachel Remen (1996)

In our experience, when students are asked why they became interested in the professions of audiology and speech-language pathology, the overwhelming response relates to a desire to help others. That is, they are "called" to this work because it provides an opportunity to use their special interests and skills to serve those in need (Sutherland-Cornett & Chabon, 1988). In Remen's discussion of the acts of serving and helping, she contends that *helping* reflects a relationship between two unequal partners because it implies that you "use your own strength to assist or support those who are weaker, and therefore may inadvertently take away from people more than we could ever give them." In contrast, *serving* is viewed as a balanced or equitable connection between individuals. Importantly, Remen observes that helping provides a feeling of satisfaction for the caregiver but serving results in a feeling of gratitude for all involved. That is, "our service serves us as well as others." As a physician and an individual with a chronic illness, she reminds us that "fixing and helping are the basis of curing, but not of healing... only service heals." This idea of serving is common to many definitions of audiology and speech-language pathology and is the theoretical concept that inspired this text. Phrases that are used by these professionals to describe their clinical practice are clinical *services, service* delivery, rehabilitative *services*, audiological *services*, and health *care*. There are many other students who, when asked what brought them to the professions, will answer that it was the expanse of the unknown, the unconfirmed, or the theoretical that motivated them, in addition to the desire to help. Individuals with language, speech, or hearing disabilities benefit substantially from the *services* provided by audiologists, speech-language pathologists, and speech-language-hearing scientists (Powers, 2000).

Audiology and speech-language pathology are two distinct service professions that are closely related. The nature of the close relationship is that they address the needs of individuals with communication disorders. Over the eons of time as humans and animals have coexisted, humans have prided themselves, have actually defined their humanness, in contrast to other species in the animal kingdom, by recognition of the existence of *language and communication*. Biologists have volumes of fascinating research studies that explore the presence and extent of animal—that is, nonhuman—communication. As fascinating as the studies are, and as sophisticated as the research findings are, apparently no animal species possesses the elaborate communication system that exists within the *Homo sapiens* species. Interpersonal communication, which occurs countless times a day, is a rather complex, primarily human, phenomenon. For example, Paul and Lourdes are discussing a movie that Lourdes is recommending that Paul see. Lourdes has an idea that she mentally converts into words and sentences. Psycholinguists refer to this cognitive process as **encoding**. The brain sends forth a motor message to the articulators (e.g., tongue, lips, teeth, soft palate), and Lourdes produces consonants and vowels in sequences that express her thoughts about the movie. The product of Lourdes's articulation is a series of acoustic signals that go out into the air and are captured and received by Paul's hearing mechanism. The acoustic signals continue along Paul's auditory transmission path to his brain, where the signals are perceived as, or interpreted into, words and sentences. Voila!—Paul has received and has perceived the message that originated with Lourdes; Paul decides to see the movie. Psycholinguists refer to the cognitive processing by which Paul was capable of receiving words and sentences and transforming them into a message with meaning as **decoding**. This processing is rather magical. Effective communication involves physical, acoustic, cognitive, linguistic, psychological, cultural, and social aspects. This is a simplistic description of the very complicated communication process. Also noteworthy is that one's gender, age, culture, ethnicity, life experiences, geography, educational level, socioeconomic level, and even occupation shape one's communication. What is perhaps most remarkable is that we learn to communicate at all and that more of us do not have communication disorders.

Who Is Served?

. . . our service serves us as well as others.

Individuals with Communication Problems

Audiology and speech-language pathology are person centered, and the persons served are many and diverse. Approximately one out of eight to ten individuals, or 46 million Americans, has communication disorders. These individuals may present a few or many abilities or disabilities and can be of any age, race, gender, sexual orientation, language, ethnic, religious, occupational, and socioeconomic group and from all geographic areas. Each person with a communication disorder is a unique combination of his or her culture, heredity, and environment. Regardless of the diagnostic label, or the severity or longevity of the speech, language, or hearing problem, the child or adult, patient or client with a communication disorder drives our service.

Over the years, the language used to describe our patients has changed to reflect our person-centered perspective on service. In the past, it was customary to refer to "anaphasic adult" or "a cerebral palsied child." Today we say instead "an adult with aphasia" or "a child with cerebral palsy." The impact of the difference is that the person is presented first, then the diagnosis. This is not just a semantic distinction; it is a philosophical orientation.

Those Interested in Serving Individuals with Communication Disorders

Audiologists and speech-language pathologists are independent and autonomous health professionals. This means that audiological services and speech-language pathology services do not need to be authorized by another professional, such as a physician. Multidisciplinary teaming, however, is an important venue for clinical practice. To ensure that patients are being treated in a holistic manner, it is often important and appropriate for speech-language pathologists and audiologists to work with other professionals. In schools, we work collaboratively with parents and guardians, classroom teachers, reading teachers, learning disability teachers, counselors, school psychologists, physical therapists, occupational therapists, ESL teachers, and social workers. In health care facilities, we work with patients' families and on multidisciplinary teams with respiratory therapists, physical therapists, occupational therapists, physicians, nutritionists, dentists, recreational therapists, nurses, case managers, and social workers.

Our Professional Service Community

The American Speech-Language-Hearing Association (ASHA) is the professional, scientific, and credentialing organization of over 135,000 audiologists, speech-language pathologists, and speech-language-hearing scientists. ASHA provides standards of professional practice and ethical conduct; publishes professional journals, accreditation standards for colleges and universities with communication sciences and disorders programs, and certification standards for individuals practicing the professions; promotes research initiatives; addresses workplace issues; lobbies federal and state governments for the benefit of our consumers and our professionals; recruits members into the professions; informs the public about the value of our professions; and addresses the challenges and needs of culturally diverse patients with disabilities and families, professionals, and students.

The National Student Speech, Language, and Hearing Association (NSSLHA) is a pre-professional membership association for students interested in the study of communication sciences and disorders. Membership in NSSLHA is available to undergraduate, graduate, and doctoral students enrolled full- or part-time in a communication sciences program or related major (www.nsshla.org).

The American Academy of Audiology (AAA) is an organization of and for audiologists. AAA has a membership of more than 11,000 audiologists and promotes quality hearing and balance care by advancing the profession of audiology through leadership, advocacy, education, public awareness, and support of research (www.audiology.org).

What Services Are Provided?

Speech-language pathologists and audiologists provide many types of clinical services. Audiologists provide diagnostic and treatment services to individuals who have hearing and balance problems. Speech-language pathologists assess and treat articulation, language, cognitive, communication, voice, fluency, and swallowing disorders. They also conduct research, teach, administer, and design or develop treatment and evaluation materials.

The "Scope of Practice in Audiology" (ASHA, 2004d) and the "Scope of Practice in Speech-Language Pathology" (ASHA, 2007) are two important reference documents that delineate the services that audiologists and speech-language pathologists perform. The services that audiologists perform include the following:

- Prevention of hearing loss and protection of hearing function
- Identification of dysfunction in hearing, balance, and related systems
- Assessment
- Rehabilitation
- Advocacy
- Consultation Education
- Research

Similarly, services that speech-language pathologists provide include the following:

- Prevention and pre-referral for disorders of speech (articulation, fluency, resonance, voice), language, cognition, feeding, and swallowing
- Screening
- Assessment/evaluation
- Consultation
- Diagnosis
- Treatment, intervention, and management
- Counseling
- Collaboration
- Documentation
- Referral

All of the above activities have the potential of making a difference for those we serve.

Where Are Services Provided?

One attractive characteristic of audiology and speech-language pathology is that they afford service providers the chance to work in any number of settings. You can find audiologists and speech-language pathologists working in schools, hospitals, clinics, rehabilitation centers, government agencies, nursing care facilities, research laboratories, and private practice. Most audiologists and speech-language pathologists provide direct clinical services in these settings. We work one-on-one and with groups of patients; we work in clinic offices, at bedsides, in classrooms, in therapy rooms, in patients' homes, in audiological booths, and in research labs.

Such a wide array of work settings offers both an opportunity and a challenge. We encourage you to acquire the knowledge and skills necessary to succeed in varied clinical settings. Many students enter graduate school with preconceived ideas about the type of setting in which they want to work upon graduation. Other students are interested in one type of setting, but once exposed to new and varied clinical settings may change their minds and choose to work in a different type of facility. This second scenario occurs quite frequently. Opportunities for audiologists and speech-language pathologists seem endless and are limited only by your individual preference and place of residence. Through corporate firms that hire rehabilitation specialists, there are possibilities for speech-language pathologists who want to travel to live and work in different cities and towns, nationally and internationally. The breadth and depth of graduate education in audiology and speech-language pathology, and national certification and state licensure standards, make changing employment settings or working in different settings possible.

When Are Services Provided?

Audiology and speech-language pathology services are initiated by referrals. Sometimes a patient refers herself, or a parent schedules an appointment for a child, or a physician refers a patient. In the schools, it is usually the classroom teacher who begins the referral process. In all these instances, there are questions and concerns, such as the following:

- Whether the person is hearing as well as he should be
- Whether the person's speech is as fluent as it can be
- Whether the child's vocabulary and sentences are as mature as they should be given the child's age
- Whether the person experiences vocal fatigue near the end of the day and is unable to produce voice any louder than a whisper
- Whether the person has difficulty swallowing
- Whether the person has had a stroke and has difficulty speaking and/or understanding others' communications
- Whether the student has difficulty with the language skills required for successful learning, such as speaking, reading, spelling, and writing passages
- Whether the child's motor development makes oral speech too difficult a task and is not understood by others
- Whether the individual is experiencing tinnitus (ringing in her ears) or vertigo (dizziness) or balance problems
- Whether the person has developed a habitually hoarse voice, has developed growths such as polyps or nodules on his vocal folds, or the like

Any of these circumstances may prompt the need for speech/language and hearing evaluations. The outcomes of these evaluations determine a diagnosis, usually the etiology or cause of the communication problem, and recommendations for speech, language, and hearing rehabilitation, if and when speech, language, and hearing services are appropriate.

One professional responsibility is the determination of whether an individual is presenting with a communication difference, not a communication disorder (refer to Chapter 4 in this text). When the person has acquired a language or dialect and is from a cultural background different from and unfamiliar to the speech-language pathologist, misdiagnoses and inappropriate professional practices can occur. Therefore, speech and language evaluations, the determination of whether speech and language treatment is needed, and speech and language intervention should be attempted with an understanding of the individual's culture and the communication standards for the cultural group. Each of the chapters in this text addresses the multicultural issues to be considered when working with patients from culturally and linguistically diverse backgrounds with communication disorders and their families.

If a person is learning English as her second language, instances of speech sound production and sentence formation, and rules of interpersonal exchanges, may differ from how communication occurs in the United States by individuals whose first language is American English. All of us develop the speech sound and syntactical rules of our communication community. A pattern of communication is not considered a disorder when communication differences are based on a person's first language or home dialect. One of the editors of this text is from North Carolina, where it is not a communication disorder for *pen* and *pin* to be pronounced the same way. One of the editors lives in Pittsburgh, Pennsylvania, where it is not a communication disorder for the plural pronoun *you* to be pronounced as *yence*. If a family has immigrated from Spain, depending upon the dialect of Spanish spoken, it may not be a lisp or an articulation disorder for its members to pronounce the *s* sound as a *th* sound. Communication differences are not communication disorders and are addressed quite differently than are communication disorders. Thus, for example, if a student has decided to seek professional assistance in order to learn English as her second or third language, the speech-language pathologist could facilitate this process, or work collaboratively with the student's classroom teacher and ESL teacher, and communicate with her family. *Language/communication education* is the process undertaken, not *communication therapy or treatment.* It is the speech-language pathologist who plays a primary role in determining when services are necessary.

If a young woman is concerned about her ability to comfortably use the speech patterns, syntax, and style of speech associated with Standard American English because she speaks a vernacular dialect of American English referred to as African American English Vernacular, she may decide to contact a speech-language pathologist. Speech-language pathologists recognize the linguistic integrity of dialects and recognize that all languages have dialects, which are rule-governed varieties of a language. A speech-language pathologist may facilitate a communication education process for this individual by clarifying those situations in which vernacular varieties of English are appropriate and situations where a standard variety of English would be appropriate, using strategies referred to as contrastive analysis. By using this strategy, the speech-language pathologist has the young woman listen to and produce, in a contrastive manner, both dialects. The Standard English dialect is most effectively taught to motivated individuals who are eager to learn more about the various patterns of English spoken in our country and to learn the appropriate use of these communication varieties. The speech-language pathologist recognizes the value of being both multilingual and multidialectal. The speech-language pathologist understands both when and how to assist an individual in using his first and second dialects or languages.

How Are Services Provided?

There are probably as many different approaches to serving those who need to and wish to change, improve, and/or control their communication or to improve their swallow and avoid aspirating as there are service providers. Treatment may take the form of specific programs, drills, and exercises; play activities and storytelling; interactive computer programs; head and body positioning; muscle relaxation or manipulation; multisensory stimulation; or counseling and guidance. Services may be provided following or in conjunction with surgery or medical or dental treatment. The speech-language pathologist and audiologist may utilize methods including augmentative and alternative communication and manual or total communication. Speech-language pathologists and audiologists may employ indirect approaches to work with the individual with the communication disorder, or indirect approaches may be used to educate, train, and counsel the family members and friends and/or staff to address the communication disorder. Some approaches are designed for children, whereas others are appropriate for adults. Treatment may be conducted on an individual basis (one speech-language pathologist or audiologist to one individual with a communication disorder) or in small or large groups; it may be offered at the educational or clinical setting and/or in natural settings such as the classroom or at home. Sessions may be conducted as often as every day or scheduled less regularly and may vary in length from 15 minutes to several hours. The variety of treatment options available suggests that no single method is appropriate for all individuals with communication disorders.

Professional audiological and speech-language pathology services may even be delivered via telecommunications technology (ASHA, 2005a, 2005c). This type of clinical practice is being referred to as *telehealth* or *telepractice*. Consultation, assessment, and intervention services can be delivered across distances by linking clinician to clinician, and clinician to patient. The rationale is that clinical services can be extended to the hard-to-reach and underserved who are often located in rural and remote locales. Telepractice addresses issues of access created by distance from available services, unavailability of specialists, and inadequate mobility.

Determinations about how service should be provided must be based on sound scientific evidence. Lubinski and Frattali (2001) describe evidence-based practice as the application of research (scientific evidence) to clinical decision making. Speech-language pathologists and audiologists consult available literature and utilize objective information to clarify and classify the communication problem and to support or validate the approaches taken to treatment. Dollaghan (2004) strongly advocates that there are two components to evidence-based practice. One component is the conscientious use of the best current research and information about the care of individual patients; the second component comes from the clinician's clinical expertise and experience. Thus, evidence-based practice is determined by the integration of clinical expertise with the best available clinical and scientific research. A third component of evidence-based practice is the views, values & beliefs of the client.

Evaluation is the first step in treatment and is systematically repeated throughout this process to identify and describe the individual's strengths and weaknesses, determine the nature and type of communication disorder, establish goals, and provide a preservice measure of the effectiveness of treatment. We serve those with communication disorders by helping them to appreciate and optimize existing communication skills, develop new skills, and reduce their communication difficulties and any negative effects these difficulties may have on their self-image, personal interactions, academic performance, and/or employment productivity.

Although the methods and format used to provide therapy may vary, what is common to all of our services is the level of importance attributed to the relationship between the individuals with communication disorders and their service providers. A relationship built on mutual respect and trust is crucial in speech-language pathology and audiology. The presence of a communication disorder involves recognition of attitudes and behaviors that create difficulties for and concerns about the individual with communication problems. The vulnerabilities that may be felt are personal and individual, so that even two people with the same or similar communication disorder will have different responses to the same treatment. It is through the relationships we build with these individuals that we understand the origin and nature of their communicative difficulties and ultimately select how best to serve them. Because of the important responsibility to ensure trust and respect in our professional relationships, we speech-language pathologists and audiologists have come to guide ourselves by the ASHA Code of Ethics. The Code of Ethics empowers speech-language pathologists and audiologists by describing the principles that direct our work and the rules, or specific statements, of what we can and cannot do to maintain the highest standards of professional conduct.

How we serve is a complicated and challenging process because it embraces a number of aspects of what people are about and because it is based on both evidence and inference about communication disorders. There are times when the speech-language pathologist or audiologist functions as a teacher, or a source of information, and other times when he or she may be a behavioral reinforcer, and still other times a listener or a counselor. The gratification that follows from serving others in our many roles as speech-language pathologists and audiologists is more than sufficient reward.

Service and Science: How? How Fast? How Often? How Much?

The use of evidence in clinical decision making, although historically important in principle, has now become central to our professional practice. In 2004, ASHA established a Joint Coordinating Committee on Evidence-Based Practice. In its official policy, this group proposed that audiologists and speech-language pathologists integrate the principles of evidence-based practice (EBP) into the clinical process (ASHA, 2005b). That same year ASHA adopted a new set of standards for clinical certification in speech-language pathology that went into effect in 2006, and in 2008, new standards became effective in audiology. Included in these certification documents is the stipulation that "the applicant (for certification) must demonstrate knowledge of processes used in research and in the integration of research principles into evidence-based clinical practice" (ASHA, 2004a, p. 6).

Inherent in the concepts of EBP and practice-based evidence (PBE) is an appreciation of the need for a combination of clinical judgments *and* clinical data. ASHA (2004b) defines EBP as "the integration of (a) clinical expertise, (b) best current evidence, and (c) client values to provide high-quality services reflecting the interests, values, needs and choices of the individuals we serve." PBE, on the other hand, refers to "a systematic collection of data about client progress, generated during treatments, to enhance the quality and outcome of care" (Burlingame, 2007). Lemoncello and Fanning (2008) view PBE as a subcomponent of EBP and suggest that each complements the other.

The privilege of serving individuals with communication disorders carries with it the responsibility to apply science to practice by seeking external evidence and systematically gathering client-specific data in the selection of treatment approaches and the evaluation of treatment efficiency, effectiveness, and effect. Nail-Chiwetalu and Bernstein-Ratner (2006) assert that EBP presupposes that clinical skills grow with the application of currently available data, not simply personal educational and clinical experience. The practice of audiology and speech-language pathology is dynamic, and training received in graduate school, as well as clinical experience garnered over time, may not provide clinicians with knowledge of the most efficacious approaches for cases that they will confront in every day practice over the span of their careers. Second, the expert clinician should consistently seek new information to improve therapeutic effectiveness. To this end, clinicians should be data seekers, data integrators, and clinical evaluators of the application of new knowledge to clinical cases. (p. 157)

In 1988, one of the authors wrote that "we wish to instill in the student clinician an understanding of the importance of scientific commitment, caring and compassion and professionalism that will evolve and grow stronger throughout his or her professional career" (Sutherland-Cornett & Chabon, 1988, p. 40). The need for a triad of interpersonal skills, theoretical knowledge, and occupational values and principles seems even more relevant to our current service orientation. This is the message of this text, and this is our hope for the future of our professions and those we serve.

Why Serve?

As authors, and as speech-language pathologists, we are eager to share with you both quantitative and qualitative data that form our "evidenced-based" substantiation of the rewards of serving individuals with communication disorders. Since 1997, ASHA has been compiling objective, quantitative data that examine the effectiveness of the work that speech-language pathologists do when serving adults in health care facilities and children in schools. This work has been conducted as well-controlled, longitudinal, and ongoing research studies. One mechanism for this research is ASHA's National Outcome Measurement System (NOMS). In 1998, ASHA established the National Center for Treatment Effectiveness in Communication Disorders, which is the adult health care component of NOMS. An example of the data is that in inpatient rehabilitation settings, speech-language pathologists treat individuals with swallowing disorders (47.7%), memory disorders (46.6%), spoken language comprehension disorders (36%), spoken language expression disorders (35.4%), attention disorders (28.8%), motor speech disorders (27.5%), reading problems (21.8%), writing problems (14.3%), pragmatics disorders (11.2%), voice disorders (6.7%), and fluency disorders (0.7%) (www.asha.org/nctecd/treatment_outcomes.htm). The mean age of the patients in this study of 2,666 patients was 69 years. The National Center for Treatment Effectiveness project indicates that patients in inpatient rehabilitation facilities improved in their functional communication as a result of the services of speech-language pathologists. Improvement in communication functioning was obtained by 90 percent of the patients with fluency disorders, 81.8 percent of the patients with motor speech disorders, 77.5 percent of the patients with voice disorders, 77.1 percent of the patients with spoken language expression disorders, 76.8 percent of the patients with pragmatic disorders, 75.6 percent of the patients with attention disorders, 74.7 percent of the patients with reading problems, 74.6 percent of the patients with swallowing disorders, 73.1 percent of the patients with memory disorders, 73 percent of the patients with writing problems, and 73 percent of the patients with spoken language comprehension disorders.

Regarding children in kindergarten to sixth grade who received speech-language pathology services in their school, the NOMS project determined that over 90 percent of teachers agree that students' speech is understood by his/her peers as a result of the students receiving speech-language pathology services. Over 80 percent of teachers felt that their students communicated their wants, needs, ideas, and concepts to others more effectively as a result of speech-language pathology services; that their students' speech less frequently attracted negative attention; and that their students spoke with less frustration. Eighty percent of teachers felt that their students were more frequent participants in classroom activities that required speech and that their students' ability to communicate in socially appropriate ways had improved. What do parents think about the speech-language pathology services their children receive in the schools? The NOMS project gathered data that revealed that 95.6 percent of the parents in the study were satisfied or strongly satisfied with the services their children received. Additionally, 91.5 percent of parents agreed or strongly agreed with this statement: "I believe that my child's communication/swallowing has improved because of the speech-language pathology services" (http://preschool.asha.org/resources/NOMS/treatment_outcomes.cfm).

Therapy works! Published clinical research studies and additional data from ASHA's NOMS project provide insight about the efficacy of treatment:

- Conture and Yaruss (2004) indicate that more than one hundred studies on adults who stutter indicate that 60 percent to 80 percent of the patients experienced significant improvement as a result of therapy. NOMS data reveal that 79 percent of adults who stutter showed improvements by undergoing therapy.

- Research suggests that at some point in their lives, 85 percent to 90 percent of children with cerebral palsy experience feeding and swallowing problems. Pediatric feeding and swallowing treatment efficacy studies present evidence that improvements in swallowing safety, such as reduced aspiration and improved nutrition, are the result of treatment. Arvedson (2004) cites that one year of intraoral therapy with children with moderate dysphagia (swallowing disorder) resulted in significant improvements in jaw stability, along with better lip closure, chewing, and oral manipulation of food.

- L. O. Ramig and Verdolini (2004) refer to NOMS data that show that the majority of patients with voice disorders demonstrated multiple levels of improvement. Voice therapy may eliminate the need for surgery or drug regimen.

- Ashford, Logemann, and McCullough (2004) refer to NOMS data that reveal that approximately 60 percent of adult patients with dysphagia who had needed an alternative method of feeding—for example, a nasogastric tube—at the beginning of therapy progressed to a level where their swallow was safe and they no longer needed an alternative feeding method because of treatment with a speech-language pathologist.

- Yorkston's (2004) examination of NOMS data on neurological motor speech disorders indicates that approximately two-thirds of adults with diseases of the central nervous system (e.g., Parkinson's disease, multiple sclerosis) who were unintelligible at the beginning of receiving speech-language pathology services progressed to a level of increased communicative independence and were intelligible to all listeners due to intervention.

- Gierut (2004) reviewed the NOMS data for children with phonological disorders. Seventy percent of preschoolers who received phonological therapy demonstrated an improvement in intelligibility and communication functioning.

- Diefendorf's (2004) examination of existing treatment efficacy data involving hearing loss reveals that early detection of hearing loss by audiologists and enrollment in audiological and speech-language pathology intervention services within the child's first year of life reduce the consequences of hearing loss—for example, reducing the delay a child may experience in language and literacy development and reducing family stress. Seewald (2004) writes, "Children whose hearing loss is identified by 3 months and who start intervention by 6 months have the same language abilities as their peers by the time they enter kindergarten."

- Weinstein (2004) examined clinical evidence that presents that one-third of adults 70 years of age have hearing loss and benefit from audiological services and the use of hearing aids. Audiologic rehabilitation promotes successful hearing aid use and improves communication and psychosocial functioning of persons with hearing loss.

- H. Goldstein and Prelock (2004) submit that children with language disorders benefit from language therapy. NOMS data show that 70 percent of preschoolers with language disorders showed improvements in language functioning in the areas of receptive language and expressive language. Their examination of over 200 clinical studies reveals that language intervention has been effective "for an overwhelming majority of participants."

Whether engaged in service to one's professional association or to the needs of those individuals and their families with communication disorders, what is clear is that serving has its own rewards.

Being an audiologist or a speech-language pathologist involves participating in mutual relationships with our patients, their families, our professional colleagues, and our professional associations that are rewarding and true partnerships. In the spirit of Remen, as audiologists and speech-language pathologists we are as served as the persons we serve.

This text has been designed to introduce, and welcome, students to the discipline of communication sciences and disorders, and, the professions, of audiology and speech-language pathology. From being a student to being an audiologist or a speech-language pathologist, you are on an exciting, interesting, and rewarding journey.

There are approximately 42 million people in the United States alone who have communication problems, and more than 100,000 professionals who are trying to help them. The arithmetic is easy. It means approximately one professionally trained helper for every 420 people who need help. Welcome to the neighborhood.

The beginning of your journey into this community is designed to give you a feel for the many professional opportunities that are out there for you, and then later, to provide you with information about the nature of their problems. It is an invitation to explore the possibilities of pursuing a career in one of the various levels of the professions that exist in the areas of communication sciences and disorders.

However, on a more personal level, you will quickly realize, as you turn page after page, that you are learning about a large number of people who are in trouble and need services. As a result, your own feelings of empathy, of walking around in their shoes, and your willingness to enter into a helping relationship start to emerge and guide you more deeply into the information that is being provided here.

As you take off on this journey, you begin to learn about some of the details of what is troubling them, and sometimes as you come face to face, you realize that, not only in this book but in your real life, you may have had contact with the pain, and frustration, and impact of their problems.

This first chapter, for the most part, deals with the professions of audiology and speech-language pathology and with the professionals. The term *multidimensional* comes to mind again and again, as you realize that communication problems can be quite complicated and embrace a number of different aspects of what people are about. As a result, those who serve these individuals also have to become multidimensional if they are going to treat the totality of these disabilities. An understanding of speech-language pathology and audiology involves learning from the disciplines of communication sciences and disorders, clinical procedures, genetics, multicultural issues, anatomy, neurology, medicine, dentistry, psychology, linguistics, and counseling.

There are times when the audiologist or speech-language pathologist functions as a teacher, or a source of information, or as an instructor; other times he or she may function as a behavioral reinforcer, and still other times as a listener, or as a counselor. Sometimes the focus is on information, sometimes on emotions and feelings, and sometimes on behavior, involving both speech and social interactions. Shifting from one function and role to another may sometimes have to occur rapidly, at different moments in his or her professional activities, depending on the needs of the situation. Whether you become an academician, an administrator, a clinician, or a researcher, you may well find yourself in different roles, fulfilling different functions and meeting different needs of the people that you work with. It is this multidimensionality that contributes to the significance and attractiveness of the variety of careers that evolve for you.

"Meaning is the antecedent of commitment, and the original meaning of our work is service. Service is not a relationship between an expert and a problem; it is a human relationship, a work of the heart and the soul" (Remen, 2001).

STUDY QUESTIONS

1. Think of an individual with a communication disorder you have read about, seen on television or in a movie, or, better yet, know personally. Describe the person's communication difficulty and those qualities you admire most about this individual.

2. Interview an audiologist or a speech-language pathologist. Ask this professional to identify the three things she or he likes best about her or his work.

3. Review a catalog of a publisher of treatment materials for individuals with communication disorders. Select products that seem to be appropriate for a preschooler, a school-age child, a young adult, and a senior citizen. Give a brief description of the products and why you would like to use them.

4. Write an ad for a job for an audiologist or a speech-language pathologist that you would like to apply for.

5. How would you change a therapy activity like storytelling for use with a preschooler, a sixth grader, and a teenager?

6. Visit an audiologist or a speech-language pathologist, tour the facility where the person works, and spend time talking with the professional about his or her career. Ask what he or she likes and dislikes about his or her career.

Chapter TWO

Development of Communication, Language, and Speech

Robert E. Owens, Jr.
State University of New York, Geneseo

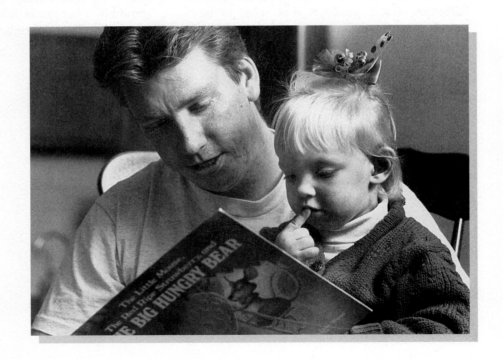

personal PERSPECTIVE

ROBERT E. OWENS, JR.

I didn't always want to be a speech-language pathologist. At first, I wanted to be a fireman. By college age, this had evolved into teacher. After Vietnam era service as a submarine officer, I began exploring the field of special education and settled on speech-language pathology. My early experiences and two years of work in the Environmental Language Program with Dr. Jim MacDonald at Ohio State University convinced me that I had chosen the right field. Nothing has happened to change my mind.

I approach each clinical language disorder case as a mystery to be unraveled and find great satisfaction when I'm a successful sleuth. I especially like the difficult clinical cases, such as those persons who are seemingly not communicating or those with multiple disabilities.

The combination of teaching, research and writing, and clinical involvement is very fulfilling. My clinical clients and college students have taught me much more than I have taught them, and my learning continues each day. For me, it's better than being a fireman.

There are several persistent myths or misconceptions about the development of communication, language, and speech. In this chapter, we shall explore the typical development of communication, language, and speech as experienced by most children in the United States. I hope to provide you with a model of development and to dispel some of the persistent myths. As we discuss development of communication, language, and speech, you may encounter several ideas that challenge your notions. That is as it should be in a text. Further study will help to clarify new questions raised.

Following is a portion of a conversation between two preschoolers:

Child 1:   (1) I'll take this one for a walk.

Child 2:   Come on.

Child 1:   (2) Coo coo. (3) You coo coo.

Child 2:   Here baby. Baby. Stop it, coo coo.

Child 1:   (4) Go to sleep now.

Child 2:   You too.

Child 1:   (5) She can't sleep next to her because she doesn't like it.

         (6) Hey, . . .

Child 2:   Why?

Child 1:   [No response]

         (7) You're not going to take a picture of us yet. (8) What?

Child 2:   Here you go.

Child 1:   (9) Coo coo.

Child 2:   This is her bottle.

Child 1:   (10) This is where the sandwich is.

Child 2:   The sandwich are in there.

Child 1:   (11) No. (12) You stupid box. (13) Let me at that one.

         (14) No, no, let me at that one.

Child 2:   Hey, coo coo. This is her bottle.

Child 1:   (15) Where's her bottle?

Child 2:   Here.

Child 1:   (16) Look at, this can come off.

Child 2:   Yeah, that can come off of that one. Hey, gonna take it off.

Child 1:   (17) I can. (18) This is the cover. (19) I got it.

Child 1 is a typical 42-month-old child. For the most part, her sentences are well formed (utterance 1) and demonstrate a variety of forms (4, 5, 7, and 15). She demonstrates morphological learning, such as third-person irregular *does* (5), contractible auxiliary or helping verb *to be* and the progressive tense ending *-ing* (7), the contractible and uncontractible *be* as a main verb (10), auxiliary verbs *will* and *can* (1 and 16), and pronouns (5, 7, and 13). In addition, she has prepositional phrases (1, 5, 7, 13, and 14) and infinitive phrases (*to* + verb) (4 and 7) and two independent clauses joined together with *because* (5). Elsewhere in the sample, she produces the complex sentence "I want to see what I look like in there."

She is able to initiate conversation and introduce topics (4) as well as respond to the utterances of her partner (5 and 15). Topics change quickly, often without signal. She can provide information to her partner, both solicited (elsewhere in the sample, she responds to the question "Baby, want your doggie?" with "No, she doesn't") and spontaneous (17), and she also is able to obtain information (15). Although there are both interruptions and lapses (between 6 and 7) common among preschoolers, she is a good conversational turn-taker. She omits shared information (11 and 17) and provides additional information (18) where needed.

Throughout the sample, the child quality of the play is evident. Both children role-play and pretend (2 and 9). Toys or objects are used symbolically to represent other objects (10).

Wow, there's a lot of language learning evident in these few short utterances. You may not even understand what some of the terms mean that I used. That's fine. You will in time. Incredibly, this child only began to produce single words 30 short months before this passage was recorded. Let's take a look at how this happens as we explore communication, language, and speech.

Communication

Communication is the process of exchanging information and ideas. An active process, it involves encoding, transmitting, and decoding intended messages. There are many means of communicating. The probability of message distortion is high, given the number of ways that a message can be formed and the connotations and perceptions of each participant. Each communication partner must be alert to the needs of the other so that messages are conveyed effectively and intended meanings preserved.

Speech and language are only a portion of communication. Other aspects of communication, shown in Figure 2.1, may enhance or even eclipse both. These aspects are **paralinguistic, nonlinguistic**, and **metalinguistic**. Paralinguistic mechanisms can change the form and meaning of a sentence by acting across individual sounds or words of a sentence. These mechanisms signal attitude or emotion and include intonation, stress, rate of delivery, and pause or hesitation. Intonation patterns include

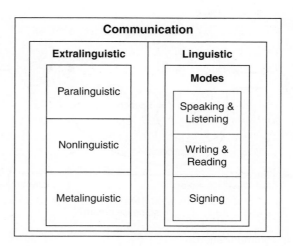

FIGURE 2.1

changes in pitch, such as a rising pitch at the end of a sentence used to signal a question. Stress is employed for emphasis. At one point, as a child, each of us firmly asserted, *I* **did** *take a bath.* Rate varies with the speaker's state of excitement, familiarity with the content, and perceived comprehension of the listener. Pauses may be used to emphasize a portion of the message or to replace it. Even young children recognize that a short maternal pause after a child's request usually signals a negative reply. Each of us has experienced the parental pause that follows, *Can Ray eat over tonight?*

Nonlinguistic cues include gestures, body posture, facial expression, eye contact, head and body movement, and physical distance or proxemics. Each of these aspects of nonlinguistic behavior can influence communication. For example, gestures tend to enhance speech and language and to set the rhythm for communication. Body posture and facial expression can convey the speaker's attitude toward a message, partner, or situation. The speaker who says, *Oh sure, I like that idea,* but who sits in a defensive, tight posture conveys a different attitude. Likewise, eye contact and physical distance can communicate the degree of involvement of two participants in the message or in the communicative interaction. A wink may convey more than a whole sentence.

Metalinguistic cues signal the status of communication based on our intuitions about the acceptability of utterances. In other words, metalinguistic skills enable us to talk about language, analyze it, think about it, separate it from its context, and judge it. Communication partners monitor both their own and their partner's communication. The focus is on what is transmitted, but also how this is accomplished.

The process of communication is illustrated in Figure 2.2. The message to be transmitted begins as a concept in the mind of the speaker. Messages rarely occur out of context, so we can assume that this concept has been influenced by preceding events and is the result of the speaker's cognitive and social knowledge. For example, the message *Yes, I'd love one* makes little sense without the context and the speaker's interpretation of that context. The concept is encoded via language into a form to be transmitted.

Rules that govern all aspects of the particular language used are employed to ensure that the message is appropriate, conveys the speaker's meaning and intention, is grammatically well formed, and contains correct sound sequences and combinations. The exact cognitive processes that accomplish this encoding are still unknown, although much of the activity occurs in the left side of the brain, using information from many other cortical areas.

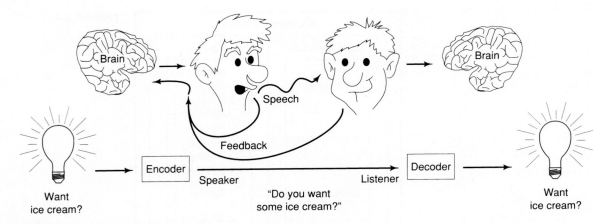

FIGURE 2.2   Process of communication.

Once the message is encoded, the speaker performs the physical act of speaking, monitoring his production via auditory and proprioceptive self-feedback—how the message sounds and feels—and visual and auditory feedback from the listener.

The listener receives the message both auditorily and visually and **decodes** it. Linguistic information is processed in the left hemisphere of the brain in most individuals. Paralinguistic and nonlinguistic information—often the bulk of the message—is processed in the right hemisphere in most. Using the message as a base, the listener draws on her linguistic, cognitive, and social knowledge to decode or interpret it. The listener may request either additional information or clarification to aid the decoding. This feedback helps the speaker sharpen the message.

Once the listener has decoded the message into the speaker's intended concept, and assuming the speaker has signaled that he is relinquishing his turn, the roles switch. The listener becomes the new speaker and will respond with an utterance that is related to that of the previous speaker.

Development of Communication

Communication appears to be present at birth. The newborn and her mother begin communicating almost immediately. The newborn will search for the human voice and demonstrate pleasure or mild surprise when she finds the face that is the sound source. Both she and her mother will do almost anything to attend to the other's face and voice.

As caregivers respond to an infant's early reflexive behaviors, the infant learns to communicate its intentions. Gradually, through repeated interactions, the infant refines these communication skills. The process is not one-sided, nor is the child a passive participant. Within the first few months of life, infants are able to discriminate contrasting phonemes, different intonational patterns, and speech from nonspeech. Infants are also able to discriminate different voices. Individual differences become evident very early, with infants differing in the amount of their attending to speech (Hampson & Nelson, 1993).

In addition, the infant learns different gaze patterns used in communication. As early as 6 weeks of age, infants are able to coordinate the amount of time spent gazing and will change their gaze patterns based on their partners' gaze (Crown, Feldstein, Jasnow, Beebe, & Jaffe, 2002). By the time the child is 3 to 4 months of age, interactions based on eye gaze form early dialogues that eventually evolve into conversational exchanges.

A relationship exists between the infant's gaze and social behavior (D'Odorico, Cassibba, & Salerni, 1997). At around 1 year of age, children look at their partners at the beginning of a vocal turn, possibly for reassurance. Six months later, they use a more adult pattern and look at their partners at the end of a turn to signal a turn shift.

The infant also learns the signal value of head movements. Both the face and the head are important for early communication because their movements are relatively advanced in their maturation and provide the bases for early communication.

Caregivers respond to these infant behaviors and treat them as meaningful social communication. The degree of caregiver responsiveness appears to be positively correlated with later language abilities. In addition, such responsiveness forges an attachment bond between mother and child that fosters communication. Mothers are able to identify consistently infant behaviors that they perceive to be communicatively important (Meadows, Elias, & Bain, 2000).

Maternal sensitivity is multifaceted and varied. Sensitive mothers vary their rate of speech based on their infants' behavior (Hane, Feldstein, & Dernetz, 2003). Over- or underresponsive moms tend to undermine attachment between themselves and their infants (Jaffe, Beebe, Feldstein, Crown, & Jasnow, 2001).

Infants receive highly selective language input within the routines of child–parent interactions. Two routines, *joint action* and *joint reference,* are particularly noteworthy. Within joint action routines, such as "peek-a-boo" and "this little piggy," children learn turn-taking skills. Mothers provide a consistent set of behaviors that enable their children to predict the outcome and later to anticipate. In turn, children learn to signal their intention to play.

Using joint reference, caregivers help their children differentiate between objects. Maternal encouragement of her infant to attend is positively related to later language development (Karrass, Braungart-Rieker, Mullins, & Lefever, 2002). The focusing of attention by both partners on objects establishes a **referent**. Once the referent has been established, mothers provide linguistic input relative to it. These comments are important for the child's later language comprehension and for early meaning development (Rollins, 2003). Maternal speech is modified systematically so that it is comprehensible to the child.

For their part, children progress from reflexive, nonintentional communication to conventional, verbal or spoken-word intentions by early in the second year of life. Three developmental stages of early communication intentions exist. Initially, the child's behaviors are undifferentiated, and his intentions unknown. Next, the child uses gestures and vocalization to express intent. Intentional vocalizations are shorter with a lower overall frequency, a different pitch shape or contour, and a greater intensity than nonintentional ones (Papaeliou, Minadakis, & Cavouras, 2002; Papaeliou & Trevarthen, 2006). This stage is significant because the child's intention to communicate is accompanied by eye contact. Finally, in the third stage, words are used to convey intentions previously expressed in gestures.

Gestures don't disappear when children begin to speak, but they do change in function (Özçaliskan & Goldin-Meadow, 2005). Increasingly, children use gestures to reinforce (*ball* + point at ball), disambiguate (*that one* + point at ball), and supplement (*push* + point at ball) speech. Two-element gestural-verbal combinations, such as pointing at a car and saying "Go," increase as a child approaches the production of two-word utterances (McEachem & Haynes, 2004).

The preschooler learns to use language, emphasis, and stress to improve her message quality. She also adjusts her manner of delivery for her prospective listener. Children as young as 3 seem to recognize the need to clarify their gestures and modify their behavior accordingly (O'Neill & Topolovec, 2000). Four-year-old children will even modify their speech and language when conversing with much younger language-learning children.

It is in the school-age period that the child makes the greatest advances in the use of the paralinguistic, nonlinguistic, and metalinguistic aspects of communication. The older child can use his communication skills to create a mood, role-play, or express sarcasm. He learns to use timing or rate to heighten his delivery or to create curiosity. Gestures are used to enhance or to add emphasis to the message. He adjusts his message and its manner of delivery to his listener and tries to predict the effects of his transmission. When conversing with peers, most teens are careful to direct their partners' attention, to give positive verbal and nonverbal feedback, and to make responses based on their partners' statements (Turkstra, Ciccia, & Seaton, 2003).

Metalinguistic abilities usually emerge after the child has mastered linguistic form. Although metalinguistic abilities appear in the preschool years, full awareness does not occur until about age 7 or 8. The preschool child tends to make judgments of utterance acceptability based on the content rather than on the grammatical structure. A 4-year-old might judge *Daddy painted a picture* as unacceptable because *Daddies don't paint pictures, pictures come from cameras*. By kindergarten, the child is just beginning to separate what is said from how it is said. The school-age child demonstrates an increasing ability to judge the grammatical acceptability of sentences, reflecting a growing knowledge of language structure.

The preschool child attempts to repair her erroneous or misinterpreted utterances and adjusts her speech and language for her intended listener. She also corrects others and comments on the effectiveness of communication. By school age, she can use intonation to signal new words introduced into the conversation; correct utterances inappropriate for the setting or specific listener; identify linguistic units, such as syllables and sentences; provide definitions; and construct humor. In addition, she is able to explain why a sentence is appropriate or impossible and how it should be interpreted. With increased skill, the child is freed from the immediate linguistic context to attend to how a message is communicated. Metalinguistic skill development is related to many factors, such as cognitive development, reading ability, academic achievement, IQ, and environmental stimulation.

In summary, the child communicates from the time of birth. Early communication does not depend on the use of language or speech. In fact, communication provides the vehicle within which initial language develops. As language skills improve, there is also a corresponding improvement in overall communication abilities.

Language

Language is a social tool, defined as a socially shared code or conventional system for representing concepts through the use of arbitrary **symbols** and rule-governed combinations of those symbols. Each language, such as English, Korean, or Farsi, has its own symbols and rules for symbol combination. **Dialects** are subcategories of these parent languages that use similar, but not identical rules. Languages exist because users have agreed on the symbols and the rules. This agreement is demonstrated through their use. Because language users can agree to follow the rules of a language, they can also agree to change the rules. New words and rules can be added, while others fall into disuse. For example, my grandmother, born in the late 1800s, called suspenders "braces," a term no longer used. Under certain circumstances, language mixing may even result in a new form of two blended languages being used in a community (Backus, 1999).

The socially shared code of symbols and rules allows language users to exchange information. Each user encodes and decodes according to his concept of a given object, event, or relationship. Thus, coding is a factor of the speaker's and listener's shared meanings, the linguistic skills of each, and the context.

Individual symbols communicate little. Most of the information is contained in symbol combinations. For example, *teacher Irene a is* seems to be a meaningless jumble of words. By shifting a few words, we can create *Irene is a teacher* or *Is Irene a teacher?* Language is this relational system, and it is the rules for these relationships that give language order and permit language to be used creatively to produce meaning. A finite set of symbols and a finite set of rules governing symbol use are used to create and interpret a seemingly infinite number of sentences. Native speakers of a language do not learn all possible word combinations. Rather, they learn the linguistic rules that enable each language user to understand and to create an infinite variety of sentences.

Components of Language

Language is a complex combination of several rule systems that can be divided into three major components: form, content, and use. *Form* includes **syntax**, **morphology**, and **phonology**, those systems that connect sounds or symbols with meaning. *Content* encompasses meaning or **semantics**, and the *use* component includes **pragmatics**. These five rule systems—syntax, morphology, phonology, semantics, and pragmatics— are the basic rule systems found in language.

The five systems are distinct, but interrelated. *Syntax* is a rule system governing the ordering of words in sentences. *Morphological rules* govern structure at the word level. For example, *dog* can be modified by the addition of *s* to form *dogs*. *Phonological rules* determine which sounds may appear together, how they will sound together, and where they may appear. For example, the plural *s* in *cats* sounds like an *s*, but on *dogs* sounds like a *z*. Some sounds may not be placed together in certain positions. There are, for example, no English words that begin with *dm*. *Semantic rules* govern meaning and the relationships between meaning units. Semantics helps language users to distinguish sense from nonsense. Finally, *pragmatics* is a set of rules for language use. These rules govern the manner of communication, how to enter and exit a conversation, adoption of roles, sequencing of sentences, and anticipation of listener needs, to name a few functions. All of these rule systems are used simultaneously in communication.

Syntax   The rules of syntax govern the form or structure of a sentence. They specify word order; sentence organization; relationships between words, word classes, or types; and other sentence units. Syntax specifies which word combinations are acceptable, or grammatical, and which are not.

Each sentence must contain a noun phrase and a verb phrase that include a noun and a verb, respectively. Therefore, a sentence must contain a noun and a verb. Within noun and verb phrases, certain word classes appear. For example, articles appear before nouns and adverbs modify verbs.

Knowledge of the language rules enables language users to understand and generate language. Thus, there is a link between language form and cognitive processing, or thought.

Morphology   Morphology, considered by some linguists to be a subcategory of syntax, is concerned with the internal organization of words. Words consist of one or more smaller units called *morphemes*. The smallest unit of grammar, a **morpheme** is indivisible without violating the meaning or producing meaningless units. For example, *dog* is a morpheme because it cannot be divided into meaningful units. Morphology enables the language user to modify word meanings and produce semantic distinctions, such as number (dog, dog*s*), verb tense (talk, talk*ed*), and possession (Mary, Mary's); extend word meanings (*dis*interested, *un*interested); and derive word classes (quick [adjective], quick*ness* [noun], quick*ly* [adverb]).

There are two varieties of morphemes, *free* and *bound*. Free morphemes can be used independently. They form words or parts of words, such as *dog, big,* and *happy*. Bound morphemes are grammatical markers that must be attached to free morphemes.

Examples include *'s, -er, un-,* and *-ly* (meaning possession, more, negative, and manner, respectively). By combining the free and bound morphemes mentioned here, we can create *dog's, bigger,* and *unhappily.*

Phonology   Each language has specific speech sounds or *phonemes* and sound combinations that are characteristic of that language. **Phonemes**, the smallest meaningful units of speech sound, are combined in specific ways to form *words.* Phonological rules govern the distribution and sequencing of phonemes within a language. Distributional rules describe which sounds can be employed in various positions in words. For example, in English, the /ŋ/ or "ny" sound found in *ring* may not appear at the beginning of a word.

Sequencing rules determine which sounds may appear in combination. For example, the word *brick* is perfectly acceptable in English. *Blick* is not an English word, but would be acceptable. *Bnick* could never be an acceptable English word. In addition, sequencing rules concern the sound modifications made when two phonemes appear next to each other. The distributional and sequencing rules may both apply. For example, the combination *nd* will not appear at the beginning of a word, but may appear elsewhere, as in *window* or *sand.*

Semantics   Meaning is a system for dividing reality into categories and units that group similar objects, actions, and relationships and distinguish dissimilar ones. Some units are mutually exclusive, such as *walk* and *ride.* A human being can't do both at once. Other units' meanings overlap somewhat, as do *walk, run,* and *jog. Semantics* is concerned with the relationship of language form to objects, events, and relationships and with words and word combinations.

Words or symbols do not represent reality, but rather each language user's ideas or concepts of reality. A concept is related to several experiences rather than to any single one. It is the result of a cognitive categorization process. Each word meaning contains two portions drawn from the concept: the semantic features and selection restrictions. *Semantic features* characterize the word. For example, the semantic features of *bachelor* include "unwed" and "male." *Selection restrictions* are based on specific features and prohibit certain word combinations as meaningless or redundant. For example, *bachelor's wife* is meaningless; *unwed bachelor* is redundant. Throughout life, language users acquire new features, delete old features, and reorganize the remainder to sharpen word meanings.

The more features two words share, the more they are alike. Words with identical or near identical features are **synonyms**. Some examples of synonyms are *big* and *large,* and *little* and *small.* Words with opposite polarity of features, or opposite meanings, are **antonyms**. Examples include *long* and *short, happy* and *sad,* and *black* and *white.*

Words may have several meanings; therefore, users must rely on additional cues, such as selection restrictions, linguistic context, and nonlinguistic context. Sentences represent a meaning greater than the sum of the individual words because they include relationships between those words that go beyond the individual symbols used.

Pragmatics   To communicate successfully, we need knowledge of social appropriateness as well as knowledge of form and content. Since language is primarily used in conversations, pragmatics or language use is concerned with discourse or conversational skills. It is the context of conversation that determines how and what the speaker chooses to say and how it is interpreted.

Language may be used to interact with others, to regulate their behavior, to try to fulfill the speaker's needs by controlling others, and so on. The linguistic code to fulfill these functions is determined primarily by the speaker's intent, but also by his perceptions of the listener, their shared cognitive and linguistic information, and the situation. Listener characteristics that influence speaker behaviors are sex, age, race, style, dialect, social status, and role.

Pragmatic rules govern sequential organization and coherence of conversations, repair of errors, role, and intentions. Organization and coherence of conversations include turn-taking; opening, maintaining, and closing a conversation; establishing and maintaining topic; and making relevant contributions to the conversation. Repair includes giving and receiving feedback. Role skills include establishing and maintaining a role and switching linguistic codes for each role. Finally, intentions are coded relative to the communicative context and the speaker's goal.

To ignore pragmatics is to remove language from its communicative context and purpose. The motivation for language use and language acquisition is effective communication. The speaker chooses the form and content that will best fulfill her intentions based on her perception of the communication situation. Thus, language is not an abstract code, but an interactive tool. A speaker's knowledge of the communication situation or context influences selection of the other aspects of language.

Summary   Language is a complex system of symbols and rules for symbol use. Native speakers must be knowledgeable about the symbols employed and the acceptable rules for use of these symbols. These rules govern concept, word, morpheme and phoneme combinations and the use of these combinations in communication. The five aspects of language that have been described in this section are interrelated and can help us understand both the communication process and language development.

Language Development

Within each of the five systems of language, development is rarely linear. At times, one aspect or a combination may be the major focus of development, as in the early stage when semantics, pragmatics, and phonology appear to be the organizing principles of child language. Rates of growth within each aspect also vary. During preschool years, the child learns numerous syntactic structures. This growth slows in the school-age years.

In the following sections, we shall explore language development within generally recognized periods of development: toddler, preschool, and school-age/adult. In the toddler period, the child concentrates on vocabulary growth based on the meanings he already possesses. Words are used to express the intentions that the child previously expressed through gestures. During the preschool period, the child concentrates on development of language form. Although this process continues during school years at a slower rate, the content and use aspects of language development become more prominent.

Infant Prelanguage   Through exposure to their native language, infants begin to recognize regularities, patterns that occur, some frequently, some less. The ability to detect patterns and to make generalizations is extremely important for symbol and rule learning (Marcus, 2001).

Babies learn the prosodic or flow patterns and phonotactic organization of their native language and use these skills to help to break into words and analyze the relative unbroken speech stream of mature speakers. Young infants are sensitive to stress and to rising and falling intonational patterns and can recognize their native language from languages with different patterns (Mehler et al., 1998; Nazzi, Bertoncini, & Mehler, 1998). Stress or emphasis patterns are another tool used by infants to determine word boundaries (Echols, Crowhurst, & Childers, 1997; Jusczyk, Houston, & Newsome, 1999b; Morgan, 1994; Morgan & Saffran, 1995).

Phonotactic organization consists of syllable structure and sound combinations. As the infant begins to recognize sound patterns, it's easier for the child to determine word boundaries. As a result, by 5 months, infants can discriminate their own language even among others with the same prosodic patterns (Bosch & Sebastián-Gallés, 1997; Nazzi, Jusczyk, & Johnson, 2000).

Extracting and reproducing individual speech sounds from the incoming speech stream is more difficult. By 8 months, children begin to store the sound patterns for words, although meaning—beyond *this-sound-pattern-goes-with-this-entity*—is not attached (Jusczyk & Hohne, 1997). By 9 months, children are using both the prosodic and the phonotactic clues to discern individual speech sounds.

Most words spoken to the infant by caregivers occur in context in the presence of entities and people to whom the caregiver refers. As a result, the infant hears the word while experiencing the entity or person. Up through age 2, comprehension is highly context-dependent (Striano, Rochat, & Legerstee, 2003).

In short, infants may use semantic, syntactic, phonological, stress-pattern, and contextual cues in combination to break the speech stream and aid interpretation. These cues are probably used flexibly depending on what's available in any given situation (Sanders & Neville, 2000). Within the speech section of this chapter, we'll explore the child's production of these words and the sounds within.

Toddler Language Development   Early language development is characterized by single-word utterances and by early multiword combinations. Learning strategies may differ from children who produce individual words, mostly nouns, to those who produce unanalyzed phrases, such as *I don't know*. These phrases, called *formulas*, represent a whole-to-parts strategy of learning that seems to be less efficient than a parts-to-whole strategy of learning words and building to longer utterances (Hickey, 1993; Pine, 1990).

Language fulfills the intentions of the child's earlier nonlinguistic communication. First words fill the roles previously served by gestures and/or vocalizations. These intentions are presented in Table 2.1. It is important to note that toddlers don't just imitate others or name objects. They use their language to influence others, to obtain information, to give information, and to engage in conversational give-and-take.

Within the stream of speech directed at the child are individual words. Toddlers seem to make six assumptions about words they hear (Golinkoff, Mervis, & Hirsh-Pasek, 1994):

Words refer to entities.

Words are extendable to similar-appearing entities.

Words refer to the whole entity, not to the parts.

Words can be grouped categorically.

Novel words go with previously unnamed entities.

Words are used consistently.

Using these assumptions, toddlers learn words and sharpen their meanings.

TABLE 2.1 Early Illocutionary Functions

Early Verbal Intentions (R. Owens, 1978; Wells, 1985)	Examples
Wanting demands	*Cookie* (Reach)
Direct request/commanding	*Help* (Hand object to or struggle)
Protesting	*No* (Push away or uncooperative)
Content questioning	*Wassat?* (Point)
Naming/labeling	*Doggie* (Point)
Statement/declaring	*Eat* (Commenting on dog barking)
Answering	*Horsie* (in response to question)
Reply	*Eat* (in response to *The doggie's hungry*)
Exclaiming	Squeal when picked up
Verbal accompaniment to action	*Uh-oh* (with spill)
Expressing state or attitude	*Tired*
Greeting/farewell	*Hi*
	Bye-bye
Repeating/practicing	*Cookie, cookie, cookie*
Calling	*Mommy*

Source: Information from *Language Development: An Introduction* (7th ed.) by R. E. Owens, Jr., 2000. Boston: Allyn and Bacon.

For toddlers, most words are learned receptively and then produced expressively, although some words may be learned in production in contexts in which they "sound right" (K. E. Nelson, 1991; K. E. Nelson, Hampson, & Shaw, 1993). In addition, comprehension seems to precede production for words that can be used in more than one context (*want, no*) but not for words that can be used in only one context, such as *bye-bye* (M. Harris, Yeeles, Chasin, & Oakley, 1995).

The comprehension–production relationship is a dynamic one that changes with a child's developmental level and with each aspect of language. The relationship changes because of different rates of development and different linguistic demands. The ability to comprehend words develops gradually and is highly context-dependent initially. By their first birthday, most infants recognize that words refer to common features across objects, such as different types of cups; can extend words to new examples; and can retain new labels for up to 24 hours (Schafer, 2005; Waxman & Booth, 2003).

Single-word comprehension continues to develop through the second year of life (Striano et al., 2003). Between 18 and 24 months, most children experience a "vocabulary spurt," especially in receptive vocabulary (Harris et al., 1995; Mervis & Bertrand, 1995). Eighteen-month-olds are capable of learning new words with as few as three exposures (Houston-Price, Plunkett, & Haris, 2005). Lexically precocious two-year-old children—those with larger vocabularies—are also grammatically precocious, with a greater range of grammatical structures and more advanced combinations (McGregor, Sheng, & Smith, 2005).

Word learning can be influenced by many variables. In general, girls seem to begin to acquire words earlier and have faster initial learning than boys (Bauer, Goldfield, & Reznick, 2002). Although having adults read to you positively affects the size of the expressive vocabulary, watching television does not have this beneficial effect (Patterson, 2002).

Regardless of the language spoken, children's early vocabularies contain relatively greater proportions of nouns than other word classes (Bornstein et al., 2004). The relative percentages of nouns decrease as vocabularies grow beyond 100 words and as children begin to use more syntax (E. Bates et al., 1994).

Phonologically, the child's first words are simple. Most contain one or two syllables; syllabic constructions usually consist of VC (vowel–consonant) (*eat*), CV (*key*), CVCV reduplicated (*mama*), or CVCV (*baby*). This syllable structure is also true for the first words of children learning Spanish (Jackson-Maldonado, Thal, Marchman, Bates, & Gutierrez-Clennan, 1993). Front consonants, such as /p/, /b/, and /m/, and back consonants, such as /g/ and /k/, predominate in both English and Spanish. The child's words are phonetic approximations of adult words.

Early word development is related to both the phonological character of the words acquired and the child's emerging phonological system. Lexical characteristics that influence linguistic processing are the word's frequency of use, the **neighborhood density**, and the phonotactic probability (Storkel & Morrisette, 2002). Frequently used words would be recognized by the child more quickly and accurately and produced more rapidly than infrequent ones.

Neighborhood density is the number of possible words that differ by one phoneme. For example, there are very few words in the neighborhood with *the*; thus, density is low. High density, or lots of neighbors, can result in more confusion and slower, less accurate recognition and production (Vitevitch, 2002; Vitevitch, Luce, & Pisoni, 1999).

Phonotactic probability is the likelihood of a sound pattern occurring. Sound-pattern probability is established for the child through experience. Common sound sequences (/st-, bl-, -ts/) are perceived and produced more quickly than less common ones (/skw-, -lf/) (Levelt & Wheeldon, 1994; Vitevitch & Luce, 1999). Words are not built phoneme by phoneme, but are perceived, learned, and produced as whole sound-patterned units (Beckman & Edwards, 2000).

Phonological development and semantics development are interdependent. The first words children produce are strongly influenced by phonology. In general, a child will avoid words that he cannot pronounce. New words are added when a child develops a "phonological template" or format for those words. For example, when a child acquires a CVC template for final plosive (/p, b, t, d, k, g/) sounds, he may add *top, pop, cat, dog, bike,* and *cake,* to name a few, but still not produce *car, knife,* or *bath.* Conversely, lexical or vocabulary development will have a strong influence on the sounds that a child produces. A child's "favorite phonemes" are usually taken from the sounds present in his first and favorite words. The child then attempts these sounds in other words.

Toddlers seem to adopt a "frame-and-slot" strategy of learning in which they acquire certain production frames or patterns and select words for expression that are similar enough in number of syllables, consonants and location, and syllable stress to fit these frames. Thus, the child integrates words and phrases from the environment with his or her own vocal patterns. This process may account for the large percentage of first words of children that contain similar sounds, sound combinations, and syllable shapes (Coady & Aslin, 2003).

The child's exact word meaning is unknown. His communication partner interprets his utterance with reference to the context and to the child's nonlinguistic behavior. Adults usually paraphrase the child's utterance as a full sentence, assuming that the child encoded the full thought, although this assumption is probably false.

The toddler operates with several constraints of attention, memory, and knowledge. In particular, she has difficulty with the organization of information for storage and later retrieval. Therefore, the child's meanings of individual words may not even overlap with the generally accepted adult meaning. More frequently, however, the child's meaning encompasses a small portion of the fuller adult definition. For example, the child might hear an adult say, *Won't fit,* when the child tries to pull her wagon through the door. She may later use the word *fit* to mean *too big or I can't do it* or as a general negation of an action. The child's sources of information are the adult's speaking in the presence of reference and the feedback the child receives for her own utterances. Thus, meaning is derived from both memory and the communication process (Levy & Nelson, 1994).

As she refines meanings, the child forms hypotheses about underlying concepts and extends her current meanings to include new examples. Through this process, she gains knowledge from examples and nonexamples of the concept. Some of her concepts are restricted, while others are extended widely. Overly restricted meanings are called *underextensions.* In contrast, *overextensions* are meanings that are too broad. Calling all men *Daddy* is an example of overextension. Toddlers seem to overextend both receptively and expressively, possibly because they fail to differentiate between basic concepts (*dog*) and categories (*animal*) (Storkel, 2002). Overextensions are common among toddlers in all languages, including those acquiring American Sign Language (Siedlecki & Bonvillian, 1998).

Children organize their early words by semantic, or meaning, categories. Within early two-word combinations, meaning is signaled by simple linear word-order patterns (see Table 2.2). Relationships are expressed by simple word-order rules rather than through abstract syntactic relationships. For example, in English the possessive function is marked by toddlers with the possessor followed by the possessed object, as in Mommy car. Other relationships depend primarily on one or two words that signal the semantic function. For example, the recurrence function is marked by a recurrent word, usually *more* or *nuther,* as in *more milk.* Although specific order will differ with the language being learned, approximately 70 percent of the two-word utterances of young language-learning children can be described by a few simple word-order rules. The child's production is the result of a complex interaction of syntactic knowledge,

TABLE 2.2   Two-Word Semantic Rules of Toddler Language

Rule	*Example*
Agent + action	Daddy eat. Mommy throw.
Action + object	Eat cookie. Throw hat.
Agent + object	Daddy cookie. Mommy hat.
Modifier + head	
Attribute	Big doggie. Little kitty.
Possessive	Daddy shoe. Mommy sock.
Recurrent	More juice. Nuther cookie.
Negative + X	No bed. All gone juice.
Introducer + X	This cup. That doggies.
X + location	Doggie bed. Throw me.

Source: Constructed from the work of Bloom (1970, 1973), Brown (1973), and Schlesinger (1971).

limited cognitive resources, communicative goals, and the structure of the conversation (Valian & Aubry, 2005).

With increasing memory and processing skills, the child is able to produce longer utterances by recombining the semantic patterns. For example, agent + action (*Mommy eat*) is combined with action + object (*eat cookie*) to produce agent + action + object (*Mommy eat cookie*). When approximately half of the child's utterances contain two words, he begins to use three-word recombinations. No new relationships are learned while the child develops skill with longer word combinations. The typical child will produce some four-word utterances by age 2. Later, when the child acquires syntactic and morphological forms, they are used to express these older semantic functions.

Children learn basic relationships between entities within the environment, and these relationships are reflected in their semantic structures. Language is used to talk about the things that they know. In other words, world knowledge precedes language. Language is grafted onto existing knowledge about the world as a means of representing that world. For example, infants demonstrate a concept of object permanence, or of the existence of an object that cannot be seen, before they express relationships such as appearance, disappearance, and nonexistence in their language.

The toddler's language knowledge is increased through the use of several learning strategies: selective imitation, evocative utterances, hypothesis testing, and interrogative utterances. Toddlers do not imitate all that they hear, and imitation is not random. In general, imitation serves to stabilize forms being learned and thus is highly selective. New information is gained by attempting new words or forms and awaiting feedback, by testing possible names, or by asking questions. Thus, on seeing a horse, the toddler might say any of the following:

Horsie.	(Evocative utterance, awaits a response)
Horsie?	(Hypothesis testing, awaits confirmation)
What? (That? Wassat?)	(Interrogative utterance, awaits answer)

Knowledge is gained in this way, not as a result of direct parental instruction.

From a developmental perspective, the role of the child's communication partners is crucial. Initially, through conversation, the child learns to understand the rules of turn-taking. A communication base is established first; then language is mapped onto this base to express the intentions the child initially expressed nonverbally through gestures.

Parents respond to early child utterances by expanding the form from the child's "Doggie bark" to "Yeah, the doggie barked," replying, imitating, or giving feedback. In addition, parents continue to provide a simplified model of adult speech. As children begin using new structures, parents systematically modify their own use of these structures. Children use those structures in their own speech that most effectively encode their intentions.

Differences in maternal speech modifications to infants reflect cultural differences (Ingram, 1995). Within the U.S. culture, race, education, and socioeconomic class each influence maternal behaviors. For example, although inner-city, working-class African-American mothers reportedly engage in vocal behavior at about the same rate as middle-class African-American mothers, the latter incorporate language more frequently in their play with their infants (Hammer & Weiss, 1999).

Preschool Language Development   Within the preschool period, major developmental emphasis centers on language form. By the time the child enters kindergarten, she has learned 90 percent of the syntax, morphology, and phonology that she will use

TABLE 2.3   Generalizations Concerning Preschool Language Development

1. American English is learned by preschoolers through conversations with caregivers, siblings, and peers.
2. Form follows function.
3. Preschool children use bootstrapping to help them learn language form.
4. Preschool children are actively involved in rule learning.
5. Complexity and utterance length are related.
6. Rule exceptions are avoided.
7. In American English, word order is a guide for construction and comprehension of sentences.
8. Deviation from or interruption of standard word order is avoided.
9. Caregivers do not directly teach, but they modify the conversation to ensure maximum child participation.
10. All aspects of language are intertwined in development.

as an adult, although she may use complex structures infrequently. In English, increases in the average length of the child's utterances, throughout most of the preschool period, correspond to increases in utterance complexity.

An in-depth description of this development is beyond the scope of this chapter. Therefore, I shall attempt to present some generalizations about preschool language development and to give examples that thoroughly demonstrate these statements. These generalizations are presented in Table 2.3.

Language Learned Through Conversation.   From birth, the child is treated as a conversational partner by her caregivers. Gradually, she becomes a fully participating one. Within these conversations, she learns new words and structures and begins to recognize the essential information needed by her partner.

Even before she could talk, the child learned turn-taking skills. Now with the help of her caregivers, she learns to take her conversational turn and still remain on the topic of discussion. By age 5, the child is able to take about a dozen turns on a single topic, although she rarely takes more than two or three (Brinton & Fujiki, 1984). A typical 3-year-old might converse as follows:

Child: I goed to gran-ma's.
Adult: Oh. Where does she live?
Child: On a farm.
Adult: That sounds neat. Does she have any animals?
Child: Horsies.
Adult: I love horses. What else?
Child: Mommy gots a new car. [Change of subject; no transition]

The child is more likely to remain on topic if engaged in sociodramatic play, describing something or some event, or solving a problem (Schober-Peterson & Johnson, 1989). The number of utterances within a turn varies with the child's intention and its desired effect on the listener (Logan, 2003).

In part, this anticipation of the effect on and the needs of the listener can be termed **presupposition**. Presupposition is the process of estimating the knowledge of the listener and the amount of information needed for comprehension. With some listeners, the child can say *Fluffy*; with others *Fluffy, my kitty*; and with still others *Fluffy, my white kitty*. As children's language matures, its use reflects better presuppositional skill.

Listener perspective is also important in the use of **deictic terms**. Deictic terms are words or phrases that can be interpreted only from the physical location of the speaker. I've seen more than one 2-year-old get paddled when mom says, "Come here" and he doesn't move. A good explanation of his nonresponsiveness may be that he's thinking "I am here," and from his perspective, he is. Other deictic terms include *this, that, I, me, you, give, take, come,* and *go*. Through conversational interchange, preschoolers gain increasing expertise in the use of these terms.

Form Follows Function.   You will recall that functions or intentions established in gestures are later filled by words when the toddler begins to talk. This is an early example of form following function. The communication function or use is established first, and then the child learns the language form to convey this function more effectively. For example, children can ask questions very early, and the function is well established. Hypothesis testing—a word stated with rising intonation, as in *Horsie?*—becomes yes/no interrogatives. Interrogative utterances—*Wassat*—become *Wh-* interrogatives (*what . . . , where . . . , who . . .*). Throughout the preschool years, interrogatives become longer, more complex, and more specific.

In yes/no interrogative development, single words become longer utterances, although the child continues to use intonation to signal a question, as in *Kitty sleeping on bed?* Around age 3, the child will use the auxiliary or helping verbs *be, do, can,* and *will* with the verb, placing them before the subject to form more adultlike interrogatives, such as *Is kitty sleeping on the bed?* (see Table 2.4). Correct inversion of the subject and the auxiliary verb varies with specific verbs (Rowland, Pine, Lieven, & Theakston, 2005). Some, such as *are, have, and do*, are significantly more difficult for children to invert than the auxiliary verbs *is* and *has*.

In similar fashion, initial *wh-* interrogatives are expanded somewhat later (Wells, 1985). *Who, which, how, when,* and *why* are added gradually to initial *wh-* words, such as *what* and *where*. Multiword *why* interrogatives, such as *why is daddy sick?*, do not appear until about age three and a half.

Negative statements offer a second example of form following function. Infants will protest over actions they do not like and may make a stronger statement by tantruming. It is not surprising then that negative words such as *no* are often present in the first 50 words of toddlers. As with interrogatives, these forms are also elaborated and made more specific throughout the preschool\period (see Table 2.4).

At first, the negative word is placed at the beginning of the utterance in forms such as *No go bye-bye, No eat yukky peas,* and *No Mommy drink juice.* Several negative words may be used interchangeably, with the child making no distinction among *no, not, don't, can't,* and *won't*. Around age 2, the child begins placing the negative element between the subject and predicate or verb, as in *Daddy don't ride bike.* Over the next few years, other negative forms, such as *isn't, aren't, doesn't, wasn't, couldn't,* and *shouldn't* are added gradually. These forms appear at about the same time that other auxiliary verbs such as *can, could, should, might,* and so on begin to occur.

Bootstrapping.   **Bootstrapping** is using what you know about language to help you comprehend and produce language, as when preschoolers use their earlier knowledge of semantics to interpret and form sentences. Before their second birthday, toddlers use forms such as *agent + action (Daddy eat)* and *action + object (Eat cookie)*. These are

TABLE 2.4 Acquisition of Sentence Forms

Approximate Age	Negative	Interrogative	Embedding	Conjoining
12–24 months	Single word *no, all gone, gone.* Negative + X. ("No eat.") *No* and *not* used interchangeably.	*Yes/no* asked with rising intonation on single word. *What* and *where.* *That* + X. *What* + noun phrase + (doing)? *Where* + noun phrase + (going)?	Prepositions *in* and *on* appear.	*And* appears. ("Coat and hat.")
24–30 months	*No, not, don't,* and *can't* used interchangeably. Negative element placed between subject and predicate.	*What* or *where* + subject + predicate.		*But, so, or,* and *if* appear.
30–36 months	*Won't* appears.	Begins to use auxiliary verbs in questions (*be, can, will, do*). ("You are going?")	Subordinate clauses appear after verbs *like, think, guess, show.* ("I know *what you like.*")	*Because* appears. Clauses joined with *and* appear (not until after 48 months do most children produce this form).
36–42 months	Adds *isn't, aren't, doesn't,* and *didn't.*	Begins to invert auxiliary verb and subject ("Are you going?"). Adds *when, how,* and *why.*		
42–48 months	Adds *wasn't, wouldn't, couldn't,* and *shouldn't.*	Adds modal auxiliary verbs (*would, could, should,* etc.). Stabilizes inverted auxiliary.	Subordinate clauses appear in object position.	Clauses joined with *if* appear.
48+ months	Adds *nobody, no one, none,* and *nothing.* Difficulty with double negatives. ("Nobody don't...")		Subordinate clauses attached to the subject. Embedding and conjoining appear within same sentence.	*When, because, but,* and *so* appear in clause joining.

expanded into *agent + action + object,* as in *Daddy eat cookie* and *Mommy throw ball.* This knowledge is used to both interpret and produce the dominant English sentence form of *subject + verb + object* (SVO). The child assumes that the first noun in the sentence is causing some action and so on. This strategy will aid in the interpretation of some, but not all English sentences. In the sentence *I am healthy,* there is no action and, therefore, no agent. Gradually, the child's inadequate strategy is expanded, new semantic classes are learned, and the child begins to use more syntactically based rules for word ordering.

Meanings first signaled by semantic word-order rules are later marked both syntactically and morphologically (see Table 2.4). For example, possession is demonstrated in two-word utterances by *possessor + possessed* as in *Mommy sock,* but by age 3, most children say *Mommy's sock.* Similarly, location is signaled by *X + location* as in *Doggie bed* and only later by the addition of prepositions, so that by age 2 children say *Doggie in bed.* In a final example, *Mommy eat cookie* (*agent + action + object*) becomes *Mommy is eating a cookie.* All essential elements are present in the semantically based structure and the grammatical markers follow. These and other morphemes may first be learned in specific constructions with particular words. For example, contracted *is* may first appear with *he* and *that* to form *he's* and *that's* (S. Wilson, 2003).

In a reverse process, syntactic structure may also be used by the child to derive word meanings (Gleitman, 1993). The syntactic context can yield valuable information about word meaning and about word membership in categories, such as verbs or nouns.

Active Involvement.   As we have seen, even toddlers do not imitate everything. Imitation is a conscious learning strategy that is selectively applied. Even imitation has its limits, however, and between 24 and 30 months of age, use of the strategy decreases. At this point in language development, the child is learning syntactic rules, and imitation is a rather inefficient learning strategy.

Preschoolers are actively analyzing incoming information, searching for patterns, hypothesizing language rules, and synthesizing their own sentences based on these rules. As a result, preschoolers often use the full form of a structure first, even though the adult model may be contracted. For example, most children will use *The doggie is running* before *The doggie's running.* Rule generalization with other forms such as the past-tense marker *-ed* can lead to use with forms that do not take this marker to produce *eated, goed,* and *sitted.* Imitation could not be used as an explanation of the origin of these forms.

One active strategy is substitution. A large number of preschool children's novel utterances differ only slightly from utterances produced previously. For example, a child says, *Where's Anna's plate?* Previously, she had said, *Where's Anna's **W**?* and *Where's **Mommy's** plate?* (Lieven, Behrens, Speares, & Tomasello, 2003, p. 340).

We might call some children "risk-takers." While some children with little knowledge of a grammatical structure make few errors because they attempt to produce it infrequently, risk-takers attempt repeatedly to produce these structures, making frequent mistakes (Rispoli, 2005).

New words are added to the child's **lexicon**—her personal dictionary—at the rate of two or three per day. Words are added rapidly by a process called **fast mapping** in which the child assumes a meaning from context and then produces the word in a similar context. Gradually, the meaning is refined. Words may be fastmapped using one or more strategies (Storkel, 2001). For example, the child may assume that the new word's definition cannot be the same as one already possessed. A second possibility is that the child uses word order and bound morphemes as clues to the meaning (Plunkett, 1993;

Samuelson & Smith, 1998). Finally, the child may use phonotactic probability or the likelihood of occurrence of different sound sequences to aid rapid recall of newly learned words.

Hypothesized meanings come from both the linguistic and the nonlinguistic context (Au, 1990; Naigles, 1990). Two strategies, *contrast* and *conventionality*, may be used to determine word meaning (Clark, 1990; Gathercole, 1989). Using a contrast strategy, the child assumes that each word is different from or contrasts with every other. This strategy occurs concurrently with the conventionality strategy in which the child assumes that a certain form will be used repeatedly to convey meaning. Using both, the child assumes that speakers will use conventional forms that clearly contrast with each other.

Complexity and Utterance Length Relationship.   As mentioned previously, there is a positive correlation between utterance length and complexity in preschool English (Rondal, Ghiotto, Bredart, & Bachelet, 1987). This association weakens later in development. More complex relationships begin to occur at about age 3.

Children begin to speak in single-word utterances, which expand at 18 months of age into two words. In quick succession, two-word utterances are combined to form three- and four-word utterances. By age 2, the preschooler is beginning to add morphological endings (*-ing, -ed*), articles (*a, the*), and auxiliary verbs (see Table 2.4).

The length–complexity relationship is also demonstrated by embedding and conjoining. **Embedding** is the placement of a phrase or clause within another clause. A phrase is a group of words that may contain a noun or a verb, but not both. Examples include prepositional phrases (*in the closet, on the table*), infinitive phrases (*to eat, to go*), and **gerunds** (*I like swimming*). A **clause** contains both a noun and a verb, called the subject and predicate, respectively. A clause can be independent, in which case it is a sentence (*I bought the toy*), or dependent (*that I saw at Smith's*) and in need of an independent clause to which to attach (*I bought the toy that I saw at Smith's*). In **conjoining**, two independent clauses are joined by a **conjunction** (*I went to school but my sister stayed home with the flu*). Obviously, the two processes of embedding and conjoining will lengthen the individual sentence and increase complexity.

Language development is not merely additive. Some complexity, such as moving auxiliary verbs (*What Mommy is eating?*) to form mature interrogatives (*What is Mommy eating?*), is achieved while not affecting utterance length.

Avoid Exceptions.   Anyone who has learned a foreign language knows that the rules are easier to learn than the exceptions. This is also true for preschoolers learning their first language. One of the first morphological endings to be learned is *-ing,* in part because there are no exceptions to the rule that action verbs—the ones most frequently used by young children—can take this ending (*eating, running, jumping*).

Preschoolers seem to follow a rule that when you find a form that works, use it. This leads to overgeneralization of the regular past-tense marker *-ed* to form *eated* and *goed* and to overuse of the conjunction *and* and the article *the.* Another interesting overgeneralization occurs between *wh-* interrogatives and embedding. You will recall that it takes some time for preschoolers to learn to invert the verb in interrogatives from *What you are doing?* to *What are you doing?* At about the same time, the child is learning to embed clauses as in the following:

I know *what you're doing.*

I remember *where we went.*

Overgeneralizing from interrogatives, the child may produce the following:

I know *what **are** you doing.*

I remember *where **did** we go.*

Although a *wh-* word is used in embedding, the intention is not to ask a question.

Finally, around age 5, the child learns several indefinite negative forms, such as *nobody, no one,* and *nothing* (see Table 2.4). Since the negative sentence form is already learned, these forms are incorporated into that form. The result is double negatives, such as *Nobody don't like me* and *I didn't get nothing.*

Word Order Is a Guide.   In English, the predominant SVO (subject–verb–object) word order is very important and can serve as a guide for sentence comprehension and formation. Sentences that deviate from this form are likely to be misinterpreted by the preschooler. When in doubt, preschoolers depend on their experience to decide the most probable meaning (Berman, 1986).

A corollary to this strategy is that the order of mention is the order of occurrence. In other words, those things mentioned first occurred first, those next occurred next, and so on. Words such as *before* and *after,* which might change that order, as in *Before you clean your room, make your bed,* are ignored. Only toward the end of the preschool period does the child attend to the specific temporal, or time, words used.

Avoid Deviation from or Interruption of Standard Word Order.   As noted previously, word order is a strong tool for comprehension and production of English syntax. Rearrangement of the words as in interrogatives or additions that may interrupt the sequence as in negatives and embeddings is resisted.

Caregivers Modify Conversations to Maximize Child Participation.   With few exceptions, parents and other caregivers of preschoolers do not formally teach language. Although they continue to provide models and to correct speech and language form occasionally, this behavior is neither preconceived nor consistent. One type of feedback caregivers use is called **reformulation**. The adult checks his or her understanding against the child's meaning by reformulating the child's utterance into what the adult thinks the child meant. In the process, the adult locates the error or errors and embeds a correction. As a result, the child hears a more conventional form for expressing his or her meaning. With preschoolers, adults reformulate more frequently than they imitate, although both forms decrease as a child passes through preschool (Chouinard & Clark, 2003).

Caregivers facilitate participation in conversations for the child. In general, caregivers discuss topics of interest to the child and encourage the child to participate by providing obvious conversational opportunities (Hoff-Ginsberg, 1990). There is a corresponding increase in the talkativeness of children. Although vocabulary growth between the ages of 1 and 3 years is positively related to the diversity of words in the mother's speech, it is not related to the overall amount of maternal talkativeness (Pan, Rowe, Singer, & Snow, 2005).

Most caregiver utterances are semantically and pragmatically contingent. Semantic contingency occurs when the speaker continues with the topic of the previous speaker. Pragmatic contingency is appropriateness of the response. For example, a topic usually receives a comment, a question usually receives an answer, and so on.

Preschoolers are encouraged to take conversational turns by the use of turnabouts by caregivers. A **turnabout** is usually a comment or reply to the child's utterance, followed by a question that serves as a cue for the child to take his turn. A series of adult turnabouts might be as follows:

Child: I got a bike for my birthday.

Adult: Oh, how special. Can you ride all by yourself?

Child: No, Daddy helps me.

Adult: That's probably good until you get used to it. Does he let go every once in a while?

Repeatedly hearing a caregiver's questions can have a beneficial effect on a preschooler's development of interrogatives (Valian & Casey, 2003).

Rather than trying to grab a turn as adults do when conversing with one another, the adult provides an opportunity for the child and a very obvious signal that it is the child's turn. The result is that the child learns to develop a topic in conversation (Foster, 1986).

All Aspects of Language Are Intertwined in Development.   It is very difficult to separate syntactic development from semantic or semantic from pragmatic. Language features are not learned in a void, but rather in a context that includes all elements of language. For example, pronouns contain semantic distinctions of number (singular, plural), person, gender, and class (subjective, objective, possessive); they contain syntactic distinctions of word order and noun–verb agreement (*I am, you are, he is*); and they contain pragmatic distinctions of role (speaker, listener, and others). Given this interdependence, it should be obvious why pronouns can be troublesome to the preschool learner.

Narratives or stories also illustrate this interrelationship. Around age 2, children begin to tell narratives (Sutton-Smith, 1986). Initially, these stories are very loose and may have no central theme. By age 3, children have acquired a sense of time or order, and events are sequenced (Sutton-Smith, 1986). Within these emerging narratives— usually telling of some incident involving himself—the child develops verb tensing; sequencing, using *and* (*then*); and descriptive terms. In addition, the child must consider the audience and the appropriate amount of information needed to convey the event.

Children use the context, past learning, and linguistic and nonlinguistic cues in both comprehension and production. When deciding on the appropriate syntactic forms, for example, young children seem to rely on all linguistic information—form, content, and use—as if unable to rely on any one form alone (Prasada & Ferenz, 2002). Even 5-year-olds depend on both linguistic and contextual information; however, by age 3, word order has become a reliable interpretive cue for the English-speaking child (Thal & Flores, 2001).

Preschool language development is also related to cognitive development. Children gain the cognitive concepts of time and place before they begin to use the prepositions that mark these concepts. Likewise, knowledge of time sequences and increased memory are required for a child to use the linguistic relationships of *before* and *after*. The child must abstract basic relationships from the physical environment and language rules from the linguistic environment. Language input is interpreted using linguistic rules that reflect the cognitive relationships.

Summary.   Within a few short years, the preschool child learns most of the conventions of language form. Development is all the more amazing when we realize the interdependence of all aspects of language and the lack of formal instruction by caregivers.

There are still important advances to be made during the school-age years. Knowledge of language use will increase. Having acquired much of the "what" of language form, the child turns to the "how" of language use.

School-Age and Adult Development   The school-age and, to a lesser extent, the adult years are characterized by growth in all aspects of language—syntax, morphology, semantics, phonology, and pragmatics. The emphasis of development differs, however, from that seen in preschool. Major developmental stress is placed on the semantics and pragmatics of language. The child learns to use existing forms to communicate more effectively. Metalinguistic abilities that enable a language user to think about and reflect on language also become more prominent during this period. In addition, the child learns new means of communication, reading and writing. The child's oral language knowledge forms a base for this new learning (V. Reed, 1986), even though this base has not completely developed and will continue to mature throughout this period.

While the changes during preschool years are rapid and dramatic, those occurring during school years are slower and more subtle. Emphasis shifts from spoken to written language in both input and output. As a result, by fourth grade the child is using reading skills to learn advanced, often specialized, vocabulary, figurative or nonliteral language, and complex forms (G. A. Miller & Gildea, 1987). The shift to reading and writing and the emphasis on more-formal language instruction require greater metalinguistic competence. In essence, written language is decontextualized or less dependent on the nonlinguistic context, requiring the user to obtain all contextual information from print, and, therefore, is more abstract. Abstract learning is also evidenced in figurative language and in linguistic ambiguities, such as jokes and puns (Nippold, 1988a, 1988b). This shift correlates with changes in cognition from concrete to abstract (Kamhi & Lee, 1988).

Adult development continues to concentrate on semantics and pragmatics, with increased vocabulary growth and versatility in use. Vocabulary growth and categorization continue throughout life. New words are added for specialized occupations, interests, and socialization. In addition, the *adult* becomes an even more adept user of language, able to adapt her language style to different social contexts and different communication goals.

In the realm of language form, school-age development consists of simultaneous expansion of existing forms and acquisition of new ones. Sentence production continues to expand during the school-age through adult years across individuals at all socioeconomic levels and of all racial/ethnic groups (H. K. Craig, Washington, & Thompson-Porter, 1998). The child's syntactic growth continues with internal sentence expansion by elaboration of the noun and verb elements, expansion of conjoining and embedding, and addition of structures such as passive voice. Most first graders do not produce adult passive sentences (*The cat was chased by the dog*), reflexive pronouns (*myself, themselves*), *because* clauses, and gerunds, and many do not comprehend the adverbial *-ly*; irregular noun and verb agreement (*The sheep **is** eating; The fish **are** eating*); several conjunctions (*though, however*); passive sentences; and several verb tenses, such as the past participle (*has eaten*) and the perfect tense (*has been* verb *-ing*). In addition, school-age children still have difficulty with some prepositions, verb tensing, and plurals.

The child's repertoire of embedded and conjoined forms increases throughout the school years. Conjoining expands with the addition of *because, so, therefore, if, but, or, when, before, and after* used to join clauses. Forms such as *although* and *therefore* are not mastered until late elementary school or early adolescence. Semantic understanding of the relations expressed by conjunctions continues to develop long after children begin to use these terms correctly in their speech (Cain, Patson, & Andrews, 2005).

Morphological and phonological development also continues beyond the preschool years. *Morphophonemic changes* are phonological or sound modifications that result when morphemes are placed together. For example, the final /k/ sound in *electric* changes to an /s/ when *-ity* is added to form *electricity*. Similarly, the vowel sound in the second syllable of *divine* shifts in *divinity*. Knowledge of vowel shifting is gained only gradually, and it is not until age 17 that most children learn to apply all the rules.

Stress or emphasis related to meaning is also learned during the school years. The stress placed on certain syllables reflects the grammatical function of the word. In English, stress varies with the relationship of two words and with a word's use as a noun or verb. For example, two words may form a phrase such as *black board* or a compound word such as *blackboard*. The speaker stresses *board* in the phrase and *black* in the compound word. In the noun *record*, emphasis is on the first syllable, while the verb *record* is pronounced with stress on the second. By age 12, most children have acquired stress contrast rules.

Although spoken language and written language have much in common, they are not just language in different forms (Kamhi & Catts, 2005). In addition to the obvious physical difference, reading and writing lack the give-and-take of conversation, are more permanent, lack the paralinguistic features (stress, intonation, fluency, etc.) of speech, have their own vocabulary and grammar, and are processed in a different manner in the brain.

The new communication means of reading and writing are taught to children during the school years, although most children begin prereading and prewriting activities prior to first grade. Gradually, the child realizes that the message is contained in the orthographic or written symbols rather than in the accompanying pictures. In his initial reading, the child concentrates on decoding single words. Only gradually does he begin to use the text as an aid for inferring meaning. In order to decode print, a child must possess both **phonological awareness** or knowledge of sounds and syllables and of the sound structure of words and **phonemic awareness** or the ability to manipulate sounds, such as blending sounds to create words or segmenting words into sounds. Phonological awareness skills also are the best predictor of spelling and ability in elementary school (Nation & Hulme, 1997). In general, children who have been exposed to a home literacy environment and to print media have better phoneme awareness, letter knowledge, and vocabulary (Foy & Mann, 2003). Between grades 4 and 8, reading shifts from decoding skill to comprehension, with increasing rates of scanning the text. Both oral language and the written context play a role in word recognition and in the ability to construct meaning from print (Gillam & Gorman, 2004). Comprehension emerges from an interaction of letters, sounds, word meanings, grammatical and contextual processes, and a reader's prior knowledge and experience (Kintsch, 1998; Sanford & Garrod, 1998; Whitehurst & Lonigan, 2001). Actively engaged, the mature reader makes hypotheses and predictions and confirms or does not confirm these.

In contrast, writing is using knowledge and new ideas combined with language knowledge to create text (Kintsch, 1998). It's a complex process that includes generating ideas, organizing and planning, acting on that plan, revising, and monitoring based on self-feedback (C. M. Scott, 2005).

In writing, the child gradually moves from drawing through "inventive" spelling to regularity as letters are matched to speech sounds. In inventive spelling, the child uses letter names and consonant sounds to spell and often includes first and last letters. For example, *say* may be spelled "SA" and *sand,* "SD." While sounds are important for spelling, the mature speller relies on a combination of memory; spelling and reading experience; phonological, semantic, and morphological knowledge; orthographic knowledge and mental grapheme representations; and analogy (Apel & Masterson, 2001). In addition, the child begins to be more aware of his reader, much as he became aware of his listener in conversations. This shift from egocentric focus to concern for the reader becomes evident around third to fourth grade. **Text generation begins with oral narratives.**

The emphasis on both reading and writing of stories requires the child to have a grasp of relational terms, such as those for time (*before, after, then, on, at*), those for space (*here, there, beside, between, left, right*), and comparative terms (*better than, almost, nearly, fewer, neither–nor, same*). These changes are reflected in the oral narratives of the child.

While the basics of reading and writing are taught in the first three grades, there is a shift in fourth grade to a reliance on the skills already established.

During the school-age period and adult years, most semantic growth focuses on increases in the size of the child's vocabulary and the specificity of definition. With age, both children and adults modify their internal definitions to specify more core defining attributes in a precise, abstract, generalized manner (C. J. Johnson & Anglin, 1995). Thus, definitions move from concrete and contextual (*My doggie hides in the closet*) to more shared (*A closet is a storage space in which we hang clothes*) to abstract and figurative (*coming out of the closet*). More than other areas of language, development of semantics varies widely with educational level, socioeconomic status, gender, age, and cultural background. The actual number of words a child knows is increased with the addition of morphological prefixes and suffixes that change word meanings (Anglin, 1995). Bound morphemes are added throughout the school years.

In school-age and adult years, definitions become more dictionarylike and conventional. Gradually, the child acquires an abstract knowledge of meaning that is independent of particular contexts or individual interpretations. Definitional skill is highly correlated with involvement in an academic culture. As a result, some working-class fourth graders outperform their parents in providing oral definitions (Kurland & Snow, 1997). During adolescence, a number of changes occur in definitions with the inclusion of category membership, the sharpening of core features of a word, and the addition of subtle aspects of meaning (Nippold, Hegel, Sohlberg, & Schwarz, 1999). The ability to provide definitions of words is related to metalinguistics, and both increase with age and educational level (Benelli, Belacchi, Gini, & Lucanggeli, 2006).

The school-age child begins to organize words in a different way than she has previously. This change has been called the **syntagmatic-paradigmatic shift** (Ervin, 1961). The earlier syntagmatic association is based on a syntactic or word-order relationship. For example, the stimulus word *girl* might elicit a child response *run*. In contrast, the later developing paradigmatic association is based on semantic attributes. In this case, the word *girl* might elicit *boy* or *woman*. The shift represents a refinement and organization of semantic features and may reflect a change in the child's general cognitive-processing strategies. The period of most rapid change occurs between the ages of 5 and 9. It is not until the adult years, however, that paradigmatic or categorical associations become consistent and fully integrated.

The school-age child also develops figurative language and uses language in a truly creative way. In **figurative language**, words are used in an imaginative sense, rather than a literal one, to create an imaginative or emotional impression. Figurative language enriches and enlivens our communication, is indicative of higher language functions, and correlates with adolescent literacy skills (Dean Qualls, O'Brien, Blood, & Scheffner Hammer, 2003). The primary types include idioms, metaphors, similes, and proverbs. *Idioms* are short expressions that have evolved through years of use and cannot be analyzed grammatically, such as *hit the roof* or *throw a party*. For preteens and adolescents, idioms that are more familiar, supported by context, and more transparent are easier to understand than those that are less familiar, out of context, and more opaque (Nippold & Taylor, 1995; Nippold, Taylor, & Baker, 1995; Spector, 1996).

Metaphors and *similes* are figures of speech in which a resemblance or comparison is implied, as in *She had a skeletal appearance*, or stated explicitly, as in *He ran like a gazelle*. Finally, *proverbs* are short, popular sayings that embody a generally accepted truth, useful thought, or advice. In general, proverbs are difficult even for adolescents to comprehend. Examples of proverbs are

Don't put all your eggs in one basket.

You can't have your cake and eat it, too.

The young school age child interprets proverbs quite literally. Some proverbs are still misinterpreted in adulthood. In general, proverbs are easier to interpret if they are concrete and familiar rather than abstract and unfamiliar (Nippold & Serajul Haq, 1996).

The area of most significant linguistic growth during the school-age and adult years is that of conversational skills, an area of pragmatics. A preschool child does not have the skill of a junior-high student. No adult is fooled by the adolescent comment *Gee, Mom, I wonder if there's skating today*. Both parties understand the request, however indirect it may be.

Successful communication involves the active involvement of both participants. Development occurs over an extended period into adolescence and adulthood with much individual variation. Some children are more effective conversationists than adults, quickly recognizing conversational breakdown and addressing it (A. H. Anderson, Clark, & Mullin, 1994). In general, the ability to detect communication breakdown improves with age. By adulthood, linguistic anomalies are detected almost instantaneously (Fodor, Ni, Crain, & Shankweiler, 1996).

During the school years, the child gains the ability to use language more subtly. To clarify messages, she must monitor and evaluate communication and the cues regarding success or failure of the communication effort. By late adolescence, the youth knows not only that a communication partner's perspective and knowledge may differ from his own, but also that it is important to consider these differences. In addition, the high schooler uses language creatively, in sarcasm, jokes, and double meanings. These begin to develop in the early school years. High schoolers make deliberate use of metaphor and can explain complex behavior and natural phenomena.

One verbal strategy used widely by adults is the **indirect request**, referring only indirectly to what the speaker wants. For example, the statement *The heater sure is working overtime* may be an indirect request for the heat to be turned down. Indirect requests represent a growing awareness of the importance of socially appropriate requests and of the communication context. In general, the 5-year-old is successful at directly asking, commanding, and forbidding. By age 7, she has greater facility with indirect forms. There is increased flexibility in indirect request forms, and the proportion of hints increases from childhood through adulthood (Ervin-Tripp, 1980).

The school-age child is able to introduce a topic into the conversation, sustain it through several turns, and close or switch the topic. These discourse skills develop only gradually through elementary school. In contrast, topics change rapidly when the conversational partner is a 3-year-old. The school-age child learns to *shadow* or to "slide" from one topic to a related one rather than making the abrupt topic changes seen in preschoolers. It is not until around age 11 that the child has the cognitive skills to sustain abstract discussions of love or peace.

As early as elementary school, the conversations of boys and girls also begin to reflect the gender differences of older children and adults. These differences can be noted in both vocabulary use and conversational style. In general, in conversations between men and women, females talk less, introduce fewer topics, avoid swearing and coarse language more, and provide more eye contact and feedback. In addition, the communication experiences and needs of adults result in many different language styles used by each person. Specific styles, often with their own vocabulary, are used in the workplace and with groups with particular interests. Conversational abilities continue to diversify and become more elaborate with age. Adolescents frequently gaze at their partners, especially during listening; nod and show neutral and positive facial expressions; and use feedback and give contingent responses (Turkstra, Ciccia, & Seaton, 2003).

Older children and adults have the linguistic skills to select from several available communication strategies that best suit a specific context. Mature language is efficient and appropriate: efficient in that words are more specifically defined and forms do not need repetition or paraphrasing to be understood; appropriate in that utterances are selected for the psychosocial dynamics of the communication situation. The less mature language user has difficulty selecting the appropriate code because she has a limited repertoire of language forms.

Both the length and the syntactic complexity of oral sentences increase into early adulthood and stabilize in middle age (Nippold, Hesketh, Duthie, & Mansfield, 2005). Although healthy adults continue to expand their language, there are subtle losses, too. Typical seniors experience some deficits in the accuracy and speed of word retrieval and naming (Nicholas, Barth, Obler, Au, & Albert, 1997). There are accompanying deficits in the ability to produce grammatically complex sentences, although there does not seem to be a loss in ability to produce simple sentences (Davidson, Zacks, & Ferreira, 2003; Kemper, Thompson, & Marquis, 2001).

Speech

Speech is a verbal means of communicating or conveying meaning. The result of specific motor behaviors, speech requires precise neuromuscular coordination. The speech mechanism and its neuromuscular control are explained in Chapter 3. Speech consists of speech-sound combinations, voice quality, intonation, and rate. Each of these components is used to modify the speech message. In face-to-face conversation, much of the message is also carried by nonspeech means, such as facial expressions and gestures.

The smallest unit of speech is the *phoneme,* a family of sounds that are close enough in perceptual qualities to be distinguished from other phonemes. Members of these families of sounds are called **allophones**. The allophones within a phoneme family differ from one another because of phonemic constraints, such as the effects of other phonemes on the sound, and production constraints, such as fatigue. Though phonemes are meaningless in and of themselves, in words they make a semantic difference. For example, the final sounds in *cat* and *cash* are perceptually different enough to signal differences of meaning. They represent two different phonemes.

Phonemes are written between slashes to distinguish them from the alphabetic, or graphemic, representations. The International Phonetic Alphabet (IPA) is used rather than the English alphabet in transcribing sounds for two reasons. First, a sound may be spelled several ways, as in *day, obey,* and *weight*. Likewise, some letters, such as *c,* can be pronounced more than one way (as an *s* or a *k*). This is especially true of vowels, such as the *e* in *be* and *bed*. Second, the pronunciation of the English alphabet cannot be applied to other languages, especially those that use a different alphabet system.

In English, phonemes are classified as vowels or consonants. *Vowels* are produced with a relatively unrestricted airflow in the vocal tract. *Consonants* require a closed or narrowly constricted passage that results in friction and air turbulence. The number of phonemes attributed to American English differs with the classification system used and the dialect of the speaker.

Phonemes can be described as being voiced or voiceless. **Voiced** phonemes are produced by phonation (vibration of the vocal folds); *voiceless* phonemes are not. All vowels in English are voiced, but consonants may be either voiced or voiceless.

Phonemic classification is based on the place of articulation and, for consonants, on the manner of articulation, usually the type of air release. In this system, vowels are described by the highest portion of the tongue, front-to-back positioning of the tongue, and lip rounding. Heights can be characterized as high, mid, or low. The location of this highest position can be described as front, central, or back. For example, a vowel can be described as high front or low back. The English vowels are displayed graphically in Figure 2.3. Words using each sound are printed next to each phoneme.

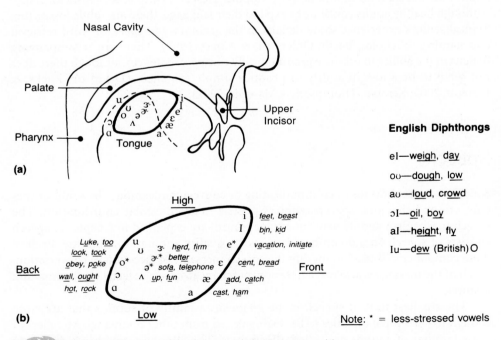

FIGURE 2.3   Classification of English vowels by tongue position.
Source: From *Language Development: An Introduction* (7th ed.), by R. E. Owens, Jr., 2010. Boston: Allyn and Bacon. Copyright 2010 by Allyn and Bacon Publishing Company. Reprinted by permission.

Lip rounding is an additional description used for vowel classification. In rounding, the lips protrude slightly, forming an "O" shape. Rounding is characteristic of some back vowels, such as the last sound in *construe*. In contrast, there is no lip rounding in *construct*.

One group of vowel-like sounds is more complex. These sounds are called **diphthongs**. A diphthong is a blend of two vowels within the same syllable. The sound begins with one vowel and glides smoothly toward another. When the word *day* is repeated slowly, the speaker can feel and hear the shift from one vowel to another at the end. The diphthongs are also presented in Figure 2.3.

Consonant descriptions presented in Table 2.5 are more complex than those for vowels and include manner of articulation, place of articulation, and voicing. *Manner* refers to the type of production, generally with respect to the release of air. The six generally recognized categories of manner follow:

- Plosive (/p/, /b/, /t/, /d/, /k/, /g/)—Complete obstruction of the airstream, with quick release accompanied by an audible escape of air; similar to an explosion.
- Fricative (/f/, /v/, /ɵ/, /ð/, /s/, /z/, /ʃ/, /ʒ/, /h/)—Narrow constriction through which the air must pass, creating a hissing noise.
- Affricative (/tʃ/, /dʒ/)—A combination that begins with a plosive followed by a fricative, as the IPA symbols suggest.
- Approximant (/w/, /j/, /r/)—Produced by the proximity of two articulators without turbulence.
- Lateral approximant (/l/)—Produced in a similar manner to an approximant with the addition of the lateral flow of the airstream.
- Nasal (/m/, /n/, /ŋ/)—Produced by incorporating resonance in the nasal cavity.

Variations result from constriction within the oral cavity.

TABLE 2.5   Traditional Classification of English Consonants

Place of Constriction	Manner of Production						
	Plosive		Fricative		Approximant†	Lateral Approximant	Nasal†
	U	V	U	V	V		V
Bilabial	p (pig)	b (big)			w (watt)		m (sum)
Labiodental			f (face)	v (vase)			
Dental			ɵ (thigh, thin)	ð (thy, this)			
Alveolar	t (tot)	d (dot)	s (seal)	z (zeal)	r (rot)	l (lot)	n (sun)
Postalveolar			ʃ (shoe, mission)	ʒ (visual, measure)			
Palatal			tʃ (choke, nature)	dʒ (joke, gentle)	j (yacht)		
Velar	k (coat)	g (goat)					ŋ (sung)
Glottal			h (happy)				

U = unvoiced; V = voiced.

†All voiced.

The place of articulation varies across the five manner categories and describes the position where the maximum constriction, either partial or complete, occurs. The eight locations are

- Bilabial (/p/, /b/, /m/)—Lips together.
- Labiodental (/f/, /v/)—Lower lip touches upper incisors.
- Dental (/θ/, /ð/)—Tongue tip protruding slightly between the lower and upper incisors.
- Alveolar (/t/, /d/, /s/, /z/, /l/, /r/, /n/)—Front of tongue to upper alveolar (gum) ridge.
- Postalveolar (/ʃ/, /ʒ/)—Tongue blade gently approximates postalveolar ridge area.
- Palatal (/j/)—Tongue blade raised to hard palate.
- Velar (/k/, /g/, /ŋ/)—Back of tongue raised to soft palate or velum.
- Glottal (/h/)—Restriction at glottis or opening to larynx.

Many English consonant sounds differ only in voicing. When two phonemes have the same manner and place of articulation, but differ in voicing, they are called **cognates**. For example, /s/ and /z/ are cognates. If you repeat the words *seal* and *zeal,* you can feel the difference at the larynx. Place and manner of articulation do not differ.

Theoretically, phonemes could be produced in almost any configuration of manner, place, and voicing. Other languages use some of the phonemes used in English, plus additional speech sounds. Some English distinctions are not present in other languages. In Spanish, for example, there is no distinction between /s/ and /z/; they are not separate phonemes. Other languages make finer distinctions that are not relevant to speakers of English (and that are, therefore, difficult for us to distinguish).

Sounds rarely occur alone in speech. Speech is a dynamic process, and movement patterns for more than one sound may occur simultaneously. This co-occurrence of production characteristics of two or more phonemes is called **coarticulation**. Coarticulation is the result of motor commands from the brain and the mechanical response of the speech muscles. Movement may occur several phonemes prior to the appearance of the phoneme associated with this movement. For example, in the word *construe,* lip rounding begins well before the /u/ sound. These anticipatory movements are a clear indication that the brain is not functioning on a phoneme level.

In a mechanical system, such as the speech mechanism, there is also built-in inertia, or drag. Muscle movements lag behind brain commands, thus continuing after the commands have ceased. The result is that the production characteristics of one phoneme may persist during production of another. For example, there is a nasalization of the /z/ in *runs* (/rvnz/) caused by the insufficient time available for the velum to return to its upward position after /n/.

Development of Speech

As he matures, the child gains increasing control of the speech mechanism and is able to produce or articulate sounds more effectively. Although he gains much motor control within the first year, the child does not achieve adultlike stability until midchildhood. In this section, we shall explore the major developmental speech changes. These and other developmental changes are presented in Table 2.6.

TABLE 2.6 Speech Development

Age	Stage	Speech	Other Development
0–1 month	Newborn	Reflexive behavior Suck–swallow pattern Nondifferentiated crying Vegetative sounds with phonation, but incomplete resonance	6–8 lbs, 17–21 in. Can't raise head when on stomach Visual and auditory preferences, best vision at 7½ in. Sensitive to volume, pitch, and duration of sound Sleeps about 70% of time
2–3 months	Cooing	Definite stop and start to oral movement Velar to uvular closure or near closure Back consonants and back and middle vowels with incomplete resonance	Holds head up briefly while on stomach or sitting supported Repeats own actions Visually searches Begins exploratory play Excited by people Social smile
4–6 months	Babbling	Greater independent control of tongue Prolonged strings of sounds More lip or labial sounds Experiments with sounds	12–16 lbs, 23–24 in. Turns head to localize sound Mouths objects Sits supported for half hour Selective attention to faces Anticipates actions Excites with game play
7–10 months	Reduplication babbling	Repetitive syllable production Increased lip control Labial and alveolar plosives /p, b, t, d/, nasals, /j/, but not fully formed	Self-feeding Progresses from creeping through crawling to standing Explores objects through manipulation Imitates others physically Gestures
11–14 months	Phonetically consistent forms and first words	Elevates tongue tip Variegated babbling Intonational patterns Phonetically consistent forms—sound–meaning relationships Predominance of /m, w, b, p/ First words primarily CV, VC, CVCV reduplicated, and CVCV	26–30 lbs, 28–30 in. Stands alone Feeds self with spoon First steps Uses trial-and-error problem solving Deferred imitation
2 years		Has acquired /p, h, w, m, b, k, g/	31–35 lbs, 32–34 in. Walks without watching feet Limited role-playing Parallel play
3 years		Has acquired /d, f, j, t, n, s/, all vowels	Short incomplete sentences 200- to 300-word vocabulary Explores by dismantling Rides tricycle Representational drawing Make-believe play Shares toys briefly Subject and verb sentences 900- to 1,000-word vocabulary

(Continued)

TABLE 2.6   (Continued)

Age	Stage	Speech	Other Development
4 years		Has acquired /v, ʃ, tʃ, z/	Walks stairs with alternating steps Categorizes Counts to 5 Role-plays Cooperative play Tells stories, asks many questions 1,500- to 1,600-word vocabulary
5 years		Has acquired /r, l, ө, ŋ, dʒ, ð/	41–45 lbs, 40–42 in. Prints simple words Time concepts of recent past and future Simple game playing 2,100- to 2,200-word vocabulary Syntactic acquisition about 90% complete
6–8 years		Has acquired /ʒ/, consonant blends	Rides bicycle Reads Enjoys action games Competitiveness Enjoys an audience 2,600-word expressive vocabulary

The Newborn   Much of the behavior of the newborn is reflexive, or beyond her immediate volitional control. The reflex of most interest for speech development is the rhythmic suck–swallow pattern, first established at 3 months prior to birth. As with other reflexes, sucking involves the midbrain and brainstem only. At birth, sucking is primarily accompanied by up-and-down jaw action. To swallow, the neonate opens her mouth slightly and protrudes and then retracts her tongue. To complete her swallow, the neonate must also close or abduct her vocal folds within the larynx to protect the lungs. Functioning and location of these structures will be described in Chapter 3.

The most common sounds made by the newborn are cries and partial vowel sounds. By the end of the first month, the cries become differentiated, and mothers can usually tell the type of cry—wet, hungry, ill—by its pattern. The noncrying sounds of the newborn include normal phonation, but lack full resonance in the oral cavity. Considerable air is emitted via the nasal cavity, and the resultant sounds are nasalized.

The newborn is capable of many types of auditory perception and can discriminate between different sound durations and loudness levels, different phonemes, and different consonants even within CVC syllables (Moon, Bever, & Fifer, 1992). Newborns are also capable of discriminating different pitches or frequencies, especially in the human speech range. In fact, neonates respond to the human voice more often and with more vigor than to other environmental sounds. This discrimination is not the same as linguistic perception, however, and does not involve sound–meaning relationships.

Cooing: 2 to 3 Months   By 2 months, the infant has developed muscle control to stop and start oral movement, though some tactile stimulation is still needed. This stage is characterized by laughter and nondistress "cooing," with near closure between the soft palate and the pharyngeal wall. The infant produces back consonants (/k, g, h/) and middle and back vowel sounds with incomplete resonance.

Babbling: 4 to 6 Months   From 4 to 6 months, the child begins to experiment with sounds and to gain increasingly independent control of the parts of the vocal mechanism. The random sounds she produces often do not appear in her native language; they often differ in some ways from the sounds of her language. During this period, Neuromuscular control moves from the back of the oral cavity to the lips. With greater control of the tongue, the infant exhibits strong tongue projection, although it will take years for her to master reliable tongue tip control. The infant is also able to use the intrinsic muscles of the tongue, rather than a whole-jaw movement, for sucking.

Speech is characterized by prolonged periods of vocalization and by strings of sounds called **babbling**. Guttural sounds, such as growling, that predominated previously tend to lessen with the appearance of labials, or lip sounds (/p, b, w, m/). Constriction abilities become more mature in the forward position of the mouth, and by 6 months, labial sounds predominate. During vocal turn-taking with a caregiver, 3-month-olds produce more speechlike syllabic vocalizations than isolated vowel sounds (Masataka, 1995).

Reduplication Babbling: 6 to 10 Months   As the infant gains increasing control of oral movements, his speech progresses to repetitive syllable production (/ba, ba/) and takes on more of the qualities of the surrounding language. By approximately 6 months of age, the infant is able to purse his lips without moving his jaw. Within 2 more months, he can keep his lips closed while chewing and swallowing. His chewing changes from vertical to the more rotary pattern found in older children and adults. In addition, the tongue intermittently can remain elevated, independent of jaw movement.

The child's consonantal repertoire is restricted initially to labial and back plosives, such as /p/, /b/, /k/, and /g/; nasals; and /j/. The phonemes are not fully formed and are produced slowly. In contrast, the resonant quality and timing of babbling more closely approximate mature speech. Long reduplicated strings of consonant–vowel syllables, such as *bababa*, are common late in this period.

The frequency of consonant appearance in babbling is reflected in the order of speech-sound acquisition later. With age, the child's babbling increasingly reflects adult speech in syllable structure and intonation. In addition, the reduplications of later babbling (*wawawawa*) often continue as the reduplications of early words (*wawa* for *water*).

The infant is able to discriminate frequency changes by 4 to 6 months of age at the latest. Intonational patterns are closely related to frequency shifts, and discrimination of this type occurs by 7 months. At about the same time, infants are able to discriminate different words.

Phonetically Consistent Forms: 11 to 14 Months   By 11 months, the infant has the neuromuscular control to bite soft, solid foods with some control. In addition, she can close her lips when swallowing liquids. Speech is characterized by variegated babbling, in which adjacent and successive syllables are not identical (/bida/). Frequently, the babbling occurs in long strings with intonational patterns that approximate adult speech. The result, an unintelligible gibberish called **jargon**, may sound like adult statements or questions.

Many speech sounds at this stage have sound–meaning relationships. These sounds, called *phonetically consistent forms* (PCFs), function as words, even though they are not based on adult words. The child may develop several PCFs before he speaks his first words. PCFs are more limited than babbling, but not as structured as adult speech. PCFs demonstrate a recognition by the child of linguistic regularities in sound–meaning relationships.

The emergence of first words or verbalizations does not signal the end of vocalizations, such as babbling, jargon, and PCFs. All three continue to be produced by the child throughout the second year of life (Robb, Bauer, & Tyler, 1994). Over time, the infant's vocalizations change and reflect changes in overall language development (Rome-Flanders & Cronk, 1995). The percentage of vocalizations and single syllables gives way to jargon and PCFs, which in turn are pushed aside for single words and multiword expressions. Although vocalizations decrease as a percentage of overall communication, the overall amount of vocalizing remains constant.

First Words and Phoneme Acquisition   With the acquisition of words, the child's sound production becomes more constrained by the words themselves. First words are determined by both the child's control of articulation and his ability to associate labels with objects.

Children's speech is a complex interaction of the ease of both production and perception of the target syllable. The success of both processes is related to the particular phonemes involved and to syllable stress and sound position within words. Initially, infant phonetic comprehension is gross or holistic perception (Walley, 1993). The child rapidly gains the perceptual skills for finer distinctions (Dollaghan, 1994). Before children can recognize words, they gain a sense of how sounds go together to form syllables of their native language (Jusczyk, 1999). Armed with these structures, the child can more easily locate word boundaries in the speech she hears. As vocabulary becomes larger, it may necessitate the ability to make finer and finer discriminations. Caregivers aid the child by naming and pointing to, holding, or manipulating novel objects to further specify the referent (Masur, 1997). As children mature, they rely more on the caregiver's language (Namy & Waxman, 1998).

The order of appearance of the first sounds children acquire (/m, w, b, p/) cannot be explained by the frequency of appearance in English. The /b/, /m/, and /w/ are the simplest consonants to produce and the easiest to perceive, so they appear first.

The relationship of speech-sound perception and production in meaningful speech is complex. The lack of agreement between studies of children's perception and production is due primarily to children's inadequate neuromuscular control, which affects their production. Children simplify their speech in systematic ways that reflect this and other processing inadequacies and the phonological rules mentioned previously.

Several studies have attempted to establish an order of acquisition of phoneme production. This order reflects the increasing speed and precision of the speech mechanism. Higher levels of neurological control and integration result in complex, integrated movements by the speech mechanism. Although the sequence of sound acquisition is not universal and differs according to the sounds used in individual languages, surprising similarity exists (Amayreh & Dyson, 1998; Paulson, 1991). We can make the following generalizations:

1. As a group, vowels are acquired before consonants. English vowels are acquired by age 3.

2. As a group, the nasals are acquired first, followed by the plosives, approximants, lateral approximants, fricatives, and affricatives.

3. As a group, the glottals are acquired first, followed by the labials, velars, alveolars, dentals, postalveolars, and palatals.

4. Sounds are first acquired in the initial position in words.

5. Consonant clusters and blends are not acquired until age 7 or 8, though some clusters appear as early as age 4. These early clusters include /s/ + nasal, /s/ + /r or l/, /s/ + stop, and stop + /r or l/ in the initial position, and nasal + stop in the final.

6. There are great individual differences, and the age of acquisition for some sounds may vary by as much as 3 years.

Although speech sounds are all acquired by early elementary school, further development may occur. Gender differences in the production of some phonemes (/f, Θ, s, ʃ/) exist as early as age 6, but are more pronounced in postpubescent adolescents and young adults, most likely reflecting vocal tract variation between men and women, although these differences decrease for adults as they age (Fox & Nissen, 2005).

The characteristics of a phoneme vary as a function of both (1) the phonetic context of the adjacent speech sounds and (2) the social factors, such as sexual orientation, class, race, regional dialect, gender, and age (Munson, Edwards, & Beckman, 2005). Adults are able to perceive speech sounds with little difficulty.

Adults' perceptual knowledge may be based on perception of very fine acoustic characteristics and on knowledge of categories of sounds. Children lack the adult ability to recognize words and sounds from different speakers, suggesting that children have incomplete auditory-perceptual knowledge (Ryalls & Pisoni, 1997).

Articulatory knowledge is knowing the movements needed to produce different speech sounds. Even adolescent speech differs from adult speech in the length of sounds and words and in characteristics that differentiate one sound from another (Lee, Potamianos, & Naryanan, 1999).

In addition to acquiring a phonetic inventory, the preschool child is developing phonological rules that govern sound distribution and sequencing. As in the other aspects of language, the child developing phonological rules progresses through a long period of language decoding and hypothesis building. Many of the phonological processes used by children are listed in Table 2.7. These *natural processes* act to simplify the speech stream for language-learning children; most are discarded or modified by age 4. Much of the child's morphological production will reflect her perception and production of phonological units.

Once the child begins babbling, the basic speech unit she uses is the consonant–vowel (CV) syllable. The child frequently attempts to simplify production by reducing words to this form or to CVCV. The final consonant may be deleted, producing a CV structure from a CVC—*ba*(/bɔ/) for ball—or followed by a vowel to produce a CVCV structure—*cake-a*(/keɪkʌ/) for cake. This process generally disappears by age 3. In addition, the child may delete unstressed syllables. For example, *away* becomes *way*. This deletion process continues until age 4. Reduplication is a third process for simplifying syllable structure. One syllable becomes similar to another in the word, resulting in the reduplicated structure. Thus, *mommie* becomes *mama* and *water* becomes *wawa*. Finally, the preschooler reduces or simplifies consonant clusters, usually by deleting one consonant. As she progresses, the child substitutes a consonant for the previously deleted one. Cluster reduction is one of the most common phonological processes, seen in the speech of Spanish-speaking Puerto Rican preschoolers also (B. A. Goldstein & Iglesias, 1996).

Assimilatory processes simplify production by permitting different sounds to be produced similarly. In general, one sound becomes similar to another in the same

TABLE 2.7   Common Phonological Processes of Preschool Children

Processes	Examples
I. Syllable structure	
Deletion of final consonants	*cu* (/kʌ/) for *cup*
Deletion of unstressed syllables	*nana* for *banana*
Reduplication	*mama, dada, wawa* (water)
Reduction of clusters	/s/ + consonant (*stop*) = delete /s/ (*top*)
II. Assimilation	*dog* becomes *gog*
III. Substitution processes	
A. Stopping: replace sound with a plosive	*this* becomes *dis*
B. Fronting	*Kenny* becomes *Tenny*
1. Replace palatals and velars with alveolars (/k/ and /g/ replaced with /t/ and /d/)	*go* becomes *do*
2. Nasals (/ŋ/ becomes /n/)	*something* becomes *somethin*
C. Liquids	
1. Gliding	*rabbit* becomes *wabbit*
2. Another liquid substitute	*girl* becomes *gau* (/gɔ/)
IV. Deletion of sounds	*balloon* becomes *ba-oon*

Source: Information from *Phonological Disability in Children,* by D. Ingram, 1976. London: Edward Arnold.

word. For example, children produce two varieties of *doggie,* one with /d/ consonants, *doddie,* the other, *goggie,* using /g/s.

Many preschoolers substitute sounds in their speech, but these substitutions are not random. In general, substitutions can be described according to the manner of production. The two most common phonological substitution rules are *stopping* and *fronting.* In stopping, a plosive phoneme is substituted for other sounds. This process is most common in the initial position in words. For example, *show* might become *tow,* *face* becomes *pace,* and *valentine* becomes *balentine.* Fronting is a tendency to replace phonemes with other phonemes produced farther forward in the mouth. Thus, /t/ and /d/ are substituted for /k/ and /g/, producing *dum* for *gum.* In conversation, it may be difficult to decipher the phonological rules a young child is using. Several processes in different aspects of language may be functioning simultaneously.

Social-indexical knowledge is knowing how linguistic variability conveys or is perceived to convey a speaker's membership in different social groups, such as working-class African Americans (Smyth, Jacobs, & Rogers, 2003). Ability to comprehend speech in an unfamiliar dialect requires great facility and develops throughout childhood (Nathan, Wells, & Donlan, 1998).

Summary

The terms *communication, language,* and *speech* describe different, but related aspects of human behavior. The potential speech-language pathologist needs to be aware of the differences among these terms and of their interrelatedness. Not all children develop communication, language, and speech in the manner described in this chapter. Much of the remainder of this text is devoted to disorders. As you proceed, you should keep the distinctions discussed in this chapter in mind and be alert to the effects of any disorder on speech, language, and communication. No doubt, as a practicing speech-language pathologist, you will someday be faced with the need to explain these terms to a client. I hope that this chapter can provide a basis for your response. I hope that I have stirred some interest in the topic of development because it is the basis for much of the therapy that you will later provide.

STUDY QUESTIONS

1. What are the differences among communication, language, and speech?

2. What is the significance of early communication development for later language development?

3. What are the characteristics of the five related aspects of language?

4. How does the overall emphasis of language development change during toddler, preschool, and school years?

5. How can we divide preschool language development? What are the changes that characterize each stage?

6. What are the discourse skills that develop during the school-age period?

7. What is the relationship between early speech mechanism development and early speech development?

SELECTED READINGS

American Academy of Pediatrics. *Parenting corner Q&A: Language delay.* Available online at www.aap.org/publiced/BR_LanguageDelay.htm.

American Speech-Language-Hearing Association. *Activities to encourage speech and language development.* Available online at www.asha.org/public/speech/development/Parent-Stim-Activities.htm.

Bochner, S., & Jones, J. (2003). *Child language development: Learning to talk.* London: Whurr Publishers.

Child Development Institute. *Language development in children.* Available online at www.childdevelopmentinfo.com/development/language_development.shtml.

Dougherty, D. P. *Developing your baby's language skills.* Available online at www.kidsgrowth.com/resources/articledetail.cfm?id=714.

Howard, M. (2004). How babies learn to talk. *Baby Talk, 69*(3), 69–72.

Nippold, M. A. (2006). *Later language development: School-age children, adolescents, and young adults* (3rd ed.). Austin, TX: PRO-ED.

Oates, J., & Grayson, A. (2004). *Cognitive and language development in children.* Malden, MA: Blackwell.

Owens, R. E. (2010). *Language development: An introduction* (7th ed.). Boston: Allyn & Bacon.

Van Hulle, C. A., et al. (2004). Genetic, environmental, and gender effects on individual differences in toddler expressive language. *Journal of Speech, Language, and Hearing Research, 47*(4), 904–12.

Chapter THREE

The Biology and Physics of Speech

Ray D. Kent
University of Wisconsin, Madison

Houri K. Vorperian
University of Wisconsin, Madison

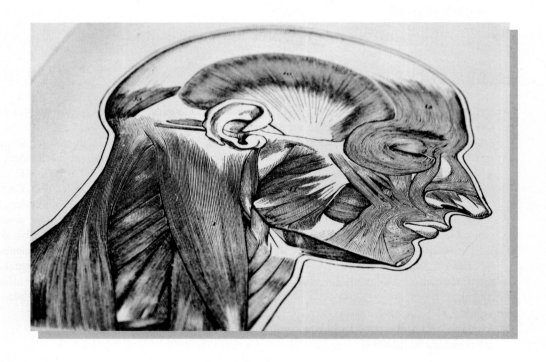

Acknowledgment: This is a revision of a chapter originally written by the late Willard Zemlin. Dr. Zemlin was an extraordinary individual whose energetic and inspired scholarship laid important foundations for the understanding of the anatomy and physiology of speech. This chapter is dedicated to his memory. This work was supported in part by Research Grants R03 DC 4362 and R01 DC006282 from the National Institute on Deafness and Other Communicative Disorders.

personal PERSPECTIVE

RAY D. KENT

The field of speech-language pathology and audiology first came to my attention when I was an undergraduate student at the University of Montana. I was interested in language, psychology, and biology, and I wanted to enter a field in which I could be of help to others. These interests and desires quickly took root in the first courses that I had in the Department of Speech Pathology and Audiology. My enthusiasm was reinforced by the faculty members I met. They had a sincere interest in their field of study, their students, and the clients they served. I earned my B.A. degree from the University of Montana and then took my M.A. and Ph.D. degrees from the University of Iowa. Then I undertook postdoctoral study at MIT so that I could learn about the application of computers to speech science. I then reversed my eastward migration and went to Wisconsin, where I accepted my first faculty position. Each step of the journey was rewarded by associations with people of exceptional caliber and dedication, including a satisfying number of students. I have been fortunate to teach and learn from many bright people who earned their degrees with me. One of them is my coauthor on this chapter.

personal PERSPECTIVE

HOURI K. VORPERIAN

As a child, I was always intrigued by my grandfather's speech. His larynx (voice box) had been surgically removed due to cancer. He used a simple electrolarynx (an external artificial sound source that sounds like a buzzer) that he placed under his chin while talking, singing, and even laughing! He had mastered the use of the electrolarynx on his own. During my undergraduate studies in biology and psychology—in particular, a course in abnormal psychology—I was introduced to the profession of speech pathology and learned about the expertise speech pathologists offer in the rehabilitation of individuals with speech and language deficits. The discipline was very appealing to me, in particular because I used to volunteer at a school for persons with disabilities and worked with many children who were either nonspeaking or dysarthric (having slurred speech) due to head injury, Down syndrome, or cerebral palsy. Having encountered many instances of communication breakdown and its unavoidable negative emotional consequences, I elected to pursue my graduate studies in speech pathology. My clinical experience was very rewarding for several years. However, my curiosity about how we perceive and produce speech led me to pursue doctoral studies in the speech sciences. I have been fortunate to complete my studies under Professor Ray Kent's mentorship. Our goal in this chapter is to provide the basis to understand speech disorders. You will note that it is important not only to understand how the typical speech apparatus works, but also to learn how it changes during the course of development from infancy to advanced age.

The primary purpose of this chapter is to describe how speech is produced. To accomplish this purpose, we must examine the biological and physical properties of speech. Speech exploits parts of the body that serve other purposes, especially the basic life processes of respiration and ingestion of food. The double function of these body parts affords an economy and efficiency.

It is easy to take speech for granted. Speech is a major part of being human and living in a social world. But for people who cannot use speech easily or successfully, life can become complicated and frustrating. To come to terms with speech disorders and to appreciate how children acquire speech, we need to know how speech is produced. This knowledge requires familiarity with the anatomy of speech (the biological structures used in speaking), the physiology of speech (the functions of the biological structures), and the acoustics of speech (the generation of speech sounds that can be heard by others). This chapter briefly covers these areas. Anatomy and physiology constitute the essential biology of speech. Acoustics is a division of physics, and this chapter considers how speech sounds are formed into a physical signal that listeners can interpret as a linguistic message.

The basic task of speech production is to select the right combination of muscles, working in the proper sequence, to produce the speech sounds needed to transmit a message. As many as 100 different muscles may be involved, and each muscle is made up of many different muscle fibers, the basic units of muscle contraction. It has been said that speech requires the use of more muscle fibers than any other routine behavior. As easy as speech may seem to be to most of us, it is actually a complex motor skill— one that children strive to learn and one that can be impaired by a variety of conditions described in the various chapters of this book.

Speech is one channel, but a very important channel, by which language can be expressed. We can also express language through written words, which is happening now with this book. Speech has a special status in language expression because it is the channel that most of us used when we first learned language as children. Reading and writing come later, and they are influenced by the early lessons learned during speech acquisition. Speech is also, for most of us, the predominant means of language expression.

The Biology of Speech: The Anatomy and Physiology of Speech Production

Basically, speech production is a joint effort of the three systems shown in Figure 3.1— respiratory, laryngeal, and articulatory—all of which serve other important functions, as noted earlier. The respiratory system provides the essential air supply for speech by generating air pressures and flows, the laryngeal system generates sound (voice or phonation) using the air supply from the lungs, and the articulatory system (or supralaryngeal system, where *supra-* means "above") serves as a resonator to form the sound energy from the larynx into recognizable speech sounds. Basically we have a chain of three processes: Energy Source (respiratory system) + Vibrator and Valve (laryngeal system) + Resonator/Shaper (articulatory system). We now take a closer look at each of these systems.

FIGURE 3.1 The three systems of speech production: articulatory, laryngeal, and respiratory. The different systems are drawn to different scales and with different orientations (e.g., the articulatory system is enlarged relative to the other two and is shown in a lateral rather than a frontal view). *Source:* From *The Speech Sciences: A Volume in the Speech Sciences,* by R. D. Kent, copyright © 1998. Reprinted with permission of Delmar, a division of Thomson Learning.

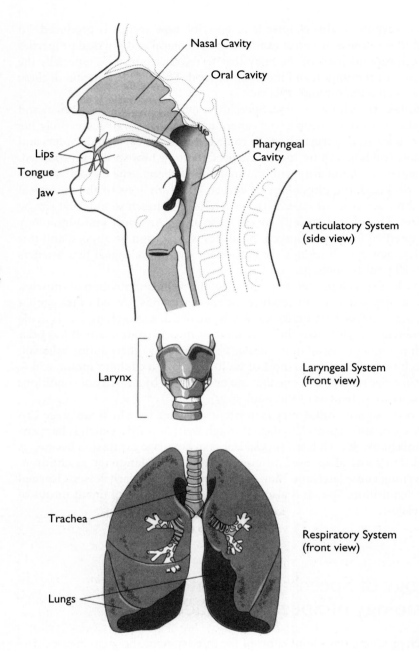

Respiratory System

We normally speak on exhaled air. The respiratory system generates the air pressures and flows that provide the basic power of speech. The actions performed on a stream of air are called **aerodynamics**, and one way of understanding speech is to view it as an aerodynamic system. The basic requirement for speech is to draw air into the lungs (an inspiratory phase) and then to release the air gradually to form the syllables of speech (an expiratory phase). It makes good sense to keep the inspiratory phase brief because no speech sounds are produced in this phase and to prolong the expiratory phase so

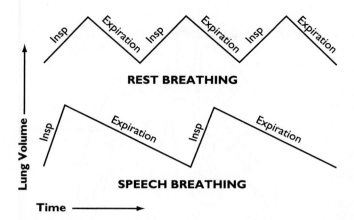

FIGURE 3.2   Schematic diagram of the inspiration (Insp) and expiration cycles during rest breathing and speech breathing. Note the prolongation of expiration for speech breathing.

that several words can be produced on a single breath. This is the essence of breathing for speech: Inspire rapidly and then regulate the expired air to produce a number of syllables and words. Inspiratory and expiratory phases are also used in ordinary breathing to maintain life, but for this purpose, the two phases tend to be nearly equal in their duration. The differences between rest breathing (such as you might do while you read this text silently to yourself) and speech breathing (such as you would do if you begin to read the text aloud) are shown schematically in Figure 3.2. Note in particular that the expiratory phase for speech is extended compared with that for rest breathing.

The respiratory rhythm of inspiration and expiration imposes on speech (and singing as well) a biologically mandatory pattern called the breath group, which is the number of syllables produced on a single expiration. When we talk or sing, we must stop to breathe. This is not true for many other kinds of movements we perform. We can wave our arms, perform keystrokes with our fingers, and move our legs quite independently of the respiratory cycle. Most people can talk on a maximal inspiration for about 20 or 30 seconds, but in ordinary conversation, we typically speak for no more than 10 seconds on a single breath.

The anatomy of respiration is shown in Figure 3.3. The **lung** (Figure 3.3a) is the main organ of respiration. The paired lungs are similar, but not identical. Air travels into and out of the lungs by means of the **trachea**, a structure composed of cartilaginous rings. The larynx is mounted on top of the trachea. The trachea divides to form **bronchial tubes** that reach into the lungs. By a series of bifurcations (successive two-way divisions), these tubes become progressively smaller and so provide air transport to and from the lung tissues (Figure 3.3b). The lungs occupy the two lateral (side-by-side) cavities of the chest (thoracic cavity) and are encased in the rib cage (Figure 3.4). The lungs can be likened to a kind of sponge that holds air. The lungs on their own do not have the power to bring air into them. They are like passive reservoirs of air, and it is the muscles of the respiratory system, working together with the bones and cartilages of the system, that act to expand or compress the chest and consequently move air into and out of the lungs. A sponge analogy illustrates the basic principles. When a sponge is compressed and then placed into a vat of water, it will absorb some water. This is rather like air flowing into the lungs, which occurs as the chest wall and abdomen expand to increase the volume of the respiratory system. When a sponge is

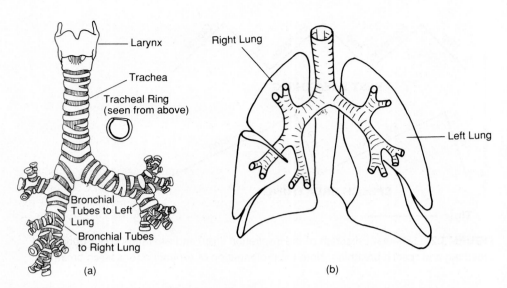

FIGURE 3.3 Partial anatomy of the respiratory system: (a) bronchial tree in relation to the lungs and (b) larynx and bronchial tree.

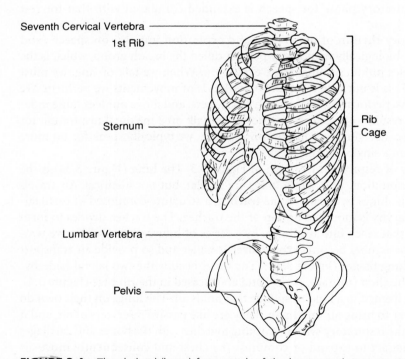

FIGURE 3.4 The skeletal (bony) framework of the lower respiratory tract and the torso. Note in particular the rib cage, which attaches at the front to the sternum and at the back to the vertebral column.

squeezed, the water in the sponge will be forced out, rather like the way in which air is squeezed out of the respiratory system when the chest wall (rib cage) and abdomen are compressed.

Many different respiratory muscles are involved in the process just described, but we can simplify the story by grouping them as (1) the **muscles of the rib cage** and (2) a single muscle called the **diaphragm**. The former are muscles that attach to the ribs and can cause the rib cage and consequently the chest wall to expand or compress. The diaphragm is a large, dome-shaped muscle that separates the thoracic cavity from the abdominal cavity. It can be likened to a flexible rubber sheet at the bottom of a glass jar. When the sheet is pulled down, air is drawn into the jar, and when the sheet is released, air is forced out. The function of these muscles can be modeled as shown in Figure 3.5. Both the diaphragm and rib cage muscles are represented by pistons that act on a bag of air (the lungs). When one or both of these act to force air out of the lungs, the air can flow out of the body through the larynx and associated airways.

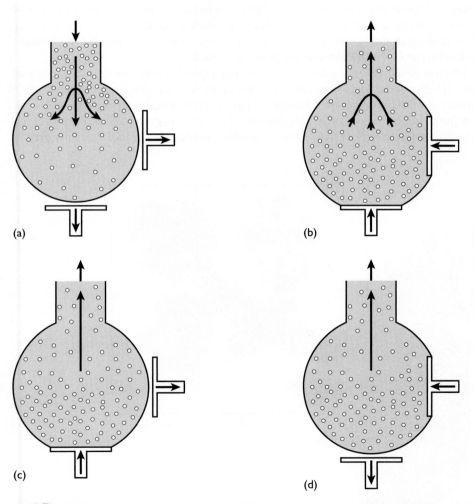

(a)

(b)

(c)

(d)

FIGURE 3.5   Schematic illustration of respiratory function, with the rib cage (side piston) and diaphragm (bottom piston) modeled as pistons and the lungs modeled as a balloon. The different actions shown in parts (a), (b), (c), and (d) are described in the text.

Figure 3.5a shows air flowing into the lungs as both pistons (diaphragm at the bottom and rib cage at the side) move outward. Figure 3.5b shows air flowing out of the lungs as both pistons move inward. Figure 3.5c and 3.5d show air flowing out of the lungs even when only one of the pistons moves inward. That is, Figure 3.5 shows in schematic fashion that the diaphragm and rib cage can move independently.

The sponge analogy has another point of relevance to the actual respiratory system. A sponge is made up of numerous tiny cavities that can hold air or water. The lungs are similar in that they contain millions of tiny air sacs called **alveoli** (plural; the singular form is **alveolus**). These are illustrated in Figure 3.6. Adults have hundreds of thousands of alveoli in each lung, but babies are born with hardly any. The alveoli are the site of gas exchange between the blood and the oxygen-rich air inspired into the lungs. If the lung tissues are stretched out to form a flat surface, their equivalent surface area is nearly equal to that of a tennis court (about 70 square meters), a large surface for gas exchange.

As noted earlier, the air that enters or escapes the lungs travels upward through the trachea and the larynx. This arrangement gives the larynx a unique opportunity to valve the airstream (close it or open it) and also to produce a vibrating sound (phonation). This sound-producing potential is used by a large number of animals, but no creature uses it with the sophistication and purpose that humans do.

During development, some aspects of respiration change, so that children and adults differ in some important respects. One example is a different rate of respiration (number of breaths per minute). Newborns have a rest breathing rate of 30 to 80 breaths per minute, but by the age of 3 years, the rate is about 20 to 30 breaths per minute, and by the age of 10 years, the rate is 17 to 22 breaths per minute. Children also use greater

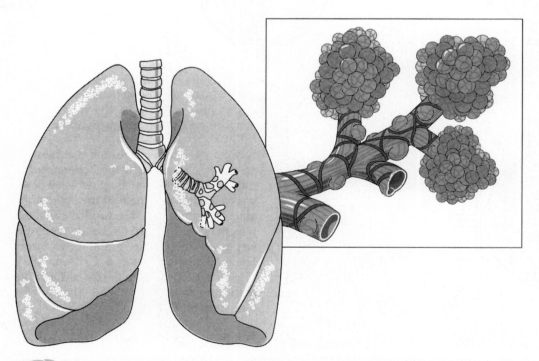

FIGURE 3.6   The lungs and, in the inset, an enlargement to show the alveolar sacs.
Source: From *The Speech Sciences: A Volume in the Speech Sciences,* by R. D. Kent, copyright © 1998. Reprinted with permission of Delmar, a division of Thomson Learning.

air pressures than adults for speaking. Such differences in function are related to anatomic differences. For example, a baby's lungs are small, and as noted earlier, they contain very few alveoli (air sacs). In addition, the airways in a baby's respiratory system have a narrow diameter, which creates more resistance to airflow.

The respiratory system changes as we age. One of the common changes is a reduction in the amount of air that can be held in the lungs. This reduction typically accompanies the change in height that is common with aging. As people age, they tend to lose stature and respiratory volume (and, in some individuals, postural changes, obesity, and physical or lifestyle changes also affect respiratory capacity). The loss of respiratory volume can become noticeable for everyday functions such as walking and even talking.

Laryngeal System

The larynx, or voice box, is an elaborate structure composed of various cartilages, muscles, and other tissues. It was noted earlier that one function of the larynx is to act as a valve that controls the flow of air into and out of the respiratory system. As an example of a nonspeech function of the larynx, suppose that you are about to pick up a heavy object. As you do so, you probably will close the laryngeal passage to maintain a rigid (air-filled) respiratory system. This is why we often grunt when we lift a heavy object. This squeezing together of the **vocal folds** is shown in Figure 3.7. The vocal folds are like muscular cushions or bands that run lengthwise from the front to the back of the larynx. If you feel the "Adam's apple" at the front of your neck, you might be able to detect a small notch at its upper boundary. The vocal folds have their frontal attachment

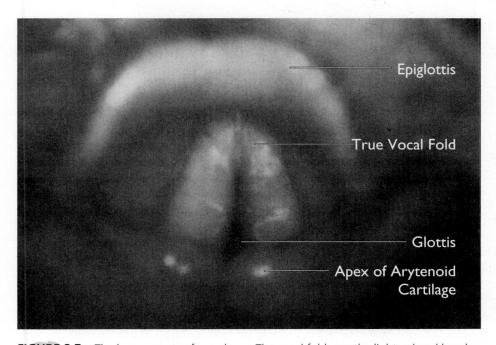

FIGURE 3.7   The larynx as seen from above. The vocal folds are the light-colored bands that form an inverted "V" in the center of the illustration.
Source: Vocal Tract Development Laboratory at the Waisman Center, University of Wisconsin-Madison.

just below this notch. Even the space between the vocal folds has its own name, the **glottis**. The epiglottis is a cartilage that can close over the entry to the elevated larynx, as it does during swallowing to prevent food from reaching this part of the respiratory airway. For ordinary breathing, the vocal folds are drawn apart so that air can move freely into and out of the lungs.

The vocal folds have a very important function in speech: They vibrate to produce sound. We refer to this sound source as **voiced speech** or **phonation**. The process is briefly as follows, with reference to Figure 3.8, which shows the vocal fold behavior during a single cycle of vibration. The respiratory system pushes air through the trachea and larynx, but the vocal folds are drawn together at the midline to form a valve (Figure 3.8, frame 1a). This valve resists the flow of air from the respiratory system. The muscle forces that draw the folds together are carefully regulated so that the air from the lungs sets the folds into a vibratory motion—a series of openings and closings that define the cycles of vibration. The air pressure beneath the folds (**subglottal air pressure**) blows the vocal folds apart (Figure 3.8, frames 3a to 3f). Once the vocal folds have been blown apart, various restoring forces, including the elasticity of the vocal folds, bring them together again (Figure 3.8, frames 4a to 5f). The force that brings the vocal folds together at the midline is called the **medial compression force**. This process repeats itself to produce voice, which is a series of opening and closing motions of the vocal

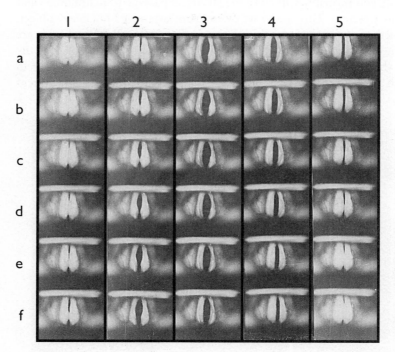

FIGURE 3.8   A single cycle of vocal vibration, photographed at 4,000 frames per second. The vocal folds are drawn together in the upper left frame (frame 1a), which is the beginning of the cycle shown here. The sequence of frames runs from the top to the bottom (a to f) of the first column, then the top to the bottom of the second column, and so on. The folds are maximally separated in the middle column and then begin to close, until they are nearly completely approximated in the frame at the lower right (frame 5f). The entire event, from closed to open to closed again, represents one complete cycle of vocal fold vibration that took about 1/140 second.
Source: Vocal Tract Development Laboratory at the Waisman Center, University of Wisconsin-Madison.

folds, as can be seen in Figure 3.8. The images of the vocal folds in Figure 3.8 were made with high-speed photography that permits observation of the vibration of the folds.

The medial compression force is carefully adjusted in relation to the subglottal air pressure. If the medial compression force is too great, the folds may not vibrate at all because the subglottal air pressure is not sufficient to blow the folds apart. Or, if the medial compression force is too small, the folds will vibrate only weakly, so that voice will barely be audible. Because most of us use our vocal folds heavily during the day, it is important that we use the right amount of muscle forces to ensure effortless and comfortable voice. Overuse of the voice, or excessive muscle force, can result in damage to the vocal folds, as discussed in another chapter of this book.

The vocal folds are the vibrating structures of the larynx, but their actions are affected by a number of cartilages and associated muscles (Figure 3.9). These complex connections are important to a detailed understanding of how the vocal folds function in speech and song. The two largest cartilages, the **thyroid** and **cricoid**, form much of the bulk of the larynx. When we view the isolated larynx, we see primarily these two cartilages. The thyroid cartilage is a relatively large structure that has an H-shape when viewed laterally (Figure 3.9b and Figure 3.9c). The cricoid cartilage (Figure 3.9a),

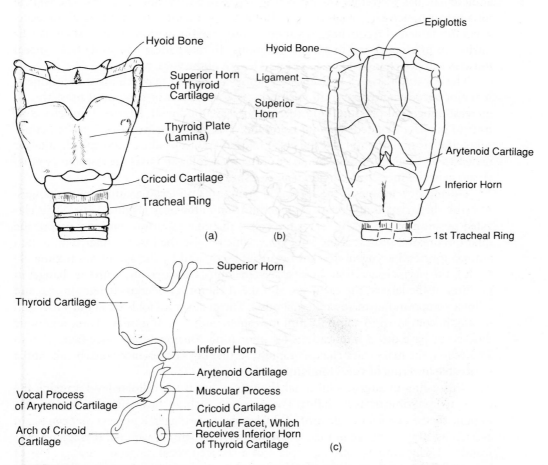

FIGURE 3.9   The cartilage framework of the larynx: (a) view from the front, (b) view from behind, and (c) exploded (separated) view from the side. Note that the arytenoid cartilages sit on top of the cricoid cartilage and the thyroid cartilage covers the cricoid–arytenoid assembly. The vocal folds attach to the vocal process of the arytenoids.

shaped like a signet ring, is positioned over the trachea. It attaches at the front to the thyroid cartilage (Figure 3.9a) and at the back to the paired **arytenoid** cartilages (Figure 3.9c). The latter are small structures shaped like a pyramid (broad base and pointed top). The arytenoid cartilages and the vocal folds are hidden inside the thyroid–cricoid framework. The vocal folds attach in the front to the thyroid cartilage and in the back to the arytenoid cartilages. Because the thyroid, cricoid, and arytenoid cartilages can move relative to another, they can act to stretch and contract the vocal folds.

With practice, the vocal folds can be exquisitely controlled so that trained singers can make precise adjustments of vocal pitch and loudness. Even for more ordinary purposes, such as conversational speech, pitch and loudness changes contribute to the effectiveness and quality of our communication. Pitch is the perceptual correlate of the physical property of frequency of vibration. Frequency is expressed in units called hertz (abbreviated Hz). One sequence of vocal fold vibration (from closed to separated and back to closed) is a cycle of vibration (an example is illustrated in Figure 3.8). As more cycles occur in a given unit of time, we hear an increase in vocal pitch. An adult male has an average vocal fundamental frequency of about 110 Hz, meaning that the vocal folds are blown apart and brought together again 110 times per second. The adult female has an average vocal fundamental frequency of about 225 Hz. The average for a baby is much higher, approximately 400 Hz. Vocal pitch (or its physical correlate, vocal fundamental frequency) is varied to produce intonation (pitch rises and falls during an utterance) and to express emotions. To make these adjustments, laryngeal muscles work to change the mass per unit length of the vocal folds.

The vocal folds work with the respiratory system to make changes in loudness. A major aerodynamic correlate of loudness is variation in subglottal pressure. To increase subglottal pressure (and thereby increase loudness), laryngeal muscles contract to increase the medial compression force. As this force increases, it takes a larger subglottal air pressure to blow the vocal folds apart. To produce loud speech, a talker increases the medial compression force of the vocal folds and uses the respiratory muscles to generate increased subglottal air pressure.

During development, the laryngeal structures undergo a number of changes. At birth, the larynx is at a relatively high position in the neck (Figure 3.10a). This elevated position of the larynx serves to protect the infant's airway and may permit the infant to breathe and eat at the same time, which is also the case for many nonhuman animal species. Laryngeal descent begins at birth, and by the age of approximately 4 years, the larynx is nearly at the level seen in adults. Concurrently with the changes in position of the larynx, the cartilages and the vocal folds undergo changes in size and cellular composition (microscopic anatomy). The infant vocal folds are about 4 to 8 mm in length, compared to about 21 mm in women and 29 mm in men. These anatomic differences have direct implications for phonation. During adolescence (ages 12.5 to 14.5 years), the male voice changes rapidly, so that boys experience voice breaks and a noticeable lowering of vocal fundamental frequency.

With aging in adults, additional changes occur at the cellular level, causing the larynx to lose some of its flexibility. These changes include the ossification (conversion to bone by the deposit of calcium) of the laryngeal cartilages, a process that can begin as early as 40 years of age in men and a decade or so later in women. If you have ever wondered why some vocalists complain of a reduced vocal range as they age, loss of laryngeal flexibility is one reason. Additional changes occur in the microscopic structure of the vocal folds. The aging changes in the larynx help to explain why we can often judge the age of a person just from the sound of the voice.

The respiratory and laryngeal systems can work together to produce voice or to generate a stream of air. But they do not in themselves produce most of the distinctive

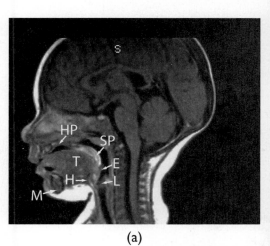
(a)

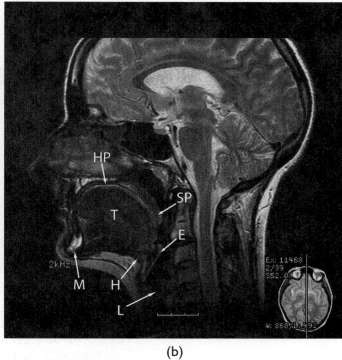
(b)

FIGURE 3.10 Magnetic resonance images of the vocal tract of (a) a newborn and (b) an adult. Note the differences in the shapes and the relative positions of the vocal tract structures as seen in this midsection view.
Key: M—mandible (jaw), T—tongue, HP—hard palate, SP—soft palate, E—epiglottis, H—hyoid bone, L—larynx.
Source: Vocal Tract Development Laboratory at the Waisman Center, University of Wisconsin-Madison.

sounds that we recognize as speech. To see how speech sounds are formed, we must look at the articulatory or resonatory system, as discussed in the next section.

Articulatory System

As we saw with the respiratory and laryngeal systems, speech production deploys the same anatomy that is used for other biological purposes. And so it is with the articulatory system, which is used not only for speech, but also for chewing, licking, swallowing, and conditioning inspired air. The articulatory system is a three-part passageway, shown initially as cavities or air spaces in Figure 3.1, but presented in more structural detail in Figures 3.10 and 3.11. The first part of this passageway, which connects directly to the laryngeal opening, is the **pharyngeal cavity**, or pharynx. The pharynx is a muscular tube formed by the pharyngeal walls and the back of the tongue. This tube can be divided into three sections: nasopharynx (near the nasal cavity), oropharynx (adjoins the oral cavity), and laryngopharynx (just above the larynx). The pharynx opens into two other passages, the **oral cavity** and the **nasal cavity**. These two cavities are separated by the hard and soft palates. The **hard palate** is an unmovable bony plate. The **soft palate** is a kind of muscular valve that can open or close the entrance into the nasal cavity. When this entrance is closed, sound energy from the larynx is directed into the oral cavity. When the entrance is open, sound energy can pass into both the oral cavity and the nasal cavity. Energy produced by phonation, therefore, can travel

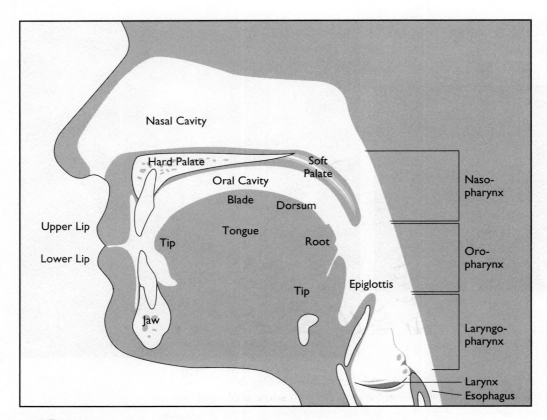

FIGURE 3.11   Midline section of the head showing the major divisions of the vocal tract, including the pharynx and the speech articulators.
From *The Speech Sciences: A Volume in the Speech Sciences,* by R. D. Kent, copyright © 1998. Reprinted with permission of Delmar, a division of Thomson Learning.

through three routes to reach the outside world: an exclusively oral route (through the mouth), an exclusively nasal route (through the nose), and a combined oral-nasal route (through both mouth and nose).

Articulation means movement. The system of speech production has several different moving parts, or **articulators**: lips (upper and lower), jaw (mandible), tongue, pharyngeal walls, and soft palate (Figure 3.10). These structures change their positions (and some change their shapes) to form the various sounds of speech. As children learn to speak, they are discovering how to move the articulators to certain positions corresponding to the sounds of the language. Before we consider how different sounds are formed, let's take a brief look at how the articulatory system develops in children and changes in advanced age. This information is a useful backdrop to a discussion of speech development in children and to certain patterns of change sometimes seen in older speakers.

During development, the structures of the **vocal tract** increase in size and change in shape. Because most of these structures reside in the skull, we first compare the adult and newborn skulls (Figure 3.12). Note that the newborn skull is not simply a miniature version of the adult skull. Rather, the newborn skull has a proportionately smaller jaw and face. The cranium (brain case) of the newborn is much closer to adult size than are the bones of the jaw and face. Turning now to the vocal tract, Figure 3.10 shows some of the anatomical differences between the infant and the adult. These anatomical differences hold implications for functional differences in articulation and

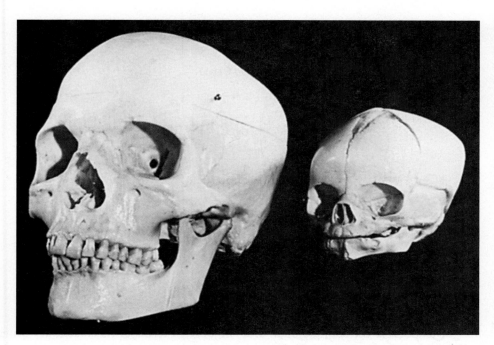

FIGURE 3.12 The skulls of an adult (left) and a newborn (right). Note the difference in the proportion of the face and the brain case.

resonance. For example, the way in which children of various linguistic backgrounds acquire speech sounds follows a fairly regular pattern, with some sounds being mastered earlier than others.

As described in an earlier section, during early childhood the larynx descends in the neck. During this same period, the root of the tongue descends into the neck to become the anterior wall of the pharynx. These changes not only increase the depth of the pharynx, but also alter the angle at which the oral and pharyngeal cavities meet. Notice from Figure 3.10 that the newborn has a gradual angle between these cavities, but the adult has an almost perpendicular angle. The illustration also shows that the tongue of the newborn nearly fills the entire oral cavity and tends to move predominantly forward and backward, rather like a piston in a cylinder. This arrangement is highly suitable for suckling. Not surprisingly, infants in the first few months of life tend to make vowel sounds with the tongue in the front of the mouth and to have relatively few consonants. By about 4 years of age, children have a vocal tract shape that it is highly similar to that in adults and also have a large set of speech sounds.

The teeth are important for eating, but they also play a role in speech. Teeth define the boundaries of oral movements and, therefore, help the child to establish control of jaw and tongue movements. The first set of teeth (primary **dentition**) begins to emerge at about 6 months of age with the eruption of the front teeth, called the incisors. The process continues until the full complement of primary teeth (20 in all) is present by the age of about 2 years. The front teeth, especially the central incisors (Figure 3.13), help in the production of noisy sounds like the *s* in the word *sass*. Most youngsters experience a change in their *s* sounds when their frontal incisors are shed. The primary teeth begin to be gradually shed at about 6 or 7 years and are replaced by the secondary dentition. The incisors are the first of the secondary dentition to appear, at about 6 or 7 years. There are 32 teeth in the full set of secondary dentition (Figure 3.13). The remaining teeth erupt over a lengthy period that is not complete until about 17 to 22 years when the "wisdom teeth" (third molars in Figure 3.13) appear.

FIGURE 3.13

Drawing of the oral cavity showing the adult (secondary) dentition along with several structures involved in speech production.

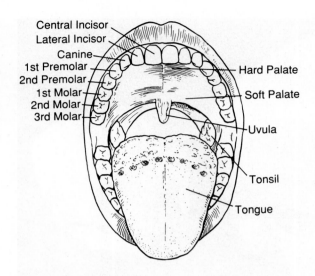

Central Incisor
Lateral Incisor
Canine
1st Premolar
2nd Premolar
1st Molar
2nd Molar
3rd Molar

Hard Palate

Soft Palate

Uvula

Tonsil

Tongue

Speech Physiology: How Speech Sounds Are Formed

Linguists describe the sound system of a language in terms of its elementary units called **phonemes**. American English has about 45 phonemes, which is about an average number compared to other languages in the world. The phonemes are divided into two major classes, **vowels** and **consonants**. Despite the widespread usage of this classification, a satisfactory definition of the terms **vowel** and **consonant** is surprisingly difficult. Generally, vowels are produced with a relatively open vocal tract (i.e., free of radical constrictions formed by the articulators), and they are associated with a resonant acoustic pattern. Vowels are usually strong sounds that dominate the loudness of speech. In contrast, consonants usually are produced with marked constrictions at some location in the vocal tract and do not have the prominent resonant quality of vowels.

The articulation of vowels can be described largely with respect to actions of the tongue and lips. Tongue position can be specified along two dimensions: front–back and low–high. As shown in Figure 3.14, all vowels can be represented as locations within a four-sided diagram called the **vowel quadrilateral**. Note that the four corners are specified with the descriptors **high front**, **low front**, **high back**, and **low back**. These four corner points correspond to the vowels in the words *heat, hat, who'd,* and *hot.* Other vowels are represented as points on the sides or in the center of the quadrilateral. Each vowel is represented by a keyword; for example, the word *heat* is a keyword for the high front vowel. Try to feel the differences in tongue position by doing the following exercises. First, say the following sequence of words: *heat, hid, hate, head, hat.* Did you feel that your tongue stayed in the front of the mouth, but gradually lowered from a high to a low position? (You may also note that your jaw lowered, which helps to lower the tongue.) Next, say *hoot, hood, hoed, hawed, hot.* This time did you feel that your tongue remained in the back of the mouth and gradually lowered across the sequence of words? To feel your tongue moving from front to center to back, say this sequence: *hate, hut, hoed.*

In addition to their tongue position, vowels are described in terms of the position of the lips. There are two basic lip configurations: rounded and unrounded. In English, only certain central and back vowels are rounded. German, French, and Swedish have rounded front vowels, but English does not.

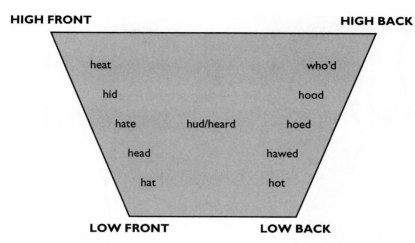

FIGURE 3.14 The vowel quadrilateral, a four-sided figure that encloses the vowel sounds. The corners are labeled high front, high back, low front, and low back, which are the primary dimensions of tongue position within the oral cavity. The different vowels are represented by keywords for the sound of each vowel.

English also has a class of sounds known as diphthongs (which literally means "two sounds"). Diphthongs are produced with a gliding change in articulatory configuration from one vowel to another. Examples of words containing diphthongs are *high, how, hay,* and *ahoy.* You can feel the diphthongal tongue movement by lightly holding a straw on your tongue as you say the word *hyoid* (which contains a sequence of two diphthongs).

Consonants are described in terms of three characteristics: **place of articulation** (where a sound is formed), **manner of articulation** (how a sound is formed), and **voicing** (whether the vocal folds are vibrating for the sound). First, we consider place of articulation. Proceeding from the front (lips) to the back (larynx), the places of articulation for American English are listed below, together with keywords for the consonants produced at each place (reference to Figure 3.11 may be helpful). For the purpose of describing place of articulation, the tongue is divided into functional parts, including the tip (the pointed forward extension), the blade (the flat section just behind the tip), and the dorsum (the broad back of the tongue). As an example of describing place of articulation, the upper and lower lips are used to form the initial sounds in the words *bay, pay,* and *may.* Say the words in each list to confirm that they are made in the same location. Refer to Figure 3.15.

1. Bilabial (upper and lower lips): first sounds in *bay, pay, may*
2. Labiodental (lower lip to upper teeth): first sounds in *van, fan*
3. Linguadental (tongue tip to upper teeth): first sounds in *this, thin*
4. Lingua-alveolar (tongue tip to the ridge just behind the upper teeth): first sounds in *dip, tip, zip, sip, nip, lip*
5. Linguapalatal (tongue blade to hard palate): first sounds in *gin, chin, shin*
6. Linguavelar (tongue back to hard or soft palate): first sounds in *gum, come;* last sounds in *bag, back, bang*
7. Glottal (vocal folds): first sound in *hay*

Next, we discuss manner of articulation, or how sounds are formed.

Stops are made with a total obstruction of the vocal tract so that airflow ceases completely for a brief time. When the obstruction is broken, the air impounded behind

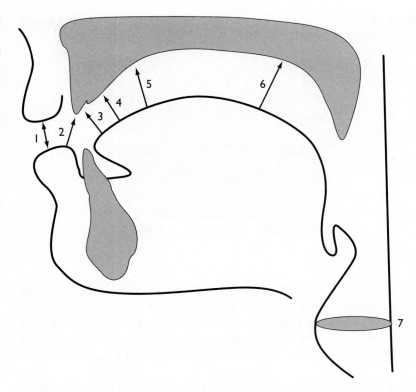

it may be released as a brief burst of air. The stops in English are the first sounds in the following words: *bill, pill, dill, till, gill, kill*.

Fricatives are produced with a narrow constriction through which the escaping air generates a noise called turbulence noise. The fricatives in English are the first sounds in the following words: *fat, vat, that, thatch, zap, sap, shack, hat*. A rarely produced fricative that occurs mostly in words borrowed from other languages is the medial sound in *azure*.

Affricates are a combination of a stop and a fricative. The affricates in English include the first sounds in these words: *gin, chin*.

Nasals involve a closure of the oral cavity, but an opening of the velopharynx, so that sound energy passes through the nasal cavity. The nasals in English are the final sounds in the following words: *ram, rain, rang*.

Glides (also called semivowels) are vowel-like sounds produced with a gradual articulatory transition from one configuration to another. The glides in English are the first sounds in the words *you* and *woo*.

Liquids are a class of two members: a **lateral** (as in the first sound in the word *law*), made with a midline closure so that air escapes laterally on either side of the midline obstruction, and a **rhotic** (as in the first sound of the word *raw*), made in several different ways, all of which produce an r-like quality.

In addition to place and manner of articulation, consonants are described with respect to voicing, or whether the vocal folds are vibrating during the production of the consonant. Sounds produced with such vibration are called *voiced*, and sounds produced without this vibration are called *voiceless*. The words in each of the following pairs differ in the voicing of the initial consonant, with the first member of each pair being voiced: (*bay, pay*), (*van, fan*), (*this, thin*), (*dip, tip*), (*zip, sip*), (*gin, shin*), (*back, pack*).

You might be able to feel the vibration of voicing if you place your fingers over your larynx as you say a prolonged zzzzzzz versus a prolonged sssssss.

Vowels and consonants combine to form various types of *syllables*. A syllable can be as simple as a single vowel or diphthong (e.g., the word *I*) or as complex as a vowel surrounded by consonant clusters (e.g., the word *strengths*). The combinatorial possibilities are remarkable. The 45 phonemes of American English can form over 4 billion arbitrary sequences of 1 to 6 members. But there are only about 100,000 possible (pronounceable in American English) one-syllable words, and, of these, only one-tenth, or about 10,000, are actual monosyllabic words. Syllables also differ in their frequency of occurrence. It has been estimated from frequency counts of ordinary speech that the 12 most frequently used of all syllables account for about a quarter of our verbal behavior, that fewer than 100 different syllables make up half of our speech, and that around 1,500 syllables are sufficient for over 90 percent of what we say.

The Neural Control System

The human nervous system is one of the most complex systems ever studied. In fact, some claim that it is the most complex system known to humans. The complexity comes about both because it contains an enormous number of **neurons** (the basic cell of the neural system)—of which there are billions, if not trillions—and because each neuron is potentially connected with hundreds of other neurons. Figure 3.16 shows the microscopic anatomy of a neuron that is the most common type within the brain and spinal cord. It is the typical neuron of the brain and spinal cord. Each neuron has three major parts: cell body, dendrite, and axon. The dendrite and axon are processes that extend from the cell body. Both the dendrite and the axon can divide to form many branches, so that a single neuron can make multiple connections to other neurons. To describe such a system in fine detail would occupy thousands of workers for thousands of years. The tasks of description and understanding become simpler if we conceptualize the system in terms of several large structures, each of which contains huge numbers of neurons. These structures are shown in Figure 3.17. Note that the brain and spinal cord together make up the **central nervous system (CNS)**. The nerves that connect the

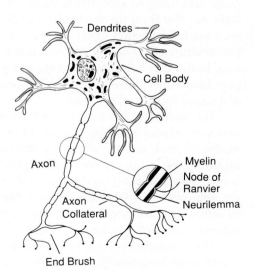

FIGURE 3.16
Schematic of a neuron, the basic unit (cell) of the nervous system.

FIGURE 3.17
Exploded side view of
the central nervous
system, showing its
major divisions.

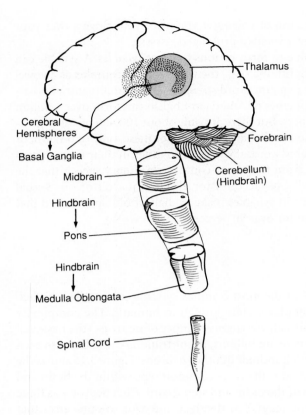

CNS to the various muscles, glands, and sensory receptors of the body constitute the **peripheral nervous system (PNS).**

The cerebral hemispheres are the two prominent, highly wrinkled half-sections that are the largest and most visible parts of the brain. Each hemisphere is covered by a thin bark of gray matter, the **cortex.** The gray color is imparted by myriads of neuron cell bodies. The cortex is often thought to be the seat of higher faculties such as language and thought. Underlying the cortex are complex webs of white matter, which takes its color from the myelin (fat) coating that insulates the axons of neurons. The axon carries the neural signal to other cells and, therefore, can be regarded as the output structure of the neuron. Also located within the cerebral hemispheres are the basal ganglia and the thalamus. These are also gray matter, for they are collections of large populations of neuron cell bodies. These structures serve important sensory (input) and motor (output) functions.

The brain stem has been likened to the stalk of a mushroom that wears the cerebral hemispheres as its cap (Figure 3.17). The brain stem consists of three portions: midbrain, pons, and medulla. These structures control a variety of basic life functions, including respiration, temperature, regulation, and appetite. The cerebellum has two hemispheres that attach to the pons at the back of the brain. Remarkably, about half of the neurons in the CNS are found in the cerebellum. The role of this neuron-rich structure is not completely understood, but it clearly has important functions in learning and controlling precise movements.

The spinal cord is the ropelike structure that runs through the center of the spinal column, reaching nearly, but not quite, to the end of the spine. In cross-section, the

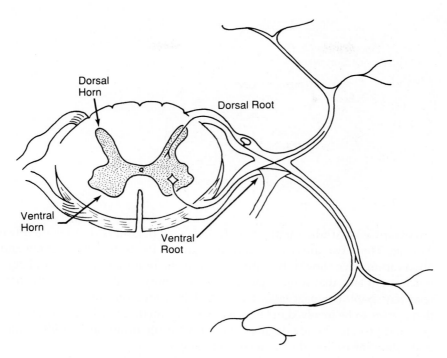

FIGURE 3.18
Cross-sectional view
of the spinal cord.

Dorsal
Horn

Dorsal Root

Ventral
Horn

Ventral
Root

spinal cord has a butterfly- or H-shaped gray interior that is surrounded by white matter (Figure 3.18). Sensory information (such as pain, touch, temperature, and joint position) enters the spinal cord by way of the dorsal (which means "back") root. Motor information that controls the muscles of the body exits the spinal cord through the ventral (which means "belly" or "front") root. The "H" shape of the gray matter has horns that carry the same names, dorsal and ventral. At its thickest, the spinal cord has the diameter of an ordinary pencil.

The neural system that controls speech is complex and not completely understood. But certain general principles are useful in developing an overview of the neural control of speech. We begin with these principles. They are **lateralization, localization,** and **contralateral innervation.**

Lateralization is the establishment of right- and left-hemisphere preferences for different functions. Especially for right-handed individuals, the left hemisphere is dominant for many (but not all) language functions. This aspect of lateralization has been known for decades, especially because of observations that injury to the left hemisphere is much more likely to result in language impairment (aphasia) than is damage to the right hemisphere. This does not mean that we should ignore the right hemisphere completely in our quest to find the neural representation of language abilities because it appears that the right hemisphere has at least some capacity for language and, in fact, may do certain kinds of language processing better than the left. One of the possible right-hemisphere advantages is the processing of the intonation (melody) of speech.

Where in the left hemisphere are language (symbol storage and manipulation) and speech (the motor expression of language) localized? Since the middle to late 1800s, language comprehension and expression have been linked to two major areas of the cerebral cortex. The area associated with comprehension is **Wernicke's area,** and the area associated with expression is **Broca's area.** Both areas take their names from

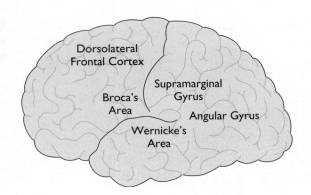

physicians who studied patients with language disorders that resulted from brain damage. These two areas are shown in Figure 3.19. Additional research and clinical observation have shown that other areas of the brain are involved in language—so much so, in fact, that some argue that massive areas of the cortex participate even in relatively simple language tasks. Figure 3.19 illustrates some of the other areas of cortex that appear to be involved in language. Modern methods of brain imaging (technologies that produce highly detailed "pictures" of the brain) are rapidly adding to the understanding of how the brain controls language.

Contralateral innervation is the principle that one side of the brain essentially controls the opposite side of the body (*contra* means "opposite"; *lateral* means "side"). That is, the muscles and sensory receptors on the right side of the body are connected primarily to the left half of the brain and vice versa. For example, a person with damage to the left brain hemisphere may have a speech disorder and a general weakness of the right side of the body (e.g., arm and leg). This principle applies even to the sense of hearing because most of the nerve fibers from one ear pass to the opposite side of the brain.

Now we look at the parts of the nervous system that are involved in the production of speech. In fact, speech is controlled by many different parts of the nervous system, as shown schematically in Figure 3.20. This figure shows how these structures are linked through pathways of motor control. The pyramidal motor pathway, usually considered the major pathway of voluntary motor control, originates in the cerebral cortex and then descends to the brain stem or spinal cord, where it connects with the cranial and spinal nerves. These peripheral nerves are the **final common pathway** by which neural commands reach muscles. But the pyramidal system does not work alone. It is assisted by the extrapyramidal motor pathway, which is a loop that connects the cerebral cortex, basal ganglia, and thalamus, as shown by the dotted line in Figure 3.20. An additional structure, the cerebellum, participates in motor control by ensuring that movements have the appropriate coordination. Figure 3.20 is a simplification in that it shows only some of the parts of the brain that are involved in controlling movement, but the illustrated structures are important particularly in the current understanding of motor control. Damage to these structures results in different movement disorders, some of which can affect speech.

The development of the brain occurs over many years and includes a number of processes. Brain development proceeds as children are acquiring language, so that neural development interacts with language acquisition. One major developmental process in neural development is the multiplication of cells to produce the enormous number of neurons (probably several trillion, but certainly billions) that are found in the human brain. Remarkably, the population of neurons may be its greatest at the gestational

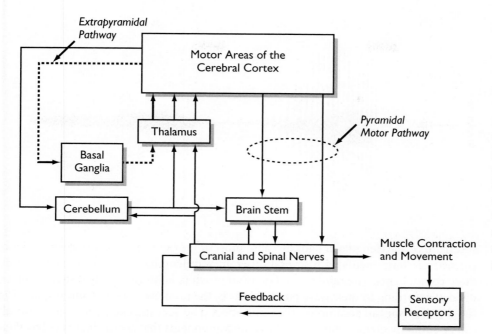

FIGURE 3.20
Schematic diagram of the motor pathways involved in the control of speech. Note in particular the pyramidal and extrapyramidal pathways as well as a neural loop involving the cerebellum. Damage to any of the structures shown can result in a speech disorder.

age of about 5 months (4 months before birth). After that age, neurons are lost faster than they are acquired, primarily because neurons that do not form synapses with other neurons are eliminated. The formation of synapses (**synaptogenesis**) is the means by which neurons form networks or functional assemblies. This process begins in the womb and apparently continues throughout life, although it is most dramatic in the very young child. Maturation of the nervous system also is signaled by **myelination**, in which the axons of many neurons are sheathed with an insulating layer of fat. This process begins in the womb and continues until early adulthood. Together with these developmental processes, there are changes in the pattern of metabolic activity in the brain that extend through childhood and most likely into early adulthood.

The Physics of Speech: Speech Acoustics

Sounds are waves—in fact, a particular kind of wave known as a longitudinal wave in which the air particles move parallel to the direction of wave movement. When we speak, the sound energy is propagated as a wave that moves through the air, eventually reaching the ears of a listener. A common way of representing this wave energy is a waveform, which is a graph of the amplitude of particle movement (vertical axis) as a function of time (horizontal axis), as shown in Figure 3.21. The waveform is a basic representation of sound energy, but it is not easily interpreted for purposes such as describing the acoustic properties of individual speech sounds. Figure 3.21 shows a waveform of speech (the word *toss*). This graph shows the amplitude of vibration as a function of time. Notice the brief noise for the *t*, the strong periodic energy for the vowel *o*, and the long noise interval for the *ss*.

An essential first step in understanding the acoustics of speech is to become familiar with the concept of a **spectrum**. A type of spectrum familiar to most people is the

FIGURE 3.21 A waveform of speech (the word *toss*). This graph shows the amplitude of vibration as a function of time. Notice the brief noise for the *t*, the strong periodic energy for the vowel *o*, and the long noise interval for the *ss*.

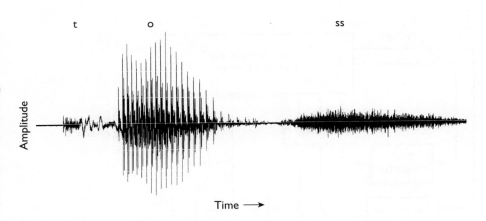

spectrum of wavelengths in light. Because most of the light in our common experience consists of components with several different wavelengths, light can be divided into these components. The rainbow is a division of white light into many different colors, divided according to their wavelengths. That is, the rainbow is a spectrum displayed in the sky. A prism can accomplish the same effect. The acoustic energy in speech sounds can be similarly divided into many different components that are distinguished by their frequencies. Some sounds have most of their energy at low frequencies, others at high frequencies, and still others at a wide range of frequencies. Listen carefully as you say the word *sound*. Does the first sound (the fricative represented by the letter *s*) seem to have a higher pitch than the vowel-like sound represented by the letters *ou*? The differences in pitch relate to the frequencies of the sounds. Generally, the higher the frequency of a sound is, the higher its pitch is judged to be. While the spectrum of light is divided into colors, the spectrum of speech sounds is represented by energy at particular frequencies or ranges of frequencies. The energy of vowels is predominantly in the lower frequencies, whereas the energy for fricative consonants, like the *s* in the word *say*, is mostly in the higher frequencies. Much as light is analyzed according to the wavelengths of its components, sound is analyzed according to its energy located at particular frequencies.

We now turn to a consideration of how the acoustical signal of speech is generated. This discussion focuses on vowels, but includes brief mention of selected consonants. We begin with a very important theory.

The Source–Filter Theory

The **source–filter theory of speech acoustics** can be stated quite simply: Energy from a sound source is modified by a resonating system (a filter) to yield the acoustic signal of speech. For vowels, the energy source usually is vocal fold vibration, and the resonating system is the vocal tract. This theoretical statement corresponds to the diagram in Figure 3.22. As shown in the figure, the vibrating vocal folds produce a sound that contains many harmonics. A harmonic is simply a whole-number multiple of a fundamental component. For the human voice, the fundamental component is the fundamental frequency of vocal fold vibration (or the number of openings and closings in every second), which averages 125 Hz for men and 225 Hz for women. The second harmonic is twice the value of the fundamental frequency, the third harmonic is three times the value, and so on. For example, the energy in a man's voice, assuming a fundamental frequency of 125 Hz, would be located at the harmonic values of 250 Hz, 375 Hz,

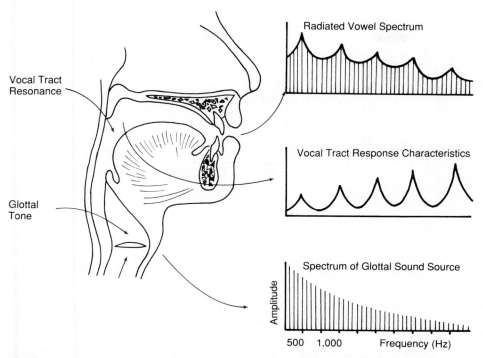

FIGURE 3.22   Schematic tracing of a radiograph (x-ray image) of a person producing a neutral vowel (one with the tongue centered in the oral cavity, so that the vocal tract has a uniform cross-section along its length from vocal folds to lips). Shown at the right side of the figure are the spectrum of the glottal sound source (the energy source), the vocal tract response characteristics (the filter), and the radiated vowel spectrum (the sound that can be heard).

500 Hz, 625 Hz, and so on. In short, the source energy generated by the vibrations of the vocal folds can be described as a harmonic spectrum in which the energy is located at integer multiples of the fundamental frequency.

The resonating system (vocal tract) acts as a filter for the sound energy produced by the source (the vocal folds). The resonator reinforces the source energy at certain frequencies (called the natural or resonance frequencies), depending on the length and shape of the vocal tract. The resonance frequencies are, therefore, the frequencies at which the harmonics of the source are reinforced. The resonance frequencies of the vocal tract are called formants. When we move our tongue, we vary the shape of the vocal tract, which in turn causes a change in its formants. The formants, then, are the filter of the source–filter theory. A filter is a system that readily passes energy at certain frequencies, but not at others. This is exactly what a resonator does. When we speak, we are using our implicit knowledge of how to shape the vocal tract to produce desired patterns of formants. Examples of the relationship between vocal tract shape and acoustic spectrum are given for three different vowels in Figure 3.23.

The source–filter theory for vowel production can be expressed this way:

Speech output = Source energy modified by the vocal tract resonances

If we consider this process in terms of an acoustic spectrum, we can say

Speech spectrum = Source spectrum modified by the resonator

FIGURE 3.23
The relationship between a vocal tract configuration and the radiated (output) spectrum for (a) a neutral vowel, (b) the vowel /i/ as in *heat*, and (c) the vowel /a/ as in *hot*.

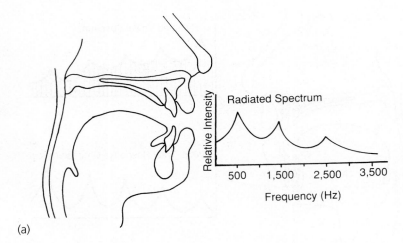

(a)

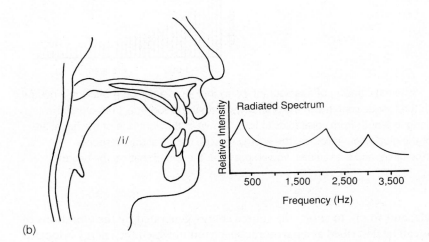

(b)

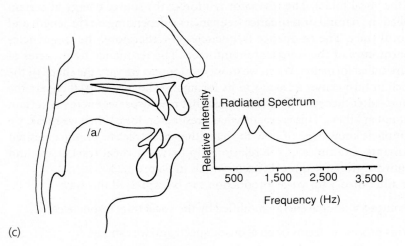

(c)

Acoustic Analysis of Speech: The Spectrogram

To see what formants look like, we need to use acoustic analysis, such as a **spectrogram**. A sample spectrogram is shown in the top part of Figure 3.24. The corresponding waveform is shown at the bottom. The spectrogram is a three-dimensional analysis printed on a two-dimensional surface. The horizontal dimension is time, the vertical dimension is frequency, and the darkness (gray scale) is intensity. With a spectrogram, a sound can be analyzed as a time–frequency–intensity pattern. The graph of intensity by frequency is a spectrum. But the spectrogram goes further to show how the spectrum changes over time, and it is this "running spectrum" feature that makes the spectrogram a useful way to understand a rapidly changing signal such as speech. Note that in Figure 3.24 the sounds of speech are represented along the horizontal axis, with time proceeding from left to right. The frequency dimension is represented along the vertical axis and covers a range from 0 to 8,000 Hz, with low frequencies at the bottom and high frequencies at the top. The horizontal grid lines represent frequency intervals of 1,000 Hz. Finally, the energy at a particular frequency–time point is represented as variations of darkness (the gray scale). This kind of analysis can be applied to many kinds of sounds, and spectrograms have been used to examine bird song, whale song, monkey calls, and human speech.

The entire spectrogram in Figure 3.24 is an analysis of the phrase "speech sounds on display." The individual speech sounds in the phrase are labeled on the spectrogram. Notice the following: Vowels are associated with high-energy dark bands that run roughly horizontally. These bands are resonances of the vocal tract—that is, **formants**.

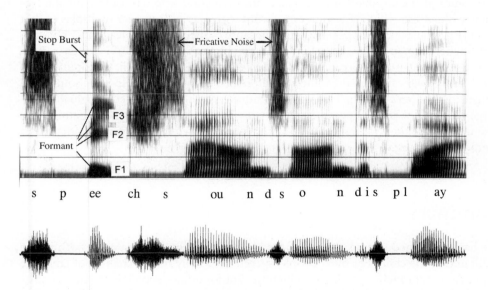

FIGURE 3.24 A spectrogram (top) and a waveform (bottom) of the phrase "speech sounds on display." Time runs from left to right on the horizontal axis. In the spectrogram, frequency runs from low to high on the vertical axis (the thin horizontal lines are divisions of 1,000 Hz, and intensity is scaled as variations in darkness). Notice that the formants (dark horizontal bands) have different patterns for the vowels represented by the letters *ee*, *ou*, *o*, *i*, and *ay*. The first three formants (F1, F2, F3) are labeled for the vowel *ee* in the word *speech*.

Several formants can be seen. The formants are designated as Fl, F2, F3, and so on, beginning with the lowest-frequency formant. Just three formants are sufficient to describe and differentiate speech sounds. Different vowels are distinguished by differences in their formant patterns. Compare the formant patterns for the vowels represented by the letters *ee*, *ou*, *o*, *i*, and *ay*. As an example of formant analysis, note that the first and second formants of the vowel *ee* in the word *speech* have frequencies of about 300 Hz for Fl and just over 2,000 Hz for F2. Vowels differ in their formant patterns, but they have in common a relatively high amount of energy. We can say that vowels are relatively high-energy sounds with a well-defined formant pattern. Now look at the noise sounds identified by the letters *s* and *ch*. These fricative and affricate sounds do not have the distinctive formant patterns of vowels, but rather a high-frequency band of noise energy. The spectrogram reveals many details about speech. For example, notice the closely spaced vertical striations that extend through each vowel segment. Each of the vertical lines represents a vocal fold pulse (a single vibration of the folds). Notice, too, that the vowels vary widely in duration. The *ou* in the word *sounds* is quite long, but the *i* in the word *display* is very short. Finally, notice that the noise interval corresponding to the *ch* in the word *speech* and the *s* in the following word *sounds* is a complex pattern with two phases of noise energy. Interestingly, the word boundary between *speech* and *sounds* occurs in the middle of this complex noise segment.

As highlighted at the conclusion of each of the three systems reviewed (respiratory, laryngeal, articulatory), there are developmental changes in each system. Similarly, the acoustic properties of speech also change during development. Children typically have a higher vocal pitch than adults, and this difference is reflected in the harmonics of the laryngeal source. For example, a child who has a fundamental frequency of 300 Hz will have a source spectrum with energy at integer multiples of that value (e.g., 300, 600, 900, 1,200 Hz). Also, because of their shorter vocal tracts, children have higher formant frequencies for vowels and higher frequencies of noise energy for their fricatives. Differences can be noted in other dimensions as well. Children usually speak at a slower rate than do adults; therefore, the durations of individual sounds are longer in children's speech. The acoustic patterns of children's speech gradually converge on those of adults' speech, so that by the age of about 16 years, the patterns are essentially adultlike with respect to vocal fundamental frequency, formant pattern, and temporal structure.

Summary

We have examined several aspects of the biology and physics of speech, both in the adult and in the child. For most people, speech is a highly robust channel of language expression that functions well over a lifetime. But for others, speech is affected by various disorders that are considered elsewhere in this book. A basic step in understanding the disorders of speech is to know how speech is produced. For this reason, the curriculum in speech-language pathology and audiology includes instruction in anatomy, physiology, physics, and psychology related to human communication. The inquiry is multidisciplinary. The understanding of even one part of speech production, such as laryngeal vibration, draws on knowledge from anatomy, physiology, aerodynamics, acoustics, and other branches of science.

STUDY QUESTIONS

1. Describe how breathing for speech differs from rest breathing. Draw a simple diagram to show how the cycle of inspiration and expiration changes as one goes from rest breathing to speech and back to rest breathing.

2. Discuss what happens in your respiratory system and larynx as you phonate a vowel sound.

3. How do consonants and vowels differ?

4. Using the information on place and manner of articulation given in this chapter, describe where and how each sound in the word *tops* is made.

5. Describe some ways in which an infant's speech production system differs from that of an adult.

6. Define the concepts of *lateralization* and *localization* in the study of brain function.

7. Referring to Figure 3.24, write a brief description of the different sounds seen in the spectrogram. For example, which sounds have mostly low-frequency energy, and which have mostly high-frequency energy?

Chapter **FOUR**

Multicultural and Multilingual Considerations

Kay T. Payne
Howard University

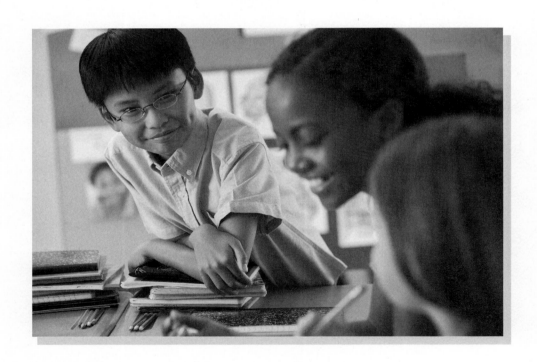

personal PERSPECTIVE

KAY T. PAYNE

When I was 12 years old, my family moved from North Carolina to New York City. I quickly discovered that there were regional and social differences of speech when my typical pronunciation of "dawg" for our family pet drew gales of laughter from the other children. Of course, their expression, which sounded something like "doo-ug," was equally humorous to me. Beyond the amusing aspects, there are many consequences to be endured for sounding different in a place where everyone else sounds alike.

My fascination for language differences led me to study languages and psychology in college. Thus, it was not difficult to select speech-language pathology as a field for master's study and sociolinguistics for doctoral study. Today I consider myself an advocate for the appreciation and preservation of social varieties of language.

As a professor of communication disorders at Howard University, I instruct students in distinguishing language differences from language disorders. There are many clients who enter the clinic to acquire Standard English as a second dialect or improve a foreign accent. Many clients exhibit influences from a different native language. Clinicians must appreciate that these individuals are not communicatively disabled. Amending true disabilities and language differences is analogous to performing cleft palate surgery and a cosmetic face lift. Similar skills are needed, but each purpose is distinct. One is necessary, while the other is optional.

I remain fascinated with the field because of its interdisciplinary nature. In distinguishing differences from disorders, the speech-language pathologist must possess the sensitivity and understanding of a linguist, psychologist, sociologist, cultural anthropologist, historian, development specialist, teacher, bilingual educator, and even political scientist. The issues relate to children as well as adults and to education as well as health. There are clinical issues as well as much research to be conducted.

Just as I was, I hope that this chapter captures your imagination and inspires you to read and develop new knowledge and thinking. Our knowledge will never be static, for languages and cultures will continually change for generations to come.

Communication is generally thought to be disordered when it deviates from the community standards enough that it (1) interferes with the transmission of messages, (2) stands out as being unusually different, or (3) produces negative feelings within the communicator. Central to this is the idea that a communication disorder can be determined only in the context of a group norm—more specifically, **speech community**. A speech community is any group of people who routinely and frequently use a shared language to interact with each other. Thus, an accurate understanding of what constitutes a communication disorder requires an understanding of the distinction between a *communication difference* and a *communication disorder*. This chapter highlights the salient issues arising from cultural and linguistic differences that can result in misdiagnosis of communication disorders.

In any geographical area, there might be several speech communities, although a common national language (English, for instance) is spoken. These varieties of the language are called *dialects*. Despite their differences, speakers of various dialects can generally communicate across speech communities. For example, New Englanders obviously can converse with Southerners.

It is also important to distinguish between *dialect* and *accent*. An **accent** refers to the phonological, idiomatic, suprasegmental, and pronunciation characteristics of spoken language. Accents are generally derived from the influence of geographical region or foreign language. Accents relate only to the surface structure of language, dialects include surface structure, **deep structure**, and rules for language use. Dialects derive from historical, social, regional, and cultural influences within the speech community. Both dialects and accents are language differences rather than disorders.

Speakers of certain dialects—usually ones thought of as nonprestigious or nonstandard—are often mistakenly perceived as having communication disorders. It is incorrect to presume that every person who speaks a dialect different from the standard has a communication disorder, even if that dialect results in breakdowns of communication, excessive audience attention, or (because of ridicule) emotional distress for the speaker. The speech-language pathologist must distinguish *differences* from *disorders* to accurately separate individuals who need speech-language pathology services from those who may need instruction in a second dialect or language. In determining the communication needs of an individual, several factors must be considered, including communication behavior, communication context, and the culture from which communication emanates.

To accurately evaluate a person's communicative behavior, it is essential to understand some basic concepts pertaining to communication, language, and culture as well as the characteristics of the dialects of American English. This information can also enhance the quality of the therapy and educational services provided to individuals with communication disabilities.

Basic Concepts Related to Culture and Language

Culture may be defined as the set of values, perceptions, beliefs, institutions, technologies, survival systems, and codes of conduct used by members of a group to ensure the acquisition and perpetuation of what *they* consider to be a high quality of life. Culture is arbitrary and changeable. Cultures overlap among one another and have internal variations. In addition, culture is learned and exists at different levels of conscious awareness. Culture should not be confused with race, nationality, religion, language, or socioeconomic status, although such groups may demonstrate a common subset of identifiable cultural behaviors. The fact is that, within any one of these groups, there is enormous internal variation.

No matter how you define it, language is a universal human phenomenon. Some form of language is used by every culture on the planet, regardless of its race, region, education, or economic or technical development. Despite the existence of thousands of languages in the world, all share a common set of universal rules. Even their patterns of acquisition are universal in some ways. Social and cultural factors universally affect the nature and use of language within human groups.

Language and culture share an intimate relationship. Although there are many more cultures than languages, the communication styles and forms adopted by a group are an important aspect of the culture. For example, proverbs, idioms, and jokes reflect beliefs and values and serve as vehicles to communicate them within the culture. Within a culture, there is usually great loyalty to the language, probably because language serves as the major unifying force for the people. Logical evidence can be seen by the fact that dialects are extremely resistant to eradication or extinction.

Sociolinguistics

The study of social and cultural influences on language use and structure falls within the domain of **sociolinguistics**. The concepts of dialects and standards are central to the understanding of sociolinguistics and its role in the study and treatment of communication disorders. A dialect is a variety of language that has developed through a complex interplay of historical, social, political, educational, and linguistic forces. In the technical sense, the term *dialect* is never used negatively, as is frequently the case with the lay public. A dialect should not be considered an inferior variety of a language, merely a different variety. In this context, *all dialects are considered to be linguistically legitimate and valid*. No dialect is intrinsically a better way of speaking the language than any other dialect.

However, despite the linguistic legitimacy of all dialects, various dialects of a language tend to assume different social, economic, political, or educational value within society. Standard dialects are those spoken by politically, socially, economically, and educationally powerful and prestigious people. It is not unusual for speakers of standard dialects to have negative attitudes toward nonstandard dialects and their speakers. These standard dialects become the de facto official versions of the language and are used in business, education, and mass media. There may be several standard dialects within a language.

In the United States, several dialects of English exist. Almost all of these varieties are identified with specific regions of the country and with certain racial, ethnic, or language groups. These dialects contain differences in phonology, semantics, discourse and pragmatics (particularly in informal situations). But it is perhaps in syntax and morphology that social attitudes regarding prestige are strongest.

Within the dialects of a language, there may be structural, stylistic, or social variations. For example, a **vernacular** or colloquial variation may be used in informal, casual, or intimate situations, but not in writing or in school. Variations in language use may occur as a function of the social situation in which communication occurs or the speech community of the participants. Thus, a particular linguistic structure may have various functions depending on the intent of the speaker. For instance, an interrogative sentence such as *Do you have the time?* is not always intended as a question, but may also be used to request the time. The selection of a specific linguistic structure, then, depends on the speaker's perception of the social situation as well as the communication intention. Finally, certain sociolinguistic variables, such as speaker, listener, audience, topic, or setting, identify the social context that may influence the usage of a particular language variety.

Six major factors typically influence the dialect acquired and the communicative behavior selected by an individual:

1. Ethnicity
2. Social class, education, and occupation
3. Geographic region
4. Context
5. Peer group identification
6. First language

Depending on an individual's language experiences and social networks, he or she may acquire the capacity to effectively speak several dialects, selecting each for use when needed. The shifting from one dialect of a language to another is called **code-switching**. Code-switching is generally determined by the preferred code of the speech community and the domain in which the communicative event is occurring.

Ethnicity

Ethnic influences on language and communication are neither biological nor genetic in nature. They are related to the cultural attitudes and values associated with a particular group and the group's linguistic history. Some linguistic forms and communicative behaviors are so characteristic of certain ethnic groups that, when used, they immediately mark the speaker either as being from that group or as having had a great deal of interaction with the group.

One must be careful, however, not to assume that ethnic group membership automatically predicts language behavior or prevents an individual from using language codes associated with other groups. To do so would be prejudicial stereotyping. In fact, many people learn the structural and functional rules of the linguistic and communicative systems of other groups. Such persons are considered **bilingual** if two languages are involved or **bidialectal** if two dialects are involved.

Social Class, Education, and Occupation

Educational achievement and occupation play a major role in determining language variety. In addition, many dimensions of language variation can be attributed to social class influences. Some research suggests that perhaps social class is more important than culture or ethnicity in shaping language development. (Hart, Bettty, & Risley, 1995; Seymour Roeper, de Villiers, & de Villiers, 2003).

It is crucial to note that social class, culture, and ethnicity do not hinder language development; however, differences are manifested in the pattern of acquisition as well as verbal usage. For example, it has been observed that Japanese mothers, emphasizing nonverbal and physical forms of communication, vocalize less to their infants than do middle-class American mothers (Van Kleeck, 1994b). Hence, Japanese children develop a pattern of silence with respect to adults. No one, of course, would infer that Japanese children are inferior in language development.

Van Kleeck (1994) discusses cultural beliefs and practices in child rearing that affect language socialization and consequently quantity and type of verbal output of children. According to van Kleeck, in order to avoid stereotypical assumptions, clinicians must consider such cultural aspects as conversational postulates (who talks to whom, what topics, what contexts, etc.), values placed upon child talk, and language-teaching beliefs. Among Native Americans, familial practices affect a child's willingness to speak, average length of utterance, response time, initiation of conversation, and turn-taking behavior. This difference may be due, in part, to a cultural view that children must develop interdependence with the family and society. In accordance with this belief, group dependence in children is facilitated by encouraging passiveness and anticipating others' needs such that little verbal interaction is required. By contrast, believing that children must develop independence, Caucasian parents encourage assertiveness, self-direction, and expression of their needs. Cultural influences on communication that differ from mainstream communication practices must be recognized when providing "clinical" services to members of various cultural groups. These differences must be respected and preserved as important characteristics of the individual.

To distinguish communication differences from communication disorders, it is necessary to have an understanding of those factors necessary for language development and the elements that enhance academic achievement. The culture of the classroom is often based on expectations of a white middle-class lifestyle. Thus, a child from a lower socioeconomic class or culturally different environment may experience difficulty in school, but have no problem in the home or community.

Geographic Region

Regional dialects are closely tied to social dialects, but are generally defined by geographic boundaries. At least ten regional dialects are recognized in the contiguous United States, including Southern, Eastern New England, Western Pennsylvania, Appalachian, Central Midland, Middle Atlantic, and New York City.

A particular speaker may choose to use a regional dialect for a variety of reasons, including local pride, local activities, or a deliberate rejection of wider affiliations. Other people may give up regionalisms because of their occupational, political, or social aspirations. Some regional dialects are viewed negatively by outsiders or by members of the upper class from the same region. Some speakers compromise by using regional dialects locally or in intimate situations and more nonregionalized dialects when they are away from home or in formal situations. Since regional dialects tend to be close to the general standard, many speakers do not find it necessary to abandon their dialect.

Context

Language may vary according to the situation and context in which it is spoken. Situational and contextual issues include occasion, purpose, spatial position of participants, and speaker's role in two-person interactions. For example, a special form of address known as *motherese* has been observed among parents, particularly mothers in addressing their children. Mothers tend to vary their pitch, intonation patterns, speed, sentence length, structure, and vocabulary when talking to their children. Some researchers have also suggested that children, like adults, vary their speech as a function of the listener. For instance, children may use a more restricted linguistic code when talking to strangers, especially if the strangers belong to an outside group. This point is of extreme importance for the speech-language pathologist who is attempting to obtain a valid language sample from a child.

Peer Group Identification

It is widely believed that linguistic behavior, particularly during childhood, is influenced by the speech community and parents. There is also strong research evidence to support the claim that the role of peers, including brothers and sisters, is of equal importance. Thus, a child with strong associations or identification with children from other speech communities might learn forms of language that are different from those of the family. In these cases, the child may use a different language or dialect for communicating with people outside the home or home community.

Several researchers stress the importance of peer influence on language during adolescence. They report that adolescents typically learn an "in-group" lingo that is primarily used by their immediate peers. Sometimes peer pressure prevails over parental standards during this period. This point often shows up in parents' complaints that they don't understand their teenage children (Owens, Metz, Hass, 2003).

Language is often an indicator of a person's age group. Language patterns of the elderly, for instance, are different in some ways from those of younger adults, which in turn vary from those of teenagers, and so on. Violations of linguistic age constraints tend to draw attention to the speaker. Thus, it is not unusual to hear pronouncements like "That boy talks like a man" or "That man sounds like a teenager."

First Language

Many individuals with a different native language learn the official language, but retain distinct vestiges of their first language. Often these persons are considered bilingual, in that they control parts or all of two languages.

Research has shown that, prior to age 3, simultaneous acquisition of two languages may occur systematically and without negative influence of one upon another (Long, 2006; McLaughlin, 2006). Successive acquisition occurs when individuals acquire a second language after the onset of development of the first language—for example, when one language is learned in the home and another at school. According to Owens (2010), learning a second language may result in modified brain organization involving right brain mechanisms not involved in single language learning. Research has shown that bilinguals are superior in some cognitive functions such as classification, memory, problem solving, and creativity (Bialystok, Luk, & Kwan, 2005; Garcia & Ortiz, 2006; Sheng, McGregor, & Mariam, 2006).

Bilingual and bidialectal persons may code-switch from one language to another depending on the social situation (Kayser, 1995b). In the process of code-switching, features of the first language are mixed with features of the second language. A person of Latino origin who speaks English, for example, might mix English and Spanish words in the same sentence: *May I have coffee con leche?* Other such speakers may have morphological differences, such as the absence of plural or possessive morphemes. Phonology and syntax in the second language may also be affected by the first language. For example, English sounds such as /v/, /ʃ/, and /ɪ/ do not occur in Spanish, and adjectives follow nouns rather than preceding them. The Spanish rules may be followed by Spanish speakers who learn English as a second language.

Social factors such as age, education, and situation influence an individual's efficiency in learning a second language. The frequency with which a person hears and interacts within the second language code and the nature of instruction in it also determine a person's skill in using the second language. If a person uses a second language more than a first language, facility in the native language might be lost if it is not reinforced at home. When a whole generation of children in a given culture moves toward usage of a second language as the preferred mode of communication, extinction of the first language is inevitable. Language extinction is occurring rapidly, for example, for several Native American and Eskimo languages in Alaska.

As you can surmise from this discussion of the social and cultural factors that influence language, no one variable operates independently of other variables. The language used during any speech event depends on the simultaneous interaction of many social, cultural, and situational factors. Therefore, no one sample of a person's speech taken from a single situation or from interaction with a single person is likely to be representative of that individual's complete linguistic repertoire. While we may be able to identify a typical speech pattern, that pattern cannot be considered the only speech variety available to that person. The speech-language pathologist must recognize an individual's potential for language variation during both assessment and intervention.

Varieties of American English

African American Vernacular English

Perhaps the most controversial and most frequently written-about dialect of American English is *African American Vernacular English (AAVE),* variously referred to as *Black English, Black Dialect, Black English Vernacular,* and *Ebonics.* Writings on this subject emerged in the sociolinguistic literature from the previous there decades.

Loosely defined, as in much of this research, AAVE may be thought of as the linguistic code used by working-class African Americans, especially for communication in informal situations within working-class African-American speech communities. Its linguistic features, like those of any other dialect, are explained on the basis of social, cultural, and historical facts, not biological differences. Speakers of AAVE are presumed to be knowledgeable in other dialects of English, notably Standard English, as demonstrated by their comprehension of these other dialects.

AAVE, like other dialects, is not exclusive of other dialects of English. In fact, linguistic analyses of transcripts of AAVE speakers show that the overwhelming majority of their utterances conform to the rules of Standard American English. In fact, only about 29 linguistic rules of AAVE that differ from Standard English have been indentified. Careful review of these linguistic rules shows considerable overlap between AAVE and several other dialects, notably Southern English and Southern White Nonstandard

English. Because of this overlap, we need to be careful not to assume that a particular linguistic feature used by African-American speakers is a feature of AAVE. African Americans in the United States have a strong historical link with the southern states, so it is not surprising that there appears to be considerable overlap between AAVE and the numerous dialects spoken in the South.

Several theories have been advanced to explain the development of AAVE. One of the most popular of these theories is the *creolist theory.* Briefly stated, the creolist position holds that AAVE is a complex hybrid involving several African languages and four main European languages—Portuguese, Dutch, French, and English. These hybrids are believed to have developed in Africa, as well as on American plantations, in the form of **pidgins** and **creoles**.

Pidgin languages develop when peoples speaking different languages come in contact with each other and have a need to find a common language, usually for commerce. Typically, a pidgin is developed by speakers of a nondominant group who are in direct contact with a dominant group that speaks another language. Good examples include the pidgins still used by many Chinese and Hawaiians. At the outset of its development, a pidgin language may be informal, consisting of single words, a simplified grammar, and many gestures.

Over time, pidgin languages may become more formal, in that vocabulary items selected primarily from the dominant language are embedded into a phonological and grammatical system derived from the nondominant language. When this happens and the pidgin is accepted as a native language, the language is referred to as *creole.* As stated earlier, extinction of the first language often occurs at this point. Eventually, as the speakers of creole languages become more assimilated into the dominant culture, creole languages tend to move toward the standard language through an intermediate stage referred to as *decreolization.*

There are some problems with the creole theory of AAVE. For instance, it tends to view the language as being European based rather than African based. Despite its problems, however, the creolist explanation of AAVE at least provides a historical orientation for the analysis and understanding of African-American speech.

English Influenced by Other Languages

The largest group in the United States today with native language influence on English consists of people from Spanish-speaking backgrounds (including Mexican Spanish, Cuban Spanish, and Puerto Rican Spanish). Tables 4.1 and 4.2 present some examples of how Spanish can interact with English phonology and syntax, respectively.

TABLE 4.1   Examples of Spanish Influence on English Phonology

Features	*Environments*	*Examples*
/ʃ/ phoneme	/tʃ/ for /ʃ/ in all positions	chair (share); watch (watsh)
/z/ phoneme	/s/ for /z/ in all positions	sip (zip); racer (razor)
/ŋ/ phoneme	/n/ for /ŋ/ in the word-final position	sin (sing)
/v/ phoneme	/b/ for /v/ in all positions	bat (vat); rabbel (ravel)
/ɵ/ phoneme	/t/ or /s/ for /ɵ/ in all positions	tin or sin (thin)
/ð/ phoneme	/d/ for /ð/ in all positions	den (then); ladder (lather)
/ɪ/ phoneme	/ɪy/ for /ɪ/ in all positions	cheap (chip)

TABLE 4.2   Examples of Spanish Influence on English Syntax

Features	*Environments*	*Examples*
Forms of *to be*	Absent in present progressive	He getting hungry (He is getting hungry).
Pronouns	Absent as subjects of sentences when subject obvious from preceding sentence	Carol left yesterday. I think is coming back tomorrow (Carol left yesterday. I think she is coming back tomorrow).
Third person (*-s*)	Absent in third-person verb agreements	He talk fast (He talks fast).
Past (*-ed*)	Absent in past-tense inflections	He walk fast yesterday (He walked fast yesterday).
Go with *to*	Future markings	He go to see the game tomorrow (He is going to see the game tomorrow).
No for *don't*	Imperatives	No do that (Don't do that).
The for possessive pronoun	With body parts	I hurt the finger (I hurt my finger).
Present-tense markings	Progressive environments	I think he come soon (I think he is coming soon).
Locative adverbs	Placed near verb	I think he putting down the rifle (I think he is putting the rifle down).

Table 4.3 presents some influences of Mandarin, Cantonese, Hmong, and Vietnamese on English phonological patterns. Cheng (1987) has also provided examples of grammatical, semantic, and pragmatic differences observed in Asians in their speaking of English.

Other Dimensions of Cultural Influences on Communication

Culture affects communication in its use as well as its function. For example, culture may have an impact on the conversational and discourse rules used by an individual speaker. These rules cover a myriad of topics:

- How to open or close a conversation
- Turn-taking during conversations
- Interruptions
- Silence as a communicative device
- Appropriate topics of conversation
- Humor and when to use it
- Nonverbal modes to accompany conversation
- Laughter as a communicative device
- Appropriate amount of speech to be used by participants
- Logical ordering of events during discourse

Narratives, the art of translating experiences into stories, are a major dimension of discourse that seems to be culture-specific. Many investigators (McCabe & Bliss, 2003) have suggested that children vary in their storytelling strategies as they do in the surface structure features of their language. These strategies are probably related to differences in conceptualization, social interaction, and problem solving.

TABLE 4.3 Phonological Patterns of Interferences

Mandarin

Consonant changes:	θ → s, ð → z, v → f
Metathesis:	r and I
Absence:	final consonants
Additions:	/ə/ in blends; blue → belue, good → gooda
Approximations:	tʃ → tç, s → ç
Shortening or lengthening of vowels:	sit → seat, eat → it

Cantonese

Consonant changes:	θ → s, z → s, v → f, v → w, ʃ → s, r → l, ee → e
Metathesis:	r and I
Absence:	final consonants
Additions:	/ə/ in blends
Vowels:	/I/, /ʌ/, /ɔ/ are difficult for Cantonese speakers

Vietnamese

Consonant changes:	θ → s, tʃ → ʃ, p → b, dʒ → ʒ, ð → d
Absence:	final consonants and consonant blends /t/, /æ/, /v/, /ə/
Vowels:	may be difficult at times

Hmong

Consonant changes:	r → l, t → θ, d → ð, b → v Voicing and devoicing of plosives
Metathesis:	w and v, r and I, k and g
Absence:	Final consonants, cluster reduction, /[ipae]/

Source: Adapted from "Cross Cultural and Linguistic Considerations in Working with Asian Populations" by L. R. L. Cheng, 1987. *Asha 29*, p. 35 (Reprinted by permission of the American Speech-Language-Hearing Association), and *Linguistically and Culturally Diverse Populations: African American and Hmong* by Wisconsin Department of Public Instruction, 1997.

Communicative strategies vary along a cultural continuum anchored by *oral strategies* at one end and *literate strategies* at the other. Oral-based cultures are thought to place value on oral narratives and poetry, while literate-based cultures are thought to value writing and speech. European-based assessments of narrative skill will systematically devalue productions by children from cultures that have different narrative values (McCabe & Bliss, 2003).

Of course, all individuals have a certain degree of control over both ends of this continuum; however, it appears that some cultures have a greater propensity for extending further into one end or the other than do other cultural groups. For example, lower- and working-class children are more likely to come to school with less mastery of the literate style of communication than are middle-class children. Schools prefer the literate style, and these lower- and working-class children are often falsely perceived as having language difficulties because they do not structure their stories in a manner prescriptively perceived as normal.

In general, *topic-centered* narratives are characterized by (1) linear presentation of tightly structured discourse on a single topic or series of closely related topics with no major shifts in perspective; (2) temporal orientation or thematic focus; (3) a high degree of thematic coherence and a clear thematic progression that begins with temporal grounding, a statement of focus, introduction of key agents, and some indication of spatial grounding; and (4) an orientation that is followed by elaboration on the topic and finishes with a punch-line resolution. The stories presume little shared knowledge between speakers and listeners and, therefore, require precise detail. They involve more telling than sharing. The topic-centered style appears to be the one most commonly used by middle-class children, possibly of all racial groups, probably because of extensive exposure to storybooks during early childhood.

Topic-associated stories tend to be a series of associated segments implicitly linked to a topic, event, or theme, but with no explicit theme or point. They typically begin with background statements and then shift across segments, with the shifts being marked by pitch and tempo indicators. Various segments are implicitly linked to a topical event or theme, although temporal orientation, location, and focus of segments often shift from one segment to the other. The links among the various segments are left for listener inference, since there is a presumed shared knowledge between speakers and listeners. Because of this presumption, these stories tend to contain less detail than topic-centered narratives. At the same time, their focus on a number of themes results in longer presentations.

Topic-associated stories are thought to be used more often by working-class children, particularly working-class African-American children. They also seem to be perfectly acceptable, understandable, and frequently used by persons who come from oral cultures, regardless of racial background.

Language Differences and Communication Disorders

The question now is "How does a knowledge of language differences contribute to the practice of speech-language pathology?" Some possible answers to this question are discussed in the following paragraphs.

Attitudes

Perhaps the most important recent contribution of sociolinguistics to the field of communication disorders has to do with attitudes toward language variation. The literature clearly suggests that speech-language pathologists must view language variety as a normal phenomenon and not necessarily as an indication of a communication problem. This is a critical prerequisite for providing clinical services that fit the language codes and expectations of clients, their parents, and their communities. ASHA's 2002 *American English Dialects: Technical Report* considers the recognition of all dialects as rule-governed linguistic systems to be an essential competence for differentiating between communication differences and communication disorders.

Definitions

Another important contribution of sociolinguistics to professional practice in communication disorders has to do with defining disordered communication. A sociocultural perspective toward communication disorders argues that all communication—normal or disordered—must be defined, studied, or discussed only in a cultural context. Since disordered communication is defined as a deviation from the norm, that norm

TABLE 4.4 Cultural Values and Beliefs Toward Health Care and Disability

	Anglo-Europeans	*American Indians*	*African Americans*	*Hispanics*	*Asians*
Health Care	Value on technology Emphasis on prevention Desire to prolong life Pharmaceutical treatments	Tribal healers Ceremonial rituals	Lack of access Home remedies Technology for trauma situations	Natural healers Spiritualists Symbolic rituals Use of amulets	Spiritual ceremonies Herbal medications Acupuncture
Causation	Individual locus of control Nonfatalistic	External locus of control Fatalistic Multiple causality Supernatural events Disturbance of balance	Punishment from deity Work of the devil Fatalistic	Works of evil Fatalistic Folk beliefs	Supernatural Focus on symptoms rather than cause Folk beliefs Punishment
Disability	Scientific causes Preventable Self-help Use of compensatory devices	Sociocultural explanation of cause	Due to misfortune Acceptance	"Act of God" Acceptance related to socioeconomic status	Viewed with considerable stigma

Source: Information from Lynch, Eleanor W. & Hanson, Marci J., *Developing Cross-Cultural Competence: A Guide for Working with Children and Their Families*, 3rd ed, 2004, Baltimore: Paul H. Brookes Publishing Co.

has to be culturally based. For example, the /s/ phoneme is typically pronounced /θ/ and other palatal sounds are dentalized in Castilian Spanish. The same would be considered as a lisp for English speakers.

There is also some evidence that societies have different values for defining normal communication and, more importantly, what to do about conditions of abnormal communication. In some societies, for example, mild deviations in communication behavior may hardly be considered cause for alarm in the context of other priorities.

Some societies feel that little or nothing should be done about a communication disorder except to keep it hidden from the public because these disorders are perceived as acts of gods or demons. In Table 4.4, Lynch & Hanson (2004) provides a broad categorization of cultural values and beliefs toward health care and disability among cultural groups.

Testing and Diagnosis

Because there are different communication rules among cultural groups, examination and diagnosis of a person with a communication disorder is much more likely to be effective if the clinician uses instruments, interpersonal interaction, testing, and interpretation of findings that are consistent with the client's cultural norms. For this reason, effective testing and diagnostic work are directly related to sensitivity and use of culturally relevant materials and clinical orientations.

Standardized Tests Speech-language pathologists rely heavily on **standardized tests** to determine the presence or absence of communication disorders. Most tests currently used in speech-language pathology are based on Northern Midland Standard English. For this reason, many of these tests, when administered and scored according to the prescribed norms, yield results that unfairly penalize speakers of nonstandard dialects. They give the inaccurate impression of communication disorder when, in fact, no pathology exists.

An example of the cultural bias can be found in tests of *auditory discrimination*. For example, a task of auditory discrimination might require a child to indicate whether the following two nonsense syllables sound alike or different: "id" /id/ and "ed" /ɛd/. The expected answer for a Standard English listener, of course, is "different." We know, however, that people tend to perceive incoming sounds according to the phonological rules of their native language. Thus, if the /ɪ/ phoneme does not exist in a particular speaker's phonological system, but the /ɛ/ does exist, she may report the word pair as "same" instead of "different."

There are seven basis types of test bias:

1. Social situational basis—lack of familiarity or conflict in the expected verbal and social interactions between the examiner and test taker

2. Value bias—mismatch between the values assumed in test items and the values of the test taker

3. Phonological bias—mismatch between the phonological rules assumed in a test item and the phonological rules of the test taker

4. Grammatical bias—mismatch between the grammatical rules assumed in a test item and the grammatical rules of the test taker

5. Vocabulary bias—mismatch between words and their use between test maker and test taker (may include underlying cognitive mismatches)

6. Pragmatic bias—mismatch between rules of communication interaction between test maker and test taker

7. Directions/format bias—confusions or misunderstandings due to the use of unfamiliar or ambiguous directions or test format

Test bias may also come from other culturally based differences in communicative style, in areas such as verbosity, the statement of obvious information, and preferred narrative style. Knowledge of sources of test bias can assist clinicians in interpreting test data, modifying existing tests, and constructing new scoring norms. Of course, the ultimate solution to this problem is the construction of tests that assess a test taker's communication skills from the vantage point of his speech community.

The use of culturally and linguistically discriminatory assessment instruments is specifically prohibited by federal mandates such as the Individuals with Disabilities Education Improvement Act (IDEA) (2004), the Bilingual Education Act of 1976, and Title VII of the Elementary and Secondary Education Act of 1965. In addition, several legal decisions have declared illegal the use of culturally and linguistically discriminatory assessment procedures for determining the presence of disabling conditions; see, for example, *Dianna v. California State Board of Education* (1973), *Mattie T. v. Halladay* (1977) in Mississippi, and *Larry P. v. Riles* (1979) in California. Thus, appropriate responses to test bias are necessary.

Two recent responses to the lack of availability of nonbiased criterion-referenced and norm-referenced tests have been introduced through the Diagnostic Evaluation of Language Variation (DELV) (Seymour, Roper, & de Villiers, 2003). Developed in response to the linguistic bias against speakers of AAVE in traditional tests, the DELV is constructed to be appropriate for speakers of any variety of English. Based on Seymour's Non-Contrastive Model, the DELV initially screens for the presence of dialect features. The formal instrument then examines only those linguistic components that are considered universal such as knowledge of subtle, abstract properties and processes that are noncontrastive for different varieties of English. Hence, the DELV can more accurately distinguish between a language difference and a language disorder.

Another response to bias against bilingual speakers is the Bilingual Verbal Ability Test (BVAT) (Munoz-Sandoval, Cummins, & Ruef, 1998). The BVAT measures linguistic competence for 17 different linguistic populations, using both English and the native language. The BVAT reduces the possibility of bias by first examining English proficiency. Incorrect items are then readministered in the native language.

An additional reasonable alternative seems to be modification of existing tests; however, clinicians must be careful that their modifications are documented valid procedures that are both culture and age appropriate. The following test modifications can be used with careful scrutiny:

Alter the scoring procedures to credit biased items
Alter biased items such as pictures and linguistic features
Allow additional time
Allow alternative responses
Eliminate biased items from the test
Elicit responses by other means than the test
Repeat test items three times to allow code-switching and check reliability
Develop additional practice items
Demonstrate desired response
Relate and reword directions
Continue testing beyond the ceiling
Allow client to explain answers
Obtain two scores, one for dialect/first language and one for Standard English

When modification of a test is selected, the following preassessment procedures are necessary:

1. Review the test to identify potentially biased items, including linguistic features, stimulus items, wording of directions, and value conflicts.
2. Review the norming statistics to determine if members of the cultural group were included in the standardization sample.
3. List all predictable responses for each potentially biased item.
4. Review the potentially biased items and predictable responses with a family member or professional member of the client's cultural group.
5. Assess the effect on scoring for the potentially biased items (i.e., total number of items, weight of each item, effect on basal or ceiling.
6. Select *one* modification from the list above to use consistently in administering the test.

During test administration, the potentially biased items should be repeated to ensure reliability of the responses. It is important to note that in test modification the norms are rendered unusable. Therefore, clinicians may not use the test norms to determine a standard score. In cases where standardized assessments are absolutely required, these may be reported in addition to the modified test results. In this case, the clinician administers both standardized and modified procedures. A language sample in a naturalistic setting should always accompany the results to cross-validate the observations. However, the mean length of utterance (MLU) should not be used as a measure of morphological development.

Following modified procedures, the evaluation report is a critical tool for the clinician. In this report, the clinician must be extremely descriptive of the assessment procedures and outcomes. The clinician must describe the exact modification procedure, provide a complete description of language characteristics, differentiate dialect features from disorder characteristics, and fully defend and justify the recommendation for the treatment decision.

Dynamic Assessment   An alternative to using standardized tests with multicultural populations is dynamic assessment. Dynamic assessment is an evaluative method based on the concept of the Zone of Proximal Development (ZPD) proposed by L. S. Vygotsky (1986). Vygotsky proposed that a child's potential for learning can be revealed by measuring the gap between independent performance and performance with adult assistance. Dynamic assessment begins with a baseline, which is the child's independent performance level. Utilizing a test–teach–retest sequence with the primary focus on the teaching phase, the aim is to examine how receptive the child is to adult mediation. During the teaching phase, the examiner is able to discern the effort required by the child to learn new material as well as the child's attention span and resilience to failure. As a result, dynamic assessment can reveal the cognitive process involved in language production and comprehension, whereas a standardized test can only compare a finite sample of language output to that of peers.

Peña, Iglesias and Lidz (2001) recommend dynamic assessment to distinguish second language development from communication disorders in bilingual children. In a study using normal and language-impaired preschoolers, the investigators observed that language-impaired children were less responsive to adult mediation and required more extensive and intensive training. Unlike the language-impaired child, a normal child displaying a communication difference due to second language acquisition will be highly receptive to adult mediation. Miller, Gillam, and Peña (2002) have developed the Dynamic Assessment and Intervention Tool, which uses narrative ability in identifying and remediating communication disorders.

Clinical Management

The speech-language pathologist can apply sociocultural principles of language and communication in the delivery of therapy and education. Significant changes in traditional approaches, however, must be considered in order for the clinician to be culturally competent.

First, the interpersonal dimension is a vital component of any type of effective clinical management of a communication disorder. For this reason, differences in the verbal and nonverbal rules used by the speech-language pathologist and the client can cause unintended episodes of insult, discomfort, or hypersensitivity, which could adversely affect the interpersonal dynamics needed for effective clinical work.

Second, knowledge of developmental patterns of a particular language or dialect can help the professional determine differences between developmental variations and pathologic deviations, the appropriate time to begin speech or language therapy for pathologic features, and the course of therapy once it has started. Taylor and Leonard (1999) provide the most comprehensive source of information on language development in various cultures of North America.

Kayser (1995a) presents some challenges to identification and treatment of language disorders in Hispanic populations. Since semilingualism may result from the acquisition process of two languages, Kayser posits that the effect of second language acquisition can often be mistaken for a language disorder.

Roseberry-McKibbin (2008) discusses the characteristics of second-language acquisition that are sometimes mistaken for language-learning disabilities.

Language interference is the term given to describe the phenomenon when a communication behavior from the first language is applied to English. For example, a Hindi-speaking child may say, "I don't know to you." It has been observed that language interference is most likely to occur in formal situations (e.g., standardized testing) and especially when English is not the language of the speaker's social milieu.

Fossilization is often idiosyncratic, thus it may or may not be observed in all bilingual speakers. Fossilization refers to the tendency of bilingual speakers to make obvious errors of translation (e.g., he for she).

Interlanguage refers to a temporary, trial-and-error period whereby a bilingual speaker makes inconsistent errors resulting from testing hypotheses about the two languages. Interlanguage is also idiosyncratic and highly variable.

Children who are becoming bilingual often display what is known as a silent period wherein they appear to be nonverbal. In actuality, there is much listening and comprehension, but little verbal output. It is believed that this is a crucial stage where children are actively learning the rules of the language. The silent period may extend up to six months.

Code-switching was discussed previously as a sociolinguistic influence on language variety. When code-switching occurs within a singular linguistic unit such as two languages in the same sentence, it may appear as a language disability. However, code-switching can be deliberate for the speaker. In addition, excessive code-switching may mean lack of competence for English, while true language ability for the first language is intact.

Occasionally, a young child may appear to have deficiencies in both the first language and English. Clinicians must be extra careful not to assume language disability. Language loss is another natural process wherein loss of skills in the first language occurs before sufficient English skills are established. Language loss occurs especially where there is no sufficient social environment for maintaining the first language.

Identification of true language disorders may be difficult, since bilingual individuals often do not have the same lexical or comprehensive proficiency in both languages. Thus, less development of the second language (English) may not be reflective of true language capacity. This fact points out the importance of language testing in the individual's dominant language and the need for more bilingual professionals.

Another challenge in identifying language disorders presented by Kayser (1995a) is the difficulty of establishing norms of language development for children developing bilingualism. Since no two children will be identical in their language proficiency and, of course, language impairments are idiosyncratic, large-group studies cannot represent the uniqueness of the individual child.

There are also unique challenges with regard to Asian populations, not the least of which is the fact of wide diversity among nationalities and cultures. With regard to terminology, reference to Asians comprises a broad spectrum of peoples, languages, and dialects. "Asian" generally denotes peoples of East Asian and Indochinese descent, specifically, Chinese, Japanese, Korean, Vietnamese, Thai, Laotian, Cambodian, and Burmese. However, the term accurately includes persons from the Indian subcontinent, the Philippines, and the Pacific Islands. Cheng and Chang (1995) attribute many of the issues of identification and management of language disorders to this diversity. Cultural differences also present challenges to professionals. According to Cheng (1995), Asians are often stereotyped as smart and hardworking; thus, exceptionalities are often not addressed by professionals. In addition, issues of cultural ambivalence and degree of acculturation add to the challenges attributed to diversity. Finally, there are issues related to inadequate education policies to address bilingualism and cultural difference that also affect the quality of services provided to Asian students.

Table 4.5 presents an overview of several multicultural populations including linguistic and cultural characteristics and relevant clinical implications.

Language Education

Language education is the term used to denote services by speech-language pathologists to children who do not have a communication disorder. Thus, language education is distinct from special education and speech therapy. In some professional settings, the speech-language pathologist may instruct speakers of nonstandard dialects in Standard English or English as a second language. This language instruction is usually targeted for speakers of AAVE.

ASHA's revised position on American English dialects permits speech-language pathologists to provide instruction for Standard English on an elective basis only. ASHA's position makes it clear that whether to receive instruction for Standard English must be a choice for the client, not the prerogative of the clinician, especially in the public school setting. To offer such instruction, ASHA asserts that the professional must be sensitive and competent in at least three areas, including

A. recognizing all American English dialects as rule-governed linguistic systems;

B. understanding the rules and linguistic features of American English dialect(s) represented by their clientele; and

C. being familiar with nondiscriminatory testing and dynamic assessment procedures, such as the following:

- identifying potential sources of test bias;

- administering and scoring standardized tests in alternative manners;

- using observation and nontraditional interview and language sampling techniques; and

- analyzing test results in light of existing information regarding dialect use.

The speech-language pathologist must bear in mind that teaching a second dialect is *not* the same as correcting a disorder. In teaching Standard English as a second dialect, the goal is to establish a parallel linguistic form to stand alongside an already

TABLE 4.5 Language and Cultural Influences and Clinical Implications

American Indians

Language Features	Cultural Influences	Clinical Implications
Navajo <ul><li>Tone and vowel length distinguish meaning</li><li>Few consonant clusters</li><li>Clusters do not occur in final position</li><li>15 sounds do not occur in English</li><li>Limited use of noun plurals; number is marked by verb</li><li>Possession is marked by pronouns affixed to nouns (e.g., girl her sweater)</li></ul> **Cherokee** <ul><li>Seven English sounds do not exist in Cherokee /b, f, j, p, r, v, and x/</li><li>/v/, which is tonal and nasalized, does not exist in English</li><li>Almost all syllables end in a vowel</li><li>g → k and d → t</li><li>Some words lack synonyms</li></ul>	<ul><li>Grandparents or extended family often care for children. Families are generally close-knit with all members working together</li><li>Respect for elders and families</li><li>Emphasis on living in harmony with nature and the environment, in addition to a strong spiritual life</li><li>Strong kinship network that emphasizes mutual support, assistance, and affection</li><li>Silence is a sign of respect for authority</li><li>Services of medicine men and traditional medicines are used to cure health concerns</li><li>May withhold information viewed as personal</li><li>Reliance on nonverbal communication</li><li>Prefer visual learning</li><li>May feel distrust of, or intimidation by public agencies</li></ul>	<ul><li>Include entire family in intervention</li><li>Develop sufficient rapport before providing service</li><li>Provide advocacy service</li><li>Become familiar with the community and culture through contact and visits</li><li>Provide treatment in small groups and allow peer assistance</li><li>Demonstrate desired responses</li><li>Allow additional time for responses</li><li>Cluster reductions and phoneme substitutions may occur</li><li>Absence of possessive and plural /s/</li></ul>

Cambodians

Language Features	Cultural Influences	Clinical Implications
<ul><li>Khmer is a nontonal language, essentially monosyllabic and uninflected</li><li>Stress is always on the second syllable</li><li>Rich system of affixes, including infixes, for derivation</li><li>Normal word order is subject–verb–object</li><li>Words change from one part of speech to another depending on context</li><li>Adjective modifiers follow the nouns</li><li>Many lexical terms derived from French</li></ul>	<ul><li>Professionals are held in high regard</li><li>Respect is expressed through nonverbal communication such as avoidance of eye contact</li><li>Respect is the cornerstone of interpersonal relationships</li><li>Extended family is an organizational power bound together by collective responsibilities and mutual obligations</li><li>Status difference between parent and child; children do not initiate conversation</li></ul>	<ul><li>High incidence of middle-ear problems</li><li>Students may not volunteer or ask questions in class</li><li>Teach recognition and production of the contrastive features of English stress, intonation, and final consonants</li><li>Difficulties with inflections, for plurals, tenses, and cases; subject–verb inversion, and use of auxiliaries, articles, pronouns, and prepositions</li></ul>

Language Features	Cultural Influences	Clinical Implications
- 50 vowels and diphthongs as compared with 14 in English - Some English consonants do not occur - 85 consonant clusters - No final clusters; only 2 fricatives - Absence of inflections for gender, number, tense, case, or voice - Interrogative sentences distinguished by question markers, not by subject–verb inversion or auxiliary verbs	- High degree of parental self-sacrifice to allow for success of children - Confucian-based culture; less likely to praise children for small achievements; focus is on overall achievement	- Placement of negative markers may be difficult - May substitute g → k, w → v, b → f, s → t, θ → s, d → t - Final consonants such as /r, d, g, s, z/ may be omitted; /b/ and /p/ imploded - Possible vowel distortions of /ɛ/, /il/, /ul/, /æ/ - The concept "special education" does not exist

Filipinos

Language Features	Cultural Influences	Clinical Implications
- Tagalog has 27 phonemes (16 consonants, 6 diphthongs, and 5 vowels) - Does not have /v, z, ð, ʤ, f, ʃ, tʃ, ʒ/ - Combination of roots and affixes determines the meaning of words - Word order in sentences is reversed compared to English - No true verb distinctions of time; either begun/not begun or completed/not completed - Verbs have the same form for singular and plural - No gender in the third-person singular pronouns. "He" and "she" are stated as "siya" - To indicate plurality "onga" is placed before the noun or by another word - Expression of possessives differs from English morphology - Freedom of word order except for pronouns	- Culture is a mosaic of Spanish, American, Chinese, Malay, Indian, and others - Child is viewed not as an individual, but as an extension of many generations - Believe that children should be protected from the environment - Believe in fatalism; it is in God's hands - Use faith healers - Important not to put people in the position to say "no" directly - Direct confrontations are avoided; indirectly deliver bad news - Negative views about the United States because of military occupation - High respect for teachers; do not question their authority	- Important to include the entire family in the clinical process - A smile and agreement from clients and parents should not be taken at face value - Considered rude to immediately start talking about business. Establish rapport! - Absence of plural morpheme "-s" - Difference in expression of possessives (i.e., "Mary's house" becomes "house of Mary") - Articles "a," "an," and "the" may be omitted - Difficult sounds for Tagalog speakers: /tʃ, ʤ, f, v, θ, ð, z, ʃ, ʒ, r, ɪ, æ, ə, ʊ ɔ, oʊ/ - Word order of sentences may be reversed - Often mix genders when referring to the same person

(Continued)

TABLE 4.5 (Continued)

Hispanics

Language Features	Cultural Influences	Clinical Implications
■ Standard Spanish has 18 phonemes and 5 primary vowels ■ Highly inflected language ■ Pro-drop language; subject pronouns are often omitted ■ Allows the construction of double negatives ■ Grammatical gender for nouns (feminine or masculine) ■ Speakers in the United States may speak different dialects; Spanish dialects can differ significantly from each other ■ Southwestern United States and Caribbean are the two most prominent ■ Lexical, phonological, and syntactical features must be considered during assessment	■ Learn better from hands-on activities and observation than verbal interactions with adults ■ Children verbally interact more often with peers or siblings ■ Adults typically neither ask children to foretell what they will do nor repeat facts ■ Children may not perform as well on tasks that target competition ■ Tend to have a more flexible attitude toward time ■ Children learn best in environments which provide frequent attention and warmth ■ Father is typically the authority figure ■ Children tend to use gestures ■ Children ascribe to a more field-sensitive cognitive style	■ Children often provide functions for objects instead of names ■ /t, d, n/ pronounced with dentilization ■ Adjectives may follow the noun (i.e., the car red) ■ Final consonants are typically devoiced (i.e., /nos/ for /noz/) ■ Adverbs often follow verbs (i.e., He drives very fast his sports car) ■ /b/ is often substituted for /v/ in all position of words ■ Superiority is described by using mas (i.e., Her brother is more big) ■ Stops are often deaspirated ■ /tʃ/ is often substituted for /ʃ/ ■ /s/ is often absent in plurals and possessives (i.e., Maria dress is pretty) ■ Silent /h/ for words that begin with /h/ ■ Schwa sound often inserted before word-initial consonant clusters beginning with /s/ ■ May substitute /j/ for /dʒ/ ■ Lexical, phonological, and syntactical features must be considered during assessment

Puerto Rican Spanish
- Deletion of final /s/
- Absence of /ð, ɵ/, final /m/, and final /t/
- Initial consonant clusters beginning with /s/ are preceded by a schwa sound
- /r/ becomes /l/ in final position of words
- Absence of consonant clusters at end of word

Mexican Spanish
- Initial /b/ substituted by /v/
- /k/ is deleted from consonant clusters in medial word position
- Final /s/ is either deleted or aspirated
- Absence of medial /d/
- /x/ is substituted by [h]

Caribbean Spanish
- /w/ is substituted by /gw/
- Flap /r/ becomes either /l/ or /i/
- Final /n/ is either deleted or substituted by /ŋ/
- /tʃ/ is substituted by /ʃ/
- /j/ is substituted by /dʒ/ or /ʒ/

Hmong

Language Features	Cultural Influences	Clinical Implications
■ Tonal language; 32 consonants, 6 vowels ■ Absence of final consonants except /ŋ/ ■ Consonant clusters in initial position only ■ Monosyllabic words ■ /z/, /θ/, /ð/, /e/, and /ɑ/ do not occur ■ Aspiration is a distinctive feature ■ Absence of copula ■ Word order is subject–verb–object, although prepositions precede nouns; adjectives follow nouns ■ Absence of plural possessive, third-person singular, and verb-tense morphemes ■ Verbs are not inflected	■ Names are important to identify ■ Indirect eye contact is a sign of respect ■ Teachers are not challenged or disputed ■ Girls marry at an early age and discontinue schooling ■ Group orientation results in lack of competitiveness, rather collaboration ■ Language differences may prevent parental assistance with homework and attendance at parent–teacher conferences ■ Birth and age records may be inaccurate ■ Belief in shamanism and natural cures	■ Ascertain how clients prefer to be addressed ■ Show interest in cultural traditions and practices ■ Encourage group participation ■ r → t, θ → t, ð → d, v → b, v → w, w → v, l → r, r → t ■ Voicing and devoicing of plosives ■ Absence of copula, auxiliaries, morphemic markers, and inflections ■ Word-order difficulties ■ Syllabification and stress modifications in pronunciation of multisyllabic words ■ Difficulty with final consonants

Koreans

Language Features	Cultural Influences	Clinical Implications
■ 29 consonant sounds; 12 vowel sounds ■ Word-initial clusters consist of obstruent + glide ■ No labiodental, interdental, or palatal fricatives ■ Fricatives and affricates do not occur in the final position ■ Bilabial nasals produced with weaker lip closure ■ Final stops nasalized before nasal sound ■ Basic word order is subject–object–verb ■ Absent plurality marker ■ Absence of definite and indefinite articles ■ Absence of relative pronouns ■ Predicates do not agree in number, person, or gender with subjects ■ Absence of word-medial or word-final clusters	■ Physical disabilities are considered to be most worthy of treatment rather than communication disorders ■ Believe that disabilities result from sins or evil deeds of ancestors ■ Family is basic societal unit and central focus of individual's life ■ Roles differ according to gender, age, and position ■ Respect for elders ■ Silence is important part of communication ■ Children are expected to be seen and not heard ■ Great respect for learning ■ Consider it rude to volunteer or ask questions in class ■ Eye contact is often avoided and considered rude ■ May be indirect in communication ■ May appear evasive and noncommittal	■ Nasalization of stops that appear before nasals (e.g., "banman" instead of "batman") ■ Substitute v → b, v → p or d → p, ʃ → s, tʃ → t, ʒ → ʤ, g → k, θ → s, or θ → t; "sanks" instead of "thanks" ■ /i/, /ɔ/, /u/, /ʌ/ vowels may be distorted ■ Plural marker in sentences not usually attached to subject, but may be added to adverbs (i.e., The cat are walking slowlys) ■ Deletion of subjects when subjects can be recovered from context ■ May sound monotonous ■ Address male of household first (however, male of household is secondary to grandparents if they are present at that time)

(Continued)

TABLE 4.5 *(Continued)*

Vietnamese

Language Features	Cultural Influences	Clinical Implications
▪ 19 total consonants; 11 vowels	▪ Consider only physical disabilities to be worthy of treatment	▪ Substitutions may be made in the initial and medial positions: tʃ → ʃ, d → z, d → ð, p → b, ʤ → d
▪ Monosyllabic with no syllables or words coarticulated with others	▪ Children expected to be seen and not heard; consider Westerners verbose	▪ Vowels may be difficult; /ɔ, æ, t, v/ may be omitted
▪ No consonant clusters	▪ Parents direct and control conversation, length of the time of talk, and topics	▪ Few consonants in final position, except /p, t, k, m, n/
▪ Tonal language (five different tones that convey differences in meaning)	▪ Parents initiate conversation, verbally explain tasks, verbally monitor children's activities, and ask factual questions	▪ Deletion of final and medial consonants and blends
▪ Monomorphemic language without inflections; grammatical meaning conveyed through word order and contextual cues	▪ Children avoid eye contact	▪ Truncating of polysyllabic words, or emphasis on the unstressed syllable
▪ Absence of past tense and plurality morphemes	▪ Consider touching on the head or slapping on the back insulting	▪ Difficulty with morphemes
▪ Adjectives and possessives usually follow the noun	▪ Interrupting conversation considered impolite	▪ Children may alter the use of articles with proper nouns and nonspecific referents ("the Nala")
▪ Absence of possessives and contractible copulas	▪ Avoid open competition and public confrontation	▪ Address the male of the household; however, males are secondary to grandparents
▪ Final consonants imploded, but not released, resulting in an inaudible sound	▪ Parents may not openly disagree with or question professionals	▪ Ease students into tasks requiring them to give opinions, form judgments, and solve problems
▪ Absence of singular present tense		
▪ Absence of propositions		

Research funded by the U.S. Department of Education, Office of Special Education Programs, Grant No. H325E990036. Acknowledgment to student investigators at Howard University: Kelly Byrd, Ivory Gleaton, Lakeesha Linning, Julie O'Donnal, Jeanette Perez, Monique Richardson, Beth Wilkinson, and Kimberly Wilson.

existing legitimate form for use in appropriate contexts. By contrast, in correcting a disorder, the goal is to eradicate an unacceptable linguistic form in favor of one that is considered normal.

Unfortunately, the decision as to whether to teach English as a second language or Standard English as a second dialect is not always clear-cut. It is one thing to determine, for instance, that a child from a Chinese family does not have the /r/ phoneme in his phonology or that a Chicano child does not have the /i/, but it is quite another matter to determine what, if anything, should be done about these dialects educationally, who should do it, and when it should be done.

Increasingly, speech-language pathologists are being requested to assume a role in providing English as a Second Language (ESL) instruction to children who are developing English proficiency. ASHA (1998) clarifies this role for clinicians in keeping with district, state, and federal regulations. Speech-language pathologists with appropriate ESL training beyond the usual academic preparation may provide the primary direct ESL instruction. However, speech-language pathologists without the requisite training can assume a collaborative consultation role along with trained ESL instructors. Requisite knowledge includes second language acquisition theory, comparative linguistics, and ESL methodologies.

New Horizons in Multicultural/ Multilingual Issues

With the increased national diversity including individuals who speak more than one language and new areas of inclusiveness such as transgender culture, new arenas for research and practice are continuously emerging. Important emerging issues are bilingual aphasia and transgender voice therapy.

Bilingual aphasia poses complex challenges for treatment and interesting questions for research. Due to the many variations of bilingual aphasia, its treatment extends the traditional protocols developed for monolingual clients; different treatment strategies may be more or less appropriate and effective (Roberts, 2001). Paradis (2004) and Fabbro (2001) document seven recovery patterns relative to bilingual proficiency; (1) parallel recovery, (2) selective aphasia, (3) differential recovery, (4) successive recovery, (5) antagonistic recovery, (6) alternating antagonism, and (7) blending recovery. Management of bilingual aphasia is complicated in that the type of recovery experienced by bilingual aphasics cannot be reliably predicted.

Thus, it is evident that special clinical skills are needed. Logically, each language must be throughly evaluated in relation to its premorbid status. Yet a limited number of translated and specially normed aphasia tests exist, and most of these are for Spanish speakers. Obviously,. there is a need to increase the number of available tests to the full variety of relevant languages.

Models of treatment and approaches are also needed to determine which languages to emphasize in therapy as well as the goals, target structures, and response criteria. According to Lorenza and Murray (2008), sufficient evidence-based research practices and experiential support are generally lacking. Moreover, the principles applied to monolingual aphasics and English language learners may be less efficient for bilingual aphasics. For example, Kiran and Edmonds (2004) and Edmonds and Kiran (2006) found that for bilingual aphasics, the weaker language produced generalization to the stronger language, an observation that contradicts widely held assumptions.

Other studies have suggested that certain abilities not typical of monolingual speakers, such as translation and metalinguistic skills, can be potential strategies for helping bilingual aphasics achieve cross-linguistic generalization (Laganaro & Overton Venet, 2001; Kohnert, 2004; Roberts, 2001; Kiran & Edmonds, 2004).

Another area that requires specific clinical skills and a high level of cultural competence is transgender voice therapy. It is important to note that the transgender male to female (MtF) and female to male (FtM) are not members of the lesbian/gay community. Voice therapy is one battery within the transition protocol. A multicultural approach is necessary because treatment involves both gender and cultural parameters. While adjustment of speech fundamental frequency is an important area for therapy, other behavioral, linguistic, and nonverbal aspects of communication must also be addressed. These include (1) resonance, (2) volume/intensity, (3) intonation, (4) speech rate, and (5) pragmatics.

Naturally, there is a cultural element to each of these parameters. For example, treatment utilizes the overlap between typical male and female speech fundamental frequencies as a target goal. However, it must be recognized that different cultures will have varying pitch gap differences; for example, Dutch male and female gaps are very close, whereas Japanese male and female gaps are much wider (Thomton, 2008). Hence, selection of treatment targets, as well as response criteria, must be culturally determined. For transgender voice therapy, language style and pragmatics are important cultural parameters, in keeping with the discussion in the earlier section on "Other Dimensions of Cultural Influences on Communication."

Summary

To avoid misdiagnosis of communication disorders, speech-language pathologists must develop skills to distinguish communication differences from disorders. A knowledge of the principles and foundations of sociolinguistics is essential. Language differences are related to social factors, including ethnicity, social class, education, occupation, geographic region, gender, social situation, peer group association, and first language.

Dialects are subvarieties of a language. Standard English is the dialect that has become the language of education and that is spoken by the middle-class, educated population. Other major dialects include African American Vernacular English, Southern English, Southern White Nonstandard English, and Appalachian English. Other varieties increasingly heard within the United States include English that is influenced by other languages.

Test bias must be considered as a possibility in distinguishing language differences from disorders. Types of test bias include situational bias, value bias, phonological bias, grammatical bias, vocabulary bias, pragmatic bias, and directions/format bias. In addition to adjusting test instruments for bias, the speech-language pathologist should consider the definition of a communication disorder from the perspective of the client's culture. For bilingual populations, the effect of first language influences on the acquisition of English must be considered.

Implications for clinical management include decisions as to whether to enroll clients in therapy, the appropriate time to begin therapy, selection of features to target in therapy, and use of the family and/or significant others. Instruction in Standard English as a Second Dialect and English as a Second Language are education issues for clinicians serving children. As the nation continues to increase in its diversity, practical and research issues continue to emerge for the profession.

STUDY QUESTIONS

1. Discuss the differences between a communication disorder and a communication difference. Select one cultural group and identify the clinical issues for assessment and treatment.

2. Define African American English Vernacular. Briefly discuss its origin and the issues surrounding its use.

3. Discuss the major factors that influence language behavior and acquisition. Which of these factors do you feel could have some impact on language difference? Defend your answer.

4. Select one cultural group and identify the phonological, morphological, and syntactic features of the native language or dialect. Select an articulation language test and describe how these features might be unfairly penalized.

5. List the clinical considerations for providing services to speakers of nonstandard dialects and speakers of English influenced by other languages.

SELECTED READINGS

Alejandro, E. B. (2002). *The Hispanic child.* Boston, MA: Allyn & Bacon.

Battle, D. E. (2002). *Communication disorders in multicultural populations* (3rd ed.). Boston, MA: Butterworth-Heinemann.

Brice, A. E. (2002). *The Hispanic child: Speech, language, culture and education.* Boston, MA: Allyn and Bacon.

Cheng, L. L. (1995). *Integrating language and learning for inclusion: An Asian-Pacific focus.* San Diego, CA: Singular Publishing Group.

Goldstein, B. (2000). *Cultural and linguistic diversity resource guide for speech-language pathologists.* San Diego, CA: Singular Publishing Group.

Kamhi, A. G., Pollock, K. E., & Harris, J. L. (1996). *Communication development and disorders in African American children: Research, assessment and intervention.* Baltimore, MD: Paul H. Brookes.

Kayser, H. (1995). *Bilingual speech-language pathology: An Hispanic focus.* San Diego, CA: Singular Publishing Group.

Langdon, H. (2008). *Assessment and intervention for communication disorders in culturally and linguistically diverse populations.* Clifton Park: Cengage Learning.

McCabe, A., & Bliss, L. S. (2003). *Patterns of narrative discourse: A multicultural, life span approach.* Boston, MA: Allyn and Bacon.

McLeod, S. (2007). *The international guide to speech acquisition.* Clifton Park: Thomson Delmar Learning.

Roseberry-McKibbin, C. (2008). *Increasing language skills of students from low income backgrounds: Practical strategies for professionals.* San Diego, CA: Plural.

Roseberry-McKibbin, C. (2008). *Multicultural students with special language needs: Practical strategies for assessment and intervention.* Oceanside, CA: Academic Communication Associates.

Taylor, O. L., & Leonard, L. B. (1999). *Language acquisition across North America: Cross-cultural and cross-linguistic perspectives.* San Diego, CA: Singular Publishing Group.

Van Keulen, J. E., Weddington, G. T., & Debose, C. E. (1998). *Speech, language, learning, and the African American child.* Boston, MA: Allyn and Bacon.

Wallace, G. (1996). Management of aphasic individuals from culturally and linguistically diverse populations. In G. Wallace (Ed.), *Adult aphasia rehabilitation.* Boston, MA: Butterworth-Heinemann.

Wisconsin Department of Public Instruction (2003). *Linguistically and culturally diverse populations: African American and Hmong.* Madison, WI: Author.

Wisconsin Department of Public Instruction. (2003). *Linguistically and culturally diverse populations: American Indian and Spanish speaking.* Madison, WI: Author.

Chapter FIVE

Genetics

Basis for Development and Disorders

Lemmietta G. McNeilly
American Speech-Language-Hearing Association

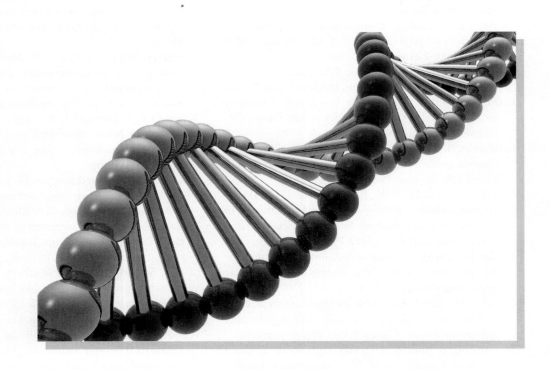

personal PERSPECTIVE

I became interested in the Human Genome Project and its implications for speech-language pathologists as a result of my clinical experiences with medically fragile children. I was selected to attend HuGemII, a train-the-trainer's summer institute, sponsored by the National Institutes of Health and Georgetown University in the summer of 1999. I became knowledgeable about a plethora of fascinating new information that revolutionized my perspective; I began "thinking genetically."

The relationship between genomics and communication behaviors interfacing with social, cultural, and environmental effects of communication disorders is intriguing to me. I have developed a course in Genetics for Communication Disorders and have modified the National Coalition for Health Professional Education in Genetics' core competencies for speech-language pathologists. I have been invited to speak with health care professionals about genetics, and I've offered workshops and seminars on the topic relative to the infusion of genomics into the curriculum for graduate programs in speech-language pathology. It is important for undergraduates, graduate students, faculty, clinicians, and researchers in the disciplines of communication sciences and disorders to be educated about genomics.

It is also critical for speech-language pathologists to become familiar with the terminology, to gain competencies in genetics, and to understand the role of geneticists and genetic counselors with families. One key point that has remained in the forefront of my mind is that genetics and environment coexist. It is important to consider the role of both environment and genetics in communication processes. Cultural values, beliefs, and practices impact the decision-making process regarding an individual's access to and acceptance of genetic information, testing, and services. Individuals from culturally and linguistically diverse backgrounds are concerned about confidentiality issues as well. I hope that at the completion of this chapter you will have a better appreciation and awareness of the importance of knowing the function of genetics in the development and disorders of speech, language, swallowing, and hearing.

Genetics is a science, and significant new information is discovered and revealed daily that requires ongoing education and research. Genetics is a prime example of the value of collaborating with health care professionals from a variety of disciplines. I challenge you to enjoy learning about genetics and to think genetically!

case study

I had the wonderful opportunity to work with a family including Maria, a beautiful 3-month-old girl with brown hair, diagnosed with Pierre Robin sequence, a genetic disorder. The parents were kind and eager to learn more about their only child's prognosis. The mother was originally from Brazil and the father was from Boston, Massachusetts, with Scottish ethnic roots. They were in their twenties and Maria was their first child. They were hoping to have three healthy children.

Case history information revealed an uneventful pregnancy with good prenatal care. However, an ultrasound was not conducted during the pregnancy. No obvious signs of problems were evident until Maria was born. She presented with a small head and lower jaw known as micrognathia. Maria's open mouth revealed a wide cleft of the hard and soft palates and upper airway obstruction. Special physicians, including neonatalogists and otolaryngologists, were consulted, and the baby was immediately rushed out of the delivery suite to be evaluated and admitted to the neonatal intensive care unit. Of course, the parents were terrified and had numerous questions about the health and well-being of their new baby girl.

After Maria's breathing and heart rate were stabilized, feeding was the next priority for her survival. As a speech-language pathologist with expertise in pediatric feeding and swallowing issues and medically fragile infants, I was a resource for the family. We were able to address Maria's feeding needs before the surgical procedure and to meet with the surgeon regarding postsurgical changes and feeding needs. I provided the parents with information about feeding strategies, developmental milestones, and access to services for Maria in the community. It was a joy to work with this delightful little girl and her family. Additionally, we discussed options for genetics testing and family planning.

Rapid advances in medical genetics continue to identify the role of genetics in communication development and disorders. Speech-language pathologists and audiologists need to be aware of the New Genetics in order to engage in competent service delivery to individuals and their families. Additionally, knowledge of how to interpret and communicate new information to families of varied cultural and linguistic backgrounds is important to professionals. Recent surveys of speech-language pathologists and audiologists revealed that they both need and want additional genetics education (McNeilly, 2001).

Birth defects are characterized by a structural, functional, or metabolic abnormality present at birth that results in physical or mental disability. There are more than 4,000 known birth defects, which may be caused by genetic or environmental factors. About 150,000 babies are born each year with birth defects.

Syndromes are a group or recognizable pattern of symptoms or abnormalities that indicate a particular trait or disease. Spectral karyotypes (Figure 5.1) are a visualization of an organism's chromosomes together, each labeled with a different color. This technique is useful for identifying chromosome abnormalities.

The Human Genome Project (HGP) began in the United States in 1990, when the National Institutes of Health and the Department of Energy joined forces with several international partners for the purpose of deciphering the massive amount of information contained in our genomes. The HGP is credited with mapping the human genome and opening doors for research that will lead to prevention and cures of many conditions, including heart disease, asthma, and cancer.

This chapter will provide an overview of genetics, genomics, terminology, and inheritance patterns. Additionally, the role of genomics in communication disorders

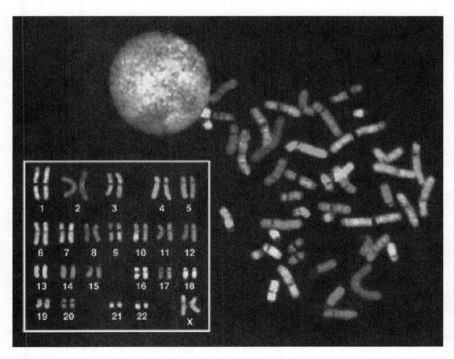

FIGURE 5.1 Spectral karyotypes.
Source: Courtesy National Human Genome Research Institute.

and the clinical competencies of genetics that speech-language pathologists need in order to provide services will be presented in this chapter. The chapter will also address the ethical, legal, and cultural implications of genomics.

Definition of Genetics versus Genomics

Genetics is a branch of biological science that studies the inheritance and function of genes. Genes are located on the 46 chromosomes and are composed of deoxyribonucleic acid (DNA) (see Figure 5.2). Genes constitute only about 3 percent of human DNA; the rest is noncoding DNA. These noncoding regions house information that determines when and where genes are active. Humans have 23 pairs of chromosomes, 22 pairs of autosomes, and 1 pair of sex chromosomes. The Y chromosome indicates a male and the X chromosome indicates a female.

Ribonucleic acid (RNA) is chemically similar to DNA except it is single-stranded, not double-stranded. It contains the base uracil instead of thymine, and it can migrate out of the nucleus. The sequences of most RNA molecules are translated to make proteins. Proteins make up essential parts of tissues and guide chemical reactions in living things. They are made of 20 different building blocks called amino acids.

The human genome is the sum of all genes and has been sequenced by the HGP. The human genome is estimated to contain 30,000 genes. Almost all of the 100 trillion cells in the human body contain a copy of the entire human genome (National Human

FIGURE 5.2   DNA.

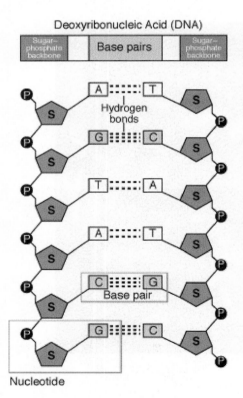

Genome Research Institute [NHGRI], 2000). Genes are involved in polypeptide synthesis, which is significant in the development of proteins. While genes get most of the attention, the proteins actually perform most life functions and make up the majority of cellular structures.

In 1953, James Watson, an American zoologist, and Francis Crick, a British bio-physicist, concluded that DNA is a double helix—that is, two spiral strands that wind around each other like a twisted rope ladder. In 2003, the finished human genome was published concurrently with the 50th anniversary of the double helix discovery (see Figure 5.3).

The human genome contains 3 billion chemical nucleotide bases—adenine, cytosine, thymine, and guanine (A, C, T, and G). The average gene consists of 3,000 bases of varying sizes.

Genomics is the study of the entire set of DNA sequences, both coding and non-coding DNA. An interesting fact is that the human genome sequence is almost 99.9 percent exactly the same in all people. The slight variations in our genomes are called single nucleotide polymorphisms, or SNPs. Scientists estimate that there are about 1.4 million locations on the genome where SNPs occur in humans. It is these small variations that contribute to individual differences. Copying errors that occur as DNA is reproduced—triggered, for example, by radiation, viruses, or toxic substances in the

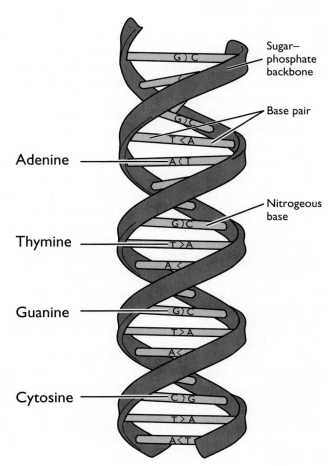

FIGURE 5.3
Double helix.

environment—can cause SNPs and other mutations. Many SNPs have no effect on cell function, but others predispose individuals to disease or influence drug responses.

Chromosome 1 is the largest human chromosome and it has the most genes—2,968. The Y chromosome has the fewest with 231 genes. Genes have been pinpointed, as have particular sequences in those genes, that are associated with numerous diseases and disorders. Scientists have identified about 3 million locations in which single-base DNA differences occur in humans. This information promises to revolutionize the processes of finding DNA sequences associated with common diseases such as cardio-vascular disease, diabetes, arthritis, and cancers. Additionally, scientists have indicated that the genetic key to human complexity does not lie in the number of human genes, but can be found in how genes' components are utilized to build different products in a process known as alternative splicing (U.S. Department of Energy, 2003).

Inheritance Patterns

There are different patterns of inheritance, including Mendelian, non-Mendelian, and multifactorial inheritance patterns. A description of each type follows.

Mendelian Inheritance

Gregor Mendel, an Austrian monk, is credited with the discovery of the basis of hered-ity in his studies of pea plants. He developed the concepts of dominant and recessive genes. Interestingly, his work went unnoticed for 30 years.

Traits are passed from each parent to each child. *Penetrance* refers to the passing of the trait from parents to child, and *expressivity* refers to how it is presented in the child. Some genes are highly penetrated and pass from mothers to all sons. Other traits are highly expressive, meaning they are seen in one child in a higher degree than they are expressed in a sibling.

Traits are inherited in two ways—recessive and dominant. A **recessive** trait is passed on to children when both parents carry the same affected gene and are, there-fore, homozygous (see Figure 5.4). When only one member of a pair of genes (i.e., an allele) is mutant, the child is a carrier of the mutation. **Dominant** inheritance occurs in children of heterozygotes, and only one parent passes the gene. The probability of expression varies depending upon whether one or both parents possess a particular trait. Sickle cell anemia, for example, is recessive. Both parents must have the gene for a child to get the disease. However, if both parents are carriers of the gene, meaning it is not expressed in them, then they have a 25 percent probability of passing the gene for the disease to a child. There is a 50 percent chance that each child will be a carrier. Thus, it is important for carrier status to be determined by couples prior to marriage if they plan to procreate.

Some disorders are linked to the X chromosome. Since males only have one X chromosome, which they inherit from their mother, this type of disorder is passed from the mother to the son and is never expressed in daughters. Daughters, however, could be carriers. It is only the mother's allele on the X chromosome that matters. Hemophilia is an example of this type of inheritance. The mother is a carrier and she passes the affected gene to her son and the disease is expressed in the son. No Y-linked disorders have been identified to date.

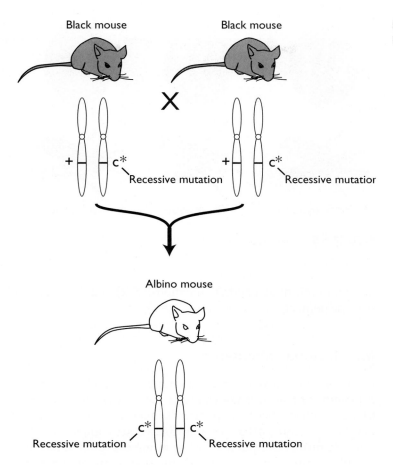

FIGURE 5.4
Recessive.

Non-Mendelian Inheritance

There are some rare cases in which both alleles of a gene are inherited from the same parent. This results in an individual with a double copy of an allele from one parent and no alleles from the other parent and is referred to as *uniparental disomy.*

Genes that are expressed exclusively from the maternally inherited allele or the paternally inherited allele are *imprinted.* For genes with imprinting, only one allele is activated, and the mutant allele will cause changes in the phenotype, or characteristics of the individual, only if it is inherited from the mother, which is maternal imprinting, or the father, which is paternal imprinting. Angelman syndrome is an example of maternal imprinting. Mental deficiency, inappropriate laughter, facial features, and absence of speech development characterize the syndrome. It is caused by maternally derived deletions on chromosome 15 and imprinting (Williams, Zori, Stone, Gray, Cantu, & Ostrer, 1990).

In rare cases, the effects of a mutation may become worse in subsequent generations. This process is known as *anticipation.* This is related usually to progressive expansion of a repeated stretch of DNA.

Mitochondrial inheritance, also referred to as cytoplasmic inheritance, is identified in both sons and daughters of an affected woman. It is not observed in an affected man that has the mutant phenotype. Due to homoplasmy, children are often more severely affected than their mother. Deafness is associated with many syndromic and

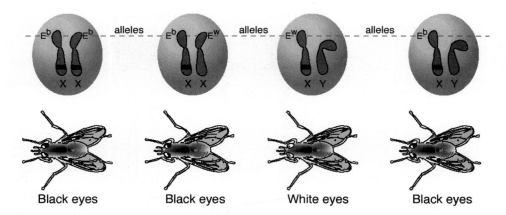

FIGURE 5.5 Phenotype.

nonsyndromic mitochondrial mutations, which may be a preeminent cause of deafness in some populations (Estivill et al., 1998).

Multifactorial Inheritance

Most communicative disorders do not have a single, clearly defined genetic etiology. A phenotype that does not exhibit a classic Mendelian inheritance pattern is said to have a complex inheritance pattern (Lander & Shrock, 1994). The inheritance patterns that occur in most heterogeneous diseases are complex and have different etiologies. They are further compounded when genotypes result in inconsistent phenotypes.

It is important that the distinction between phenotype and genotype is understood. **Phenotypes** refer to the characteristics that are displayed in an individual, including physical and behavioral characteristics that are produced by the interaction of the genotype and the environment. Phenotypes are specific to individuals (see Figure 5.5).

Genotypes include both expressed genes and unexpressed genomes. Since the environments of twins vary, the phenotypic behaviors and characteristics displayed in each twin may be quite different; however, the genotypes are the same.

Genotypes may be altered or mutated, which results in permanent changes. Mutations can be expressed as positive or negative. Each time genes are passed from one generation to the next some alterations occur. Some mutations become extinct and other mutations may actually aid the evolutionary process.

Genetic Testing

There are many different types of genetic tests and they are utilized for a variety of purposes. Gene tests can be used to diagnose disease, confirm diagnoses, provide prognostic information about the course of disease, confirm the existence of a disease in an individual who is symptom free, and predict the risk of future disease in healthy individuals or their progeny. Gene tests also have some limitations. Some tests may not detect every mutation associated with a particular condition and the ones that are detected may present different risks to different individuals and populations. Tests may reveal information about the risk of future disease, which can result in emotional and psychological effects on the individuals. Other issues that impact gene tests include regulations of laboratory quality assurance, availability of testing for rare diseases, and education of health care providers and patients about correct interpretation and risks.

Qualified professionals, including medical geneticists and genetic counselors, can adequately interpret the results of genetic tests. They are trained to diagnose and explain disorders and to review available options for testing and treatment, and they can provide emotional support to individuals (USDOE, 2003). The following tests are currently being used: FISH, PCR, Northern blot, and Southern blot.

It is important to understand how chromosomes are visualized when reading the results of genetic tests. Karyotypes are the chromosomal complement of an individual, including the number of chromosomes and any abnormalities. The term is also used to refer to a profile of an individual's chromosomes (see Figure 5.6). The place on a chromosome where a specific gene is located is referred to as the locus. It is a kind of address for the gene. (The plural is *loci*, not "locuses.") Chromosomes have a short arm and a long arm, referred to respectively as *p* and *q* arms.

Fluorescence in Situ Hybridization (FISH) is a process by which chromosomes or portions of chromosomes are vividly painted with fluorescent molecules. This technique is useful for identifying chromosomal abnormalities and mapping genes (see Figure 5.7).

Polymerase chain reaction (PCR) is a relatively inexpensive, quick molecular procedure. It utilizes small amounts of DNA, as small as a single cell, for analysis. It can also extract DNA from old samples, hair, and cells obtained from cheek swabs (see Figure 5.8).

The *Northern blot* technique is applied to RNA to determine if a gene contained within one's genome actually transcribes a agene product as examined in a specific tissue (Shprintzen, 1997). *Southern blot* is a technique used to identify and locate DNA sequences that are complementary to another piece of DNA called a probe. Lymphocytes, white blood cells, are the source of DNA utilized in this procedure.

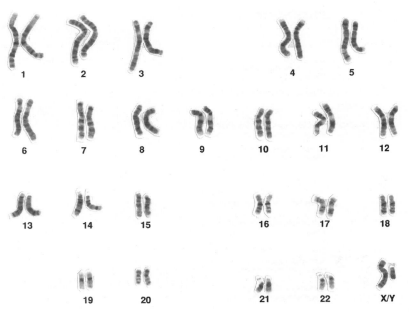

FIGURE 5.6
Karyotypes.
Source: Courtesy National Human Genome Research Institute.

FIGURE 5.7   FISH.
Source: Courtesy National Human Genome Research Institute.

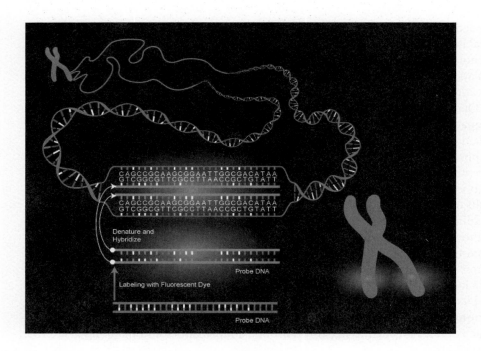

FIGURE 5.8   PCR.

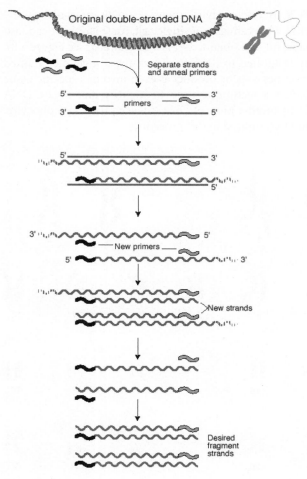

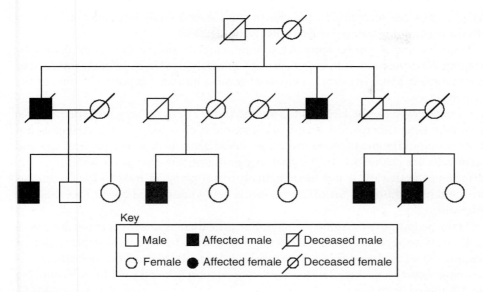

Key

☐ Male	■ Affected male	⊘ Deceased male
○ Female	● Affected female	⊘ Deceased female

FIGURE 5.9   Pedigree.

Genetic Counseling

Certified genetic counselors are trained to provide information about genetic tests, syndromes, diseases, and inheritance patterns. They provide both pre- and posttest counseling to individuals and their families. Speech-language pathologists should avail themselves of genetic counselors in their communities and make referrals as indicated.

Genetic counselors and clinical geneticists construct pedigrees when an individual is considering genetic testing. A pedigree is a simplified diagram of a family's genealogy that shows family members' relationships to each other and how a particular trait or disease has been inherited. The pedigree allows the plotting of information regarding at least three generations of the proband's family (the proband is the individual that presents to the genetic counselor). The symbols used are standardized and displayed in Figure 5.9.

There are uncertainties associated with gene tests for susceptibilities and complex conditions (e.g., heart disease) linked to multiple genes and gene–environment interactions. This leads to a number of important questions: Should testing be performed when no treatment is available? Should parents have the right to have their minor children tested for adult-onset diseases? Are genetic tests reliable and interpretable by the medical community? The answers will vary from individual to individual.

Gene Therapy

Gene-based therapy may lead to more precise therapeutic treatments. Knowledge of the genome can be utilized to develop medications that treat patients and reduce the side effects experienced by them. Additionally, gene therapy can replace the protein that genes give rise to. It may be possible to administer a small molecule that interacts with the protein to repair or replace cells (NHGRI, 2000).

Gene therapy is a novel approach to treat, cure, or ultimately prevent disease by changing the expression of a person's genes. Gene therapy is in its infancy, and current gene therapy is primarily experimental, with most human clinical trials only in the research stages.

Gene therapy can be targeted to somatic (body) or germ (egg and sperm) cells. In somatic gene therapy, the recipient's genome is changed, but the change is not passed along to the next generation. In germline gene therapy, the parent's egg and sperm cells are changed with the goal of passing on the changes to the offspring. Germline gene therapy is not being actively investigated, at least in larger animals and humans, although a lot of discussion is being conducted about its value and desirability.

Many people falsely assume that germline gene therapy already is being done with regularity. News reports of parents selecting a genetically tested egg for implantation or choosing the sex of their unborn child may lead the public to think that gene therapy is occurring. Actually, in these cases, genetic information is being used for selection. No cells are altered or changed.

Genomic Applications

Many human diseases and defects are caused either directly or indirectly by genetic abnormalities. Sickle cell anemia, for example, is caused by a change in just one nucleotide out of 6 billion. Specific genes have been associated with breast cancer and deafness. The analysis of the genomes of disease-causing microbes, viruses, and insects, such as the human malaria parasite and its carrier, the Anopheles mosquito, is helping in the development of new prevention and treatment strategies. Microbes are nature's simplest and most abundant organisms and can thrive under extreme conditions of heat, cold, pressure, and even radiation. By studying their genomes, scientists hope to find ways to use bacteria and other microorganisms to solve a variety of environmental problems, develop new energy sources, and improve industrial processes. Some microbes can convert a wide range of organic and inorganic materials into renewable energy (USDOE, 2003).

Of all the branches of science, genetics is the most self-reflective; not without coincidence, it is also the most universal. We all like to think about who we are, where we came from, and how we are related to others, sometimes even a little too much.

Role of Genetics in Human Development

The HGP facilitates the fast pace of discoveries regarding the genetic basis of a large number of disorders. These include diseases caused by changes in single genes as well as more common diseases like cancer, Alzheimer's disease, diabetes, and heart disease where several genes in interaction with environmental factors influence who develops a disease and when.

Connecting a gene with a disease was a slow, arduous, painstaking, and frequently imprecise process before the advent of the HGP. In 1989, geneticists had tracked down only four genes associated with disease by sorting through heredity. By 1998, the same list included more than 100 genes. A gene for Parkinson's disease was mapped in only 9 days, and precisely described within 9 months. Instead of restricting their studies to conditions caused by mutations in single genes, scientists can now study the genetic basis for complex diseases, like diabetes and Alzheimer's disease, that involve several genes.

The Gene Expression Nervous System Atlas (GENSAT) is one of the first large-scale efforts to look at where specific genes are expressed in the brain and spinal cord. GENSAT builds on the information generated by the HGP. It helps investigators understand which genes are critical in the nervous system and how they function. This project allows the viewing of images of gene expression within living brain cells. It will facilitate the understanding of many processes, including where neurotransmitters are expressed in the brain. Additionally, results of the study will facilitate investigations into the function of both normal and diseased brains. All of the information from the project is publicly available to other researchers. The National Institute of Neurological Disorders and Stroke (NINDS) funds the project.

New Genetics

The term *New Genetics* refers to research and clinical applications based upon the human genome. It allows researchers and clinicians to employ strategies that were impossible prior to the mapping and sequencing of the human genome.

Human Genome

The rapid progress in genome science and a glimpse into its potential applications have spurred observers to predict that biology will be the foremost science of the twenty-first century. Technology and resources generated by the HGP and other genomic research are having major impacts on research across the life sciences. The biotechnology industry employed 250,000 Biotech Industry org website in 2006. Revenues for 2005 totaled more than $50.7 billion (Biotechnology Industry Organization, www.bio.org). Some of the current and potential applications of genome research follow. Additional studies and public discussions are necessary to validate and implement some of these applications.

In Molecular Medicine

- Improve diagnosis of disease
- Detect genetic predispositions to disease
- Create drugs based on molecular information

- Use gene therapy and control systems as drugs
- Design "custom drugs" based on individual genetic profiles

Microbial Genomics

- Rapidly detect and treat pathogens (disease-causing microbes) in clinical practice
- Develop new energy sources (biofuels)
- Monitor environments to detect pollutants
- Protect citizenry from biological and chemical warfare
- Clean up toxic waste safely and efficiently

Risk Assessment

- Evaluate the health risks faced by individuals who may be exposed to radiation (including low levels in industrial areas) and to cancer-causing chemicals and toxins

Bioarchaeology, Anthropology, Evolution, and Human Migration

- Study evolution through germline mutations in lineages
- Study migration of different population groups based on maternal genetic inheritance
- Study mutations on the Y chromosome to trace lineage and migration of males
- Compare breakpoints in the evolution of mutations with ages of populations and historical events

DNA Identification

- Identify potential suspects whose DNA may match evidence left at crime scenes
- Exonerate persons wrongly accused of crimes
- Identify crime, catastrophe, and other victims
- Establish paternity and other family relationships
- Identify endangered and protected species as an aid to wildlife officials (could be used for prosecuting poachers)
- Detect bacteria and other organisms that may pollute air, water, soil, and food
- Match organ donors with recipients in transplant programs
- Determine pedigree for seed or livestock breeds
- Authenticate consumables such as caviar and wine

Agriculture, Livestock Breeding, and Bioprocessing

- Grow disease-, insect-, and drought-resistant crops
- Breed healthier, more productive, disease-resistant farm animals
- Grow more nutritious produce
- Develop biopesticides
- Incorporate edible vaccines into food products
- Develop new environmental cleanup uses for plants like tobacco

(www.ornl.gov/sci/techresources/Human_Genome/publicat/primer2001/7.shtml)

Human Genetic Variation and Health

One of the benefits of understanding human genetic variation is its practical value for understanding and promoting health as well as understanding and battling disease. Almost all human diseases have a genetic component. In some diseases, such as Huntington's and Tay-Sachs, the genetic component is very large. In other diseases, such as cancer, diabetes, and heart disease, the genetic component is smaller. In fact, we do not typically think of these diseases as "genetic diseases" because we inherit not the certainty of developing a disease, but only a predisposition to developing it (Genes, Environment, and Human Behavior Biological Sciences Curriculum Study, 2000) (see Figure 5.10).

Genetics and Communication Disorders

Historically, the single-gene disorders that result in genetic disorders characterized by communication disorders have been studied and reported in the literature. Some of these disorders include Angelman syndrome, Beckwith-Wiedemann syndrome, de Lange syndrome, Epstein syndrome, Escobar syndrome, Pierre Robin syndrome, Sotos syndrome, and Sturge-Weber syndrome.

The mapping of the human genome has facilitated the investigation of multifactorial genetic conditions related to the speech and language phenotypes. Studies in the areas of speech include molecular genetics of familial laryngeal paralysis, speech delay

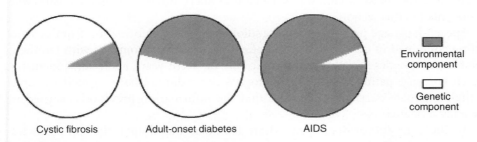

Cystic fibrosis   Adult-onset diabetes   AIDS

Environmental component

Genetic component

FIGURE 5.10 Genetic components of human diseases.

of unknown etiology, genetic markers in severe phonology disorders, and the FOX-p2 gene. Linguistic studies include investigation of the phenotype in familial dyslexia and the gene–environment interaction of specific language impairments in twins. There are several studies investigating the genetic link to autism, which has a strong linguistic component. Additionally, some studies are investigating the genetic link to reading and language processing.

Several studies are investigating the characteristics of genes in hearing loss. Several genes have been linked to hearing loss: Connexin-26 is one of the most studied genes related to hearing loss. There is a need for additional research in the areas of swallowing, fluency, and voice disorders as well.

Social and Behavioral Research

The Social and Behavioral Research Branch (SBRB) is a branch of the NHGRI. The focus of the SBRB is the development of cutting-edge approaches to translating the discoveries from the HGP into interventions for promoting health and presenting disease and for counseling patients and families dealing with the impact of genetic disorders. The SBRB is located within the Division of Intramural Research (DIR) at the NHGRI. Additionally, this branch investigates the complex social, ethical, and public-policy impact of genomic research.

The research portfolio of the SBRB encompasses four conceptual domains:

- Testing the effectiveness of communications strategies aimed at relaying genetic risks
- Developing and evaluating behavioral interventions
- Translating genomic discoveries to clinical practice
- Understanding the social, ethical, and policy implications of genomic research

Infusion of Genomics into Speech-Language Pathology

The advances in the HGP will impact services provided by speech-language pathologists to culturally diverse infants and toddlers who present with communication disorders. Genomics, cultural issues, clinical intervention, and research issues will be presented in this section.

Speech-language pathologists and audiologists utilize information from genetic testing contained in case histories and often discuss referral options with families. The field of genetics has advanced significantly in recent years, and many practicing speech-language pathologists and audiologists either did not have a genetics course in their graduate curriculum or, find that the information previously learned is currently outdated.

In 2001, the author developed a draft document based upon the competencies endorsed by the National Coalition for Health Professional Education in Genetics (NCHPEG), a consortium of more than a hundred organizations involved in health care. The scientific discoveries from the study of genetics have provided information with potential for tremendous influence on health care. Understanding the role genetics plays in health and disease provides the means to integrate such information into diagnosis, prevention, and treatment of many communication disorders.

Genetic discoveries exist in mainstream health care. Patients are beginning to ask providers about genetic services. Ultimately, speech language pathologists, regardless of specialty area, role, or practice setting, will face questions about the implications of genetics for their patients. The fast pace of genetic advances and the paucity of professional training in genetics leave many providers without up-to-date answers for their patients.

The Core Competency and Curriculum Working Group of NCHPEG recommended that all health professionals possess the following core competencies in genetics to enable them to integrate genetics effectively and responsibly into their current practice. Competency represents the minimum knowledge/skills/attitudes necessary for health professionals (in, e.g., medicine, nursing, allied health, public health, dentistry, psychology, speech-language pathology) to provide care to their patients that involves awareness of genetic issues and concerns. The recommendations provided by NCHPEG are a useful tool for organizing the teaching of basic genetics in many educational settings and have been modified for speech-language pathology.

Implementation of Clinical Competencies

The impetus for developing a list of ideal competencies related to genetics was to encourage speech-language pathologists to integrate genetics knowledge, skills, and attitudes into routine clinical practice in order to provide effective service delivery to individuals and families.

Each speech-language pathologist should appreciate the limitations of their own genetics expertise, understand the social and psychological implications of genetic services, and know how and when to make referrals to genetics professionals.

It is essential that individuals responsible for continuing education, curriculum development, licensure, certification, and accreditation in speech-language pathology consider adopting these recommendations and integrating genetics content into ongoing education. These competencies provide direction for curriculum content that can be utilized in the design of seminars, workshops, and academic preparation. There is a need for commitment on the part of all educators to incorporate genetic information into all levels of professional education. Enhanced genetics competency will help speech-language pathologists meet changing health care system demands and promote human benefit as a result of genetic scientific discoveries. Academic faculty need to be educated about the New genetics and how the knowledge, skills, and competencies may be infused into the curricula for graduate programs in speech-language pathology. Although this may appear challenging, it is important to prepare for the reality of tomorrow and not only for the needs of today.

Speech-language pathology curricula can infuse genetics into the content of several existing courses, including the basic sciences, craniofacial anomalies, and the clinical practicum. Additionally, new courses could be developed to address the ethical and social implications of genetics as they relate to the professions of speech-language pathology and audiology. A variety of educational models and mediums can be used, including Internet-based courses and interdisciplinary courses.

In the clinical practicum, students can practice obtaining family histories and getting information that covers at least three generations. They also can become familiar with referral sources and diagnostics available in the local community. Other elements of clinical education should include how to work with teams and collaborate with genetics professionals, clinical application of information about genetic syndromes and disorders, and infusion of genetics into clinical practice—specifically, prevention, diagnostics, and intervention.

Research that addresses the genetic components of communication disorders is also expanding. Surveys of speech-language pathologists have been conducted regarding preparation in and knowledge of genetics, and the results support the need for continuing education in genetics. Additionally, research regarding specific diseases and conditions with traditional genetic links is expanding to address multifactorial conditions. Clinical research focuses on the genetic aspects of communicative disorders as well as the impact of genetics in the prevention, and diagnosis of and intervention in communication disorders. It is important for speech-language pathologists to collaborate with other health care professionals and geneticists to conduct research.

Ethical, Legal, and Cultural Implications

There are several ethical, legal, and social issues that arise from the explosion of genetics research. NHGRI has dedicated funds through its Ethical, Legal, and Social Implications (ELSI) research program. The ELSI program priorities are as follows:

- Intellectual Property Issues Surrounding Access to and Use of Genetic Information
- Ethical, Legal and Social Factors that Influence the Translation of Genetic Information to Improved Human Health
- Issues Surrounding the Conduct of Genetic Research
- Issues Surrounding the Use of Genetic Information and Technologies in non-Health Care Settings
- The Impact of Genomics on Concepts of Race, Ethnicity, Kinship and Individual and Group Identity
- The Implications, for Both Individuals and Society, of Uncovering Genomic Contributions to Human Traits and Behaviors
- How Different Individuals, Cultures and Religious Traditions View the Ethical Boundaries for the Uses of Genomics (http://www.genome.gov/1000618 The Ethical, Legal & Social Implications (ELSI) Research Program)

Societal Concerns Arising from the New Genetics

The advances in genomic information will continually impact individuals in all facets of society. Fairness in the use of genetic information by insurers, employers, courts, schools, adoption agencies, and the military, among others, is a primary concern: Who should have access to personal genetic information, and how will it be used? Privacy and confidentiality of genetic information are another concern: Who owns and controls genetic information? Psychological impact and stigmatization due to an individual's genetic differences are yet another concern: How does personal genetic information affect an individual and society's perceptions of that individual? How does genomic information affect members of minority communities?

It is important to consider some reproductive issues including adequate informed consent for complex and potentially controversial procedures as well as the use of genetic information in reproductive decision making and reproductive rights: Do health care personnel properly counsel parents about the risks and limitations of genetic technology? How reliable and useful is fetal genetic testing? What are the larger societal issues raised by new reproductive technologies? These are critical questions to consider.

Clinical issues exist, including the education of doctors and other health service providers, patients, and the general public about genetic capabilities, scientific limitations, and social risks; and the implementation of standards and quality-control measures in testing procedures: How will genetic tests be evaluated and regulated for accuracy, reliability, and utility? How do we prepare health care professionals to utilize New Genetics? How do we prepare the public to make informed choices? It is of critical importance for us as a society to balance current scientific limitations and social risk with long-term benefits.

Conceptual and philosophical implications regarding human responsibility, free will versus genetic determinism, and concepts of health and disease have arisen: Do people's genes make them behave in a particular way? Can people always control their behavior? What is considered acceptable diversity? Where is the line between medical treatment and enhancement?

Health and environmental issues have arisen concerning genetically modified (GM) foods and microbes: Are GM foods and other products safe for humans and the environment? How will these technologies affect developing nations' dependence on the West?

Regarding the commercialization of products including property rights (patents, copyrights, and trade secrets) and accessibility of data and materials, a couple of questions are posed: Who owns genes and other pieces of DNA? Will patenting DNA sequences limit their accessibility and development into useful products? (www.ornl.gov/sci/techresources/Human_Genome/elsi/elsi.shtml)

Summary

Speech-language pathologists treat children and adults living with varied conditions that impact their ability to communicate. Most, if not all, conditions have a genetic link, although some of the linkages have not yet been identified. Therefore, it is imperative that students and practicing speech-language pathologists receive education about genetics and resources for connecting with professionals trained in genetics. Speech-language pathologists must acquire this new knowledge and apply it in translational research as well as in assessment and intervention strategies. Translational research involves applying what is learned in laboratories to clinical settings; it serves as a bridge.

Understanding the role genetics plays in health and disease provides the means to integrate such information into diagnosis, prevention, and treatment of many communication disorders.

Ultimately, speech-language pathologists, regardless of specialty area, role, or practice setting, will face questions about the implications of genetics for patients. The fast pace of genetic advances and the paucity of professional training in genetics leave many providers without up-to-date answers for their patients.

Speech-language pathologists involved in the direct provision of services to children receiving genetic services will require additional training to achieve an appropriate level of competency. Indeed, there are a number of examples of specific recommendations for genetic skill training for those in disciplines that require specialized knowledge of genetics, including pediatricians, nurses, nutritionists, and social workers. The NCHPEG core competencies have been modified by McNeilly (2001) for speech-language pathologists.

The actual clinical practice is an excellent opportunity to identify clinical placements that will provide students with the opportunity to collaborate with interdisciplinary teams that include a genetics professional. Additionally, students could be advised to select placements that provide them with evaluation and treatment hours across the life cycle.

Ethical, legal, and social implications of genetics are integral components of research, education, and clinical practice for speech-language pathologists. These issues and how they interface with cultural values, beliefs, and practices for consumers and clinicians were also addressed in this chapter.

case study

A patient with hypernasal speech secondary to a cleft palate was referred for a speech evaluation. A speech-language pathologist participating in a multidisciplinary cleft palate team was asked to determine if the patient required speech therapy, pharyngeal flap surgery, or prosthetic management. The speech-language pathologist performed a complete speech assessment and requested nasopharyngoscopic and videofluoroscopic studies to evaluate the velopharyngeal mechanism. In collaboration with the other team members, the speech-language pathologist determined that speech therapy would not positively affect the velopharyngeal insufficiency and recommended to the patient that a pharyngeal flap be completed first and speech assessment after surgery.

A geneticist or dysmorphologist never saw the patient. As a result, the examining professionals missed a number of anomalies, including a small ear tag, mild asymmetry of the ears, a small cyst in the left eye, and mild mandibular asymmetry. Furthermore, an audiogram was not completed prior to surgery. If the audiogram had been obtained, it would have revealed that the patient had a 40 dB conductive hearing loss in the right ear, but no evidence of middle-ear fluid. Additional assessment would have revealed a malformation of the ossicles and an abnormal middle-ear space.

The patient actually had oculo-auriculo-vertebral dysplasia (OAV) (also known as hemifacial microsomia). Other clinical findings in OAV are cervical spine malformation, vertebral fusion, hemi vertebrae, hypoplastic (underdeveloped) vertebrae, and an occipitalized atlas. During surgery, the patient's neck was hyperextended to position the mouth appropriately to perform the pharyngeal flap. This patient had an occipitalized atlas and fusion of C1 and C2. Because of fusion, the neck did not hyperextend easily, so the surgeon was more vigorous than usual in manipulating the head. This resulted in severe quadriplegic paralysis.

STUDY QUESTIONS

1. Describe the important value that a geneticist or genetics counselor would have provided the team.

2. What are the ethical issues presented in this case, particularly for the speech-language pathologist?

3. What are the options for the family regarding the severe quadriplegic paralysis that resulted based on incomplete information prior to the surgery?

4. Explore genetics websites and review published articles to determine which chromosomes have been identified that relate to specific communication disorders in speech, language, swallowing, and hearing.

5. Describe the roles of penetrance and expressivity in recessive and dominant inheritance patterns.

6. How might knowledge of the mistreatment of participants in the Tuskegee Syphilis Study impact an African-American male's decision to seek genetic counseling and testing that is offered by the employer?

7. As a student studying communication disorders, describe some of the specific knowledge, skills, and attitudes about genetics that are required to provide families with current and accurate information about the role of genetics in communication disorders.

SELECTED READINGS

Baker, Catherine, (n.d.). *Your genes, your choices.* Washington. DC: AAAS Directorate for Education and Human Resources.

A dictionary of genetics. (2002). Oxford, England: Oxford University Press, www.oup.com/us (promo number 23847).

Genomic medicine: Articles from the New England Journal of Medicine. (2004). www.press.jhu.edu.

GlaxoSmithKline. *Basic human genetics elearning program* [CD], www.gsk.com.

Human Genome Project. (2001). *Exploring our molecular selves* [online multimedia educational kit]. www.genome.gov/Pages?EducationKit/.

Primer: Genomics and its impact on science and society: The Human Genome Project and beyond. (March 2003).

The science behind the Human Genome Project: Basic genetics, genome draft sequence, and post-genome science. www.ornl.gov/sci/techresources/Human_Genome/project/info.shtml

WEBSITES OF INTEREST

www.genome.gov
These website for the National Human Genome Research Institute provides teaching resources, summaries of current research, and glossaries.

www.nchpeg.org
The National Coalition for Health Professional Education in Genetics is an interdisciplinary organization that promotes information about human genetics nationally.

www.doegenomes.org
This site describes genomic research programs funded by the Department of Energy, publications, research summaries, media, and much more.

www2a.cdc.gov/genomics/GDPQueryTool/frmQueryBasicPage.asp
The Centers for Disease Control's: Genomics and Disease Prevention Information System provides access to resources for guiding public health research, policy, and practice using genetic information to improve health and prevent disease.

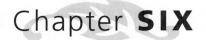
Articulatory and Phonological Disorders

Richard G. Schwartz
City University of New York

Klara Marton
City University of New York

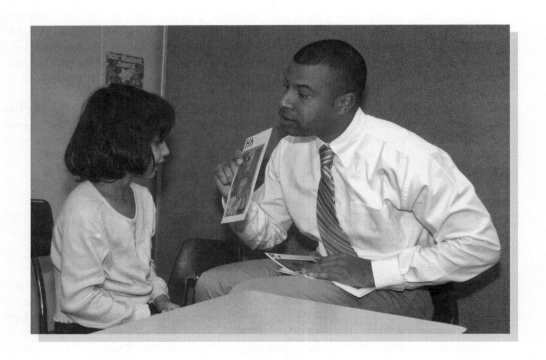

personal PERSPECTIVE

RICHARD G. SCHWARTZ

My interest during high school in the biological bases of development led me to major in psychology with the goal of teaching and doing research. Once I took an introductory course in linguistics, my interests in speech perception broadened to include language acquisition, with a focus on phonology. I was convinced that there were a number of important, basic research questions that had yet to be addressed. Research concerning the nature of children's speech and language disorders would lead to a better understanding of these disorders as well as to advances in assessment and intervention. The timing was ideal. The modern era of normal language acquisition research was just beginning. Aspects of linguistic theory such as distinctive features had just been applied to articulation disorders, and phonological rules and processes were first being used to describe phonological disorders in children. One topic in which I became interested was the relationship between phonology and other components of language in normal and disordered language acquisition. Phonology has an impact on vocabulary, language processing, and sentence structure in normal and disordered children. My continuing interest in phonology is understanding its role in language acquisition and disorders. Early in my career, I used language samples and experiments in which children learned novel words to study production and perception. Currently, I am using computer-controlled auditory language processing tasks, eye-tracking, and electrophysiology to study the underlying processing and to examine the underlying neurobiology of phonological acquisition and disorders.

personal PERSPECTIVE

KLARA MARTON

I approached the field of speech-language pathology in a spiral way. I received my B.A. in special education with a specialty track in education of children with hearing impairment. At that time, in my native Hungary all schools for children with hearing impairment provided oral education. We did not learn sign language and the children in the schools were not supposed to use it. Of course, they did. I was fascinated by their communication. During my practicum, I often asked the students after class to teach me some signs. This was our "secret" language outside the classroom. Prior to completing my M.A. in psychology, I received a research fellowship from the Hungarian Academy of Sciences. My research focused on communication development in children with cerebral palsy. None of the children I worked with could use oral language for communication. I went to Germany to study different augmentative and alternative communication methods. During that trip, I learned more "secret" languages such as Bliss symbols and other pictographic systems. As the result of my clinical experiences and my studies in psychology, I became interested in the relationship between language and cognition. First, I completed a doctorate in developmental psychology, and then I received a Ph.D. in speech and hearing sciences. My interest in understanding how the different cognitive mechanisms affect language acquisition led me to my current research, working memory and executive functions in children with language impairment. This is a dynamically developing area, and it is wonderful to see how the integration of knowledge from various disciplines multiplies our understanding of language development and disorders.

Introduction

Phonology is the communicative link that allows language speakers and listeners to encode and decode the intention, meaning, and structure of language. All languages have phonology, whether the language is manual, like American Sign Language, or oral. In a manual language, phonology includes the configuration, sequence, speed, and rhythm of hand movements produced by the "speaker" and perceived visually by the "listener." In an oral language, phonology includes the configuration, sequence, speed, and rhythm of oral, vocal, and respiratory movements produced by the speaker and heard by the listener. Another way to think of this is that phonology is the notes (e.g., consonants, vowels, and syllables), measures (words and phrases), and melody (rhythm and prosody) of the language song. Importantly, phonology also includes a mental representation of the categories, patterns, rules, and constraints of human sound systems and the specific features of the child's language(s).

Phonology differs from other aspects of language in that, besides the structural and cognitive dimensions that characterize syntax, semantics, and morphology, there are motor (e.g., speech) and sensory (e.g., auditory) components. This unique feature of phonology is reflected in the variety of theories of speech production, speech perception, and phonology as well as in the approaches to the assessment of and intervention for disorders. Phonology, like other parts of language, includes things that we cannot observe directly—our general and specific knowledge of language. Furthermore, phonology interacts with other components of speech and language in ways that become readily apparent in some disorders.

Speech-language pathologists and audiologists historically used the term **articulation** to describe the development and disorders of the speech sound system. Articulation refers to the motor movements involved in speech production. This reflected the theoretical view of phonology prominent in our field during the first half of the 20th century. Phonology, like other aspects of language, was viewed as a series of units—in this case, consonants and vowels—produced by motor gestures and strung together one after another. Even articulation is no longer viewed as separate groups of movements to produce a sequence of individual consonants or vowels. There is much more involved in the speech sound system and its development than just the movements of articulators or their mastery. The units of phonology range in size from phonetic features that describe articulatory movements (e.g., the vibration of the vocal folds) to segments (consonants and vowels) to larger units (syllables, words, phrases) in which the focus is on the rhythm (stress pattern).

The term *articulation* is still used, but **phonology** subsumes articulation. Phonology includes broader aspects of speech production and speech perception along with the cognitive-linguistic aspects of the speech sound system. This seems like a simple change in terminology, but there are important theoretical and clinical implications. It reflects a clinically useful distinction between phonetic components of the speech sound system, which include peripheral motor-speech production and auditory perception, and phonology, which includes mental representations, categories, and rules or constraints. The phonetic components may be viewed as the form of speech, whereas phonology represents the cognitive-linguistic functions of speech-language.

An important part of language acquisition is learning the sounds, rules or patterns, and rhythm specific to the language of the environment. Children learn that English doesn't have sounds produced at the very back of the throat or the clicks characteristic of some other languages. They also have to learn that, in English, no words begin with "shl" and that most English words have stress on the first syllable. Importantly, phonology influences the order and ease of acquisition of some other language features. For example, early in development, a word that shares phonological characteristics with the words already in a child's vocabulary is more readily acquired. Later in development, the mental storage of words is organized into "neighborhoods" of phonologically similar words. Stressed syllables in certain positions of words or phrases are easier to learn, perceive, and produce. Learning to read and write also depends on phonological knowledge concerning the correspondence between written (orthographic) characters and sounds as well as the phonological structure of words.

Although general information about the sequence and timetable of normal phonological acquisition is very important, there are many significant individual differences. Two types of differences—dialect and the acquisition of more than one language, either simultaneously or sequentially—affect many children and adults. Dialects are variations within a language that are common to a geographic region or to an identifiable group. Actually, all versions of a language are dialects. Despite the fact that one version may be referred to as "standard," the value attached to one dialect over another is purely social. All dialects are spoken with various accents. Accents refer to the manner of pronunciation. Accents are reflected in vowels, in some consonants, and in rhythm. Children who acquire a second language before age 12 are more likely to do so with a native-like accent than are children who acquire a second language after that age. Most of the information we have about phonology and phonological development concerns individuals who speak a single language. However, individuals who speak more than one language or dialect are the norm throughout most of the world—and increasingly so in the United States.

Most children acquire the phonology of their first language without direct instruction and without any difficulty. As discussed in Chapter 2, this is a gradual process that begins with speech perception and early vocalizations. The perception of speech begins before birth. During the first 6 months of life, speech perception is quite general, and children are sensitive to differences that are important across many languages. Beginning at 6 months of age, children's perceptual sensitivity narrows to focus on those features that are important in the language of their environment. The same is true of their vocalizations. Early meaningful speech is characterized by certain types and patterns of errors that disappear gradually. Once children reach school age, their phonology changes because of further maturation and because they learn to read and write. These changes permit the acquisition of complex, formal phonological rules.

A phonological disorder is the most common problem for the 15 percent of all children who have a primary or a secondary (to some other condition) communication disorder. Hearing impairments interfere with speech perception, causing some of these disorders. Others are caused by deviations in the speech production mechanism (e.g., cleft palate), in the development of complex motor behaviors (e.g., speech), or in the neural control of the speech mechanism (e.g., developmental apraxia). Some are secondary to general developmental disabilities (e.g., Down syndrome or autism). Finally, there are disorders in which the child's phonology may be organized differently than those of peers with no apparent physical basis. These disorders may be manifested in speech production, speech perception, or both. For example, a child may have a phonology without final consonants: this would be fine if the child were acquiring a language that typically does not have word-final consonants (Spanish or Italian), but is a disorder for a child acquiring English. In some cases, these disorders may be part of a broader language deficit. Children and adults who have already mastered part or all of the target speech sound system may acquire speech sound disorders as the result of strokes, head injury, or other neurological disorders.

The Nature of Phonological Disorders

A phonological disorder can be defined as a significant deficit in speech production, in speech perception, or in the organization of phonology in comparison to a child's peers. The discrepancy may be identified initially by a parent, by other caretakers, by a teacher, by peers, or by other significant individuals in the child's life. A speech-language pathologist confirms the disorder with standardized and nonstandardized assessment methods. The source of normative data is an important consideration. Those who select the child's peers for purposes of comparison must take into account characteristics of the child's language environment (e.g., dialect) and must recognize the issues facing bilingual children in both their first and their second languages (see Chapter 4). For example, a child from Boston who does not say /r/ in certain contexts (e.g., car) is not considered disordered because most people around the child speak the same way. Similarly, a child who speaks African American Vernacular English may, consistent with her dialect, say ghos rather than ghost. This is not an error, but simply a characteristic of the child's dialect. A Spanish-speaking child who is learning English as a second language may confuse p/b, t/d, and k/g because voicing is different in Spanish than in English.

A second consideration in identifying a phonological disorder is defining what constitutes a "significant" deficit. The criteria for making this determination range from a subjective judgment that the child may be at risk socially or educationally to evidence-based judgments that the child's speech abilities are not comparable to those of her peers. Even the mildest of impairments may interfere with communication and social interaction because the listener focuses on how something is said rather than on the message. Listeners may be unable to understand the child or may judge the child's speech as defective or immature.

Children with phonological disorders are not all alike in the nature and the extent of their disability. They vary in the severity of their disorder, with some children exhibiting a small number of errors (e.g., an 8-year-old child who produces [w] in place of [r] or [th] in place of [s]) and other children producing only parts of the words (e.g., a 4-year child who omits consonants at the ends of words and some whole syllables, a 5-year-old child who produces [t] instead of a number of different sounds).

The range of severity may also be described by the ease or difficulty with which listeners can understand what the child says. This is called **intelligibility**. Intelligibility is an important functional measure because the goal of speech is communication.

We can also describe disorders in terms of their cause or etiology. Speech-language pathologists distinguish between disorders that have an identifiable physical cause and those that have no identifiable physical cause. These are called, respectively, **organic** and **functional**. Organic disorders are attributable to physical conditions such as the inappropriate passage of air through the nose when producing sounds such as /b/ or /s/ in children with a cleft palate or velopharyngeal insufficiency (VPI) or the omission of consonants at the ends of words because of a hearing loss that precludes hearing these sounds. Functional disorders involve a pattern of speech errors in the absence of any observable physical abnormality. This distinction helps to describe, but it may not be useful for assessment and intervention. All such disorders have some biological bases; phonological disorders (C. M. Stein et al., 2004) are genetically transmitted like other communication disorders (see Chapter 5). Children with functional language impairments differ from typically developing peers in their brain responses to language.

FIGURE 6.1

Schematic diagram of the speech sound system.

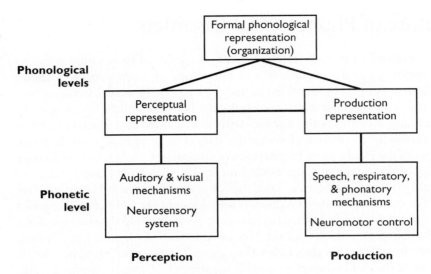

One alternative is to distinguish between *phonetic* disorders and *phonological* disorders. In Figure 6.1, the phonological system is divided into three levels: (1) audition-motor speech production, (2) representation, and (3) organization. The first is the phonetic level. The latter two are the **phonological levels**. The phonetic level and the representations can be further divided into two components: input or perception, and output or production. Each component of the figure may be thought of as representing a type of speech sound disorder. For example, a child may have errors that are the result of some deficiency at the **phonetic level** in the motor production system or in the neuromotor control system. This would include speech disorders that are the result of neurological impairments (e.g., **dysarthria** or **apraxia**, discussed in Chapter 10), speech disorders that are the result of physical anomalies (e.g., cleft palate or inadequate velopharyngeal closure, discussed in Chapter 9), and speech disorders that may be the result of deficits in motor learning (e.g., isolated errors in individual sound production, such as distortions). On the perception side of the phonetic level, we might see deficits attributable to hearing losses or other perceptual deficits. For example, a child with a hearing loss affecting high frequencies might have difficulty producing fricative sounds because of their high-frequency components. This group of disorders might be called articulation disorders.

The phonological levels include the cognitive-linguistic components of the speech sound system. One level includes specific representations of sounds, syllables, words, or phrases either in the form of some acoustic information, based on perception, or in the form of motor plans for speech production. The uppermost level includes more general, abstract representations reflecting constraints (e.g., permissible or preferred syllable structures in English) and rules that result in certain changes (e.g., changing the [k] to an [s] when <u>ity</u> is added to <u>electric</u>). Disorders in this aspect of the speech sound system are characterized by (1) widespread error patterns (e.g., the omission of final consonants in words, the substitution of one group of sounds for another); (2) severe limitations in the range of sounds produced (e.g., the child produces [t] in place of a wide variety of consonants); (3) limitations in the syllable structures produced (e.g., only words or phrases with an unstressed syllable followed by a stressed syllable—*a book*—or isolated stressed syllables—*bug*—are produced correctly); (4) errors reflecting sound and syllable structure interactions (e.g., all words end with [s]); or (5) the influence of one sound on the other sounds in a word (e.g., the consonants are produced so that they are identical or nearly identical, as when <u>sick</u> is produced as [kIk]).

This categorization scheme incorporates the traditional distinction between functional and organic articulation disorders, but differs in two important ways. Functional phonetic production or perception disorders involving isolated errors with otherwise intact phonological levels are grouped with organically based disorders. Also, some disorders that are organic in origin (e.g., cleft palate and severe hearing impairment) affect phonology and are grouped with functional phonological disorders. Beginning phonological development with a physical disability prevents the child from forming typical phonological categories or rules (e.g., the distinction between oral and nasal consonants). Even when the palate is closed or amplification is provided, partially or completely resolving the organic impairment the deviant phonology remains. Thus, the primary distinction between disorder types is the presence or absence of accurate phonological knowledge on which errors are based. This grouping better reflects commonalities within these groups for treatment and assessment.

Another consideration in characterizing phonological disorders is whether other aspects of language are also impaired. Although some children may have isolated phonological disorders, such disorders co-occur with syntactic and morphological deficits in many children (e.g., R. Paul & Shriberg, 1982: Shriberg & Austin, 1998). Many children who are identified as having syntactic deficits (i.e., short utterance lengths) or morphological deficits (e.g., omitted verb endings) also exhibit speech sound errors. Conversely, many children initially identified as having phonological disorders, on closer examination, also have morphological or syntactic deficits. Assessment of language should not be limited to the component that is most obviously disordered. There are three groups of children with phonological disorders: (1) children who have a generalized language disorder, (2) children who have a phonological disorder that directly affects their production or perception of other features of language such as morphology (e.g., children who omit final consonants, including plural or unstressed syllables), and (3) children who have a disorder limited exclusively to their phonology.

A final topic is the relationship between the errors in disordered children's speech and the errors that occur in typically developing children. The question is whether these errors differ; whether the errors are comparable, but just occur later in children with disorders; or whether the errors are comparable, but more frequent in children with disorders (Ingram, 1976). Part of the answer lies in determining whether phonological disorders reflect a delay or a deviation in development. Few errors are seen in the speech of disordered children that are radically different from those seen in typically developing children. This is not surprising because there are only so many variations possible, given the speech mechanism, auditory system, and underlying neurobiology. However, two differences, both attributable to the pace of development in children with disorders, are noteworthy. Children with phonological disorders frequently make unusual errors outside those generally seen in typically developing children. For example, a single sound may be substituted for a wide variety of unrelated targets, or there may simply be unusual substitution patterns. The slow pace of development in these children means the error patterns last longer and thus make these patterns easier to recognize. When we look more carefully, we find the same "unusual" errors in typically developing children (L. Leonard, 1985). The second phenomenon is the co-occurrence of patterns of errors that would typically not be present at the same point in development. For example, children under 3 years of age may omit final consonants when they are still producing predominantly single-syllable words. In a disordered child, final consonant omission or unstressed syllable omission persists through a longer period of development and thus affects more-advanced word forms.

Determinants of Phonological Disorders

Several important linguistic and nonlinguistic factors are related to typical and atypical phonological development. Such information can guide assessment and help us to predict the course of a child's phonological development. Finally, these factors sometimes identify special populations of children who have phonological impairments with unique characteristics that require specialized assessment and intervention techniques.

Motor Abilities

Speech uses the same physical structures as breathing, chewing, swallowing, and other nonspeech oral motor movements. Speech and nonspeech oral motor movements also share neurobiological structures and pathways for sensation, feedback, and movement. However, the neural control of speech involves additional cortical pathways that are not engaged by nonspeech oral motor functions.

General motor abilities (e.g., walking, coordination) are unrelated to speech production, except in generalized neuromuscular disorders such as cerebral palsy (Winitz, 1969). Oral motor abilities are related to speech abilities in a complex fashion. Even rapid alternating movements for certain speech sound sequences, called **diadochokinesis**, are not reliable predictors of speech production. *Diadochokinesis*, which has been the subject of a great deal of research and is often used in assessment, is the movement involved in rapidly saying a series of syllables (e.g., [pʌ, tʌ, kʌ]). Some speech production problems may be revealed in this task. However, the relationship between the rate of producing these syllables and articulatory abilities is unclear. Some people with normal speech production are slower than individuals with disorders. Individuals with speech disorders may be slower because they are more conscious about their speech and about making errors. The relationship between oral motor movements for basic nonspeech functions (e.g., blowing, kissing, swallowing) and speech is even less clear. Intuitively, we think there should be a relationship because they use the same structures and because physiological functions seem to overlap. However, research indicates that speech and nonspeech oral motor behaviors are not related (Moore & Ruark, 1996). There is no evidence that work on nonspeech oral motor abilities has any impact on speech abilities. Speech-language pathologists, however, often work on children's nonspeech oral motor abilities with the goal of improving their speech production. This illustrates the importance of evidence-based practice.

The relationship between speech and nonspeech also comes into play in a condition called **tongue thrust**. Infants and young children swallow by bringing the tongue against the hard palate and pushing the food or liquid forward, instead of propelling food or liquid toward the back of the mouth. Although there is no research evidence, some speech-language pathologists assume that older children with this pattern are delayed in their swallowing development. Tongue thrust is frequently associated with errors in producing [s] and [z] and with dental malocclusion. However, because there is no evidence of a causal relationship, speech-language pathologists do not perform tongue thrust therapy to correct these speech errors. Instead, therapy focuses on the speech errors. Speech-language pathologists do provide intervention for swallowing disorders (dysphagia) and for feeding disorders in children and adults.

One final issue concerning motor abilities is specific to speech. Some children who have phonological disorders seem to have particular difficulty in the motor production of speech. Their speech disorders are typically severe and are resistant to therapy. These children are said to have **developmental apraxia of speech (DAS)** or **developmental verbal apraxia** (see Chapter 10). As with adults diagnosed with *apraxia*, the assumed underlying difficulty involves the sequencing of motor movements to produce speech sounds or syllables. Children identified as having this disorder, however, have not lost any ability due to neurological damage; the disorder is developmental. Speech is characterized by syllable omissions, consonant substitutions, and vowel errors comparable to those seen in other children with phonological disorders. These errors are inconsistent, suggesting that underlying phonological knowledge is intact, but that the implementation of this knowledge in speech production is impaired. Some, but not all, of these children often have difficulty in performing nonspeech oral motor activities. They typically make slow progress in therapy and have difficulty following instructions for sound production. A large-scale, systematic investigation has brought into question many of the assumptions regarding these children (Shriberg, Aram, & Kwiatkowski, 1997a, 1997b, 1997c). These children have a phonological disorder (not a motor planning disorder) characterized by inappropriate stress or prosody that appears to be transmitted genetically. The atypical stress patterns, which previously were not considered systematically, can account for the segmental errors and their apparent inconsistency.

Speech Perception and Hearing

Because the acquisition of phonology directly depends on exposure to the language of the environment, normal hearing is crucial. Phonological deficits in children with hearing impairments vary with the type and the severity of the hearing loss, the child's age when it occurs, the child's age when intervention (e.g., amplification, speech [lip] reading) begins, and the child's ability to utilize residual hearing (see Chapters 17 and 18). Because of all these factors, it is difficult to generalize about phonological acquisition in children with hearing impairments. However, aspects of speech that are least visible (e.g., vowels, nasal versus non-nasal sounds, [r] and [I]) and that are least salient perceptually (e.g., unstressed syllables, voiceless fricatives, voiceless vowels) and prosody pose challenges for these children. The earlier children are diagnosed and are provided with amplification, the better the speech and language outcome. Many children with severe to profound hearing loss now receive **cochlear implants**. These are surgically implanted devices designed to provide electrical stimulation to the auditory nerve through the cochlea. The most remarkable application of cochlear implants is for children who are congenitally deaf or have lost hearing at a very early age. Such children now routinely receive implants before age 2, with some children receiving implants as early as 12 months. Cochlear implants and hearing aids must be accompanied by intensive therapy to achieve maximum success. For infants and toddlers who receive amplification, the goal is to help them create a phonology and lexicon as rapidly as possible.

Other children with hearing impairments are those with chronic **otitis media (OM)**. This is an infection of the middle ear that is often accompanied by fluid (effusion), resulting in a conductive hearing loss. Clinicians often note that many children with language disorders (particularly phonological disorders) have histories of repeated episodes of OM. Otitis media may be a causal factor in some phonological disorders and language impairments. However, research is complicated because these episodes may differ in their severity and their impact on hearing. The fact that many children have such a history without any obvious negative effects on their speech and language development clouds the picture. Another problem with research in this area is that many episodes go undetected. Despite this controversy, the risk of a speech delay for a 3-year-old child with a history of chronic OM with effusion and an average hearing level above 20 decibel between 12 and 18 months of age is 33 percent (Shriberg, Friel-Patti, Flipsen, & Brown, 2000). In a large longitudinal study of 150 children (R. G. Schwartz, Mody, & Petinou, 1998), children (0–12 months) who had frequent episodes of OM produced more consonants that are more visible (e.g., [b], [p]) than consonants that are less visible (e.g., [t], [d]) than did children without this history. At 2 years, these children had greater difficulty producing words or syllables with final consonants than did children who did not have frequent middle-ear infections.

Speech perception in children with normal hearing has a less clear relationship to speech production. Though it seems safe to assume that perception is better than production, this is not always true. Some perceptual errors may cause production errors, and sometimes production appears to be accurate with inaccurate auditory perception (e.g., when there is visible information such as [b], [p], or [m]). When perception testing focuses on the child's specific production errors, approximately a third of the children tested evidenced errors in discriminating their error production from the target (Locke, 1980b). It does not mean that the misperception caused the production error or that remediating perception for these children should be the primary focus of intervention, but it should be considered in intervention planning.

Speech perception, as measured by discrimination (i.e., judging whether two syllables are the same or different), identification of speech sounds, or judgment of syllable sequence, appears to be related to children's overall language abilities. Children with language disorders (including phonological disorders) typically have difficulty in such tasks. However, the specific nature of perception deficits and their relationship to language acquisition remain controversial.

Dentition

The relationship between dentition and speech production has often been overestimated. Studies of normal speakers indicate that the articulatory mechanism is highly adaptable. We can produce reasonably intelligible speech while chewing gum, while chewing food, and even after receiving local anesthetic at the dentist. Therefore, minor dental abnormalities rarely cause significant deviations in speech production. Severe dental abnormalities resulting from malocclusion or from deviations in jaw alignment, however, may lead to speech errors. This may be important for children with cleft palate and other craniofacial anomalies when dentition is severely affected.

Oral Mechanism

Adequate oral structure and physiology along with adequate respiration are required for speech production and for phonological acquisition. A variety of physical and physiological deviations in the mechanism for speech production may occur. The most common group of deviations is the result of craniofacial anomalies referred to commonly as cleft palate (see Chapter 9). The phonological deficits associated with cleft palate include hypernasality, nasal emission, and poor production of sounds that depend on intra-oral breath pressure (stops and fricatives). Some children with cleft palate incorrectly produce sounds at the back of the oral cavity, in the pharynx, or at the glottis to compensate for their inability to produce these sounds at the appropriate place of articulation. These error patterns are complicated further by the fact that almost all of these children have chronic OM with effusion accompanied by hearing loss.

Intelligence and General Development

For many decades, children and adults with intellectual disability have been described generally as having speech that is imprecise, slow, and inaccurate with inappropriate rhythm. In adults with intellectual impairment, consonant omissions are the most common phonological error, and although errors are inconsistent (i.e., target sounds are produced correctly on occasion), the error types are similar to those of children with phonological impairments (Shriberg & Widder, 1990). Because of the inconsistencies, the cause is not likely to be a deficit in the motor execution of speech production. Instead, the errors are the result of cognitive limitations in one of the stages of speech production.

One special subgroup of children with developmental disabilities is those with **Down syndrome.** In Down syndrome, there is a complex interaction of motor deficits that affect speech production, perceptual limitations attributable to a very high incidence of chronic OM with effusion along with transient hearing loss, and phonological acquisition that reflects their developmental delay. In particular, these children are delayed in the onset of canonical babbling. Their early vocal behavior suggests a high degree of variability with some particular difficulties with high/low distinctions in vowels and front/back distinctions in consonants and vowels in speech production. A variety of speech disorders are common among individuals with developmental disabilities of unknown origin. Some of these disorders appear to have a neurological basis and are dysarthrias or apraxia (see Chapter 10). These disabilities may also be associated with genetic syndromes, some of which also involve hearing impairment.

A final group of children has Pervasive Developmental Disabilities (PDD), also referred to as autism spectrum disorders. This is a category of severe developmental impairment affecting social, cognitive, language, and communicative abilities. Children vary widely in their degree of impairment and their specific behavioral symptoms. The vast majority of these children have moderate to severe cognitive and linguistic deficits and may not have basic, functional language skills. Approximately 20 percent of these children do have IQs within the average range and functional language (American Psychiatric Association, 1994). These children are "high functioning" or have a related disorder called Asperger's Syndrome. A number of these children and adults have residual articulation errors indicating earlier phonological impairments, inappropriate stress, fluency, and resonance (Shriberg, McSweeney, Kiln, & Cohen, 2001). The latter errors appear to co-occur with limitation in pragmatic skills and sentence formulation.

Language

As discussed above, phonology is an integral part of language and is related to other language components. Infants rely on prosodic and segmental information in the speech of adults to identify word and syntactic phrase boundaries. There is an interaction between phonology and other language components in their synchronous development. Young children who are Late Talkers or have identifiable syntactic deficits (low mean length of utterance) are likely to have comparably delayed phonological abilities. Children with Specific Language Impairment have deficits in the perception of grammatical morphemes (e.g., third-person singular, past-tense endings) that may underlie their deficits in syntax and morphology (L. Leonard, 1998). In other children, the acquisition of morphology is impaired because of a phonological deficit that affects certain segments (e.g., [s], [z]), final consonants in general, or unstressed syllables (R. Paul & Shriberg, 1982; Shriberg & Austin, 1998; Shriberg, Tomblin, & McSweeney, 1999).

Complexity is another aspect of this relationship. Length and structural complexity determine what children produce under certain circumstances. As syntactic complexity increases, children may revert to simpler phonological forms, and errors may increase. Increases in phonological complexity may result in decreases in syntactic complexity or decreases in syntactic errors. Accuracy of production in children less than 3 years of age also appears to be influenced by the syntactic category of words. Nouns are produced more accurately than are verbs, perhaps because of the conceptual complexity.

There also is an interaction between pragmatics and phonology involving the distinction between **new information** (changing aspects of a situation or things that are not known to the listener) and **old information** (static aspects of a situation or things that are known to the listener). Children produce words that refer to new information more accurately than they do words that refer to old information. This is also true for adults. In conversation, the first production of a word is longer in duration and is produced more clearly than subsequent productions of that word.

Although syntax and phonology may be closely related in development, intervention for syntactic disorders does not lead to spontaneous improvements in phonology (M. Fey et al., 1992). Children with syntactic and phonological deficits need intervention that focuses on each component of language.

Reading

The emergence of literacy involves learning an orthographic (i.e., alphabetic) system for writing and reading that corresponds to oral phonology, learning a set of words that can be recognized on sight, and learning strategies to read words that are not recognized on sight (see Chapter 13). In a general sense, all aspects of phonology are prerequisites for reading. A child cannot learn about sound–letter correspondences without certain basic knowledge about consonants, vowels, syllable structure, phonological rules, or constraints. Although children acquire phonology without being able to express this knowledge consciously, reading is more directly dependent on **metaphonological** abilities (also referred to as **phonological awareness**).

Metaphonological abilities are a subset of metalinguistic abilities. Metalinguistics is the aspect of language that includes the general ability to make judgments about language (e.g., whether sentences are grammatical or not) and to perform tasks that require conscious examination of language (e.g., providing synonyms). In phonology, this includes tasks that require children to provide rhymes, to identify beginning and ending sounds of words, to break words into syllables, and to pronounce words without beginning (e.g., slip—"lip") or ending (boat—"bow") sounds. Performance on metaphonological tasks predicts later reading and writing abilities. Phonological working (or short-term) memory is also related to reading abilities and to spoken language performance. Phonological working memory is often measured with nonword repetition. In this task, children are asked to repeat nonsense words of increasing length (one to four syllables). By 5 years of age, children can repeat most two-syllable words correctly, but even 7-year-old children may have some difficulty with longer words. When children are asked to repeat a list of phonologically similar (e.g., rhyming) words, they have more difficulty producing the list accurately than they do a list of phonologically dissimilar words (Marton, Schwartz, & Braun, 2005).

Phonologically related reading disabilities, termed **dyslexia**, are language-based disorders. Children with dyslexia have great difficulty with metaphonological tasks. They also may have syntactic and speech perception deficits. Even if they have compensated for these deficits in oral language, children with phonological disorders are likely to demonstrate reading impairments.

Assessment

There are different steps in assessment. **Screening** is used to determine whether there is reason to suspect a disorder. **Identification** involves the use of norm-referenced tests and other measures to determine whether or not a child who failed a screening actually has a phonological disorder. Once that determination is made, a **diagnosis** involves specifying the nature of the disorder, its severity, the prognosis, and the recommended course of treatment. It is important to focus on those aspects of a child's phonology that will be most relevant for intervention. Each assessment procedure should be undertaken with a specific intervention goal in mind. Phonological assessment is an ongoing process that is not limited to a single diagnostic session. The initial assessment provides a starting point for intervention, with information added as intervention proceeds.

Screening

A number of screening instruments are commercially available. Typically, they include the sounds that children are most likely to produce incorrectly and are most predictive of the presence of a phonological disorder. The stimuli may be pictures, single words that the child imitates, sentences or passages that are read, or a set of questions that the child must answer. Some commercially available screening tests have norms and cutoff scores. An alternative method is to elicit a short sample of spontaneous speech by asking a child to tell a story (e.g., a favorite movie or book) or to relate an event (e.g., a birthday party). Clinicians then determine whether a given child has passed or failed the screening. They also make judgments about the number and type of errors and overall intelligibility in light of their knowledge of typical development. Clinicians may also consider concerns expressed by parents or teachers, the types of errors (some errors are less likely to disappear without intervention), the consistency of errors, and the child's ability to correct errors with some minimal instruction. Children who fail the screening are referred for further testing. Children with a small number of potentially developmental errors may be rescreened after 6 months.

Screening tests sometime yield *false positives*, children who fail the screening, but who do not have a phonological disorder, and *false negatives*, children who pass the screening test, but who actually have a phonological disorder. Screening tests also can be characterized in terms of their sensitivity and specificity. Sensitivity is the success rate in identifying all of the children who truly have a disorder, whereas specificity is the success rate in identifying only the children with disorders (no typically developing children fail by mistake). Ideally, a test will have high sensitivity and high specificity, but for screening, when we do not want to miss any children with a disorder, sensitivity takes on greater importance.

Case History   The child's developmental and family history is an important facet of assessment. Parents, other caretakers, and other informants (siblings, other relatives, and teachers) provide information regarding pre- and postnatal history. This information includes the ages at which the child achieved general developmental milestones; the general history of the child's language development; the child's vocabulary, which can be assessed at early ages using a checklist; and factors that might have had an influence on the child's linguistic or nonlinguistic development. Potential signs of related motor or sensory deficits are important. For example, feeding difficulties for an infant may be indicative of velopharyngeal insufficiency or a neuromotor disorder. A history of chronic OM is also noteworthy. It is important to obtain a description of the nature, the course, and the extent of the child's disorder; the impact on the child's communication; the emotional reactions to the disorder; and the response of peers and family members. Finally, it is useful to know whether the family has a history of such disorders. Phonological disorders are genetically transmitted (e.g., Shriberg, 1991; Stein et al., 2004). Although this will not influence intervention for a child who is being assessed, it may alert the speech-language pathologist to the possibility that other, younger family members may be affected.

Sampling and Analyzing Children's Speech

The central element in assessing a child's phonology is a speech sample. This section discusses articulation tests, spontaneous and elicited sampling procedures, sample recording and transcription, and sample analysis.

Standardized Tests   The most widely used means of collecting a speech sample is a commercially available, standardized test. Many tests include normative data. The typical format involves asking a child to name a series of pictures (*What's this?*) or complete phrases ("You brush your _____." "teeth"). The target words included on these tests represent the various consonants, consonant clusters, and, sometimes, vowels in word-initial, word-medial, and word-final positions. One widely used test of articulation is the Goldman-Fristoe Test of Articulation–2 (Goldman & Fristoe, 2000), but there are many others (H. B. Fisher & Logemann, 1971; Fudala, 1970; Pendergast, Dickey, Selmar, & Soder, 1969; M. C. Templin & Darley, 1969). These tests all have distinct characteristics. For example, the Goldman-Fristoe–2 tests more than one target sound per item. It includes a test of stimulability, which examines how the child produces sounds in error with varying levels of instruction, and a story-retelling task, which elicits a sample of connected speech with pictures. A number of tests provide sentences that can be read by older children or adults. Most tests focus on individual errors, characterized as **omissions**, **substitutions** of one sound for another, **additions** of sounds, and **distortions** in which sounds are produced incorrectly. These tests provide a standardized, efficient, and convenient way to sample a child's speech. They are particularly important for children whose spontaneous speech is unintelligible.

Like standardized tests for other components of children's language, many tests are limited in their structure and content. Normative data are often based on too few children or on children who are not comparable to the child being tested. For example, normative data collected in a small city may not be applicable to a child from an inner-city school who speaks a different dialect. Even with a large set of representative normative data (e.g., the Goldman-Fristoe–2), the child's performance is compared to a general population instead of children from the same language group.

These tests may also not be the best way to examine a child's phonology in detail. Because most of these tests focus on single words, they do not provide information about connected speech. The target words also have some limitations. Most are nouns, which young children produce more accurately than verbs. The words are often complex (e.g., [s] in the middle of the word <u>Christmas</u>), and sometimes the target sound is tested as a grammatical morpheme (e.g., [z] as a plural in the word <u>matches</u>). These are not typically the contexts in which children first produce sounds. Sometimes the test words (e.g., <u>valentine</u> for [v]) yield residual errors. Many children continue to say *balentine* long after they produce a [v] correctly in other words. Also, these tests examine only a given segment in initial, medial, and final word position. This does not provide a full sample of the child's production, underlying knowledge, or production consistency. Such detailed information is important for planning therapy. Most of these tests do not systematically test vowels, which is a problem area for some children. Finally, these tests do not sample speech in a natural communicative situation.

Despite all of these limitations, articulation tests are a valuable method of collecting an initial speech sample. Recognizing their limitations enables clinicians to supplement the information they provide so that intervention can be better planned.

One way to expand the information provided by a standardized test is to analyze all aspects of the child's production of each word on this test rather than just the target sound or sounds. The Khan-Lewis Phonological Analysis (Kahn & Lewis, 1986) takes the results of the Goldman-Fristoe and provides a method for examining phonological processes. The Assessment of Phonological Processes–Revised (Hodson, 1986a) uses an articulation test format with objects rather than pictures and addresses the limitations in pattern analyses of previous tests. A Spanish version is also available. By completely transcribing children's productions of the single words on an articulation test and by analyzing the patterns of errors across words, clinicians can expand the scope and increase the utility of the information obtained from these tests.

Spontaneous Sample   A sample of spontaneous speech is the most useful source of information for phonological analysis and for intervention planning. A sampling session must be carefully organized. For young children, we use age-appropriate toys and books to facilitate play and conversation. Other individuals (e.g., siblings, peers, parents) may facilitate spontaneous speech. The people interacting with the child should minimize their talking and provide the child with opportunities to talk, using open-ended questions and comments (*What do you think will happen next?*). Older children may just be engaged in conversation. The sample should include ample opportunities for children to produce a range of sounds in a variety of phonetic and communicative contexts. The speech-language pathologist can accomplish this by her choice of books, toys, and topics. The session should also be planned so that the sample can be used to analyze aspects of language other than phonology (see Table 6.1).

There are varying views about how long a sample should be. For phonological analysis, it should be at least 100 utterances for children with a mean length of utterance (MLU) of 3.0 or below. For children with higher MLUs, including 250–300 different words should be sufficient. Spontaneous speech is more representative of the child's typical speech outside the clinic. It also permits more detailed analysis. If the child is unintelligible or is reluctant to talk, more-structured approaches (e.g., story

TABLE 6.1   A Portion of a Sample from Alicia (3;2)

Target Word	Adult Version	Child's Production
1. house	haʊs	hʌ
2. telephone	tɛlɛfoʊn	tɛpo
3. cup	kʌp	kʌ
4. momma	mama	mama
5. spoon	spun	puː
6. eat cookie	it kʊki	iː tʊti
7. banana	bənænə	nænə
8. car go	kar goʊ	da doʊ
9. chicken	tʃɪkən	tʌː
10. Kiss baby	kɪs beɪbi	tɪ beɪbi
11. Doggie go	dɔgi goʊ	dɔdi doʊ
12. Duck go bye bye	dʌk goʊ baɪbaɪ	dʌ do baɪbaɪ
13. Daddy eat soup	dædi it sup	dædi iː tu
14. drink water	drɪŋk wɔtⁿ	diː wɔ
15. helicopter	hɛlɪkaptⁿ	kʌː
16. drink juice	drɪʌk dʒus	diː duː
17. stove	stoʊv	toʊ
18. rabbit	ræbɪt	wæː
19. see	si	ti
20. zoo	zu	du
21. elephant	ɛləfənt	ɛfən
22. paper	peɪpe	peɪ
23. that	ðæt	dæ
24. carrot	kærət	kæː
25. spaghetti	spəgɛti	gɛti
26. two books	tu bʊks	tu bʌː
27. bath hot	bæθ hat	bæː haː
28. thumb	θʌm	tʌm
29. throw ball	θroʊ bɔl	toʊ bɔː
30. goodnight moon	gʊdnaɪt mun	naɪː muː
31. jump	dʒʌmp	dʌm
32. baby sleep	beɪbi slip	beɪbi tiː

retelling) are needed. The clinician can create stories, use books, or use stories on standard tests such as the Goldman-Fristoe–2 for this purpose.

Elicited Sample   Probes examine certain aspects of phonology in greater depth. For example, a list of words (or pictures) with various final consonants could be used to examine final consonant production. Similarly, a list of minimal pairs (e.g., thick–sick) could be used to examine a child's error production with the intended target. Elicited samples along with a spontaneous sample can provide a **baseline** (an initial measurement before intervention begins).

Sample Recording and Transcription   Collecting a carefully recorded sample is the first step. The sample is then transcribed using the International Phonetic Alphabet (see Chapter 2). These symbols provide a standardized way of characterizing speech production because the same sound can be spelled in different ways (e.g., [s] can be spelled as "s" or "c") and letters can have multiple pronunciations (e.g., "c" can be said as [s] or [k]). It is also important for bilingual individuals because *letters* are pronounced differently across languages. Clinicians use diacritic (more detailed) symbols for errors that cannot be transcribed as another consonant or vowel (e.g., distortions). Transcription can influence analysis. Clinicians sometimes must decide whether to transcribe an error as a diacritic or another sound (e.g., is [s] produced with the tongue protruding slightly transcribed as a [θ] or as a fronted [s]?). The clinician's belief whether the error is phonetic (an alternative production of /s/) or a production of another sound category ([θ]) determines the transcription. The way speech is transcribed can make a difference in diagnosis and intervention.

Sample Analysis   Analyses can be divided into two general groups, independent and relational (Stoel-Gammon & Dunn, 1985). Independent analyses examine a child's productions as an independent system, ignoring the accuracy of these productions in relation to the targets. These analyses include a listing of the consonants, consonant clusters, vowels, syllable structures, and stress patterns produced by the child, which is called a *phonetic inventory* (see Table 6.2). Sometimes the sounds that are missing from the child's inventory are the most important information. Recent advances in phonological theories, called nonlinear phonology (Bernhardt & Stoel-Gammon, 1994;

TABLE 6.2   Summary of Sample Analyses

Analysis	*Purpose*	*Procedure*
Phonetic Inventory	Describe consonants, vowels, clusters, syllable structures, word structures, and patterns in the child's productions, independent of the adult targets.	List and calculate the frequency of consonants, vowels, and clusters by word position and the syllable structures produced. Note gaps in the child's inventory and constraints.
Selection Characteristics	Describe the segments and syllable structures of the adult words attempted by the child.	List the consonants, vowels, and syllable structures of the adult target forms. Note gaps and constraints.
Individual Errors	Identify and describe the child's segmental errors.	List and count the number and type of segmental and syllable errors (substitutions, omissions, additions).
Error Patterns	Identify and describe the error patterns in the child's speech.	List and calculate the frequency of error patterns (processes, rules, constraints). Infer limitations in the child's underlying representation.
Variability	Describe the consistency of the child's productions.	Calculate the consistency of the child's production of given words. Calculate the consistency of error patterns.

FIGURE 6.2
Levels of
phonological
representation.

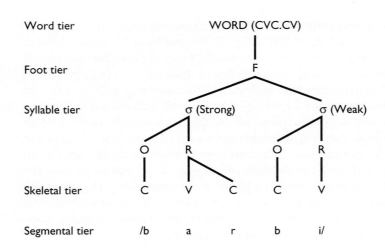

Word tier — WORD (CVC.CV)

Foot tier — F

Syllable tier — σ (Strong)   σ (Weak)

O   R   O   R

Skeletal tier — C   V   C   C   V

Segmental tier — /b   a   r   b   i/

R. Schwartz, 1992), have added important dimensions to this analysis. For example, by organizing a feature analysis in a developmental hierarchy, intervention goals emerge naturally. Another analysis examines the interaction among phonology levels (see Figure 6.2) such as the distribution of the child's production of consonants according to syllable and word position.

Sounds can also be analyzed to determine whether they are in contrast (i.e., change the meaning of words). Children may have different groups of sounds that contrast. Instead of six separate stops (/b/, /p/, /d/, /t/, /g/, /k/), a child may have only three (/b/, /p/, /t/), with all nonlabial stops produced as /t/. Intraword variability examines the consistency of word productions. The characteristics of the adult words that the child attempts are examined in a selectivity analysis.

Relational analyses examine the relationship between the child's production and the adult target. Traditionally, errors have been categorized as substitutions, omissions, additions, and distortions. However, it is more effective and efficient to identify patterns of errors and focus intervention on eliminating these patterns. The most commonly used method to describe error patterns is phonological process analysis. Nonlinear phonology and optimality theory (Barlow, 2001–2002) provide some other approaches. There are several procedures for phonological process analysis: Natural Process Analysis (Shriberg & Kwiatkowski, 1980), Procedures for the Phonological Analysis of Children's Language (Ingram, 1981), and Phonological Assessment of Child Speech (Grunwell, 1985). There are also computerized analyses including PEPPER (Shriberg, 1986), LIPP (Oller & Delgado, 1991), Computerized Profiling (Long, 2003), and CAPP (Hodson, 1986b).

For some children, phonological process analysis provides an adequate description of their error patterns. For other children, their error patterns do not fit phonological processes (e.g., L. Leonard, 1985; Stemberger, 1988). For example, some children have a sound preference (e.g., substituting [t] for a variety of other sounds); a positional constraint (e.g., some sounds appear in only the syllable-initial position); a contextual constraint (e.g., a velar consonant occurs only with mid or back vowels and an alveolar consonant only with high vowels); patterns that extend across words (e.g., assimilation or resyllabification—the final consonant of one word is added to the beginning of the next word); or a single production pattern for most words (e.g., [s] as the final segment in many words).

TABLE 6.3   Examples of Some Common Phonological Processes

Phonological Process	Target Word	Example
Substitution Processes		
Stopping	see	[ti]
Gliding	red	[lɛd]
Nasalization	bow	[noʊ]
Fronting	cow	[taʊ]
Backing	tea	[ki]
Neutralization	bye	[baɪ]
Denasalization	me	[bi]
Glottal replacement	bike	[baɪʔ]
Assimilation Processes[a]		
Progressive	dog	[dɔd]
Regressive	dog	[gɔg]
Syllable Structure Processes		
Unstressed syllable deletion	telephone	[tɛfoʊn]
Reduplication	cake	[keke]
Cluster reduction[a]	blue	[bu]
Final consonant omission	dog	[dɔ]

Note: Though the above examples illustrate a single error in each word, productions in which children make more than a single error in each word are common.

[a]Many clinicians and researchers subdivide cluster reduction according to the type of cluster (e.g., /s/ cluster reduction—**spoon** [pun]) and assimilation according to the influencing sound (e.g., labial assimilation—**boat** [boʊb].

Advances in phonological theories (Barlow, 2001–2002; Barlow & Gierut, 1999; Bernhardt & Stoel-Gammon, 1994; Schwartz, 1992) provide alternative descriptions. Final consonant omission may indicate a representation of word structure without final consonants (like in Spanish) rather than a rule or process that deletes final consonants from an underlying representation. This could also be explained by a constraint (filter) that blocks final consonant production. If [t] is produced as the final consonant of most words, it may be the "default" word-final consonant. Analyses may also examine the stress patterns of words and phrases and the influence of stress on sound production. Apparent inconsistencies may be explained by stress patterns (e.g., fricatives are accurate only in stressed syllables). These newer theories also suggest analyses in which matches and mismatches between the child's production and the target are identified and counted for features, segments (consonants and vowels), syllable shapes, and segment position in words and in syllables (see Table 6.3).

The overall goal of sample analysis is to infer the child's underlying knowledge of phonology, perceptual abilities, and phonetic production abilities (e.g., McGregor & Schwartz, 1992). In combination with data from other methods, this will determine the approach to intervention (see Table 6.4).

Perception Testing

Several tests of speech perception are commercially available. Audiologists and speech-language pathologists also use these tests as part of larger test batteries to identify **central auditory processing disorders (CAPDs)**. These disorders may be more accurately considered impairments in the auditory perception and processing of phonetic, phonological, or linguistic information. The diagnosis of these disorders involves a variety of complex perceptual tasks. One test requires a child to select a picture in an array in response to a spoken word to determine minimal-pair discrimination (e.g., *coat* vs. *goat*). These tests include a large number of items, comparable to an articulation test, and provide a general speech discrimination score. These tests do not reveal the role of perception in a child's specific errors (Locke, 1980a). Some children with phonological disorders have perceptual deficits, whereas others do not. As yet, we can only speculate what signs might indicate a perceptually based disorder. Some indications might be a history of OM, the omission of unstressed syllables or less salient consonants (final consonants, unvoiced stops), and a collapsed class of segments (e.g., all fricatives are produced as [θ]).

The Speech Production-Perception Test (Locke, 1980b) uses a more focused approach. The child is asked to judge the appropriateness of a label for a picture. For example, when shown a picture of the sun, the child would be asked, "Is this a sun?" "Is this a tun?" "Is this a fun?"

Oral Mechanism Examination

Oral mechanism examinations determine whether there are any physical or physiological conditions that may account for the child's phonological disorder. The first step is to form an overall impression of the child's oral and facial structure and breathing patterns. Atypical breathing patterns, facial musculature deviations, any asymmetry of muscle tone, and an abnormal facial structure that reflects jaw and dental alignment are noted. The next step is to examine the dentition and the palate. The palate is examined to identify the general height of the palatal vault along with the status of the hard palate (anterior two-thirds), the soft palate (posterior third), the tongue, and the buccal cavity (inside of the cheeks). Any of the following are noted: muscular or structural asymmetry, dental abnormalities, unusual appearance of the tongue, bifid uvula (the uvula is heart shaped with a notch in the middle or actually divided into two pieces), fistulae (i.e., holes) in the hard palate, a translucent hard palate, a bluish line in the middle of the hard palate, or an exceptionally short soft palate coupled with a deep pharynx. These findings may indicate neuromotor disorders or structural abnormalities that require a referral to other professionals.

The final step is a functional evaluation of the speech mechanism in speech and nonspeech activities. Velar movement is assessed by asking the child to produce a vowel such as [a] while the clinician watches the velar and pharyngeal wall movement. The movement should be symmetrical and appear to be sufficient to achieve velopharyngeal closure, with no audible nasality or nasal emission of air. Children should also be able to open, close, and purse their lips. The tongue is examined to determine the adequacy and range of movement. This examination can be supplemented by instrumental analyses of nasal versus oral air emission, respiration, and vocal fold function. Serious abnormalities may indicate the need for referrals to other professionals including dentists, otolaryngologists, and neurologists.

Audiological Testing

Any child being evaluated for a phonological disorder should receive a complete audiological evaluation (see Chapter 9). A speech-language pathologist can begin this process by administering a pure tone screening and a **tympanometry** screening for middle-ear function. Additional tests may include air and bone conduction thresholds for pure tones and thresholds for speech. Special methods are used for testing younger children and infants. Discrimination testing by an audiologist may not be possible, as many of these tests require production, which may be confounded by the child's phonological disorder.

Stimulability

The goal of **stimulability** testing is to determine how readily the child can produce an acceptable version of a target. Clinicians provide the child with an imitative model, some visual cues, physical cues, and instructions about the correct production of the child's error sounds. These are organized so that there is a sequence from least to most cues. Clinicians also use a sequence of easiest to most difficult in which they test stimulability first in isolated continuant sounds (e.g., vowels or [s]) or syllables and then in words and phrases. Word and phrase testing may be ordered by complexity (e.g., length or number of syllables) and stressed versus unstressed syllable contexts. If a child is stimulable for a sound, it is a positive prognostic indicator; intervention for stimulable sounds will be easier or maybe even unnecessary. However, accurate production in imitation or in response to instructions reflects phonetic level abilities rather than phonological representation, knowledge, and organization.

Determining Intelligibility

Intelligibility is the ease with which listeners can understand an individual's speech. Most frequently, clinicians make subjective judgments of intelligibility on a scale (e.g., poor or low, fair, moderate, high). Intelligibility also may be more systematically described in terms of the number of words or sentences correctly identified or understood by a listener under various conditions. There are several dimensions that can vary in the sample used for intelligibility assessment: (1) the selection of the words or sentences from either a set that is known (also called closed) or one that is unknown (also called open) to the listener, (2) the content and complexity of the words or sentences, and (3) the degree of context (e.g., redundancy in the sentence or in the nonlinguistic context) available to the listener. One approach is to put approximately thirty written words or pictures on slips of paper and have the child select and produce 10 to 20 words. The 30 words can be selected so that they reflect the child's error patterns (e.g., with the same or similar final consonants). An intelligibility score can then be calculated as the proportion of words identified correctly by the listener, who does not know the target. Intelligibility assessment can serve as a measure of the functional effects of a phonological disorder or the functional outcome of intervention.

The Process of Assessment

Following a screening failure, assessment begins with a case history and a brief observation of the child's speech. An articulation test may then be administered along with other standardized tests. The remainder of the session is devoted to the collection of a

TABLE 6.4   Summary of Assessment Information and Intervention Goals for Child₁ (Alicia)

Chronological Age: 4;2

Audiological Status: Normal hearing bilaterally; history of otitis media

Oral Structure and Function: Normal

Overall Language Status: Comprehension within normal limits for age; probable syntactic disorder (limited utterance length and complexity); absence of grammatical morphemes; limited vocabulary; pronoun errors.

Spontaneous Sample (see Table 6.1): Limited phonetic inventory. Most adult words attempted are limited to two syllables with few longer targets. Multiple errors including final consonant omission, stopping, unstressed syllable omission, gliding, cluster simplification, vowel neutralization, assimilation, and some reduplication. Fricatives and affricates are consistently produced as stops. [I] and [r] are consistently produced as [j] and [w], respectively. Frequently unintelligible to examiner, but parents are able to interpret.

Stimulability: Some correct productions of final consonants [n], [p], and [t] when initial and final consonants are identical. Fricatives and affricates are not stimulable.

Speech Perception: Speech perception generally accurate.

Summary: Severe phonological disorder and language disorder affecting syntax and morphosyntax.

Initial Goals: Establish production of final consonants in single-syllable words. Expand phonetic inventory by establishing affricates with the expectation that fricatives will improve. Expand inventory of multisyllable words. Work on expanding utterance length, adding vocabulary, and establishing grammatical morphemes.

sample of the child's spontaneous speech, an oral mechanism examination, and an audiological evaluation. As necessary, other testing, including in-depth probes of speech perception and speech production, are conducted. Finally, the speech-language pathologist prepares a written report of the assessment that includes a determination of whether the child has a phonological disorder, a summary of the analyses of samples obtained through the various means described, a summary of the supplemental tests, a statement of prognosis, and recommendations for intervention. Table 6.4 presents a summary of assessment information for a child.

Determining the Presence of a Disorder

There is no single criterion for determining whether a child has a phonological disorder. Clinicians use information about typical development to make this determination. A number of normative data sets are available (e.g., Sander, 1972; Smit, Hand, Freilinger, & Bernthal, 1990; M. Templin, 1957). Although they provide important information, they may be misleading (e.g., Smit, 1986). Furthermore, they are just lists of ages at which consonants appear to be produced correctly; they are not a complete picture of phonological development. A child who falls into the lowest 10 percent (10th percentile) of her peers on some phonology measure, who falls more than one standard deviation below the mean (i.e., average) for her age (this puts the child in approximately the lowest 15%), or who falls at least 6 months below the phonological acquisition norms for her age (see Chapter 2) is judged to have a phonological disorder. Clinicians avoid using the last of these criteria, referred to as **age-referenced norms**. A 6-month deficit in a 3-year-old means something very different than a 6-month deficit in a 7-year-old. The child's intelligibility also may play a role in this decision. Finally, stimulability may influence the clinician's decision. If a child is highly stimulable for the sounds in error, the child could be monitored before enrollment in intervention.

Dialect and Exposure to Other Languages

A critical step in the assessment is the consideration of the dialect or language characteristics of the child's environment. Increasingly, speech-language pathologists work with children who are acquiring English as a second language or simultaneously with other languages, a regional dialect of English, or African American Vernacular English. It is important to distinguish among speech characteristics that are attributable to the child's language environment and those that are characteristic of a disorder. Many simplifications normally occur in conversational speech (e.g., leaving off [d] at the end of and or changing [ŋ] at the end of ing to [n]). In some cases, production characteristics attributable to the environment may also be targeted for intervention (e.g., to improve English production accuracy in bilinguals or to reduce an accent). In the case of dialect, some adults or parents may decide it is desirable to establish Standard English production for use in some communicative situations. There are a number of published lists of dialect and bilingual speech characteristics (e.g., Kamhi, Pollock, & Harris, 1996; R. Owens, 2010). Developmental norms are not currently available. The clinician's task is to distinguish between production characteristics that are part of the child's dialect or other language and errors. Clinicians adjust scores on standardized tests so that dialect characteristics are not counted as errors. Speech samples from caregivers, siblings, or peers may be useful in understanding the child's language environment.

Choosing Intervention Goals

Intervention goals are directly linked to the clinician's theoretical framework. For example, in an articulation framework, goals focus on correct production of individual segments. In a phonological process framework, goals focus on the elimination of error patterns (i.e., phonological processes). In other frameworks, goals address the alteration of underlying knowledge and representation. For example, the goal might be to change the boundaries of sound classes (e.g., to establish six distinctly produced consonants) or to change rules (e.g., to eliminate a rule that deletes word-final consonants). In more recent theories (e.g., nonlinear phonology), intervention goals include feature additions by establishing new consonants in the child's phonetic inventory, different syllable structure representations (e.g., syllable and word structures that end in consonants), or new associations between syllable structures and segments. An important distinction in goal selection is the difference between outcomes and efficacy (Gierut, 1998, 2001). Although all of the treatments discussed in the following sections have been demonstrated to be effective in changing children's speech (outcome), less information is available about their relative efficiency (efficacy). One goal selection approach that has yielded strong evidence of efficacy involves the choice of later acquired, nonstimulable, linguistically complex, and never accurate sounds as the targets of choice (Gierut, 1998, 2001).

Intervention

Using information gathered during assessment, speech-language pathologists select specific short-term and long-term goals that can be measured. Intervention is generally divided into two general components: (1) establishment and (2) cognitive change or generalization. In establishment, the goal is to ensure that the child is able to produce and to perceive accurately the sounds, syllables, or structures in error. In cognitive change or generalization, the goal is to ensure that changes effected in establishment become an integral part of the child's phonology. Establishment techniques are generally consistent across approaches, but other components of intervention vary.

Establishment

The first step is to find facilitating contexts in which the child can produce the targets. For example, a child who substitutes velar sounds for alveolars may be more likely to produce alveolars in words with high front vowels. Stressed syllables are more likely to facilitate correct production than are unstressed syllables.

Clinicians sometimes intervene more directly to achieve initial target production. Phonetic placement approaches are used in which clinicians give more direct instructions for articulator placement for sound production. This is best suited to older children who are able to comprehend such instructions. For younger children, visual aids or mirrors may be helpful. Clinicians sometimes use **successive approximations** to achieve correct production gradually, such as moving from an [l], which the child can produce, or from a growling sound to an [r] (see Bernthal & Bankson, 1998; N. Creaghead, Newman, & Secord, 1989; Shriberg, 1975). Perception training to distinguish the target sound from the error is an integral part of some intervention approaches. Consider a 6-year-old child who substitutes [θ] for [s] and [ð] for [z]. Perception testing revealed that this child also failed to discriminate thick and sick. Initial sessions were devoted to eliciting approximations or correct productions of [s] and [z] by having the child keep her tongue behind the teeth, look in a mirror, and place her finger on her lips. For perception, we used activities in which the child had to discriminate between and then categorize *noisy* syllables ([s] or [z]) and *quiet* syllables ([θ] and [ð]). Once the child reached a level of 60 percent correct in syllables, the segments were considered to be established.

Some intervention approaches described below directly address this initial stage of therapy. Intervention procedures also typically share some of the general steps that are illustrated in Table 6.5. Beyond this stage, intervention approaches may differ markedly. An overview of some specific approaches follows. The selected readings provide more detailed descriptions.

Articulation Approaches

Articulation approaches focus on motor production, employing imitation, shaping, or successive approximations, and reinforcement for desired responses. One longstanding method is the traditional approach (M. Powers, 1971; Van Riper & Emerick, 1984), which includes two components, *ear* or perceptual training and production training. Perceptual training includes a series of levels: labeling the target sound (*identification*), identifying the presence and location of the sound (*isolation*), receiving intensive exposure to the target sound (*stimulation*), and discriminating the target

TABLE 6.5   General Organizational Steps in Intervention

Establishment

1. Imitative production of target sounds (initial and final position) in simple words with and then without cues
2. Discrimination of target sounds from error productions in initial and final position of simple words (one syllable)

Spontaneous and elicited production of targets in words

1. Simple words
   a. Facilitating contexts with frequent models of correct target production
   b. Nonfacilitating contexts with frequent models of correct targets
   c. Reduction of models in both contexts
2. Complex words (two or more syllables)
   a. Facilitating contexts with frequent models of correct target production
   b. Nonfacilitating contexts with frequent models of correct targets
   c. Reduction of models in both contexts
3. Discrimination of the child's correct and incorrect productions

Production of targets in more complex utterances

1. Set carrier phrases (e.g., "I see a _____) with frequent models
2. Simple spontaneous utterances with frequent models
3. Reduced frequency of models
4. Discrimination of the child's correct and incorrect productions

Generalization

1. Controlled discourse (e.g., storytelling or story retelling) with clinician designed to frequently include targets
2. Introduction of other conversational partners and settings
3. Reduction of target frequency and increased spontaneity of discourse
4. Further work on self-monitoring and self-correction skills

---

sound from the error (*discrimination*). Once perceptual training is complete, the next step is production training. Production training begins with the target segment in isolation or in a syllable and moves progressively to simple word contexts, phrases and sentences, controlled conversation, and spontaneous speech.

The multiple phonemic approach (R. McCabe & Bradley, 1975) has several components that focus on multiple errors, and each component is divided into detailed steps. The principal components are **Establishment**, which focuses on the elicitation of target sounds in isolation; **Transfer**, in which the child moves from establishment to production in conversational speech; and **Maintenance**, which addresses production in conversational speech within and outside the clinic. This approach is unique in its focus on multiple targets, in the detailed activities and techniques within each component, and in the data-keeping scheme provided.

Many other articulation-oriented approaches are available. Some rely on various forms of stimulus generalization (e.g., McLean, Raymore, Long, & Brown, 1976; Weston & Irwin, 1971) or other behavioral principles. Such approaches may be particularly effective for children who have a small number of errors that do not seem to reflect underlying deficits in phonology. Clinicians have had some success in treating phonological disorders involving deficits at the level of representation or underlying knowledge. However, this is incidental to these intervention approaches, as their focus is on articulation.

There is evidence that substantial gains may be achieved for some children through discrimination training alone (Winitz, 1989). This phonological approach emphasizes the discrimination of minimal pairs of words and the establishment of consonant contrasts through discrimination training.

Phonological Approaches

Phonological approaches differ from articulation approaches in their emphasis on changing the patterns of errors or underlying knowledge. For a child who does not produce word-final consonants and who substitutes stops for fricatives, therapy would focus on the acquisition of consonants in the word-final position and on the establishment of the features that distinguish stops from fricatives.

The earliest phonological approaches organized treatment in terms of distinctive features (e.g., McReynolds & Bennett, 1972). The idea was that establishing voicing in one pair of contrasting segments would generalize to other pairs. Weiner and Bankson (1978) suggested establishing a conceptual understanding of the feature contrast (e.g., air blowing vs. puffs of air for continuant vs. noncontinuant sounds).

The cycles approach (Hodson & Paden, 1991) focuses on the elimination of multiple phonological processes. It is based on some key assumptions: Phonological acquisition is gradual, children acquire phonology through listening, sound production can be facilitated by selecting appropriate phonetic contexts, children establish auditory and kinesthetic connections with new speech patterns, and children have a natural tendency to generalize. A number of phonological processes are simultaneously targeted for intervention. Each process is worked on for a period of time, and the full set is called a cycle. There are no criteria that must be reached before progressing to the next goal. Instead, if the child does not reach the critera for the goals in a cycle, the cycle is begun again. To start each session, the clinician and the child review words containing target sounds from the prior session. This is followed by auditory bombardment, in which the clinician reads a list of words in isolation and sentences containing the target sound. Mild amplification using an auditory trainer is recommended. Five words are identified for production practice, and these are incorporated into a variety of games and activities. A probe determines the target for the next session, and that target is introduced at the end of the session. An important part of this approach is the home program. Caretakers are asked to present the *auditory bombardment* list and elicit the production practice words once a day.

One other commonly used method is the minimal pair or contrast approach (Elbert, Rockman, & Saltzman, 1980; Weiner, 1981). This focuses on minimal word pairs that contrast in the target and the child's error (e.g., bow and boat for a child who deletes consonants at the ends of words). Perception and production activities can be organized around sets of these pairs. Other activities such as grouping or categorizing activities that highlight phonological characteristics may also be effective; Metaphon therapy (Howell & Dean, 1994) formalizes that idea. Intervention research (Tyler, Edwards, & Saxman, 1987) has demonstrated that both the minimal pair and the cycles approaches are effective.

Studies have used an evidence-based practice framework to examine the effectiveness of different intervention methods. The majority have focused on phonological awareness (e.g., Justice & Pullen, 2003; Pokorni, Worthington, & Jamison, 2004). For kindergarten children, Ladders to Literacy (Notari-Syverson, O'Connor, & Vadasy, 1998) and Sound Foundations (Byrne & Fielding-Barnsley, 1991) yield immediate and long-term improvements in phonological awareness (Justice & Pullen, 2003).

Several intervention methods have been compared to determine their effectiveness for specific phonological awareness skills, such as consonant blending and segmenting (Pokorni et al., 2004). The Lindamood Phoneme Sequencing Program for Reading, Spelling, and Speech (LiPS; Lindamood & Lindamood, 1998) is more effective than the other selected methods in improving children's ability to blend phonemes. Children also made significant gains in segmenting with this. A. G. Kamhi (2006) defined treatment efficiency as gaining something for free. According to this idea, the most efficient methods are the ones that lead to a high degree of generalization. Gierut's complexity approach (Gierut, 2005) is an effective method for facilitating generalization (e.g., targeting affricates improved fricative production, working on clusters improved the production of singletons).

Frequency and Organization of Therapy

There are diverse views about the ideal schedule of therapy sessions. Two sessions per week of at least 30 minutes is a common minimum, though there is no evidence that this is ideal. More sessions and longer sessions may be necessary for children with a more severe disorder. This may include both group and individual sessions. In whole language approaches (e.g., Hoffman, 1990; Schory, 1990), intervention is often integrated with the child's regular classroom activities. This can also be accomplished in conversational contexts within small groups and in individual therapy. Therapy can be divided into blocks of time, dictated by school schedules or defined by the clinician to facilitate and to organize intervention or to organize the measurement of progress.

The general organization of therapy involves sequencing multiple goals. Several factors have been used to prioritize goals: (1) the order of typical acquisition (i.e., earlier developing aspects of phonology are targeted first), (2) impact on intelligibility (i.e., frequently occurring sounds or omitted sounds), and (3) occasionally correct (variable) or stimulable sounds. Until recently, clinicians assumed that they should work first on early acquired, stimulable, and inconsistently produced sounds. However, the strong research evidence indicates that complexity should be the basis of goal selection (Gierut, 2001). The most efficacious approach is to choose sounds that are most complex: (1) 0 percent accurate, (2) nonstimulable, (3) later acquired, and (4) linguistically complex.

There are three basic schemes for organizing multiple goals (M. Fey, 1986). The first is a sequential approach, in which the clinician works on one goal until the child reaches a preset criterion. Then the next goal is the focus of intervention and so on. An alternative is to address a group of selected goals simultaneously with some time devoted to each until the criterion is reached for each of these goals. The final possibility is the cyclical approach (Hodson & Paden, 1991) described earlier. The clinician cycles through the set of goals again until the child reaches the selected criterion on each goal. The last of these approaches more closely resembles typical acquisition.

Measuring Change

Change is measured in many ways, from counting correct responses during therapy activities to counting correct productions in spontaneous speech. The choice of measurement context, among other variables, depends on the nature of the intervention, the intended purpose of the measurement, and the stage of intervention. Often speech-language pathologists use probes composed of approximately twenty elicited items (typically words) that have not been part of therapy activities. To determine whether a child should be dismissed from therapy, clinicians examine production in spontaneous speech.

The **criteria** for movement across stages of intervention and for dismissal are an important facet of measuring change. Because we attempt to establish mastery, a criterion of 80 percent or even 90 percent correct is often required. However, this ignores the likelihood that once the child begins to change, she will continue to consolidate this new knowledge and accuracy will increase without additional therapy. If we use 60 percent and speech production remains at this level or deteriorates, intervention can be reinstated. Dismissal from therapy should occur when all goals have reached this point as measured in spontaneous speech. The ability to self-correct errors may also be considered. This certainly would be a sign of the child's ability to make additional gains without further intervention.

A final issue is whether observed changes are attributable to the intervention or to development that is independent of intervention. One approach is a *multiple baseline design*. The clinician chooses one or more **target goals**, which are the focus of intervention; **control goals** that are not likely to be affected by the intervention; and **generalization goals** that will not receive direct intervention, but should benefit indirectly. For example, eliminating fricative omission might be a target goal, eliminating final consonant omission might be a generalization goal (e.g., as fricatives in the final position are established, other final consonants might begin to appear), and eliminating the substitution of glides for liquids might be the control goal. Before intervention begins, probes determine the baseline performance on each goal. These baseline probes are readministered periodically during intervention, and the child's progress is tracked. If the intervention is responsible for change, the performance on the target goal should improve sharply, the improvement on the generalization goal should be more gradual, and development on the control goal should be minimal. Without this approach, clinicians cannot be certain whether the intervention caused the changes observed.

Intervention Settings

Intervention for phonological disorders has traditionally taken place in individual sessions. However, small- or large-group therapy may be used as the sole mode of service delivery or in conjunction with individual therapy. There are no published studies of the relative efficacy of individual versus group therapy. Both have advantages. Individual intervention provides an opportunity to establish structural aspects of language such as phonology that may be more difficult to establish in groups. Group therapy provides an opportunity to address intervention targets in communicative contexts with the child's peers, provides correct models from their peers (in a heterogeneous group, children have different error patterns), and offers the potential to link intervention goals in whole-language approaches. Each intervention mode also has some drawbacks. In individual sessions, it is more difficult to introduce varied communicative contexts, limiting generalization. In groups, it may be difficult for children to extract the structural targets. A hybrid approach may be the ideal solution.

One additional intervention setting is the home, with the parents acting as intervention agents. This may not be appropriate for all children and their parents. But it can be the primary approach for children under 3 or a valuable supplement to intervention in the clinic or at school.

Regardless of the approach, effective activities must have several characteristics. The tasks must be interesting and engaging, while eliciting perception and production responses. Early in intervention, the child should have opportunities to succeed. Thus, the tasks must provide the child with opportunities to hear correct productions. Over the course of intervention, this support is gradually reduced, and activities more closely resemble natural communicative situations.

Generalization

Children are very successful in achieving establishment of the correct production and perception of targets in single words. They also successfully generalize these gains to words and phrases that were not included in intervention activities. This is accomplished by including a variety of stimuli in intervention activities. However, the goal of generalization to communicative settings, particularly outside the clinic, is often more difficult to achieve. One challenge is achieving naturalness in intervention (Fey, 1986). There are three dimensions of naturalness. Activities may range from the most natural, daily activities, to the least natural, drill. The physical context may be manipulated from the least natural, the clinic; to the middle, the school; to the most natural, the child's home. Finally, the naturalness of the interactor or social context may vary, with the clinician being the least natural interactor, the teacher being somewhat more natural, and parents, siblings, or peers providing the most natural social context. If therapy becomes more natural as it proceeds, generalization will be facilitated.

Summary

The last several decades have seen significant changes in the assessment and remediation of phonological disorders, reflecting changes in phonological theories and phonological acquisition. One major theme has been an expansion of our understanding of early perception and production in the general context of language acquisition. Two implications are the importance of early intervention and the integration of phonology with other aspects of language. As current theories evolve in the future and their clinical applications become clear, speech-language pathologists will develop more-inclusive and more-effective procedures that will further increase the accuracy of assessment and the efficacy of intervention for these disorders.

case study

Alicia came to a speech-language pathologist because her parents had concerns about the length and complexity of Alicia's sentences, her vocabulary size, and the intelligibility of her speech. Other relatives, her preschool teacher, and aides characterized her speech as difficult to understand and as immature in comparison to her peers. She was 4;2 at the time of the initial evaluation.

Alicia's parents reported that her prenatal and postnatal developmental history was unremarkable with two exceptions. She had repeated episodes of bilateral middle-ear infections during her second year of life that were treated initially with antibiotics and subsequently with pressure equalization tubes at 2 years of age. Her language development has been slow compared to that of her sister, who is 2 years older. Alicia's parents also reported a late onset of identifiable words (18 months) and a late onset of initial word combinations (30 months).

A spontaneous sample of Alicia's language collected with her parents and older sister revealed a limited set of sounds in Alicia's speech. Overall, she produced relatively few consonants and none at the ends of words. Fricative and affricate sounds were produced as stops. [l] was produced as [j] and [r] was produced as [w] and were not stimulable. Unstressed syllables were often omitted. Words in phrases were often produced with assimilation (consonants were repeated across words). Her language production was difficult to evaluate because utterances of more than two words were unintelligible and grammatical morphemes such as past tense, plurals, and third-person singular markings were absent. She also didn't produce articles. However, standardized testing revealed that Alicia's language comprehension was appropriate for her age. Her hearing was normal and her nonverbal IQ was within normal limits. Alicia was diagnosed as having a Specific Language Impairment with a severe phonological disorder.

Alicia was enrolled in a half-day preschool for children with language impairments. The preschool provided large- and small-group activities, with a strong language emphasis. In addition, Alicia received three 20-minute periods of individual therapy per day. By midyear, she was producing a number of final consonants and some fricatives. In addition, she had begun producing some unstressed syllables in words and in phrases. Assimilation in phrases was virtually eliminated. Her MLU seemed to be only slightly below what would be expected for her age level. By the end of the school year, most grammatical morphemes were present at least some of the time; most final consonants were produced correctly on occasion. Some fricatives were produced correctly. Final consonants were correct in many words, and most morphological endings were correctly produced. Her one- and two-word productions were all intelligible, but sentence productions were still often difficult to understand. There were some residual errors ([l], [r], affricates, consonant clusters) in single words. Alicia continued to receive therapy in kindergarten the following fall. The focus of therapy was on residual errors and continued generalization of gains to spontaneous speech, on some errors in her language production (e.g., pronouns), and on the production and comprehension of complex sentences.

STUDY QUESTIONS

1. How is phonology related to other aspects of language?

2. Discuss how the following factors may impact production accuracy: the length of the word, the position of the target sound in the word, the syllable structure, and the syllable stress.

3. Describe the difference between speech disorder and language disorder. Provide an example of each as well as an example of a condition that is characterized by both speech and language disorder.

4. What are the components of a complete phonological assessment, and how do you decide what to analyze?

5. How does intervention reflect current theories of phonology?

6. How can we differentiate among different types of speech sound disorders, and what are the implications for intervention?

SELECTED READINGS

Ball, M., & Kent, R. (1997). *The new phonologies: Developments in clinical linguistics.* San Diego, CA: Singular.

Barlow, J. (2001–2002). Clinical forum: Recent advances in phonology: Theory and treatment: Parts I and II. *Language, Speech, and Hearing Services in the Schools, 32,* 225–228; *33,* 4–8.

Bauman-Waengler, J. (2007). *Articulatory and phonological impairments: A clinical focus* (3rd ed.). Boston, MA: Allyn & Bacon.

Bernthal, J., Bankson, N., & Flipsen, P. (2009). *Articulation and phonological disorders* (6th ed.). Boston, MA: Allyn & Bacon.

Ferguson, C., Menn, L., & Stoel-Gammon, C. (1992). *Phonological development: Models, research, implications.* Timonium, MD: York Press.

Fey, M., Edwards, M. L., Elbert, M., Hodson, B., Hoffman, P., Kamhi, A., & Schwartz, R. (1992). Clinical forum: Issues in phonological assessment and treatment. *Language, Speech, and Hearing Services in the Schools, 23,* 224–282.

Kamhi, A. G., & Pollock, K. E. (Eds.). (2005). *Phonological disorders in children: Clinical decision making in assessment and intervention* (Communication and Language Intervention Series). Baltimore, MD: Paul H. Brookes.

Stockman, I. (1996). Phonological development and disorders in African American Children. In A. Kamhi, K. Pollock, & J. Harris (Eds.), *Communicative development and disorders in African American children: Research, assessment, and intervention* (pp. 117–154). Baltimore, MD: Paul H. Brookes.

WEBSITES OF INTEREST

www.waisman.wisc.edu/phonology/Index.htm
   The Child Phonology Project, University of Wisconsin, Madison. Director, Lawrence D. Shriberg. This website includes information concerning a longstanding research and clinical center for the study, assessment, and treatment of phonological disorders.

www.computerizedprofiling.org
   Computerized Profiling is a program for the analysis of children's speech and language samples. The program may be downloaded for free. It contains a phonological analysis as well as analyses of other components of language.

www.apraxia-kids.org/index.html
   This website, maintained by a private organization for parents and professionals, provides information concerning developmental apraxia and phonological disorders.

weston.ruter.net/projects/ipa-chart/view/keyboard
   This website contains interactive charts of the International Phonetic Alphabet with a keyboard to use.

Chapter SEVEN

Stuttering and Other Disorders of Fluency

Peter R. Ramig
University of Colorado at Boulder

Ryan Pollard
University of Colorado at Boulder

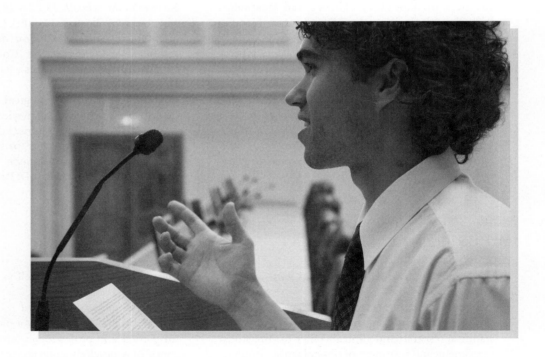

Acknowledgment: Drs. Ramig and Pollard wish to acknowledge Dr. George Shames's invaluable contribution to the previous seven editions of this chapter. Dr. Shames continues to serve at one of the editors for this new edition of *Human Communication Disorders*, but no longer coauthors this chapter.

personal PERSPECTIVE

PETER R. RAMIG

My stuttering impacted my life from the time of onset at age 3. I have memories of feeling bewildered and frightened because I so often struggled when I spoke. I remember experiencing feelings of embarrassment, frustration, and shame in elementary school, junior high, and high school and during my undergraduate college years. Frequently, I avoided words as I spoke, replacing one difficult-to-say word with a word of similar meaning that began with an easier-to-say sound. I also changed logical word sequence in sentences in order to try to talk around the words I knew I would stutter, often resulting in an illogical and difficult-to-understand message. I was on guard when I spoke, gingerly choosing my words, often avoiding speaking situations completely. After all, I felt if I chose my speaking situations carefully, I would avoid ridicule and embarrassment.

Most of us know that decisions we make can impact our life significantly. A decision I made to conceal my stuttering had a tremendous impact on my life in 1966 at the age of 19. The Vietnam War was in its early stages and escalating rapidly, in turn requiring a rapid buildup in U.S. forces. Although I was enrolled in college, I was not attending full-time because it was necessary for me to work to support myself. However, because I was only 19 years old, I mistakenly thought I would not have to worry about induction for another year or two. That miscalculation was my first big mistake! Before I knew it, I received a draft notice from Uncle Sam to report for induction in six weeks. Upon reporting for the routine examination in the neighboring town of Milwaukee, I was given a questionnaire form to answer regarding my physical and psychological health. Although I was a healthy young man overall, I checked off on the form that I stuttered. Consequently, at the end of the physical examination I was called to appear before the examining psychiatrist who began to question me about my stuttering. I was about to make my second big mistake. Because I was so embarrassed to stutter openly, I did what I always did: I gingerly "danced" around my stuttering by avoiding words and circumlocuting, creating the misperception that I was a fairly fluent speaker. After a few minutes of interaction, the psychiatrist looked up at me and said, "Son, stuttering is a very good reason to avoid the military, if you stuttered, but you don't stutter much at all! I think you'll do fine in the army!"

If I had let my real stuttering show as I spoke to the psychiatrist, I am convinced I would have been excused from serving in the military during a time of growing unrest in U.S. history, the Vietnam Era. I did not want to serve in the military at the time because I had plans to earn a college degree and because I felt the Vietnam conflict was not a good reason to wage war. However, even though I knew I could probably be exempted from military service due to my stuttering, I was still too embarrassed to forthrightly expose it face-to-face with the examining psychiatrist.

As a result, I was inducted that day into the military. My next surprise was that I was not drafted into the army; instead, I became one of the first Marine Corps draftees since the Korean War. Although it was highly unusual for the Marine Corps to draft, such action was initiated periodically in times of conflict and military buildup. Of the 2 years I spent in the Marines, 14 months were spent in Vietnam, an experience that to this day has dramatically changed and impacted my life.

After my 2 years in the Marine Corps, I once again enrolled in college, where I was fortunate to meet two knowledgeable speech-language pathologists, both of whom were persons who stuttered and had learned through expert help to speak much more fluently. They both helped me understand, confront, and control my stuttering. They were great role models. Thanks to their expertise, understanding, and caring, I learned to communicate more fluently without the avoidance, tension, and struggle that had maintained and fueled my stuttering since childhood. Their help gave me the confidence and strong desire to pursue graduate school. I then earned a master's degree in speech-language pathology at the University of Wisconsin–Madison and a doctorate in the same field at Purdue University, where it specialized in the area of stuttering.

My choice to pursue stuttering within the field of speech-language pathology was a major life-impacting decision that I have not regretted. My earlier work in the public schools as a speech-language clinician and my 20 years to date as professor of speech-language pathology at the University of Colorado have been most gratifying. The balance I have been able to maintain in my teaching and research and my treatment of scores of children and adults who stutter has been a most enjoyable way to earn a living. My hope is that I have been able to enrich the lives of my students and clients in the same way my professors and speech clinicians enriched mine.

personal PERSPECTIVE

RYAN POLLARD

I don't remember ever speaking normally. My parents tell me that I began to stutter at age 4, so there must have been a couple fluent years in there, but they're lost to me now. For as far back as I can recall, talking to others was always a struggle.

This would have been a revelation to most people who knew me growing up, as I was able to conceal my disorder fairly well. By all outward appearances, I was a typical, happy kid. I got good grades in school, played several sports throughout the year, was outgoing, and had many friends. Everyone knew I stuttered, of course, but no one said much about it, and it didn't seem to keep me from living a full life. But looks can be deceiving. Stuttering, perhaps more so than any other speech disorder, proves that old adage: Over time, it can become infinitely more than the noticeable repetitions and blocks and stumbled words that occur in one's speech.

And so it was for me.

As I neared the end of high school, I had become the epitome of what stuttering can do to a person if left unchecked and allowed to follow its natural, insidious course. I employed a huge arsenal of tricks and avoidances to get through the day, carefully evading any situation where I might stutter and be marked as abnormal. This method of communicating continued as I entered the University of Northern Colorado and began my undergraduate degree in psychology. I chose that major because phobias, obsessions, distorted thoughts—maybe one of my textbooks would help me understand why I couldn't talk right. Deep down I knew I would never be able to be a clinical psychologist with such a severe stutter as mine, but I ignored that looming reality as best I could. In some indeterminate future, I would do something about my speech, but not now. I managed to graduate magna cum laude, having never raised my hand or given an oral presentation in class. I still feel like there should have some sort of asterisk on my diploma, acknowledging that feat.

After college, I found myself with a degree I was unable to use. How could I interview for a decent job if I couldn't pick up the phone to schedule a meeting? There was graduate school, but how could I become a psychologist when I was afraid to talk to clients and their families? Suddenly, the real world hit me like a brick wall, and I discovered that I was frightfully unequipped to function in it. Years of failing to deal with my stuttering had finally caught up with me. Not able to do anything else, I mopped floors and cleaned rooms at a hospital—a janitor with a college degree. I knew that, if I didn't do something soon, I would spend the rest of my life there or in some other unfulfilling job. It was at this point, at age 22, that I decided the time had come to quit running and confront this thing at last.

I enrolled in stuttering therapy (my mom had to make the phone call) and spent the next 2 years learning how to control my speech rather than continuing to allow it to control me. This period of my life was an unheaval in every sense of the word. To my astonishment, I learned that I could analyze and change my stuttering behaviors, replacing them with a far more normal way of speaking. I came to understand that stuttering was something I did rather than an inscrutable force against which I was helpless. I gradually gained confidence and a new sense of what was possible; it was as if a door opened and the world lay before me. Naturally, I started considering previously barred careers.

I looked into how to pursue my interests—history, anthropology, journalism, travel writing, even film. About a year into stuttering treatment, I realized that it was an appealing career option as well. It occurred to me that the disorder that had caused me so much pain, that I had always hated so vehemently, was also the thing about which I was most passionate. If I could harness that zeal and become the therapist, then perhaps I could help others as I had been helped. What could be more rewarding? I didn't know it at the time, but I was following a well-worn path in the field of stuttering: the client who becomes the clinician.

That was several years ago. Since then, I have enrolled in a doctoral program at the University of Colorado, learned a great deal more about fluency disorders and other fascinating areas of speech-language pathology, and am about to embark on a career as a stuttering researcher and therapist. I can only shake my head and smile when I think about what that fearful boy and adolescent I was not so long ago would have thought if he had been told what would one day become of him.

The fluency disorder of stuttering is a complicated, multidimensional communication problem. There is an overt, easy-to-see, easy-to-hear side of the problem. But there is also a covert, private side of the problem involving the feelings of the person who stutters, the feelings of his listeners and family, and often their attempts to deny the problem's existence. There is a mutual self-consciousness or concern that develops and is expressed, sometimes subtly and sometimes blatantly. Persons who stutter and their listeners engage in a type of conspiracy of silence about stuttering, with each often helping the other to avoid a confrontation, acknowledgment, and acceptance of this problem. Society's penalties for stuttering, though unintentional, are often quite harsh and intolerant, as well as intolerable.

One of the most difficult aspects of this problem is not knowing with any confidence what causes stuttering and, hence, being left with the unanswered questions *Where did it come from?* and *Why me?* In spite of not knowing the exact cause of stuttering, children, adults, and their families have been helped a great deal with this problem by professional speech-language pathologists who understand its development and treatment. It is hoped this chapter on stuttering will provide the information and insights needed to better understand the complex disorder of stuttering.

Stuttering is the major subcategory of fluency disorders seen in both children and adults and is emphasized in this chapter. It is a problem for approximately 1 percent of the population, over 2 million children and adults in the United States. The latest statistics reveal that in some locales in the United States, prevalence is as high as 2.1 percent. Prevalence data outside of the United States range up to 4.7 percent in the British West Indies (Bloodstein, 1995). About 85 percent of all cases of stuttering start during the preschool years. Boys outnumber girls who stutter by a ratio of 4 to 1. But a study of African Americans by Goldman (1967) showed a ratio of 2 to 1, males over females, suggesting the influence of cultural effects on this problem.

Types, Descriptions, and Definitions of Various Disfluency Types

In addition to stuttering, the most common disorder of fluency, there are several other problems that may interfere with a person's ability to produce ongoing fluent speech. Each problem, thought to have different causes not yet fully understood by researchers, is briefly defined and described as follows (see Figure 7.1):

1. **Stuttering** usually begins in early childhood and is the most common disorder of fluency.
    I. It is defined as (a) disruption in the fluency of verbal expression, which is (b) characterized by involuntary, audible, or silent repetitions or prolongations in the utterance of short elements—namely, sounds, syllables, and words of one syllable. These disruptions (c) usually occur frequently or are marked in character and (d) are not readily controllable.
    II. Sometimes the disruptions are (e) accompanied by accessory activities involving the speech apparatus, related or unrelated body structures, or stereotyped speech utterances. These activities give the appearance of being speech-related struggle.

III. Also, there are (f) indications or reports of the presence of an emotional state ranging from a general condition of "excitement" or "tension" to more-specific emotions of a negative nature such as fear, embarrassment, irritation, or the like. (Wingate, 1964, p. 489)

Although there may be strong emotional and psychological components, these are viewed by most authorities as resulting from embarrassment, frustration, and shame—the common by-products of the stuttering experience. We favor the above definition of stuttering because it incorporates several important factors such as stuttering behaviors, reactions, and feelings.

The longer stuttering persists, the more likely it is that associated emotional problems will develop. As listeners react to a child developing stuttering speech, the child also reacts to his speech and to the reactions of others. He may feel embarrassed, guilty, frustrated, or angry. Many people who stutter come to feel helpless, which often damages their sense of personal value. Stuttering frequently leads to confusion and to social and emotional conflicts for the child or adult speaker and for his family, friends, teachers, and anyone else who interacts with him. Thus, the normal disfluency that is a relatively simple and effortless developmental milestone can be transformed into a serious social, emotional, and communicative disability. It can profoundly affect an individual's self-concept, sense of worth, goals, aspirations, expectations, and basic style of coping with life.

Some people who stutter may respond to their problem by being overaggressive, denying its existence, projecting reactions in listeners, or feeling anxious and timid. They often avoid talking or any social circumstances in which talking is expected, to the point of socially isolating themselves. A child's potential for an education, occupation, and fulfilling social and emotional life can be seriously reduced by long-term, persistent stuttering. Stuttering can easily become the focal point around which a person and his family organize their lives. The speech-language pathologist, therefore, must address this problem within all of the individual's developmental, familial, and social contexts.

Stuttering affects the fluent, smooth, and effortless flow of words emitted by a speaker and has long been recognized as a problem. This complex and unusual disorder has perplexed its victims and their families, as well as professionals, from the days of Moses and Demosthenes to the present. Although a great deal of research has been conducted on people who stutter, we still do not know its cause.

People who stutter present a wide variety of symptoms, both visible and hidden. Overtly, they may repeat sounds or words; prevent their vocal cords from vibrating, resulting in a block or absence of sound; or prolong sounds abnormally. In addition, they may show secondary behaviors, such as eye blinking, head jerking, or facial grimaces. Many people who stutter show a great deal of muscular tension and forcing when they try to speak. Covertly, they may substitute words, talk indirectly around a topic, or reply with incorrect information to avoid certain words. We must be careful not to categorize a stuttering problem as mild, moderate, or severe based on overt behavior alone. A person who stutters with only covert behaviors may have as many difficulties as one who has an overtly severe problem. Although other people may not recognize the person as a disfluent speaker, he may be avoiding speaking situations or may be giving incorrect information to avoid stuttering. For example, people who stutter have reported giving a false name when asked, ordering hamburger when they

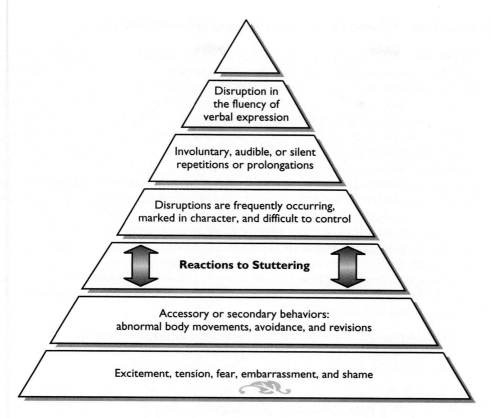

FIGURE 7.1
Stuttering behavior.

wanted steak, and answering *I don't know* to questions as simple as *What is your address?* The problem of stuttering can have an extreme effect on a person's life, whether or not the problem appears severe on the surface.

2. Acquired organic or neurological stuttering is a common problem that usually occurs suddenly as a result of trauma to the brain that is caused, for example, by stroke, auto accident, projectile wound, brain disease, or intake of drugs. Usually, this type of fluency problem is not associated with a past history of stuttering.

3. Psychogenic stuttering is rare and reportedly occurs as a result of an emotionally or psychologically traumatic experience. Although this type of fluency disorder has been cited in the literature, the authors have witnessed only a couple of clients out of over a thousand who were suspected of stuttering as a result of emotional or psychological trauma.

4. **Cluttering** is a less common fluency disorder that begins in childhood. It is defined as follows:

> Cluttering is a disorder of both speech and language processing resulting in rapid, disrhythmic, sporadic, unorganized, and frequently unintelligible speech. Accelerated speech is not always present, but an impairment in formulating language almost always is. (D. A. Daly, 1992, p. 107)

In contrast to persons who stutter, many persons who clutter are also said to struggle academically and are unaware of how unintelligible and abnormal their speech sounds to their listener.

Examples of Some Phenomena Associated with Stuttering

The disorder of stuttering has intrigued scholars for centuries. For example, research over the decades has shown (1) there are several conditions of speaking in which stuttering is suddenly reduced or absent; (2) stuttering occurs nearly equally between the sexes in the early years of childhood; however, males eventually come to greatly outnumber females in the adolescent and adult years; (3) stuttering occurs more often in children who are twins; (4) the onset of stuttering usually occurs in early childhood, between the ages of 2 and 5, a time when the child is stringing many words together to speak in phrases or sentences; (5) in approximately 40 to 60 percent of those who stutter, there is a paternal or maternal relative who stutters or has recovered from stuttering; (6) there are several conditions or speaking situations wherein stuttering increases; and (7) stuttering occurs more in children who are bilingual. (See Figure 7.2.)

Contemporary theories that attempt to explain the cause of stuttering need to address the many conditions of speaking when most stutterers stutter significantly less or not at all. Such speaking events are referred as *fluency-enhancing conditions* or *novel conditions*. W. Johnson and Rosen (1937) identified scores of such speaking conditions. Several of those eliciting the greatest reduction in stuttering have been examined by researchers and include the following:

singing, reading in chorus or unison with another person, speaking at a whisper, speaking to young children, speaking under the influence of a loud masking noise, speaking at a higher or lower than normal pitch, speaking in a

FIGURE 7.2

Phenomena associated with stuttering.

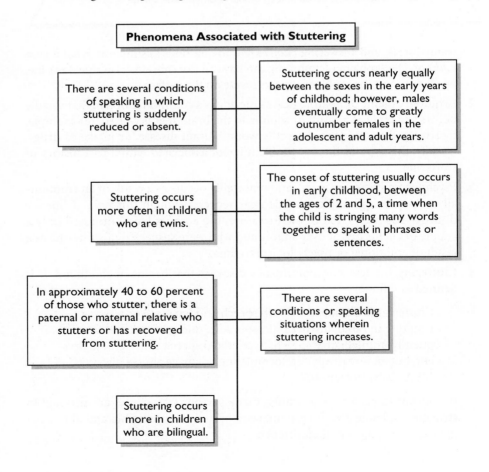

monotone, speaking to the rhythmic beat of a metronome and speaking under the influence of delayed auditory feedback.

All of the aforementioned fluency-enhancing conditions appear to facilitate a physical change in the manner of the speech of the person who stutters. For example, several of the conditions induce the person who stutters to speak more slowly, allowing more time for the complex motoric action of respiration, vocalization, and articulation. Several other conditions create an increase or decrease in loudness and pitch. In all of these fluency-creating conditions, the person who stutters is induced to change his manner of speaking or forces himself to consciously alter the usual manner of speaking to comply with the examiner's instructions to speak at a different pitch, in a whisper, and so on. Some researchers have speculated that such a physical change in vocalization somehow overrides the stuttering trigger, otherwise evident during normal speech. It is important for contemporary theorists of stuttering to attempt to account for the significant increase in fluency experienced by the vast majority of persons who stutter as they speak in these conditions. These phenomena represent one of the few ways in which persons who stutter respond similarly.

Males Who Stutter Eventually Outnumber Females   For nearly a century, it has been well established that more males stutter than females. The gender ratio has stood at approximately three to five males for every female who stutters (Bloodstein & Bernstein Ratner, 2007; Van Riper, 1982). While this is true in later childhood and adulthood, it is not the whole story. The reality is that in early childhood, near the time of stuttering onset, the gender ratio is almost equal (Kloth, Janssen, Kraaimaat, & Brutten, 1995; Yairi, 1983). Males gradually come to outnumber females because young girls are more likely to spontaneously recover. Why the later gender imbalance occurs is unknown. However, researchers have offered several possibilities: (1) The inherited genetic predisposition to stutter may be stronger and more enduring in males, (2) environmental expectations of males may differ and result in males being more likely to continue stuttering past early childhood, and (3) because males have been shown to exhibit more language and articulation problems compared to females, males may also be more susceptible to stuttering persistence.

Twins Have a Higher Prevalence of Stuttering   A child has a greater chance of stuttering if he or she is a twin. Although identical or monozygotic twins show a greater percentage of stuttering in both children, nonidentical or fraternal twins show more of a tendency for only one of the children to stutter. Twin studies tend to support the increasingly popular view that a predisposition for stuttering may be genetically transmitted. In contrast to this view, others postulate that stuttering in twins could result from a slowness in maturation in early development.

Stuttering Usually Begins When the Child Strings Words Together   Stuttering in most children does not begin as they are learning their first words. Instead, the onset is often associated with the child speaking in longer phrases or sentences, usually between ages 2 and 5 (Bloodstein, 1995; Shapiro, 1999), an age range indicative of more complex speech and language development. Although empirical evidence is lacking as to why this is the case, there is speculation as to why onset occurs at a later stage of language development. First, combining words may increase stress to the child's cognitive and/or motor system, creating a breakdown manifested as stuttering behaviors. The cause of stuttering or the *stuttering trigger* may already be present, but is not *pulled* until a certain amount of stress is introduced to the system, which may be the case when speech and language become more complex. Another possibility pertains to the child's negative reaction to otherwise more normal mistakes he naturally makes as speech and language become more complex. The child's stress reactions to what may only be normal nonfluencies may further tense the complex, finely tuned muscles of respiration, phonation, and articulation, creating an exacerbation of the stuttering. This may result in even more frustration, tension, and subsequent stuttering. Although some cases of adult onset of stuttering have been reported, very few persons begin stuttering in adulthood (Van Riper, 1982).

Stuttering Increases in Several Situations   Silverman (2004) outlines several conditions or situations known to be associated with an increase in stuttering severity. Some examples are speaking on the telephone, to large audiences, and to authority figures. Others include telling jokes, saying one's name, and speaking in any situation when speaking fluently is of the utmost importance to the person who stutters. Although Silverman identified other conditions or situations, the previous examples are some of the more common ones. The possible reasons that these conditions seem to elicit more stuttering are logical, but still speculative. Specifically, many of these speaking events represent situations in which the person has stuttered before, often resulting in embarrassment and shame. Remembering this, the person who stutters begins to view speaking in that situation with apprehension, fear, and trepidation. These feelings are likely to increase stress and, as a result, muscular tension, which appears to maintain and often exacerbate stuttering. In this scenario, facing situations in which the person anticipates and fears stuttering tends to lead to more stuttering, creating a vicious cycle of continued anticipation, tension, and consequent stuttering.

More Stuttering Is Found in Children Who Are Bilingual   The higher percentage of stuttering noted in bilingual children may result from "syntactic overload" (Karniol, 1992), or the extra linguistic demands experienced by children learning more than one language. This possibility is further postulated by Benstein Ratner and Benitez (1985) in the discussion in their article on the impact of syntax in the development of stuttering. In short, the learning of language requires an incredibly complex and not fully understood synergy of motor and cognitive interaction and cooperation. Logically then, learning two languages may place increasingly heavy demands on those syntactic systems of young children addressed both by Karniol and by Benstein Ratner and Benitez.

Young children who are expected to speak more than one language tend to be at greater risk for stuttering. Possible reasons for this may include the greater demand placed on the child's motor and cognitive systems. Many experts feel the learning of one language places great demands on a child, so the learning of two or more languages places extreme and unrealistic demands on the functioning systems of children. In turn, the extreme demands on the child's system may cause breakdown manifested as stuttering.

Famous People

There are hundreds of famous people past and present whose lives have been impacted by living with a significant problem of stuttering (see posters from the National

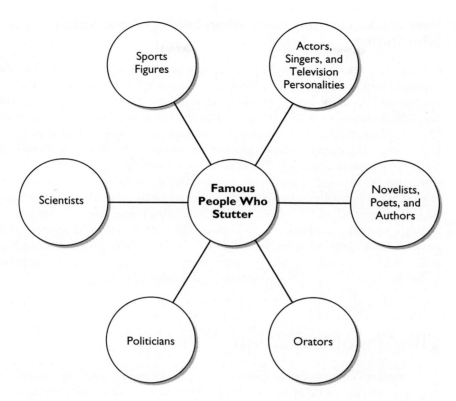

FIGURE 7.3
Famous people who stutter.

Stuttering Association and the Stuttering Foundation). Following are examples of such persons and the origin of their prominence (see Figure 7.3).

1. *Actors, singers, and television personalities:* Nicolas Brendon, James Earl Jones, Peggy Lipton, Robert Merrill, Marilyn Monroe, Anthony Quinn, Eric Roberts, "Scatman" John Larkin, Carly Simon, James Stewart, John Stossel, Mel Tillis, John Lee Hooker, John Melendez, Sam Neill, Jack Paar, and Tom Sizemore.

2. *Novelists, poets, and authors:* Lewis Carroll, Richard Condon, Washington Irving, Henry James, Somerset Maugham, Alan Rabinowitz, Neville Shute, and John Updike.

3. *Orators:* Aristotle and Demosthenes.

4. *Politicians:* Joseph Biden, King George VI of England, Winston Churchill, Claudius, Lenin, Theodore Roosevelt, George Washington, and Frank Wolf.

5. *Scientists:* Charles Darwin and Isaac Newton.

6. *Sport figures:* Lester Hayes, Ron Harper, Bo Jackson, Tommy John, Ben Johnson, Pat Leahy, Bob Love, Greg Luganis, Ken Venturi, Chris Zorich, Robin "Hurricane" Carter, Antonio Dixon, Kenyon Martin, Adrian Peterson, Darren Sproles, Herschel Walker and Tiger Woods.

7. *Other prominent persons:* Aesop, Clara Barton, P. F. Bentley, Erasmus, Henry Mather, and Moses.

Evident by this list is the abundance of accomplished, famous people whose lives have been influenced by stuttering. It is hoped this impressive group should serve to encourage all who stutter to pursue their life interests and dreams.

How Should Listeners React When Talking with a Person Who Stutters?

Often people ask, "What should I do or say when I talk with someone who stutters?" "Should I look away when he is repeating or blocking?" "If I know the word she is stuck on, should I say it for her?" "Should I make affirming comments, such as, 'Take your time,' 'Slow down,' or 'Take a breath'?" The answer to these questions is a resounding "No!" Understandably, well-meaning listeners are often uncomfortable in hearing and seeing someone struggle as he speaks and are unsure as to what they should do or say while the person is stuttering. The best advice we can give is to do what you would do when you are having courteous conversations with normal speakers during your daily routine. That is, maintain normal eye contact and wait patiently for the person to finish before responding. Of course, you will be waiting longer, but do what you do when having a normal conversation with anyone. Although you may be uncomfortable, the person who is stuttering is probably far more so. He is feeling frustrated, embarrassed, and possibly ashamed, but your patience portrays you as an understanding person who knows how to interact with a person struggling with a disability.

Theories of Causation

As with other communication disorders, we can generally classify the numerous theories of stuttering as being based on inheritance, child development, neurosis, and learning and conditioning. These categories of theories overlap somewhat, and a specific theory may fit into more than one category (see Figure 7.4).

Cerebral Dominance Theory

Dysphemic theories view stuttering as a symptom of some inner, underlying, complicating neurophysiological or biological disorder. The Orton-Travis theory of cerebral dominance (Orton & Travis, 1929) is one of the better-known dysphemic theories of the cause of stuttering. It states that a child is predisposed to stutter because neither side of the brain is dominant in controlling the motor activities involved in talking. This theory was of great interest to researchers for many years, eventually falling out of favor due to equivocal research evidence. More recently, however, positron emission tomography (PET) and

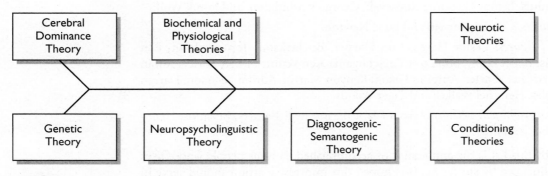

FIGURE 7.4   Theories of causation.

other types of brain imaging research have revealed differences in the brain activity of persons who stutter as compared to that of normal speakers. This recent research has generated renewed interest in this theory and the possibility of a lack of brain dominance or of competing cerebral hemispheres in persons who stutter.

Biochemical and Physiological Theories

West (1958) also viewed stuttering as involving an inherited predisposition. He felt that it was primarily a convulsive disorder, related to epilepsy, with instances of stuttering being seizures that could be triggered by emotional stress. West related his theory to a blood–sugar imbalance observed in persons who stutter while they were stuttering. This theory in particular is associated with a great deal of research on basal metabolism, blood chemistry, brain waves, twinning, and neurophysiological correlates to stuttering.

Related theories have been developed by M. R. Adams (1978); Perkins, Ruder, Johnson, and Michael (1976); and M. Wingate (1969). These researchers discuss the physiological and aerodynamic events occurring in the vocal tract during speech and view stuttering as problems with phonation, respiration, and articulation. Adams, Perkins and colleagues, and Wingate separately discuss the problem in terms of phonetic transitions that make it difficult for the person who stutters to start, time, and sustain airflow and voicing in coordination with articulation. Freeman and Ushijima (1978) suggest both discoordination and excessive tension in the laryngeal area as factors in stuttering, while Conture, McCall, and Brewer (1977) suggest that persons who stutter mismanage their laryngeal activity and that "laryngeal stuttering" covaries with "oral stuttering."

Genetic Theory

It is pointless to attribute the development of any complex trait or behavior solely to the effects of genetics or the environment because all traits develop in some context. Given that the genetic and environmental factors interact, the question is how to determine the relative contributions of each—in this instance, to the problem of stuttering (Kidd, 1977). We have not yet been able to identify or locate a single gene to account for all stuttering, as it is more likely that a number of genes contribute to the manifestation of the disorder. Even as specific genes are located and examined, determining their contribution to the development of stuttering remains difficult because of confounding environmental factors. We do have, however, research models that have been applied to the data on the concentration of stuttering in families. Those data sometimes enable us to predict stuttering and suggest that there may be an important genetic basis for this problem. There is little doubt that stuttering runs in families, and it is logical to conclude that a genetic component influences it (Felsenfeld, 1997). As a result, more empirical genetic research is necessary to increase our understanding of this complex, multidimensional problem. However, because of the methodological complexity of genetic research, investigators who focus on stuttering are often discouraged from conducting this line of study.

Neuropsycholinguistic Theory

In 1991, Perkins, Kent, and Curlee proposed their theory of neuropsycholinguistic function in stuttering. This comprehensive theory addresses the production of fluent speech, stuttered speech, and nonstuttered speech disruptions. Specifically, the production of stuttered speech requires two components called the linguistic or symbol system and the paralinguistic or signal system, each said to be processed separately in the brain and then eventually channeled into a common output system. To produce fluent speech, both components must be synchronously timed and integrated as they converge into the common system. If the components are not in synchrony, a breakdown in fluency results. However, this breakdown is experienced as a loss of control—a true moment of stuttering—by the speaker only if the added factor of time pressure is present. The authors define time pressure as "the speaker's need to begin, continue, or accelerate an utterance." If time pressure is lacking, the resulting breakdown is merely a fleeting nonstuttered disfluency of the kind that most fluent speakers experience now and then.

Another comprehensive neuropsycholinguistic theory was developed by Postma and Kolk (1993). In their view, stuttering stems from a disturbed interaction between phonological encoding (i.e., constructing the phonetic plan for utterances) and verbal self-monitoring (i.e., checking for errors and correcting them if necessary). The monitoring system fasely detects "errors" and then attempts to self-correct by halting or stalling execution of ongoing speech, resulting in stuttering. Future research that addresses the hypotheses of these theorists is needed to determine the strength of their models.

Diagnosogenic-Semantogenic Theory

From 1940 through 1970, perhaps the most widely embraced theory of the cause of stuttering was Wendell Johnson's diagnosogenic-semantogenic theory (Johnson, 1938, 1942, 1944, 1961). This theory has been called a developmental theory (Ainsworth, 1945) and an "anticipatory struggle" theory (Bloodstein, 1995). Following his research and interviews with parents of young stuttering and nonstuttering children, Johnson stated:

> Practically every case of stuttering was originally diagnosed . . . by usually one or both of the child's parents. What these laymen had diagnosed as stuttering was by and large indistinguishable from the hesitation and repetitions known to be characteristic of the normal speech of young children. . . . Stuttering as a definite disorder was found to occur, not before being diagnosed, but after being diagnosed. (1944, pp. 330ff)

In Johnson's view, this diagnosis by the parents creates an environment of "difference" and "handicap." The child soon begins to speak abnormally in response to the parents' anxieties, pressures, help, criticisms, and corrections. Both child and parents respond to the idea of handicap more than to the child's speaking behavior. As Johnson stated so aptly, stuttering begins not in the child's mouth, but in the parent's ear.

This theory inspired a great deal of research. We have a large amount of evidence showing that most normal young children exhibit disfluent speech (D. M. Davis, 1939, 1940; Winitz, 1961). We also know that parents of persons who stutter are sometimes anxious and perfectionistic and have high standards; however, there is some question about the dynamics of the "original diagnosis" (Bloodstein, 1995). And there are serious questions about whether calling attention to disfluency necessarily results in an increase in its frequency (M. Wingate, 1959).

Neurotic Theories

The neurotic theories of the causes of stuttering focus on a number of different personality and psychological attributes of stutterers. Through observation, interviews, projective tests, and paper-and-pencil tests, attempts have been made to understand the personality, psychodynamics, social adjustment, and inner, unconscious needs of the person who stutters. Stuttering has been viewed as a need for oral gratification, a need for anal gratification, a covert expression of hostility, an inhibition of threatening feelings and messages, a fear of castration, repressed aggression and hostility, a device for gaining attention and sympathy, and an excuse for failure. According to these theories, stuttering can become a well-integrated, purposeful defense against some threatening idea. From a psychoanalytic point of view, stuttering acts as a mechanism to repress unwanted or threatening feelings (Abbott, 1947; Barbara, 1954; Travis, 1957).

The reader should know that neurological, genetic, and behavioral findings of the past several decades have largely discredited these views. Many neurotic theories were popularized in the heyday of psychoanalysis and have since been shown to be poorly supported by scientific evidence; therefore, they are not well regarded by most professionals in the field of stuttering today.

Conditioning Theories

Any reader who has taken an introductory psychology course will be familiar with the two mechanisms of associative learning; *classical* and *operant conditioning*. *Classical conditioning* involves pairing an unconditioned stimulus, such as a bowl of food that evokes a physical response, with a neutral stimulus, such as a bell that does not evoke a response. When these two stimuli are repeatedly paired, they eventually become associated with each other, and the organism comes to produce a behavioral response to the formerly neutral stimulus. When applied to stuttering, classical conditioning theories do an excellent job of explaining how the disorder can worsen over time. These theories suggest that early breakdowns in speech fluency gradually become associated with the speaker's anxiety about talking. The embarrassment and shame that naturally result from stuttering (the *unconditioned stimulus*) become linked to the listener or setting or word that evoked no reaction in the beginning (the *neutral stimulus*). After some time, the person will stutter in any anxiety-provoking situation that has caused him trouble in the past; the stuttering becomes classically conditioned. Brutten and Shoemaker (1967) formulated a two-factor theory of stuttering based on learning principles. They theorized that most speech disruptions are triggered by autonomic fear reactions, which are classically conditioned responses to factors that have precipitated stuttering in the past: specific environments, individuals, conversation topics, and so on. They view the nonspeech behaviors of persons who stutter (the muscular tension, blinking eyes, grimaces, etc.) as being operantly conditioned behaviors designed to avoid or escape from moments of stuttering.

Operant conditioning involves modifying a behavior through consequences that occur immediately after it. Behaviors can be encouraged through *reinforcement*, or they can be lessened through *punishment* (it is important to remember that punishment in this context does not necessarily imply something negative; it is merely a consequence that causes a decrease in a behavior). Flanagan, Goldiamond, and Azrin (1958) demonstrated that stuttering responded very predictably to procedures that rewarded or discouraged the behavior, showing that it could be increased or decreased in the laboratory as a function of its consequences. As an example of this principle in action, a child can be made to stutter less often if his fluent speech is rewarded with a token such as a sticker (*reinforcement*) or if he is asked to go back and correct a disfluency (*punishment*).

Focus of Contemporary Research in Stuttering

We have highlighted several theories of stuttering causality put forward by researchers over the years. Each one is supported by varying degrees of evidence and offers insights into the complex and often puzzling nature of the disorder. Collectively, the theories have focused on such factors as articulatory control, inheritance, language abilities, familial dynamics, and learned behaviors. All of these are important contributors to any person's particular stuttering pattern and rightfully continue to be studied by modern researchers. However, at the vanguard of current research into the underlying cause(s) of stuttering are two areas: neuroimaging and early childhood stuttering.

Contemporary neuroimaging research has allowed scientists to probe speech-relevant areas using powerful technologies that measure neural activity and intake detailed images of the brain. There is a great deal of evidence showing differences between persons who stutter and fluent speakers. Since we cannot relate all of the relevant information on this topic, the interested reader is encouraged to read the following papers: Alm (2004); Chang, Erickson, Ambrose, Hasegowa-Johnson, and Ludlaw (2008), and Pollard, Ellis, Finan, and Ramig (2009). This is exciting research that is helping establish a strong base of physiological evidence against which to test past and present theories of stuttering.

The results from these efforts have shed much light on the neural correlates of stuttering. For instance, compared to controls, persons who stutter reliably show differences in the structure and function of brain regions that process auditory input, including one's own speech. Regarding the cerebral dominance theory mentioned earlier, current research suggests that many persons who stutter do in fact have atypical lateralization for speech and language processes, relying more heavily on right-sided areas than their fluent counterparts. Those who stutter also appear to have impaired communication between speech-language brain regions as well as abnormal anatomy of those structures. There is recent neurological evidence to corroborate the behavioral deficits in phonation, breathing, and articulation found by previous researchers. This newer evidence has shown abnormalities in brain regions that coordinate speech movements, such as the inferior frontal cortex and the cerebellum. Lastly, linguistic theories of stuttering have received some neurological support through modern findings indicating that brain regions controlling certain aspects of language like sentence processing and lexical access may function differently in persons who stutter.

Research on the onset of stuttering has also been a hot topic in recent years. To quote two prominent experts in this area, "Although stuttering affects a substantial number of people across a wide age range . . . it is a disorder that triumphs in early childhood" (Yairi & Ambrose, 2005, p. 6). Indeed, considering how many more children show signs of stuttering than adults, it is surprising how little we know about the disorder near its onset. Research on early childhood stuttering is currently focused on exploring issues of temperament, distinguishing stuttering warning signs from typical speech and language development, and differentiating between children who will recover and those who are more likely to persist.

As one might expect, these two areas of inquiry are interconnected. Nearly all of the neurological research on stuttering has been performed on adults, leaving questions related to early childhood stuttering largely unanswered for the moment. We still know very little about the nervous systems of children who stutter. Do their brains resemble those of adult persons who stutter, or are developmental and/or practice-induced changes responsible for the differences seen in recent studies? These questions are beginning to be addressed as neuroimaging techniques improve and interest in early childhood stuttering grows.

The Speech-Language Pathologist's Role in Treating Persons Who Stutter Who Come from Different Cultural and Ethnic Backgrounds

Every person is a unique individual. As speech-language clinicians, we must be aware not only of the speech and/or language concerns of our clients, but also of differences they may bring related to their cultural and ethnic background. The best rapport and treatment efficacy are built by the professional who takes the time to learn of differences so as to best interact and relate to the client.

Battle (1998) lists several very important factors to consider when treating persons from different cultural and ethnic backgrounds (see Figure 7.5). These factors also apply to clinicians in their treatment of persons who stutter who come from culturally and ethnically diverse backgrounds. Battle cautions readers to consider the following:

1. Use the name that the culture uses to describe its members. For example, use Chinese when referring to a client from China, not Asian or Oriental.

2. When describing a person who is nonwhite, avoid overgeneralizing by using a term such as *minority*. This term may not be understood by its intended meaning of coming from a population of less than 50 percent. In contrast, it could be interpreted to mean something more demeaning.

3. Do not use terms such as *culturally deprived* or *culturally disadvantaged*, which may have negative connotations to the person coming from a diverse cultural or ethnic background.

4. Be aware of the role of appropriate styles of greeting, the role of touch, and the role of distance between persons when communicating. In some cultures, violation of these styles may place barriers between communicators.

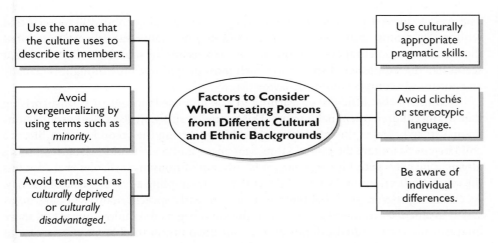

FIGURE 7.5

Factors to consider when treating persons from different cultural or ethnic backgrounds.

   5. Avoid using clichés or language that may be interpreted as reinforcing ethnic stereotypes.

   6. Be aware of individual differences and avoid using stereotypic language that implies people from a specific culture are alike.

When the clinician is not aware of the above factors described by Battle, the efficacy of intervention may be limited or nonexistent.

Shames (1989) reports that "therapy often becomes an intercultural collision of values, attitudes, expectations, and definitions." According to Leith and Mims (1975), misunderstanding cultural differences leads to a high early termination rate for African Americans treated for stuttering. Further, Taylor (1986a) reports that there is a tendency for a large percentage of cultural and ethnic populations who stutter to not seek treatment at all.

How stuttering and the person who stutters are perceived in his culture often impacts treatment efficacy. For example, African-American culture places importance on verbal ability (Leith & Mims, 1975). Those with less proficiency are often viewed with intolerance by their peers. This may be why Leith and Mims found that African-American persons who stutter often attempt to hide and mask their stuttering more than do their Caucasian counterparts, who, in comparison, generally tended to stutter more overtly and speak more often. This finding suggests that stuttering in African-American cultures may be viewed with less tolerance than in the Caucasian community.

Bloodstein (1995) presents the prevalence of stuttering in schoolchildren in other countries. His review of the literature reveals a higher percentage of reported stuttering in some cultures as compared to others. For example, more cases of stuttering are seen in children living in Belgium, Tasmania, Bulgaria, and the British West Indies. In contrast, he reported substantially less stuttering in Denmark, Vienna, Prague, and the United States. Why these differences occur is unknown; however, some researchers speculate that factors such as socioeconomic status, home environment, and genetics may intermingle to play a contributing role in the differences in the prevalence of stuttering in some cultures.

Normal Disfluency

The average speaker produces 14 phonemes per second, using about 100 muscles that require 100 motor units apiece. Lenneberg (1967) has conservatively estimated that there are 140,000 neural events required for each second of speech production. What seems like the simple act of speech to which most people give little thought is actually an enormously complex motor behavior.

Because of the difficulty of learning to talk and use language, it is unsurprising that young children often make errors. This normal disfluency, also called normal nonfluency, may begin in the infant's early babbling. During the second year of life, the child begins to imitate the rate, rhythm, sequences, and melody of his language, using *jargon* as he plays with his voice. Jargon is a stream of nonsense syllables that contains the correct inflections and stress of the language, resembling adult patterns of fluency. As children progress from babbling to jargon to early speech, many will have occasional disfluencies in their speech. When the child begins to employ longer and more linguistically complicated utterances, it is not uncommon to observe an increase in these normal nonfluencies. This typically occurs around the ages of 2 and 3 years and is characterized by an increase in revisions, pauses, and effortless repetitions of words and syllables. Most children will go through a period of disfluency as they grapple with learning the challenging motor and linguistic skills necessary for speech. The length of this process varies from child to child—lasting weeks, months, or longer and decreasing significantly as they develop. It is important to state, however, that normal nonfluencies persist to at least a nominal degree in all people regardless of age.

The Development of Stuttering

Bloodstein (1960a, 1960b) describes four developmental phases of stuttering (see Figure 7.6). These phases may overlap, and there is a great deal of individual variation. In its earliest phase, phase 1, the stuttering is episodic, occurring most often when the child is upset, has a great deal to say, or is under pressure to communicate. The stuttering is characterized mostly by repetitions of words or syllables at the beginning of an utterance, on function as well as content words. In this phase, the child usually shows little concern about or reaction to the speech disfluencies.

In phase 2, the stuttering has become more chronic, and the child thinks of himself as a person who stutters. The stuttering occurs on the major parts of speech, increasing under conditions of excitement or rapid speech. The child still shows little concern about his difficulties in talking. This phase is usually characteristic of elementary school children.

In phase 3, the stuttering may vary with specific situations. The child who stutters may regard certain sounds and words as more difficult than others. He may avoid saying certain words and substitute easier words in their place. There is little avoidance of talking situations and no outward evidence of embarrassment. The child may show the beginnings of anticipatory stuttering, however, and react with irritation to his difficulty.

In phase 4, the person who stutters fearfully anticipates stuttering; fears words, sounds, and situations; makes frequent word substitutions; avoids speech situations; and feels afraid, embarrassed, and helpless. This phase is usually seen in late adolescence and adulthood.

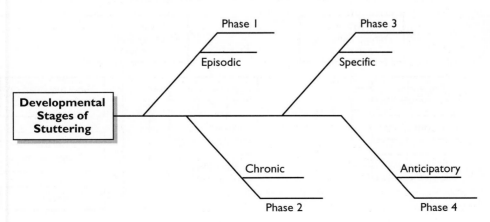

FIGURE 7.6
Developmental stages of stuttering.

The Powerful Need to Avoid Stuttering

As the reader now knows, the experience of stuttering often has a significantly negative impact on the life and the feelings of the person who stutters. The feelings of frustration, embarrassment, fear of speaking, and shame at not being able to say what one wants to say when one wants to say it can cause a person to feel less competent, alone, abnormal, misunderstood, and bewildered. All and all, it makes a person feel different, a feeling we all find unacceptable.

As a result of this experience, stutterers do what anyone would do to try to escape an unpleasant experience: The feelings of frustration, embarrassment, fear of speaking, and shame at not being able to say what one wants to say when one wants to say it can take a huge emotional toll. They can make a person feel incompetent, alone, and bewildered. Altogether, stuttering makes a person feel different and separated from his peers; a feeling we all find unacceptable. Although it is understandable why stutterers want to avoid the negative experiences and feelings associated with stuttering, it is, unfortunately, that which they do to avoid unpleasantness that can actually maintain and even worsen the problem. The avoidances they use, also called *accessory* or *secondary* strategies, are learned behaviors that result from their often fruitless attempts to avoid the blocking and repeating and prolonging of sounds, syllables, and words. It's these that make up the stuttering and are considered the *core behaviors* (see Figure 7.7), or the behaviors that many researchers feel are the direct result of the neurological cause of stuttering. The accessory, or secondary, strategies are those avoidances that stutterers then adopt (learn) in their attempts to lessen or avoid the negative experience of stuttering. Typically, most young children beginning to stutter do not begin to use these learned patterns until they begin to react to the core behaviors they are experiencing.

Van Riper (1973) described several types of avoidance used by children and adults who stutter. Some of the more common ones are as follows:

> **Postponement** is a temporal delay used by the person who stutters as he or she attempts to speak. This delay takes the form of vocal behaviors (e.g., "Um-um-um-um-um-um let's go to the movie") or nonvocal behaviors (e.g., moving the head back and forth several times prior to beginning the first word of a sentence).

FIGURE 7.7

Stuttering behaviors.

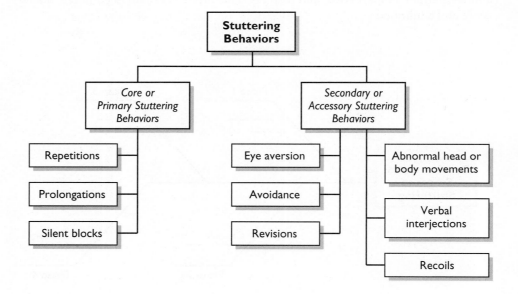

Another example of a postponement behavior could be "Tony and I . . . Tony and I . . . Tony and I . . . Tony and I . . . Tony . . . Tony . . . um . . . ah . . . ah went to Aspen this . . . um . . . um . . . weekend." Postponements, like all avoidance patterns, occur because of the anxiety and fear felt when stuttering is anticipated or when in the actual moment of blocking, repeating, or prolonging.

Starters are another form of trick or avoidance. They can take the form of postponements, but differ some in that they are used to facilitate movement or release from a stuttering block, while postponements are used to try not to stutter. So this type of learned avoidance pattern typically occurs once the stutterer is already in the throes of stuttering. Often the person attempts to time trying to say a word with a sudden movement of the body such as a head or jaw jerk, or he may use stereotyped utterances to get a running start on a difficult word.

Substitution, another type of behavior used to avoid or minimize stuttering, involves replacing one word with another. This strategy of using a synonyn is usually implemented in attempts to completely avoid anticipated or upcoming stuttering, but may also be used as a way of trying to get out of stuttering as it is happening.

Circumlocution is another common strategy wherein the person uses additional words and/or rearranges word order in attempts to get around anticipated or actual in-the-moment stuttering. For example, if a person wants to say, "I want to go shopping with Tanya today," he may, in attempts to "dance" around stuttering, say something that might sound illogical like this: "Today, you know, I and Tanya shop we went over there at the mall."

All of the foregoing reactions are common strategies that the person who stutters uses in response to the anticipation of stuttering or the actual occurrence of stuttering. They are used in an attempt to minimize or completely avoid the unpleasantness of being disfluent. Unfortunately, more often than not, these learned attempts to lessen the amount and severity of stuttering do the opposite, actually increasing the stuttering as well as the appearance of abnormality to the listener.

The Assessment Process

There is no one right way to assess a stuttering problem. The choice of tactics will vary with the problems presented by the person who stutters. These may vary from person to person, with the theoretical and professional training of the speech-language pathologist and with the interpersonal styles of both participants.

The diagnosis of stuttering requires a sensitivity to many factors. Diagnosis is not just a determination that a child repeats words or parts of words, hesitates, or prolongs or struggles with a sound. It is also important to determine the history of these patterns, their severity compared to typically fluent children, and their consistency across different situations. This information will help to differentiate between normal disfluency and stuttering.

Distinguishing between these two clinical entities is the major task of the diagnostician. During speech development, it is expected that young children will exhibit breaks in the rhythm of their speech, resulting in various forms of disfluency. This is a normal aspect of learning to talk and is not a problem requiring professional intervention. But differentiating between normal disfluency and true stuttering can be difficult. For instance, a child's disfluency may be associated with environmental pressure at home. In this case, the differentiating factors may reside in the child's home environment, and the clinician would need to assess that setting. A child should not be expected to outgrow a highly pressurized environment, and in these cases, professional intervention focused on reducing exacerbating stress at home may be warranted.

There are many protocols for examining the characteristics of a child's speech that help the clinician discriminate stuttering from normal disfluency. M. R. Adams (1980) states that the child who can be considered normally disfluent has nine or fewer disfluencies per 100 words uttered, primarily emits whole-word and phrase repetitions as well as revisions, shows no effort or tension when initiating an utterance, and does not substitute the schwa for the appropriate vowel in part–word repetitions (e.g., says *buh-buh-baby* rather than *ba-ba-baby*).

Curlee (1980), in a review that cited Van Riper (1982), suggested the following criteria as indicative of a stuttering problem:

1. Part–word repetitions of two or more units per repetition on 2 percent or more of the words uttered; an increased tempo of repetitions and use of the schwa for vowels in the word as well as vocal tension.

2. Prolongations longer than 1 second on 2 percent or more of the words uttered; abrupt termination of prolongations and increases in pitch and loudness.

3. Involuntary blockings or hesitations longer than 2 seconds in the flow of speech.

4. Body movements, eye blinks, lip and jaw tremors, and signs of struggle that are associated with disfluencies.

5. Emotional reactions and avoidance behaviors associated with speaking.

6. Use of speech as a reason for poor performance.

7. Variations in frequency and severity of speech disruptions with changes in speaking situations.

These seven criteria have generally been employed, and one or more of these behaviors are commonly observed and differentiate stuttering from normal disfluency.

P. R. Ramig (1994), in his handouts to parents and teachers, lists nine observable danger or warning signs in a child exhibiting disfluent speech (see Figure 7.8). He feels

FIGURE 7.8

Stuttering warning signs.

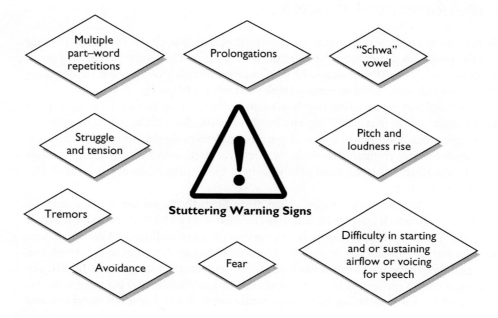

Multiple part–word repetitions

Prolongations

"Schwa" vowel

Struggle and tension

Pitch and loudness rise

Tremors

Stuttering Warning Signs

Avoidance

Fear

Difficulty in starting and or sustaining airflow or voicing for speech observation of one or more of these signs necessitates evaluation of the child by a speech-language pathologist knowledgeable in stuttering. His strict criteria are based on the belief that proper identification of the child at an early age is essential to preventing what could otherwise develop into a disabling, lifelong stuttering problem. Ramig emphasizes the necessity for intervening with the parents and child before the child's stuttering becomes characterized by persistent struggle and tension and the youngster begins to view himself as a person who is different from other children. Similarity exists between Van Riper's suggestions cited by Curlee (1980) and the following list offered by Ramig:

Stuttering Danger or Warning Signs

1. *Multiple part–word repetitions*—repeating the first letter or syllable of a word, such as *t-t-t-table* or *ta-ta-ta-table.*

2. *Prolongations*—stretching out a sound, such as *r———abbit.*

3. *"Schwa" vowel*—inserting a weak, neutral (schwa in German) vowel, such as *buh-buh-buh-baby* in place of *bay-bay-bay-baby.*

4. *Struggle and tension*—struggling and forcing in attempts to speak, especially at the beginning of sentences. Muscular tension may be apparent in the lip and neck area as the child attempts to talk, and actual ongoing speech may sound strained or tense.

5. *Pitch and loudness rise*—pitch and volume increase momentarily while repeating and/or prolonging sounds, syllables, or words.

6. *Tremors*—fleeting quivering of the lips and/or tongue may occur as the child blocks, repeats, or prolongs sounds or syllables.

7. *Avoidance*—as the child becomes more concerned and frustrated by his speech, he may display an unusual number of pauses; substitutions of words; interjection of extraneous sounds, words, or phrases; and avoidance of talking.

8. *Fear*—as the child becomes more aware of and embarrassed by his speech, he may begin to display an expression of fear as he anticipates or experiences stuttering.

9. *Difficulty in starting and/or sustaining airflow or voicing for speech*—heard most often as the child begins to speak at the beginning of sentences or after natural pause boundaries within sentences. Breathing may be irregular, and speech may occur in spurts as the child struggles to keep his voice "on."

It is common to hear clinicians ask questions such as the following:

- In your own words can you tell me why you are here today?
- What aspects of Jason's speech concern you the most?
- When did you first notice he was stuttering?
- What did you hear that made you realize it was stuttering?
- How did he then, and does he now, react to stuttering?
- How did you and other family members react?
- Do any other family members stutter?

These are examples of questions asked during an initial evaluation of stuttering. They are intended to tap an important source of information: the observations that parents make during daily contact with their child. While parents are an excellent source of information about a child's stuttering patterns, direct observation of the child must also be included in any assessment. With direct observation, we need not worry about the memory lapses of parents, their distortions of the extent of the problem, or intervening theoretical interpretations by previous speech-language pathologists. However, if we limit our assessment to merely observing current behaviors, we might lose the overall historical development of the problem and long-term patterns of behaving, feeling, and interacting. This is why both sources of information are needed to provide a more complete picture of the disorder.

Even with information gleaned from direct observation and parents' recollections, any assessment procedure is at best a short-term compromise. Since we cannot observe everything that is currently happening or go back in time to watch the problem develop, we try to sample as best we can the client's and family's behaviors, interactions, and personalities during the brief evaluation session. We do this with direct observation, interviews, and tests, trying to capture representative and pertinent dimensions of the problem. Most of the time, this process of substituting small snapshots for long-term observation is recognized as a necessary compromise. Good speech-language pathologists view assessment as a long-term, ongoing process, continuing after the initial visit and into therapy. They incorporate what is learned initially with information gained during the therapy process.

Description of the Problem and Baseline Measurement

The evaluation of the person who stutters includes two components: (1) a description of the disordered behaviors and (2) an assessment of the impact of stuttering on the person's life. The first category can be tackled through objective measures of the person's speech patterns. Many clinicians tally the frequency and type of disfluencies exhibited during spontaneous speech and oral reading. Other behavioral baselines include measures of speech rate and naturalness as well as counts and descriptions of secondary symptoms such as head jerks, eye movements, and tension in the speech muscles. These measurements combine to give us a picture of the overt severity of the problem that can be transferred to a rating scale and categorized with terms like *mild*, *moderate*, or *severe*.

The covert, or hidden, components of stuttering can often impact the person's life as much as or more than the surface speech behaviors we observe. To get at these factors, the clinician must use other instruments. The interview is the primary method for gathering information about the client's history and current functioning. An interview with the client or family is intended to provide useful information about how stuttering has impacted the client's social, school, and/or vocational life as well as his self-concept. The interview will also include a general medical history and many questions related to the client's or parents' perception of the stuttering problem. These questions might include the following: What behaviors do you call stuttering? Why do you think you stutter? In what situations do you have the most difficulty with stuttering? There are also several questionnaires the clinician can use to probe the largely unobservable symptoms of stuttering. These symptoms include the client's emotional and cognitive reactions to stuttering or his expectancy to stutter, secret avoidance patterns, and quality-of-life issues.

The baseline data should be used throughout the therapy process to monitor the effectiveness of the treatment. Since accurate progress monitoring is an important part of treating any communication disorder, it is crucial that the clinician be conscientious and thorough when collecting these data.

Prognosis and Treatment Plan

Once the clinician has a good estimate of the totality of the stuttering disorder, she can use the baseline measures to help determine the client's prognosis. Questions about prognosis are usually some of the first ones raised by prospective clients or their parents. Although questions about the chances of success and the length and cost of therapy are of vital importance to most people seeking stuttering therapy, they are often difficult to answer with any precision. Each person will progress through the therapeutic process differently. Generally, the longer the person has been stuttering and the more stuttering has become incorporated into his identity, the more tentative the prognosis, as years of struggling with the disorder often leave one with deeply ingrained patterns of behaving and thinking that are resistant to change. However, a sense of self-determination, tolerance of stress, willingness to take risks, and supportive home environment all bode well for a positive outcome.

During the assessment, the clinician determines a general treatment plan. For some younger children, she may plan to spend a great deal of time with the parents in the home and clinic. The goal may be to alter the child's environment rather than directly treating the child. For others, she may implement both environmental manipulation and direct treatment of the child's speech. For older clients, the primary and secondary symptoms of stuttering will need to be targeted directly, and often emotional and cognitive aspects of stuttering will have to be addressed as well. Regardless of the client's age, the professional should describe the proposed treatment outline as completely as possible, allowing the client (or the parents) the opportunity to make an informed decision as to whether to enroll in therapy.

Therapy for Stuttering

There are probably as many perspectives toward therapy for stuttering as toward its causation. Some of our ideas have changed, while others have remained fairly constant over time. As you might expect, the ideas that have remained constant are generally those that have proved to be effective. In general, the approach to treatment will depend first and foremost on the age of the person who stutters; different techniques are often used for young children who are just developing the problem than for adolescents and adults who have had fluency problems (and often unsuccessful therapy) for years.

In our discussion of treatment, we will first briefly describe the major schools of thought on treating children and adults who stutter: (1) fluency-shaping therapy, (2) stuttering modification therapy, (3) integration of fluency-shaping and stuttering modification therapies, (4) electronic devices, and (5) parent-directed intervention (see Figure 7.9).

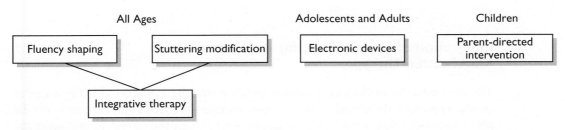

FIGURE 7.9 Types of treatment available for stuttering.

Fluency-Shaping Therapy

This type of treatment involves decreasing the occurrence of stuttered speech. The major goal is for the client to learn to speak more fluently (see Figures 7.10 and 7.11). One way to accomplish this goal is to structure treatment so the client produces short utterances that are free of stuttering, typically at the syllable or one-word level at first. The clinician reinforces the fluency and seeks to eliminate the stuttering. As the client becomes more successful, the complexity and length of the utterances are increased. Fluency-shaping strategies aim to alter the client's habitual speech patterns in ways that are incompatible with stuttering. This can be accomplished through learning to easily and slowly turn on the vocal folds, properly manage one's breath stream before and during the act of speaking, gently use the articulators, and dramatically reduce one's rate of speech. The slow, sometimes robotic-sounding speech resulting from these procedures is then gradually shaped to approximate more-normal-sounding speech. With guidance from the clinician, the client finally begins to generalize his fluency to the outside world and use it in everyday life.

Stuttering Modification Therapy

In this approach to treatment, the client learns to stutter in an easier, more controlled manner (see Figures 7.10 and 7.11). Rather than attempting to eliminate stuttering, the major goals are for the client to confront fears and avoidances, modify his disfluencies so that they are less conspicuous, and maintain control of his speech during instances of stuttering. The focus of this therapy is on changing not only how one stutters, but also how one reacts to stuttering. This is accomplished through directly targeting the feelings of anxiety, embarrassment, and frustration that exacerbate the stuttering problem. A common method for lessening these contributing factors is called desensitization. Desensitization is a systematic process whereby feared situations are confronted so that one's tolerance of stress can be increased. This can be done through myriad activities, including disclosing to others that you are a stutterer and are working on your speech, choosing to stutter on purpose (i.e., pseudostuttering), and maintaining eye contact during instances of stuttering. Along with improving how the client handles stress, other techniques are taught that help the client learn to stutter in a less abnormal fashion. Such techniques include putting slow, controlled repetitions into one's speech (i.e., easy bouncing); drawing out a sound with no tension (i.e., prolongation); holding onto a moment of stuttering long enough to gain control and move forward with speech (pullout); and repeating a stuttered word by saying it over again in a smooth, controlled fashion (i.e., cancellation/self-correction). As with fluency-shaping treatments, the clinician will aid the client in transferring his newly learned skills from the clinic room out into the real world, with the ultimate goal that the client will be able to manage his speech on his own.

Integration of Fluency-Shaping and Stuttering Modification Therapies

The most effective method of treatment is the one that best suits the client's particular needs. Therefore, the clinician who focuses on one approach exclusively may not be able to provide what is most appropriate for every client she serves. To best serve the widest variety of clients, what is often required is flexibility in treatment design.

One way to be a more adaptable clinician is to integrate fluency-shaping and stuttering modification procedures. Integrative therapy enables the clinician to draw on different aspects from both therapies, depending on the needs of the client (E. B. Cooper & Cooper, 1985; Guitar, 2005; P. R. Ramig & Bennett, 1997). For instance, some clients respond very well to highly structured therapy regimens or prefer using less conspicuous strategies for managing their disfluencies that draw little attention to their disorder. Others may favor a looser therapy protocol, or they may thrive on confrontative activities and prefer using more overt techniques that "advertise" their stuttering. Integrating components of both therapy approaches is becoming more common as clinicians learn the limitations of operating from the perspective that one approach works, or ought to work, for all persons who stutter.

Electronic Devices

There is a long history of using electronic devices to help reduce stuttering. These devices create several types of fluency-enhancing conditions mentioned earlier in the chapter, including delayed auditory feedback, frequency-altered feedback, masking noise, and rhythmic sound. For decades, such devices were useful in the therapy room as adjuncts to stuttering treatment. They were quite large and heavy, however, and often incorporated attached cords and wires, neck bands, or headphones. The cumbersome nature of these earlier machines made their use outside of the clinic unfeasible, as most stutterers reacted negatively to such conspicuous fluency aides.

Several smaller electronic devices have appeared on the market more recently. The most widely known and well researched of these modern fluency aides is the SpeechEasy, introduced in 2001. The SpeechEasy is very small, resembling a digital hearing aid, and it delivers delayed auditory feedback and frequency-altered feedback simultaneously. This causes wearers to essentially hear their voice echoed back to them at an altered pitch. Recent longitudinal research on the SpeechEasy has shown it to be effective in everyday life for some people who stutter (e.g., O'Donnell, Armson, & Kiefte, 2008; Pollard et al., 2009); however, the success figures reported to date by researchers are less than those reported by the developers. It does work for some people by lessening their stuttering and/or increasing their confidence when speaking.

Unfortunately, aside from having clients personally try them out, there is currently no reliable method to determine who might benefit from the SpeechEasy or other electronic devices. What we do know is that some people who stutter find these devices to be more helpful than other, more traditional stuttering therapies they have experienced. Generally, electronic aids should be considered as a viable treatment option for clients who (1) have stuttered for a significant period of time and continue to struggle with the disorder, (2) have a history of unsuccessful stuttering treatment, (3) have busy schedules that preclude regular clinical contact, or (4) live in rural areas where gaining access to a speech-language pathologist is difficult or impossible. If a client decides to pursue this option, it is crucial that he or she undergo an evaluation and fitting by a certified speech-language pathologist who has been trained to fit the device.

Parent-Directed Intervention

As implied by the name, parent-directed programs rely on the parents to provide treatment to their child once they have been trained to do so by a certified speech-language pathologist. The best-known parent-directed intervention for children is the Lidcombe

FIGURE 7.10
Components of fluency-shaping and stuttering modification therapies.

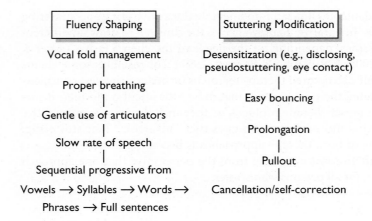

Fluency Shaping

Vocal fold management
|
Proper breathing
|
Gentle use of articulators
|
Slow rate of speech
|
Sequential progressive from

Vowels → Syllables → Words →
Phrases → Full sentences

Stuttering Modification

Desensitization (e.g., disclosing, pseudostuttering, eye contact)
|
Easy bouncing
|
Prolongation
|
Pullout
|
Cancellation/self-correction

FIGURE 7.11
General goals of the two major approaches to stuttering treatment.

Fluency Shaping

– Learn to speak more fluently (i.e., talk without stuttering).
– Establish a basic form of fluency in the clinical setting, reinforce it, and gradually modify it to approximate normal-sounding speech.

Stuttering Modification

– Learn to stutter in an easier, more controlled manner.
– Maintain conscious control of one's speech mechanism during a moment of stuttering.
– Confront tears and extinguish avoidances.

Program, an individualized behavioral approach to stuttering treatment developed by Onslow, Packman, and Harrison (2003). What is most unique about this program is that the parents do the treatment, not the clinician. It is a program that focuses only on stuttering children 6 years of age and younger. Its developers view it as neither a fluency-shaping nor a modification approach, nor an integration of the two treatments. Rather, the primary goal of the Lidcombe Program is to completely rid the child of stuttering. To some, this goal may sound exaggerated and unrealistic; however, as with many other intervention programs focusing only on very young stuttering children, it is not unrealistic to expect this outcome for many.

Intervention for the Young Developing Person Who Stutters

Therapeutic strategies for the preschooler developing stuttering have generally had high success rates. This is likely due to two important factors: (1) Most young children showing signs of stuttering will spontaneously recover on their own, irrespective of treatment, and (2) children just beginning to stutter typically do not display the secondary emotional and cognitive symptoms that aggravate the problem and make it more resistant to treatment. The approaches to intervention for early stuttering fall into the categories of indirect and direct therapy.

Indirect Therapy   While there is some ambiguity in the field of fluency disorders around indirect and direct therapy, we can say that, generally, indirect treatment occurs outside the therapy room and involves decreasing or eliminating stuttering in ways that do not explicitly call the child's attention to his own speech. This can be accomplished through manipulating the child's environment and advising the parents and family on how they can change their interactions with the child to better facilitate fluency in everyday life. With direct treatment, the clinician (or the parents under the guidance of the clinician) regularly sees the child for treatment. This can mean working with the child in a caring and supportive manner to actively his speech patterns, or it can mean modeling fluent speech patterns for the child to follow without his knowledge.

Environmental Manipulation.   Environmental manipulation is a procedure that focuses on altering variables in the child's environmental that are thought to maintain the stuttering. Through observing the child at home and conducting parent and family conferences, the speech-language pathologist tries to identify these factors and change the environment so that they no longer perpetuate the problem. A critical variable when dealing with young children is always the family—which can either reinforce or counteract the efforts of the clinician. Variables that can contribute to stuttering in young children include the following:

1. Increased excitement level in the home
2. Fast-paced activity
3. Communicative stress
4. Social or emotional deprivation
5. Sibling rivalry or competition for talking time
6. Excessive speech interruptions and talking attempts aborted by family members
7. Standards and expectations that are unrealistically high
8. Inconsistent discipline
9. Too much or too little structure for acceptable child behavior
10. Lack of availability of parents
11. Excessive pressure to talk perform
12. Arguing and hostility among members of the family
13. Negative verbal interactions between the child and the family
14. Use of the child as a scapegoat or displacement of family problems onto the child
15. Use of a faster-than-normal speaking rate by one or both parents

Clearly, the list could be much longer. Each of these variables could be potent in maintaining stuttering. And each, if reversed, could help eliminate stuttering. By helping a family become aware of these elements and their effects on the child's fluency, helping each family member to determine his or her own individual influence, and establishing a high priority for changing the child's environment, the speech-language pathologist may be able to reduce or eliminate the stuttering. But to accomplish this, the family has to agree on the goal—to eliminate the child's stuttering. The needs of each of the family members and their direct influences on the child's fluency have to be reconciled with the process of changing the family environment. Often this process opens up new and unexpected problems that relate to the child's speech. It may also lead to interpersonal or psychological problems of the family. The speech-language pathologist should be prepared to deal with these problems or refer the family for appropriate intervention, such as family therapy, marital counseling, or psychological therapy.

Direct Therapy   Direct therapy includes any type of intervention in which the child is taught to alter the way in which he speaks. This kind of treatment is usually carried out within the clinic room by a speech-language pathologist, but can also be administered by the parents during the child's day-to-day life (as with the Lidcombe Program). Regardless of who inhabits the role of therapist, the child could be given a model of what easy, fluent speech sounds like; asked to imitate more fluent ways of speaking; or asked to correct a *disfluency*. The therapist may model a slow rate of speech for the child to copy, giving it an age-appropriate name like "turtle talk." She may openly acknowledge her own disfluencies that she inserts into her speech, calling it "bumpy speech." The child may be asked to imitate the therapist's disfluencies, catch the therapist when her speech gets bumpy, and eventually catch himself when his own speech is disfluent. The child may also be asked to use "stretchy speech" to prolong sounds out in a smooth, relaxed manner. Sometimes the therapist may request that the child say a stuttered word or sentence again by asking him. "Can you say that again using your smooth speech?"

Whatever the specific techniques employed, it is critical when directly working on a young child's stuttering to always maintain an atmosphere of acceptance and good humor. Stuttering treatment should never punitive to the child or become a negative experience, as that can lead to emotional reactivity and physiological arousal that can make the stuttering worse and, ultimately, more difficult to eradicate.

Parent and Family Counseling.   We have just seen that many aspects of the child's environment cut to the core of the family and its individual members. Identifying and ultimately changing some family behavior patterns might well require a close and caring counseling relationship for the group as a whole as well as for its individual members. To meet the final goal, the needs of the family as well as the child must be considered. Parent and family counseling is designed to help family members to understand how their behaviors and feelings interact with those of the person who stutters and to recognize, accept, and act on these feelings.

In some instances, the speech-language pathologist may feel that the speech of the child is within the boundaries of normal disfluency, but the anxieties and concerns of the parents persist. Parent concern is then a legitimate target for therapeutic intervention. The parents, not the child, can become the clients.

Interviewing and counseling skills—as well as knowledge of stuttering, child management, and family dynamics—are prerequisites for this type of therapeutic intervention. The combination of parent and family counseling with environment manipulation and, in some cases, direct treatment of the child probably represents the highest rate of therapeutic success for the problem of stuttering. This success may be due to the short history of the child's stuttering problem and its early form and development.

Therapy for Advanced Stuttering

Advanced stuttering is usually more difficult to treat than early stuttering. Generally, the longer a person has lived with the disorder, the harder it will be to change the behaviors and attitudes that have developed over years of struggling to communicate.

Most people with advanced stuttering have evolved a repertoire of coping strategies to try to handle the problem, and their efforts to talk often include excessive muscular tension, fragmented sentences, and extraneous facial and body movements. They have become painfully aware of their abnormal speech and of others' reactions to it. Given the behavioral and emotional complexities of a problem that feeds on itself, it is unsurprising that therapies for advanced stuttering have vacillated among the mysterious, the complicated, and the straightforward.

Historically, many well-intentioned, but misguided tactics have been used to treat advanced stuttering. These have included putting stones in one's mouth, having surgery to cut the frenulum beneath the tongue, waving one's hand rhythmically in the air, "chewing" one's breath stream, reciting superstitious incantations, and undergoing electric shock. More-modern therapy attempts have involved biofeedback, psychotherapy, counseling, desensitization, deliberate easy stuttering, speech restructuring exercises, and behavioral conditioning techniques. Unfortunately, there is not space within this chapter to discuss these different therapeutic approaches. What the reader should know is that variations in how the problem is treated are in large part due to how stuttering is viewed theoretically by the clinician. If stuttering is seen as a symptom of anxiety, then therapy will focus on reducing anxiety and increasing one's tolerance of stress. If stuttering is seen as an anticipatory struggle, then therapy will deal with the stutterer's expectancies prior to speaking. If it is viewed as being a learned behavior, then treatment will deal with components of the behavioral conditioning model.

General Goals of Therapy   Regardless of the specific methods used, all of the therapies for advanced stuttering share a concern for helping the client learn to communicate effectively and change the quality of his interpersonal relationships. Fluency-shaping therapies take more of a top-down approach to accomplishing these goals. They tend to focus on fine-tuning the mechanics of speech production rather than targeting the emotional and cognitive components of stuttering that maintain the problem. The idea is that, by removing the stuttered speech and allowing the client to accumulate more and more talking time that is free of stuttering, the person's expectations should eventually change from anticipating stuttering to anticipating fluency. This should result in a reduction of speech-related fears and greater comfort in social interactions. Essentially, decrease the stuttering and the emotional and cognitive factors will resolve themselves.

Stuttering modification therapies take a bottom-up approach to attaining the two major goals of treatment. Their primary target is the maladaptive, often distorted attitudes and thoughts that underlie much of the person's disfluent speech and serve to perpetuate the stuttering. This type of treatment allows the client to confront feared situations, such as using the telephone or initiating conversations. Clients work on eliminating behaviors designed to avoid stuttering, as well as abnormal facial and body movements that distract, through strategies like voluntary stuttering and easy controlled stuttering. The philosophy is essentially this: Decrease the fear of stuttering and instill a sense of control over one's speech, and the stuttering will subside dramatically.

Transfer and Maintenance   As many stuttering therapists and clients who have been through treatment know, it is relatively easy to reduce stuttering in the therapy room. Some people have dubbed such circumscribed improvements "clinic room fluency," meaning that genuine, lasting gains have not been made until the skills learned in the clinic can be reliably transferred into the outside world. Often the courage and resolve that operate in the therapy room have to be gingerly moved into real-life situations. This can be a difficult task for some people who stutter. The clinician may have to accompany the individual at first as he engages in real-world encounters using his newly learned communication techniques. Gradually, as the client experiences more successes while speaking to waiters, salespeople, cashiers, and the like, it will become less daunting to carry over skills that were first mastered within the therapy room.

Maintenance refers either to the continued emission of target behaviors or to the continuing experience of desirable feelings and social patters that were acquired during formal therapy. Once stuttering treatment has come to an end, the client needs to maintain the gains that were made during treatment. To do this, he must possess durable patterns of speaking and dealing effectively with disfluencies that can be used across a variety of situations. While very few people with advanced stuttering will ever be completely rid of the disorder, many are able to leave treatment and go on to lead lives in which their disorder plays a negligible role. Unfortunately, research tells us that relapse occurs with alarming and discouraging frequency following most therapies for advanced stuttering. This means that many clients eventually return to their pre-therapy state or substitute new, undesirable behaviors for their old ones. While this is disheartening prospect, it is not inevitable, and much can be done to combat it. For instance, the likelihood of relapse can be decreased if clients are taught how to identify and manage the recurrence of old avoidance patterns and fear responses to stuttering. Clients also need to possess practical techniques for dealing with disfluencies that will inevitably arise after treatment. Building a client's desire and ability to self-monitor their speech on a daily basis also supports long-term success. The clinician who incorporates those components into her therapy is ensuring that the client leaves her care well fortified for the challenges that await all people who stutter.

Prevention

More researchers have begun to examine the issue of prevention of stuttering. Unlike the medical sciences, we cannot immunize children against developing stuttering. From a humanitarian and ethical standpoint, we cannot attempt to cause a child to stutter (even if we knew how) because we are not certain that we could reverse the process. Direct research on the prevention of a problem that may have an environmental base is extremely difficult to conduct. Except for the genetic theory of stuttering, however, most theories imply a message of prevention.

As stated in the previous paragraph, preventing stuttering from occurring continues to be a puzzling problem to many researchers; however, preventing its continuation into adolescence and adulthood has now become a realistic focus of many clinicians and researchers (e.g., Dell, 1996; P. R. Ramig, 1993; P. R. Ramig & Bennett, 1995; Shapiro, 1999; Shine, 1980). Experienced clinicians report that their early intervention focus with children who stutter and/or their families has been the crucial element for pulling the child out of stuttering, thus preventing a problem that, for some, was otherwise destined to become a lifelong frustration.

case study LAURA

When she first came to the clinic, Laura was 30 years old. She was a college graduate, trained as an occupational therapist. She had been married for 10 years and had three children, aged 8, 5, and 2 years. Her husband was a young, successful attorney with offices in a large eastern city some 30 miles from the small urban community in which the family resided. Laura had worked, but never as an occupational therapist. Before her marriage, she had worked for a short time on an assembly line in a factory and as a waitress while in college. She had applied for a job as an occupational therapist only once and was turned down, she felt, because of her speech. She never again applied for such a position. Laura was graceful, poised, mature, and articulate; she would be considered an attractive and sensitive person. She had an open and ready smile for her children and her husband, and an easy and comfortable manner with them. During her first interview, however, we could see the traces of sadness in her face and eyes. She projected a sense of helplessness that elicited a great deal of nurturing from those around her. Two years before, soon after the birth of her third child, she had become extremely depressed and attempted to commit suicide, but it was considered more of a gesture than a bona fide attempt. Her psychiatric therapy was brief and apparently successful. Laura attributed her depression in part to having a severe stuttering problem.

As she related the history of her stuttering, she openly cried when recalling how, in her childhood, her parents had forbidden her to talk when guests were in the home. Her embarrassment, sadness, and anger over these thoughts overwhelmed her. Wherever she went, she carried little index cards on which she had written brief messages as substitutes for oral communication, in case she needed information, was lost, or was in an emergency situation that required communication. She reported that on one occasion, in an airport, she had wandered around for 30 minutes trying to locate a gate and flight without talking or asking for help. She had finally found her destination in silence. She tearfully stated that, because she stuttered, she could never say thank you to people, who, as a result, thought she was rude, aloof, or ungrateful. She never used the phone; depended on her husband for talking, shopping, and so on; and constantly stayed at her husband's side during social outings. She felt she was a failure as the wife of a professional and as a mother. She recognized her overdependence on others and how she had benefited from her own posture of helplessness.

She reported several previous encounters with therapy for her problem. These ranged from parent counseling, psychiatric therapy, and hypnosis to more-traditional speech therapy in schools, hospitals, and universities. She had been in and out of therapy for about twenty five years. Although her hopes for help had been dashed many times, and she carried the scars of many years of disappointment and futility, she was still more hopeful than skeptical. She came in for her initial interview literally pleading for freedom from her agonies, both public and private, about her stuttering.

One could not help but be impressed with her motivation, need for support, and fragility as she was about to initiate still another duel with her problem. It was with this awareness of her and a sense of our own responsibility that we joined her in this clinical relationship.

The brief case report that you just read may seem unusually dramatic. After all, a disorder of fluency—in this case, stuttering—is not typically a matter of life and death. But it is most certainly a matter of the quality of life. Volumes could be filled with horror stories associated with the problem of stuttering. This problem can eat away at one's sense of well-being, personal adequacy, and confidence. The longer it persists, the more it feeds on itself, as people who stutter attempt to hide their problem to avoid social stigma and embarrassment. The joys of life, communicating with other human beings, sharing oneself intimately with loved ones, accepting and valuing oneself—the things that fluent speakers take for granted in their daily lives—can be major crises for a person who stutters. His circumstances at times appear to have no exit, and he often gives up all hope for ever reversing this problem. We see people who are literally choking on their own helplessness.

Some Final Thoughts by a Prodigy of Stuttering

After studying the disorder of stuttering for more than seventy years, the late Dr. Charles Van Riper, considered by many to be the world's leading authority on stuttering, offered in a 1990 article what he referred to as his "final conclusions about stuttering." They are as follows:

- That stuttering is essentially a neuromuscular disorder whose core consists of tiny lags and disruptions in the timing of the complicated movements required for speech.

- That the usual response to these lags is an automatic part–word repetition or prolongation.

- That some children, because of heredity or as yet unknown brain pathology, have more of these than others do.

- That most children who begin to stutter become fluent perhaps because of maturation or because they do not react to their lags, repetitions, or prolongations by struggle or avoidance.

- That those who do struggle or avoid because of frustration or penalties will probably continue to stutter all the rest of their lives no matter what kind of therapy they receive.

- That these struggle and avoidance behaviors are learned and can be modified and unlearned though the lags cannot.

- That the goal of therapy for the confirmed stutterer should not be a reduction in the number of dysfluencies or zero stuttering. Fluency-enhancing procedures can easily result in stutter-free speech temporarily, but maintaining it is almost impossible. The stutterer already knows how to be fluent. What he doesn't know is how to stutter. He can be taught to stutter so easily and briefly that he can have very adequate communication skills. Moreover, when he discovers he can stutter without struggle or avoidance most of his frustration and other negative emotion will subside. (pp. 317–318)

Van Riper's conclusions and his wisdom should not be ignored or dismissed. However, any statement about the cause or treatment of stuttering must account for its variability of form (its many symptoms and behaviors), the sex ratio, and its manipulability, both short- and long-term. It must also reconcile the numerous speaking conditions under which it is reduced or absent as well as increased.

Van Riper offers one type of definition and cause that logically leads to a particular strategy of treatment. But he does not offer data that reconcile the variations of the problem among people who stutter with the implied inevitability, permanence, and nonmanipulativeness of the problem inherent in his observations and conclusions. We need a logic that reconciles these variabilities among persons who stutter.

One such logic may integrate the dynamic and complicated interactions between inheritance factors (and, therefore, all physiologically based predispositions to stutter) and environmental factors.

Another possible logic is one that may offer the variability of stuttering as a dimension of its inherited predisposition. A third logic may offer that there are many different types of people who stutter and different types of stuttering and that their only commonality is the label they carry.

There may be as many different types of persons who stutter as there are different types of people. Each may respond in his own unique way, each with a different outcome relative to the way he talks, feels, believes, and interacts with people and society.

For some persons who stutter, learning to stutter briefly and easily may well be the answer for adequate communication, while for others, the answer may be speech that is more free of stuttering.

Summary

The problem of stuttering continues to present a number of challenges to theorists, researchers, speech-language pathologists, and persons who stutter themselves. The cause of the problem is still not clear. As a result, prevention has received less attention than warranted. The problem has had a history of controversy and inconsistency. Experts have argued and disagreed over its theory, causation, definition, dynamics, measurement, and clinical management. Emerging from all this controversy, however, has been a history of growth and improvement. Some parts of the problem are obvious and available for all to see; other parts are hidden and private. There are many facets to its study, understanding, and management. We can look at its behavioral, physiological, emotional, and interactional components. As these various components of the problem are conceptualized, integrated, and related to broader perspectives in the cognitive, developmental, behavioral, and biomedical sciences, the potential for the ultimate resolution of the problem is accordingly enhanced.

In the study of the problem of stuttering, we must not forget the person who stutters and the daily impact this complex disorder can have. We have tried in this chapter to impress upon our reader the very real human impact. We have learned that for many persons who stutter, effective treatment necessitates providing the client with fluency-shaping skills to replace their stuttering with fluency. For many others, we have learned it is necessary to teach confrontation and modification of the stuttering moment, allowing the client to control how he manifests stuttering. Yet for many other persons who stutter, integrating fluency-shaping and modification techniques may be crucial to successful treatment.

Working with children and adults who stutter can be challenging because of the pervasive personal impact of the disorder on the person. However, we also feel helping those who stutter can be among the most rewarding accomplishments experienced by speech-language clinicians. Many children and adults have experienced dramatic, positive life changes through the help of proficient clinicians of stuttering. As a result, many of those once disabled by their stuttering have learned to become more fluent and more communicative, enabling themselves to experience life without continued disability.

Websites and Mailing Information on Stuttering

The reader is cautioned against assuming that all website information pertaining to the topic of stuttering is presented by certified or professional speech-language pathologists. Certain information on stuttering is offered by persons presenting their own solution to stuttering and information that supports their selling of devices or programs that many professional speech-language pathologists knowledgeable of stuttering may not endorse. Terminology used by website advertisers—such as "stop stuttering," "alleviate stuttering," and "stutter no more"—is misleading because it implies their techniques or devices erase the problem of adult stuttering. The truth is that adult stuttering is rarely cured, as in completely eradicated. The reader is advised to proceed through the vast world of the Internet carefully and with caution and to be alert to those who use it in a manner that could be viewed as exploitive of persons suffering from this embarrassing and frustrating disorder.

The following organizations are located in the United States and can aid the interested consumer in learning more about the nature of stuttering and available services for the treatment of child and adult stuttering. Some of these organizations sell low-cost books, videos, brochures, and so on pertaining to stuttering.

American Speech-Language-Hearing Association, 10801 Rockville Pike, Rockville, MD 20852-3279 www.asha.org/public/speech/disorders/stuttering.htm (phone 800-498-2071)

Friends: The National Association of Young People Who Stutter, 38 South Oyster Bay Road, Syosset, NY 11791, www.friendswhostutter.org (phone 866-866-8335)

Friends Who Stutter, www.friendswhostutter.org

National Stuttering Association, 119 W, 40th Street, 14th Floor, New York, NY 10018, www.nsastutter.org (phone 800-937-8888)

The Stuttering Foundation, 3100 Walnut Grove Road, Suite 603, P.O. Box 11749, Memphis, TN 38111, www.stutteringhelp.org (phone 800-992-9392)

The Stuttering Homepage, created and maintained by Judith Kuster (judith.kuster@mnsu.edu), www.mnsu.edu/comdis/kuster/stutter.html

National Institute on Deafness and Other Communication Disorders, 1 Communication Avenue, Bethesda, MD 20892, www.nidcd.nih.gov/health/voice/stutter.asp (phone 800-241-1044)

STUDY QUESTIONS

1. Discuss the ways in which a theory of the origins and dynamics of stuttering contributes to the management of stuttering.

2. How does therapy for early, preschool stages of stuttering differ from therapy for advanced stuttering in adults?

3. Choose two famous people who have experienced stuttering and give a brief biography of their life.

4. Explore the websites listed above and describe what each site presents regarding stuttering.

PROJECTS

1. Contact the director of a self-help support group in your area for persons who stutter and ask for permission to attend a meeting. Document in writing the format of the meeting, the approximate ages of the attendees, and the topics of discussion. (1) Pay particular attention to attendee reports of types of therapies they are undergoing or have received, and (2) try to gain an understanding of the ways stuttering has impacted their lives.

2. View the movies *A Fish Called Wanda Pan's Labyrinth*, and *My Cousin Vinny*. Report on the depiction of the character in each movie who stutters. How were they treated in each of the movies, and how did the nonstuttering characters in the movies react to them when they stuttered? Compare and contrast the three movies regarding the depiction of the stuttering character in each. As a result of watching these three movies, how might average movie viewers be influenced in ways they view a person who stutters? Do you think the average moviegoer would view a person who stutters in a positive or negative light? Why?

SELECTED READINGS

Bloodstein, O., & Bernstein Ratner, N. (2007). *A handbook on stuttering* (6th ed.). San Diego, CA: Singular.

Conture, E. G., & Curlee, R. F. (2007). *Stuttering and related disorders of fluency* (3rd ed.). New York, NY: Thieme Medical Publishers.

Curlee, R. F., & Siegel, G. M. (Eds.). (1997). *Nature and treatment of stuttering: New directions* (2nd ed.). Boston, MA: Allyn and Bacon.

Hulit, L. M. (1996). *Straight talk on stuttering.* Springfield, IL: Charles Thomas.

Manning, W. H. (2009). *Clinical decision making in fluency disorders* (2nd ed.). San Diego, CA: Singular.

Myers, F. L., & St. Louis, K. O. (Eds.). (1992). *Cluttering: A clinical perspective.* Leicester, England: Far Communications.

Silverman, F. H. (2004). *Stuttering and other fluency disorders.* Long Grove, IL: Waveland Press.

Williams, D. F. (2006). *Stuttering recovery: Personal and empirical perspectives.* Mahwah, NJ: Waveland Press.

Chapter EIGHT

Voice Disorders

Christine Sapienza
University of Florida

Douglas M. Hicks
Cleveland Clinic Foundation

Bari Hoffman Ruddy
University of Central Florida

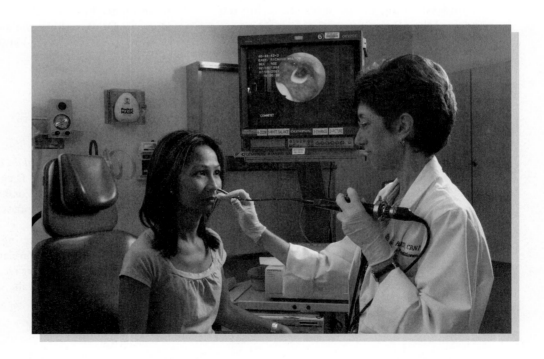

personal PERSPECTIVE

CHRISTINE SAPIENZA

I was born and raised in Buffalo, New York. My parents never went to college; however, my father became a successful computer software and hardware analyst in the banking industry. It was him that I turned to when I was trying to decide what to major in during college at the State University of New York in Buffalo. Before speaking with him, I entered my freshman year majoring in Physical Education. As a high school athlete, that was what I was most comfortable with. Yet, from an intellectual standpoint, I didn't feel challenged and came home confused. I knew that I didn't want my college experience to last more than 4 years; I had better things to do than spend a "lifetime" in school. When I approached my dad with the many career options I had selected from the college handbook as potential jobs, he would offer both the positive and the negative aspects of each. At one point, I said, "How about Speech Pathology?" He said it looked like an intensive program and that the terminating degree was a master's degree. The program looked interesting to me, yet I was less than eager about having to spend 6 years to obtain the required master's degree to practice. Despite my reservations, I decided to sit in on some of the introductory courses during the second semester of my freshman year. It was then that I took Anatomy and Physiology with Dr. Elaine Stathopoulos. Her course fascinated me. It was easy to understand, and she was enthusiastic about her field and dedicated to her research in speech science. I was immediately hooked by such motivation.

When I left SUNY Buffalo to pursue an Assistant Professor position at the University of Florida, I wanted to combine my knowledge of speech science and physiology with clinical practice. The study of the larynx and the respiratory system and its interaction with the etiology of voice disorders fascinated me. I was extremely fortunate to have time with Dr. G. Paul Moore at the University of Florida. He taught me so much about the larynx, the history of laryngology, and voice study. I have now been at the University of Florida for 11 years and have met wonderful people there as well as around the world who have assisted me in studying the voice, its normal production, the nature of disordered voice, and the outcomes of treatment. It has been a very rewarding and fun ride, and I look forward to many more enriching years and giving back to my Ph.D. students what was given to me by the mentors who took the time to educate and train me.

personal PERSPECTIVE

DOUGLAS M. HICKS

Reflecting on my life's journey creates some wonder as to my present career. My earliest (and still private) passion was operating heavy construction vehicles; college held little excitement. However, as early as my freshman year, I met the first of three professional mentors who have greatly influenced what I now do professionally. My undergraduate advisor, Dr. James Rea, was a speech-language pathologist with a passion for clinical care who urged me into the field. My doctoral advisor, Dr. Robert Coleman, introduced me to the challenge of performing arts medicine, a subspecialty in voice disorders, that continues to be a driving clinical/research interest. Former coauthor of this chapter, Dr. Paul Moore, provided me with fruitful collaboration (research and clinical) for almost a decade while I was a professor at the University of Florida. He taught me much about the wonder of the "ultimate instrument," the larynx. After more than a quarter of a century, I have been privileged to work with fine colleagues from various institutions; to teach numerous students from undergraduate to doctoral levels; to uncover some of the mystery of our invisible instrument, the larynx; and to be influenced by decades of patients for whom I have provided care.

I owe each of my mentors an ongoing debt of gratitude.

personal PERSPECTIVE

BARI HOFFMAN RUDDY

My path to my chosen profession was not direct. That is, I did not begin my college experience with a major in communication sciences and disorders in mind. Rather, I began my academic pursuits as a vocal performance major. Growing up in Jupiter, Florida, I enjoyed singing and entertaining, studied classical and musical theater, and participated in community theater and choir, but it always had a strong interest in science and medicine. As I completed my first year in college, I grew disinterested in pursuing vocal performance as a major and began my search for a new one. I was fortunate at the time to seek advice and mentorship from faculty who have become lifelong mentors and friends. Without the strong guidance and support of Drs. David Ingram and Thomas Mullin at the University of Central Florida, I would not have had the opportunities afforded to me in the area of voice science, clinical voice care, and rehabilitation of performance voices. I quickly learned that my background in the performing arts would provide an excellent foundation for learning and training in clinical voice care. Later, during my undergraduate training, I was invited to volunteer and participate in an apprenticeship at a local ear, nose, and throat medical practice that housed a state-of-the-art voice care center. This experience confirmed for me that I had chosen the right course of study. One might say that I had happened upon a perfect combination of both my personal interests and my areas of professional study. And because of this experience, once again, I had the good fortune of meeting another lifelong mentor, Jeffrey J. Lehman, M.D., a laryngologist at The Ear Nose and Throat Surgical Associates (who provided a collaborative environment in which I have had the privilege of practicing for over 10 years). Although pursuing a doctoral degree was not my intent when I began my college experience, the collective mentoring of these distinguished colleagues led me to the laboratory doorsteps of Dr. Christine Sapienza at the University of Florida. My experience in her lab and as a student at the University of Florida was exciting and challenging, shaping my clinical and research skills and leading me to my current career path. My work, which I truly enjoy, combines a perfect combination of teaching and clinical service delivery, affording me the opportunity to bring real-life case examples into the classroom setting.

Description of Voice Disorders

Etiology

Voice problems can impair both speaking and singing. There are three main categories of voice disorders: functional, organic, and neurological. Each type has a different cause and results in different symptoms presented by the patient as well as distinct treatment options that are used to rehabilitate the voice disorder. The specific types of disorders that fall into each of these categories are described later in this chapter. Functional voice disorders are typically the result of particular behaviors a person is doing or a reaction to some organic disease or traumatic event that has placed the larynx in a less than optimal condition: for example, when the physical education teacher has to use her voice loudly to be heard in the gymnasium or the patient must strain the muscles of his larynx because of damage that occurred to one or both of the vocal folds during an operative procedure. Organic voice disorders are caused by some physical condition that has impacted the structure and/or function of the larynx. Neurological voice disorders are a result of an impairment to either the central nervous system (brain and spinal cord) or the peripheral nervous system (cranial nerves). Voice disorders exist among persons of all ages and sometimes are seriously disabling. You hear deviations in people's voices all around you. Start listening to the voice quality produced by some of your acquaintances, or the waitress who serves your lunch, or the store clerks at the mall, or the athletes and broadcasters during interviews on radio or TV, or your own teachers/ professors. Many will have some variety of voice quality deviations.

Characteristics

Voice problems occur when there is difficulty initiating or controlling the voice. As a result, the pitch, loudness, and/or quality suffers. Vocal pitch is controlled by how fast the vocal folds vibrate. Deviations in vocal pitch result in voice that is too high or too low and that does not meet your expectation of the type of voice that should be produced. Another symptom of a voice disorder may be associated with vocal loudness. The loudness level of some voices is too weak; other voices are too loud. Still others have voice quality deviations such as hoarseness or nasality. These kinds of deviations to the pitch, loudness, and quality of the voice are classified as voice disorders. These problems sometimes exist by themselves, but frequently they are combined with other voice or speech problems to form a complex communication disorder. A speech-language pathologist is the person who must be prepared to manage each or all, regardless of their combinations.

Prevalence

Although establishing any percentage is arbitrary, clinical experience suggests a reasonable estimate falls between 6 and 10 percent. Voice disorders can occur in both children and adults, but are recognized more frequently in the adult population. Since these problems rarely interfere with understanding what is said, laypeople pay relatively little attention to most of them. One probable reason is that temporary conditions such as colds, laryngitis, and other upper-respiratory disturbances that cause voice disturbances are so common they are not a source of concern. Unfortunately, the chronic and sometimes serious diseases that affect the same areas and cause the same types of vocal deviations also tend to be ignored. It pays to be cautious and recommend that a person seek an evaluation if the condition lasts for more than a week.

The study and treatment of voice is different from the study and treatment of speech disorders. This has resulted from technological advances that have allowed us to examine the larynx and determine what is causing the voice quality to be different from normal.

Differentiating the Normal from the Abnormal Voice

A voice—whether it is good, poor, or in between—tends to be identified with the person who uses it. For example, there are famous singers who use a deviant voice quality as a trademark. A contrasting attitude is found universally among persons who depend on their voices in their work, like telemarketers, teachers, lawyers, politicians, clerical personnel, and preachers. Each person perceives the severity of a voice disorder differently, and whether a person seeks an evaluation or treatment will depend on how much the voice disorder is affecting daily functioning.

How can voice disorders be recognized? How are they determined? And when is it time to manage them and prescribe treatment? Perhaps the easiest way to get at the question is to try to define the normal voice. Defining normal is difficult because every person has a model of what he or she believes to be the ideal voice quality. Our experience tells us that there are many normal voices. We distinguish the voices of babies, children, adolescents, adult men and women, and aged men and women. Each of these groups has distinctive vocal characteristics. They are different from each other, yet they are normal as long as they meet our expectations for the group. On the other hand, when the pitch, loudness, or quality of a voice differs from that which is customary in the voices of others of the same age, sex, or cultural background, we classify it as deviant or defective. Obviously, the listener's personal criteria, which are derived from training and experience, are the bases for these judgments. Almost everyone will consider an extremely hoarse voice to be defective, but there are many degrees of hoarseness. Where on the continuum from a severely defective voice quality to an excellent voice quality would a particular voice be placed? The listener must make the judgment. Though everyone has a set of criteria for vocal excellence, your evaluation skills will improve with training. Consequently, it is essential that people dealing with speech-language pathology learn to listen definitively. And the listener is first you, the speech-language pathologist; then the patient; and finally others such as the patient's family, friends, and coworkers. There are instruments now available that assist listening by objectively measuring pitch, loudness, and some aspects of quality. These instruments are discussed later in the section on instrumentation.

Assessment

Voice of Subsystems

Understanding the structure and function of the larynx is essential for persons involved in the training or remediation of voice. Read Chapter 3 carefully and note particularly the sections on respiration and phonation. Respiration is critical for providing the power source for vocal fold initiation, and the structures of the larynx modify vocal fold movement in a complex and finely tuned manner. When assessing a person with a voice disorder, it is important not only to examine the function of the larynx, but also to examine the way in which the person is breathing and to consider if there are any breathing problems (asthma, chronic obstructive pulmonary disease) that may be contributing to difficulties with his voice. The manner of articulation can also influence voice production, as can deviant anatomy of the structures in the oral and/or nasal cavities. Assessment of voice requires the clinician to examine breathing, voice, and articulation in order to accurately diagnose the problem.

Breathing

There are many pieces of instrumentation that can be used to assess pulmonary function. Speech-language pathologists may not have access to all of the equipment, but can then rely on the help of respiratory therapists and medical staff in pulmonary medicine if serious question arises about a patient's pulmonary health. If you find yourself not in a setting such as this, there are still ways to assess someone's breathing. First, ask questions about pulmonary health. Ask questions about history of smoking and history of lung problems (cancer, emphysema, asthma) and questions about how breathless the patient feels when walking, talking, and walking and talking. Ask how her breathing feels after walking 100 feet or climbing some stairs. Ask if she feels like she runs out of air when talking. Sometimes it's difficult to determine if the feelings of breathlessness are due to pulmonary issues or due to the larynx not functioning properly. Using thorough interviewing strategies and then carefully examining the larynx together with a thorough account of the patient's medical history should give enough information to differentiate a pulmonary problem from a voice problem. And, if you're still not sure, then make an appropriate referral to a pulmonologist or general physician.

The Voice Disorder

The speech-language pathologist's major objective is to provide effective therapy that will enable individuals with a voice problem to speak more normally or will allow them to function adequately in their daily living. To develop rational therapy, the speech-language pathologist must understand the structure and function of the vocal mechanism and the disorders that may impair that mechanism. The process is best accomplished in conjunction with medical specialists who provide the diagnosis of disordered structure and function of the larynx. Starting therapy without a diagnosis is a lot like starting on an automobile trip in a strange place without a map. It is unethical for a speech-language pathologist to initiate voice therapy without a laryngeal examination and medical diagnosis made. The procedures of assessment and diagnosis of voice disorders are not codified into one best system, but a plan that works reasonably well can be described as having five steps: (1) listening; (2) asking questions—that is, obtaining a history; (3) looking; (4) seeking the help of specialists in other fields as necessary; and (5) assembling the data and establishing a diagnosis, prognosis, and recommendations.

Listening

Earlier in this chapter, you were urged to listen to the voices of your associates and people in your community and to your own voice. The speech-language pathologist's most useful skill is the ability to hear the voice and its associated variations. This capacity enables the speech pathologist to recognize when the pitch goes upward or downward in reference to the musical scale, when the sound is loud or soft, and when the voice quality deviates from normal. This ability to hear, however, does not enable us to measure how much change or deviation is present, and it does not enable us to remember the exact vocal sounds over a period of time. There are a number of manufactured instruments on the market that will precisely display pitch (frequency), loudness (intensity), breath flow, duration, and some of the components of quality to aid the clinician and the client in both diagnosis and therapy (Baken, 1987; Bless & Hicks, 1996; Colton & Casper, 1990; Hirano, 1981; Stemple, 1984). Most of these instruments allow measurement, which means that changes over time can be monitored and compared. The amount of vocal improvement or regression reveals the effectiveness of therapy or, possibly, the progression of disease. New instruments are being developed, and many of them are related to computers. There is not enough space to adequately describe them here, but this fact is not detrimental at this stage in your training. How should you go about listening to a voice that may be atypical? You should listen to a variety of samples to assess its conversational characteristics, customary pitch and pitch range, usual loudness, and phonatory and resonance qualities. A simple method is to listen to a voice that you have recorded. This procedure not only gives you an opportunity to hear the voice in its customary state, but also establishes a permanent record for reference. By the time the speech-language pathologist has heard the voice samples from preliminary conversations and during the recording, he should be able to describe the major features of the problem and its probable source—that is, the larynx, resonance areas, or both. Any other deviations in speaking, such as articulatory abnormalities, should also be noted.

Looking

Usually, what you hear is not an adequate basis for assessment; observation of the structures that produce the voice is also necessary. The voice that comes from a person's larynx is only as good as the motions and adjustments of the structures that produce the voice, like the breathing mechanism and the vocal folds. The vocal folds cannot be seen when looking directly into a person's mouth. Therefore, assessment of the laryngeal structure and function is completed by using imaging techniques. Imaging techniques are referred to as *endoscopy*, which means "viewing the inside of" the body. Laryngeal endoscopy means viewing the larynx. To view the larynx, an endoscope can be placed in the mouth or through the nose, referred to as oral endoscopy and transnasal endoscopy, respectively. Each procedure has its pros and cons and is used for different reasons. When a clearer, more magnified image of the vocal folds is needed, the oral endoscope is used, and when assessment of the vocal folds during more dynamic tasks such as speaking or singing is required, the transnasal endoscope is used. Look carefully at the vocal fold images in this chapter. Self-observation of the structures used in speaking is a first step toward diagnostic observation of persons with voice and speech problems.

Case History

The case history is the clinicians opportunity to explore the nature and time line of the patients's symptoms. Gathering a thorough history contributes greatly to the planning and conduct of the voice treatment program. In those instances for which the cause of the problem is obvious, such as an accident, surgery, or a specific disease, the collection of background data will concentrate primarily on the patient's current symptoms and attitudes about the problem, expressed need for remedial help, motivation, and capacity to undertake a rehabilitation program. When the cause of the vocal difficulty is not evident, however, careful questioning is essential. The speech-language pathologist attempts to obtain the following five types of information: (1) the individual's opinion of the nature and seriousness of the problem; (2) the start and course of development of the problem, including previous treatment; (3) an overview of the medical and health history; (4) family structure and interrelationships; and (5) history of voice and speech disorders. Answers to questions about these five areas will tell how precisely the child or adult perceives the problem as compared with what the examiner has heard and seen. They will also reveal the length of time the disorder has been present, plus the suddenness or gradualness of onset.

Learning about previous rehabilition experience will give insight into the concern for the problem felt by the person and the family. The medical and health history, particularly before and around the time the voice problem seemed to begin, may reveal not just the diseases that could have influenced voice production, but also the feelings of the family toward the person and the problem. The family structure, including the number of siblings, the position of a child in the sequence of children, and the stability of the family, will reveal the presence or absence of verbal competition and compatibility and/or emotional factors that could be contributors to the problem. When voice disorders are apparently present from birth, as evident in the cry sound or stridulous breathing, the cause may be developmental lag, structural abnormality, or disease. The developmental and structural deviations may be inherited, and questioning sometimes reveals voice problems elsewhere in the family. Obtaining a thorough case history requires broad knowledge about voice disorders and skill in developing questions. It can be facilitated by careful reading of the pertinent books listed at the end of the chapter. Questioning is an art that improves with self-evaluated experience.

Referral

As has been learned, voice disorders have different and often quite complicated causes. This chapter has suggested that the causes may be found in heredity, disease, injury, learning ability, family structure, environmental models, or a combination. While speech-language pathologists are required to know the potential significance of etiologic factors, they are not qualified to explore all of them. Fortunately, there are skillful professional colleagues in special areas of medicine, psychology, and education who are ready to help. Frequently, a complete diagnosis of a voice disorder cannot be made until one or more of the specialists have contributed to the evaluation.

Defining Pitch, Loudness, Voice Quality, and Resonance

Pitch/Frequency

Frequency is a physical concept that indicates the number of vibrations within a period of time. Pitch is the perceptual correlate that relates to frequency of vibration. When a tone goes from a lower to a higher pitch on a musical scale, the vibrator, whether violin string, clarinet reed, or vocal folds, increases its frequency. Frequency, when referring to sound, is a physical concept that indicates the number of vibrations within a period of time. The pitch of the voice is raised when the vocal folds are elongated. This adjustment accomplishes two changes. First, it increases the tension or elasticity (which is defined as the relative speed of return of an object to its position of rest after it has been displaced). Second, elongation reduces the mass of the vocal folds at all points along their length. Lengthening the vibrator to raise pitch may seem at first to contradict the idea that a shorter vibrator produces a higher frequency. When the vocal folds are elongated, however, the increased tension and reduced mass counter the length factor and cause a higher frequency. You can observe the same phenomenon by stretching and plucking a rubber band. Fundamental frequency can be measured with a number of devices. Currently, there are many pieces of instrumentation that are commercially available that enable a speech-language pathologist to measure this parameter easily. A list of pertinent websites for companies that market such instrumentation can be found at the end of the chapter.

Loudness/Amplitude

Loudness is a perceptual correlate that relates to the amplitude of air-molecule motion against the eardrum. When the sound wave, which is represented by the forward and backward movement of the air molecules, displaces the ear drum a greater distance, the sound is louder. Variation in sound amplitude is generated by a combination of breath pressure and manner of vocal fold vibration. When the air pressure developed by the lungs is relatively large and the resistance to glottal opening is substantial, the air is released in brief spurts that have both high velocity and high volume. When a high-energy pulse hits the air above the glottis, it moves the molecules a greater distance than when the pulse has a lower-volume velocity combination. This greater distance is in effect a greater amplitude, which is propagated in the sound wave and heard as a louder sound. The loudness of the voice influences the vibratory pattern of the vocal folds. For example, when a person talks louder, the frequency of the voice is higher. The loudness level that is produced by a speaker can also affect a listener's perception of the vocal quality. When assessing a patient's voice, it is important to measure or control for the loudness levels that the person is speaking at, particularly when trying to document when improvement has been made with a particular intervention technique.

Quality/Complexity

The quality of voice cannot be completely separated from pitch and loudness, but the word *quality* designates the audible features of a voice that distinguish it from another voice when both are at the same pitch and loudness. The perceptual concept of quality relates to spectral characteristics of the voice and has a parallel physical representation in the complexity of the sound wave. Almost all the sounds we hear are complex sounds. An uncomplex, single, or pure tone is the kind that comes from a tuning fork or pure-tone audiometer. When two or more tuning forks are sounded at the same time, the combined sound is complex. There are many other complex sounds, some of which contain noise. In technical use, noise is complex sound composed of irregular vibrations, to which a pure pitch cannot be assigned. Some of these are the normal fricative speech sounds such as /f, v, s, z/. Noise is also a frequent component of hoarse and breathy voices, caused by the aperiodic vibration of the vocal folds. If several tuning forks are sounding and another is added, the quality of the sound will change. The quality of the sound will also change if one or more of the forks are made to produce a louder sound. The complex sound that is voice is determined by the way the glottal pulse is released and the modifications of that pulse sound in the pharynx, mouth, and nose. Not all of the vibratory factors are known, but we have reason to believe that the speed of opening and closing of the vocal folds during vibration, the length of the closed phase in the vibration cycle, and the undulatory configurations of the vocal fold margins influence the number and intensity of the tones within the spectrum.

Resonance

A process called resonance modifies the sound generated in the larynx. As sound passes through the upper vocal tract, some of the tones are enhanced and others are suppressed. Each vowel requires a unique positioning of the tongue and other structures; that is, the /i/ sound in *see* cannot be made when the mouth and tongue are adjusted for /a/ as in *father*. Sometimes the structures are impaired by paralysis or physical deformity, which alters the resonance patterns and creates speech or voice disorders. Today there are computerized software/hardware packages that allow the voice signal to be displayed so that the resonant frequency components of the vocal tract can be analyzed. The distinction between phonation and resonance is illustrated by the fact that a person may have the larynx removed and still learn to speak. The requirement for speech without a larynx is a sound source that can substitute for the larynx. Any complex sound in the voice range that can be put into the mouth or pharynx will form intelligible speech when you perform the customary articulatory movements and adjustments. Therefore, the larynx or an artificial means of producing sound is considered the source of speech. The articulators (e.g., mouth structures, pharynx) are considered the filter, which shapes the sound into a perceptual speech signal.

General Classification of Voice Problems

Functional Voice Disorders

Voice problems that occur when there is no observable disease or structural defect are presumed to be psychosocial problems or situations that cause atypical behavior of the voice-producing mechanism. Aphonia may occur when a person does not want to speak or sing; however, nonorganic aphonia and dysphonia are more apt to be unconsciously related to stress and anxiety. Emotional problems associated with overwhelming situations at home or at work or school may incapacitate the laryngeal functions enough to prevent phonation. There are other instances when a true temporary laryngeal disease creates an aphonia that persists after full biological function has been restored. Possibly the aphonia provides a protection or relief somewhere in the individual's life and is, therefore, extended. Some voices are aphonic all the time, but that degree of voicelessness is rare. Usually, aphonia is intermittent; the voice often alternates irregularly between aphonia and dysphonia, which may be breathy-sounding or hoarse. The implication is that the laryngeal conditions that contribute to one type of voice may also cause others when subtle changes in breath flow or muscle contractions occur. Dysphonia of the breathy type, which signals vocal fold vibration without a closed phase, may also be associated with home or work environments where an extremely quiet voice is required. This type of speaking can easily become habitual. Young women in high school and college who try to emulate actresses and entertainers may develop a similar condition and voice. In our culture, the breathy, low-pitched, female voice is often interpreted as sexy. Another type of functional dysphonia occurs when the vocal folds are squeezed together so tightly that they cannot vibrate normally. The adjustment resembles the laryngeal closure in the first stage of a cough. When overadduction occurs, the vocal sound may be quite hoarse and low-pitched, as heard in some of the stereotyped gang bosses shown in films. Occasionally, the ventricular folds are adducted more or less completely and forced to vibrate. The voice usually is quite hoarse. The several forms of hoarseness associated with excessive closure of the glottis are called hyperfunctional dysphonia in the literature (Boone & McFarlane, 1994; Froeschels, 1952), many of which are a result of overuse or a misuse of the laryngeal mechanism (referred to as phonotrauma).

Organic Voice Disorders

Many voice disorders are caused by organic impairments. Treatment of the impairment is usually the responsibility of medical specialties such as otolaryngology, endocrinology, or neurology. If a person with a voice disorder comes to a speech-language pathologist for assistance without previous attention by a physician, the individual with the problem must be referred for proper medical diagnosis and appropriate treatment. Subsequently, if voice therapy is indicated, the speech-language pathologist should relate the plan for the rehabilitation voice program to both the underlying problem and the medical treatment used. Consequently, the speech-language pathologist must have a basic knowledge of the common diseases, disabilities, and medical treatments related to the voice-producing mechanism and is considered an integral part of the medical team. Some examples of organic voice disorders include laryngitis, tumors, Papillomata, vocal fold bowing, and arthritis, among others. The role of the speech pathologist in managing organic voice disorders is to assist in the evaluation of the disorder, administration of voice therapy prior to a necessary surgical procedure, and/or administration of voice therapy following a laryngeal surgical procedure.

Neurological Voice Disorders

Neurological voice disorders are caused by either central or peripheral nervous system impairment. Vocal fold paralysis is one example of a neurological voice disorder. Adductor vocal fold paralysis is a common neurological cause for the failure of one or both of the vocal folds to close the glottis completely (see Figure 8.1). This condition usually results from impairment of the nerve supply, which causes the muscle to lose its ability to contract; consequently, the structures to which paralyzed muscles are attached cannot be moved voluntarily. In unilateral adductor paralysis, the healthy fold usually can approach its paralyzed mate and thereby narrow the space between the vocal folds enough to cause the air stream to set the folds vibrating; however, it is dependent on the position of the paralyzed vocal fold. The closer the two vocal folds are to each other, the greater the ability of the two vocal folds to close. The result will be a louder and less breathy voice. In bilateral abductor vocal fold paralysis, both folds often rest closer to each other, which provides the condition for an almost normal voice. Unfortunately, the airway is usually compromised, breathing becomes difficult,

FIGURE 8.1 Vocal
fold paralysis, pre-
and postthyroplasty.
Source: Photo courtesy
of The Ear Nose and
Surgical Associates,
Winter Park, FL, Jeffrey
Lehman, M.D.

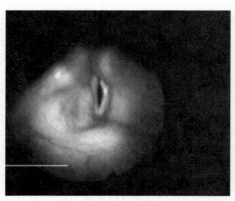

Vocal fold paralysis

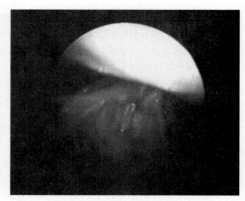

Vocal fold paralysis following intervention

and surgical intervention is necessary to ensure an airway. One of the surgical procedures for adductor paralysis is called thyroplasty. With thyroplasty, the surgeon uses a
silicone shunt to move the paralyzed vocal fold closer to midline so the glottis can close
more completely. Other conditions such as ankylosis, or impairment of arytenoid
movement resulting from stiffness or fixation at the cricoarytenoid joint, can be
another cause for incomplete glottal closure and a breathy voice. Differentiating ankylosis from vocal fold paralysis is necessary so an appropriate treatment plan can be developed. If cancer, arthritis, or some other inflammatory joint disease prevents adduction
and abduction, the function of the impaired larynx is essentially the same as that
accompanying paralysis. The amount of glottal opening varies among individuals, and
the severity of the vocal deviations corresponds to the degree of opening. In order to
determine if it is the laryngeal muscle that is impaired versus the arytenoids joint, electromyographic analysis is typically required. Other neurologic voice disorders can occur
in isolation (such as spasmodic dysphonia) or as a symptom of a larger disease process
(such as Parkinson's disease, mysthenia gravis, and amyotrophic lateral sclerosis).

Trauma and Surgical Modification

Occasionally, movements of one or both arytenoid cartilages are limited or prevented
by trauma. If the cartilages of the larynx are fractured or dislocated in an automobile
or motorcycle accident, they may heal in such a way that normal motion is not possible. The accompanying voice, of course, varies with the type and extent of the physical
alteration. The trauma problem is illustrated by the case of an 18-year-old student who
was in a motorcycle accident. He was riding through a forest at dusk when he struck a
chain that had been stretched across the trail at neck height. His larynx was crushed,
but surgeons realigned the broken cartilages and placed a special splint called a stent
into the larynx to support the parts while they healed. After the stent was removed,
both vocal folds remained in lateral positions, causing a wide-open glottis and total
aphonia. Some months later, the right vocal fold regained the ability to adduct and
abduct normally, but the left arytenoid cartilage and vocal fold remained somewhat
lateralized. With the restoration of a partial glottal closure, some vibration could be
achieved, producing a weak and breathy, but functional voice. A similar case occurred
in which the larynx was crushed so severely it could not be preserved. Consequently, a
total laryngectomy (surgical removal of the larynx) was performed. This young man

developed excellent esophageal speech. Additional information about speech without a larynx can be found later in the chapter.

Examples of Vocal Fold Pathologies

Protruding Masses

Protruding masses and localized lesions can frequently impair glottal adjustment and have a local influence on one or both vocal folds sufficient to cause voice abnormalities. Earlier in this chapter, we mentioned that roughness could be caused by random variations in the consecutive vibrations of the vocal folds. One cause for this vibration is abnormal increase or decrease in the size or mass of one or both vocal folds. Aronson (1990) summarized the effects of mass lesions: Mass lesions of the vocal folds produce one or more of the following pathologic changes:

1. Increased mass or bulk of the vocal folds or immediately surrounding tissues
2. Altered vocal fold shape
3. Restricted vocal fold mobility
4. Changed vocal fold tension
5. Modified size or shape, or both, of the glottic, supraglottic, or infraglottic airway
6. Vocal folds prevented from approximating completely along their anteroposterior margins
7. Resulting excessive tightness of approximation

   What are these masses that can influence the vocal folds, their vibration, and the voice? A few of the common ones need to be well understood by the speech-language pathologist. You must always remember, however, that an abnormal voice and the aberrant vibrations associated with it can have a variety of causes. You cannot diagnose a specific disease by the sound of the voice. A mass on a vocal fold exerts its influence variably according to its location, size, and firmness (see Figure 8.2). Diagnosis is left to the

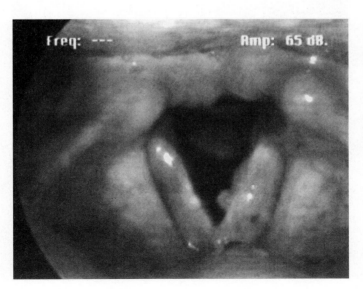

FIGURE 8.2 Vocal fold carcinoma. Middle-aged adult male with a history of smoking.
Source: Photo courtesy of The Ear Nose and Surgical Associates, Winter Park, FL, Jeffrey Lehman, M.D.

medical team, of which you are a part. You will assist the medical team by offering your opinions of how the symptoms suggest a particular etiology, or cause of the problem.

Tumors

Tumors usually come to mind first when you think about mass lesions of the vocal folds, but what is a tumor? A tumor is defined as a "neoplasm; a new growth of tissue in which the multiplication of cells is uncontrolled and progressive" (*Dorland's,* 1988). Tumors can be either benign or malignant. A benign tumor is one that is "not malignant, not recurrent, favorable for recovery" (*Dorland's,* 1988). Malignant means "tending to become progressively worse and to result in death; having the properties of invasion and metastasis" (the disease migrates from one location to another and establishes itself in the new location) (*Dorland's,* 1988).

Polyps

A polyp is a benign tumor commonly found in the larynx (see Figure 8.3). This term is also broad in its meaning. *Polyp* is a general descriptive term used with reference to any "protruding growth from mucous membrane" (*Dorland's,* 1988). It may be broad-based (sessile) or attached by a stalk (pedunculated). If a polyp protrudes from the glottal border of a vocal fold, it tends to interfere with contact between the folds during vibration. The result may be breathiness in the voice. If the polyp is large, it may rest partially on the opposite vocal fold, where it interferes with vibration. It may become an auxiliary vibrator contributing to hoarseness or roughness.

Vocal Fold Nodules

Vocal nodules are sometimes referred to as singer's nodes or screamer's nodes. Vocal nodules are usually small, sessile, slightly pink or grayish white protrusions located bilaterally, opposite each other, at the junction of the anterior and middle thirds of the

FIGURE 8.3
Hemorrhagic vocal polyp.
Source: Photo courtesy of The Ear Nose and Surgical Associates, Winter Park, FL, Jeffrey Lehman, M.D.

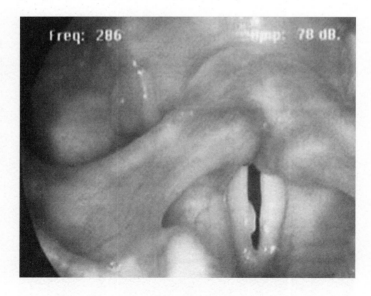

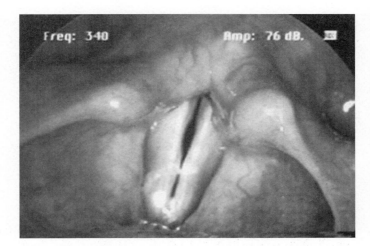

FIGURE 8.4 Vocal fold nodules. Well-defined vocal nodules in a 24-year-old female teacher who has a history of chronic sinus infections and tonsilitis.
Source: Photo courtesy of The Ear Nose and Surgical Associates, Winter Park, FL, Jeffrey Lehman, M.D.

entire length of the vocal folds (see Figure 8.4). This position is the same as the midpoint of the membranous section of the vocal folds. The location of the nodules identifies the place where the vocal folds strike each other most vigorously during vocal fold vibration, particularly in females. Vocal fold nodules develop in people who use their voices excessively. The excessive use causes swelling that reduces the flexibility of the vocal folds, tends to increase their contact at the swollen areas, and may also prevent total glottal closure. Swelling usually disappears in 24 to 36 hours with rest and moderate use. When vocal use continues, however, as with people who talk excessively, yell often, or sing abusively (as in some popular entertainment groups), the swelling persists, tissue changes occur, and the traumatized area becomes organized, circumscribed, and protuberant.

The vocal behaviors associated with vocal nodules can be caused by both psychological and social factors. Children with vocal nodules may have a younger sibling who fights verbally with his brothers and sisters. They are usually competitive, aggressive, interested in sports, and vocally loud and have some personality adjustment problems. Aronson (1990) observes that the factors related to vocal nodules in children are basically similar to those in adults, such as being overly active, both physically and vocally.

Papillomata

The laryngeal papilloma is caused by exposure to the human papilloma virus (HPV). Papillomata can occur in children (called Juvinile) and adults. There are two types of papillomata; one is hard, the other soft (*papilla* means nipplelike). An example of a hard papilloma is the common wart. Soft papillomata do not look like warts, but instead tend to be glistening, pinkish white, and irregular. These lesions arise from the mucous membranes and may be found in the pharynx, in the trachea, and at other sites, including the larynx. "Papillomata are common benign neoplasms of childhood and occur between the first and eighth years of life, although they are most common between ages 4 and 6 years" (Aronson, 1990, p. 56). When these lesions are located on the vocal folds, they usually cause dysphonia; the type and severity of the voice deviation are related to the size and location of the lesion (see Figure 8.5).

FIGURE 8.5

Papilloma in the anterior portion of the vocal folds.

Source: Photo courtesy of The Ear Nose and Throat Surgical Associates, Winter Park, FL, Jeffrey Lehman, M.D.

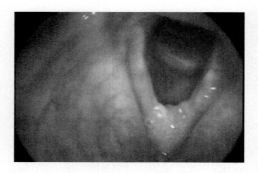

Carcinoma

A carcinoma (a type of cancer) is a malignant tumor and is indeed a threat to life. It can grow on one or both vocal folds and affect their vibration much as do polyps or papillomata. It is not possible to distinguish among carcinoma, polyps, papillomata, and the like by the sounds produced, although depending on the extent of the lesion the voice will sound more or less hoarse/harsh (see Figure 8.6). The cause of carcinoma is not known, but there is a well-established positive statistical relationship between laryngeal cancer and smoking. The chance of developing laryngeal cancer is increased substantially when alcohol is combined with smoking (Snidecor, 1962, 1971; Webb & Irving, 1964; Wynder, Covey, Mabuchi, & Mushinski, 1976). Carcinoma, which is a cancer that develops from surface tissue, may grow subtly in the larynx and not become apparent until it produces a change in the voice. This vocal change often appears early in the course of the disease and provides an opportunity for early, and frequently successful, treatment. Therapy is the responsibility of physicians, but their treatment may leave a condition that requires the services of a speech-language pathologist. This is addressed later in the section of the chapter on laryngectomy.

Edema

Edema is swelling caused by excessive fluid in the tissue (see Figure 8.7). Its presence in the larynx signals a number of possible problems, including vocal abuse (-*itis* means inflammation), localized diseases, and systemic disorders such as allergic reactions and endocrine disturbances. Even normal phenomena related to hormonal changes during pregnancy or menses can create edema. The amount of swelling can vary from minimal to extensive, involving one or both entire vocal folds. When it is minimal, it may lower the pitch slightly as the result of increased mass and change in the manner in

FIGURE 8.6

Source: Photo courtesy of The Ear Nose and Throat Surgical Associates, Winter Park, FL, Jeffrey Lehman, M.D.

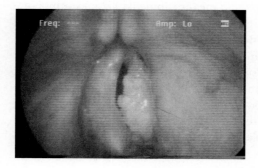

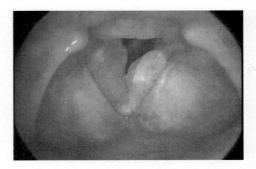

FIGURE 8.7 Severe vocal fold edema from a 35-year-old female with a 15-year history of smoking and reflux.
Source: Photo courtesy of The Ear Nose and Throat Surgical Associates, Winter Park, FL, Jeffrey Lehman, M.D.

which the vocal folds vibrate. When swelling increases moderately, it can cause some changes in the vibration sequences, leading to hoarseness. When edema becomes so extensive that the vocal folds are greatly enlarged, the arytenoid cartilages may be prevented from closing, which could cause a breathy hoarseness. With this degree of swelling, the vocal folds may also be pressed together so tightly that they cannot vibrate. Edema is not a disease, but a symptom that can be caused by various factors. Sometimes edema is present in those who smoke and may be a precursory sign that alerts the clinician to begin to counsel the patient on the adverse side effects of smoking with regard to laryngeal health.

Contact Ulcer Granuloma

Contact ulcers, or granulomata, are benign growths that can result from three causes:

1. Laryngopharyngeal reflax irritation
2. Intubation trauma
3. Phonotrauma

Vigorous glottal closure, mechanical trauma, and/or chemical explosure can traumatize the mucosal covering of the vocal processes or other contacting areas of the arytenoids, causing an ulcer (a sore) to form on one or both cartilages. If the inflammation continues, granulation tissue develops on the ulcer. The granulation may become large enough to prevent complete glottal closure (see Figure 8.8). This granulation tissue is referred to as a contact granuloma. There is recent evidence that gastric reflux is a predisposing factor (Aronson, 1990; Cherry & Margulies, 1968; Chodosh, 1977; Delahunty & Cherry, 1968; Koufman, 1991), and this cause needs to be differentially identified, since it is due not to vocal behaviors alone, but also to physical reasons.

Laryngeal Web

Laryngeal web refers to a membrane extending usually from one vocal fold to the other. It may occur also at the level of the false vocal folds or below the glottis. It can be either congenital or composed of scar tissue resulting from injury or surgical procedures. Webs can vary in size from a small bit of tissue to a membrane that completely occupies the glottal space. When the web is extensive, it will impair breathing and require surgical intervention. When it is smaller, it may cause stridulous breathing

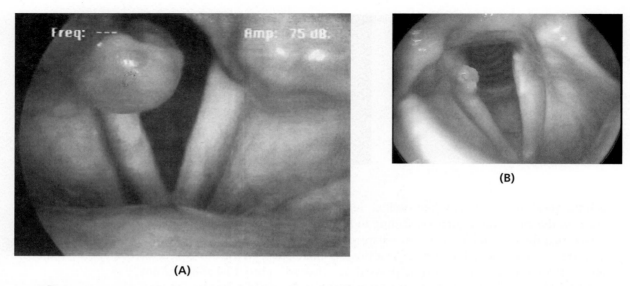

(A)

FIGURE 8.8 Contact granuloma. **(A)** Forty-two-year-old female teacher with a history of gastro-esophageal reflux. **(B)** Twenty-nine-year-old male restaurant manager with a history of laryngopharyngeal reflux disease.
Source: Photos courtesy of The Ear Nose and Surgical Associates, Winter Park, FL, Jeffrey Lehman, M.D.

or hoarseness, or even aphonia (see Figure 8.9). The presence of the smallest congenital webs may not become apparent until a child attempts to talk. The voice may be hoarse and have a higher than normal pitch. This condition is another in which the laryngeal surgeon and speech-language pathologist must work together. The effects of a laryngeal web and other problems are illustrated in the case of an 11-year-old boy in the fourth grade who had hypernasality and a high-pitched voice. The other children called him "Squeaky" as a result of his unusual voice and ridiculed him. The hypernasality reduced his intelligibility somewhat and contributed to his communication problem. All these conditions led to withdrawal from his schoolmates and reclusiveness. Several physicians examined the child over a period of years. They reported a bifid uvula (divided into two parts) and a normal larynx. The probable cause for the nasality was recognized as the uvular defect, but the speech-language pathologist who worked with the boy became convinced that there was also some laryngeal abnormality causing the high pitch. She arranged for another laryngeal examination. On this attempt, a small web was exposed anteriorly between the

FIGURE 8.9
Laryngeal web. **(A)** Adult laryngeal web after multiple surgeries to remove laryngeal papillomata. **(B)** Pediatric laryngeal web.
Source: Photos courtesy of The Ear Nose and Throat Surgical Associates, Winter Park, FL, Jeffrey Lehman, M.D.

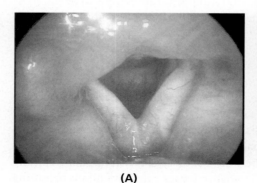

(A)

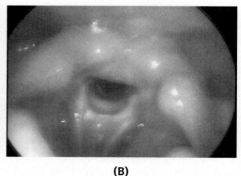

(B)

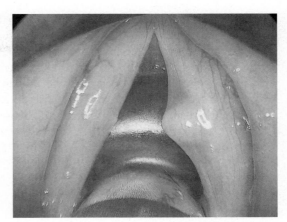

FIGURE 8.10
Cyst, shown under direct laryngoscopy prior to surgical removal.
Source: Photo courtesy of The Ear Nose and Throat Surgical Associates, Winter Park, FL, Jeffrey Lehman, M.D.

true vocal folds. Appropriate surgical procedures eliminated the web and provided the basis for a normal voice, which the speech-language pathologist was able to help the boy develop and stabilize. The hypernasality was reduced through speech therapy, and the boy's socialization and personality markedly improved.

Cysts

A cyst is "any closed cavity or sac, normal or abnormal, lined by epithelium, and especially one that contains a liquid or semisolid material" (*Dorland's,* 1988). Cysts can be caused by phonotraumatic behavior or the blockage of glands. Sometimes cysts develop on a true vocal fold (see Figure 8.10). When a cyst is on the glottal border, the voice is usually hoarse, breathy, and weak, similar to that heard with a polyp or other protrusion into the glottal space. The effects of a cyst range from mild to severe depending on the size and firmness of the cyst.

Additional information can be collected during the assessment of voice disorders. With technological advance, the field of voice has developed instrumental measures of voice production that provide an objective means of documenting the function of the voice. This chapter does not allow for particular details about instrumentation, such as their pros and cons, to be discussed. A general overview of the categories of measurement is included.

Collecting and Assessing the Data About the Voice

Instrumental assessment of the voice involves three main levels: imaging, aerodynamics, and acoustics. Imaging provides the speech-language pathologist with a visual record of the laryngeal structure. When coupled with videostroboscopy, the function of the vocal folds can be assessed. See Selected Readings for more information on this topic. Aerodynamics is a method that allows the examiner to gain information about how the upper airway modulates the airstream to form the phonetic segments of speech. Aerodynamic parameters primarily measure pressures and airflows. From these measures, calculations of laryngeal airway resistance can be made (e.g. Smitheran & Hixon, 1981). Clinically, these measures tell the clinician about the valving characteristics of the vocal folds. Instruments provide a way to objectively document changes in vocal fold structure and function with intervention. One of the liabilities of using instrumental analysis and commercially available techniques is the tendency to forget there is a theoretical basis to the measures that are made. Furthermore, not all of the measures available on a software program are applicable to or valid for the examination of your patient. And, finally, for pediatric patients in particular, there may not be a normative database with which to compare your results. Careful consideration of all of these factors is warranted when evaluating your patient with a voice problem. In that way, instrumental tools can be used to their greatest capabilities.

Summary and Diagnosis

The cause of voice disorders can usually be determined when the description of the vocal sound is evaluated along with observations made by the speech-language pathologist and physician and with information from the history. Of course, during the voice evaluation, the examiner constantly relates what is heard with what is seen and reported, so that establishing a diagnosis may not require a separate, formal assembly process. When referral data are not available at the time of vocal assessment and several persons are involved in the evaluation, a systematic amalgamation of information is desirable. The first focus is on a description of the voice and an indication of its relative severity; second, a statement should be made of pertinent medical, social, and psychological information; third, an opinion should be stated that indicates the probable causal chain. Finally, the speech-language pathologist should be prepared to provide a statement of prognosis (projection of future outcome both with and without treatment) and recommendations. The case study presented on pages 234–236 illustrates a typical summary and diagnosis.

Intervention for Voice Disorders

Voice Therapy

The real reason for learning about voice disorders and their causes is to help prevent or remedy these disorders. We have seen that voice problems almost always occur when the vocal folds vibrate abnormally. The altered vibration can be caused either by organic/neurological changes affecting the size, shape, texture, tonicity, and position of the critical structures or by learned changes, which can also determine position as well as dimensions and contractile tensions in the antagonistic muscle groups. The organic changes originate in disease, heredity, injury, and aging; the learned changes are based on speech models, personal beliefs, and methods of adjustment to environmental requirements and stresses. Obviously, the organic and nonorganic causes are frequently intertwined. Whenever possible, therapy is directed toward the underlying factors that caused the problems. Sometimes the direct causes are no longer active or are not amenable to change. Consequently, therapy must often be directed partly or entirely to symptoms. Unfortunately, the term *voice therapy* is synonymous with voice exercises. Voice exercises are important, but they constitute only a small part of voice therapy. One of the major objectives of this chapter is to stress that vocal rehabilitation is an overall process affecting the individual's health and lifestyle as well as the voice itself.

Therapy for voice disorders combines three distinct, but interdependent procedures (referred to as combined modality management). One is medical, which includes surgery, radiation, medication, and psychiatry; the second is environmental, which encompasses both modification of the environment for the benefit of the child or adult and the related program of helping the individual adjust to the environment; the third is direct vocal rehabilitation, which includes use of training activities designed to promote predictable change in specific voice aspects. Therapy approaches should be chosen not because of their popularity, but because of their known effectiveness and efficacy (Pannebacker, 1998). A technical report written by an ASHA committee and a committee from the American Academy of Otolaryngology-Head and Neck Surgery (AAO-HNS) in 2005 detailed the use of voice therapy in the treatment of dysphonia (http:www.asha.org/docs/html/TR2005-00158.html). This report summarizes the studies that provide evidence for use with a variety of patient populations and can be used as a reference source for providing evidence for treatment choices both as an independent treatment and within a combined modality paradigm, particularly in combination with surgical techniques.

Medical Approach

Surgical treatment may completely eliminate a voice problem, or it may unavoidably leave an impaired structure and a voice defect. In all situations, voice rehabilitation can help the person to achieve maximum effectiveness with the structures that remain to achieve a functional voice. Medications and other nonsurgical techniques may help cure a disease or bring a condition such as an allergic response under control, thereby restoring physical vigor or reducing swelling. This kind of aid provides a more normal vocal mechanism and the possibility of a normal voice.

Environmental Approach

Earlier in this chapter, we suggested that school or employment and living environments sometimes cause people to use their voices excessively or traumatically and thereby create behavioral or organic changes in the larynx that produce voice disorders. Environments may also contain physical irritants or allergens that are detrimental to the larynx and consequently cause problems. Voice therapy must consider and, when possible, help the individual manage these damaging factors. One procedure that can be used when appropriate is consultation with the family, teachers, or employer to explain the effects of these factors and to gain cooperation in reducing the factors that are taking their toll on the laryngeal structures. Air pollution from particulates, dust, pollen, and the like can often be reduced by the use of air conditioners or masks.

Direct Approach

Many and varied activities can be used by the speech-language pathologist working directly with a person who has a voice disorder. These procedures constitute the therapy of the clinical sessions and transition into independent practice and daily use of the voice. For convenience, the activities are grouped under the following seven headings, listed alphabetically: listening skills, mental hygiene, physical hygiene, posture and movement, regulation of breathing for voice, relaxation, and voice training. Entire books have been written on each of these seven items; the discussion here is limited to the concepts involved.

Listening Skills   Most of us do not hear our own voices as others hear them when we speak or sing. We are almost always surprised when we hear a recording of our voices for the first time. Teaching a person to listen is an important and early step in voice rehabilitation. Motivation for this step is based on the premise that therapy will ultimately be less effective if the patient is unable to determine when and in what way the voice is defective. The process should be systematic and usually begins with pitch recognition and discrimination. Identifying pitch differences can be followed by attempts by the child or adult to match them. A great number of recorded instrumental and animal sounds can be introduced when recognition deficits are severe.

Mental Hygiene   This old-fashioned term, which has been replaced in current literature by *mental health,* is used here intentionally to parallel the concept of physical hygiene. It implies healthy thinking and the means of both achieving and maintaining it. Everyone must confront problems and decisions, and some form of resolution is always made, whether appropriate or inappropriate. When people have a way to resolve difficulties, they do it easily and appropriately. When they do not have a normal or acceptable solution, they may acquire some substitute such as withdrawal, aggressive behavior, worrying, or a voice disorder. Many people with voice disorders do not understand what is happening in the larynx when they produce deviant sounds. They also do not readily associate their vocal disorders with their anxieties and frustrations. Careful explanations using diagrams, photographs, and models or other illustrations when appropriate often help people to understand their problem. Detailed descriptions also provide insight that can lead to modified behavior or relief of anxiety about possible disease. The person who is worried or anxious about her voice or state of health will tend to be hypertense and will have poor control over her voice.

Careful, sympathetic, unhurried listening by the speech-language pathologist is advocated. When the person learns that what he says is held in strict confidence, he may reveal worries, frustrations, and anxieties that adversely affect his life and his voice. Many of these problems are not deep-seated or of long duration, but they can interfere with the restoration of a normal voice. With proper management by the speech-language pathologist, the basic problems can often be talked through with relief and voice restoration.

You may wonder about the appropriateness of using interviewing, counseling, and guidance techniques in therapy for voice disorders. This concern is appropriate because it should encourage you to seek instruction in these techniques in clinical psychology. They are essential. Aronson (1990) expressed the need in the following statement:

> Any in-depth study of voice disorders forces us to conclude that so long as clinicians obtain privileged information from patients; so long as people have voice problems because of life stress and interpersonal conflict; so long as voice disorders produce anxiety, depression, embarrassment, and self-consciousness; so long as patients need a sympathetic person with whom they can discuss their distress, will speech pathologists need to consider their training incomplete until they have learned the basic skills of psychologic interviewing and counseling.

Physical Hygiene   Good physical hygiene encompasses those activities and practices that promote good physical health. The presumptions underlying our emphasis on physical well-being are that healthy people learn more easily, their muscles respond more readily, they have greater stamina, and their respiratory system is more efficient. Conversely, muscles that have lost tonus and strength as the result of sedentary living, poor diet, or illness are less capable of performing properly than when they were strong and in good condition. Voices of weakened or ill persons reflect their disabilities. The speech-language pathologist can contribute to the health of the child or adult by encouraging a proper diet and hydration, adequate rest, and sufficient exercise. Many persons with voice disorders, particularly functional disorders, are not aware of the potential relationship of the voice to physical health. This is an important concept, particularly in light of the fact that we are living longer.

Posture and Movement   Good posture could be considered an aspect of physical hygiene, but it is so vital in voice therapy that it deserves special emphasis. The term *good posture* as used here means maximum efficiency in body movement and positioning. It does not mean a rigid military position. People who have sedentary occupations without compensatory physical activity typically lose strength in the muscles of the abdomen, back, and legs. This weakening allows the anterior abdominal wall to protrude and the shoulders to droop forward. When these persons stand or walk, a rounded upper back, forward head carriage, and forward curving of the lumbar spine often accompany the abdominal protrusion and shoulder droop. This postural change tends to interfere with respiratory efficiency. The speech-language pathologist can help people improve posture by encouraging them to institute a physical education program at a local physical fitness center or at least to do routine daily calisthenics at home. Poor posture and reduced tonus of the skeletal muscles cannot be identified as a direct cause of voice disorders, but attention to this factor certainly will augment the remedial process.

Regulation of Breathing for Voice   Sometimes voice problems are caused by or related to the amount of lung pressure, airflow, and manner of breathing. The movements of the body mechanisms that control breathing can be modified; breathing for speaking and singing can be made more efficient through training. The literature in the area of voice and diction is rich with guidance and exercises.

Relaxation   Many voice problems are associated with too much tension in the muscles used in speaking, a condition that is often found in other muscles throughout the body. Earlier in the chapter, we referred to stressful situations causing excess muscle tension. The resolution of conditions causing anxiety and worry is certainly important in reducing such tension, but the satisfactory management of psychogenic factors often is not possible. The reduction of psychological and social pressures may leave a void. Consequently, direct and specific training in relaxation is usually helpful and often necessary in the management of a variety of voice problems. There are many procedures in use today through which people try to achieve a state of relaxation. For general purposes, relaxation is defined as the absence of muscle contraction. The techniques commonly used to achieve relaxation can be grouped into four categories: (1) meditation and/or deep breathing, (2) biofeedback, (3) suggestion, and (4) muscle sense with voluntary reduction of contraction (5) and manual laryngeal relaxation.

Meditation techniques emphasize quiet surroundings and a mental state of peacefulness and calm. Deep breathing and various postures are often employed to help achieve the desired state. Biofeedback makes use of the phenomenon of electrical activity in muscles, which is directly proportional to the degree of muscle contraction. When sensors (small electrodes) are placed on the skin (usually the forehead) and the sensed excitation is amplified and connected to a meter or other responder, an individual can be informed visually or audibly of the extent of muscle contraction. This feedback monitoring allows the person to learn how to reduce undesirable muscle contraction. Relaxation by suggestion is an old procedure that depends on imagination. The person pictures herself in a quiet, peaceful place or imagines her arms, legs, hands, feet, and so forth as being either heavy or light. Often an instructor who is guiding the relaxation procedure heightens the effect of suggestion by directing attention to, for example, heaviness in the arms and legs, while speaking in a quiet, monotonous voice. The fourth listed technique, which teaches the person to become aware of muscle contraction and to release the tension, is called progressive relaxation and is associated most closely with Edmund Jacobson (1976). Jacobson developed a systematic procedure in which each of the major muscles of the Jacobson muscle groups is contracted, one at a time in a progressive sequence, usually beginning with the arms, so that the sensation of the particular contraction can be identified and voluntarily released. As a person practices relaxation, the amount of tension progressively diminishes; practice facilitates relaxation. A refinement of total body relaxation is called differential relaxation. In this process, the individual learns to recognize and release muscle contractions in a limited area such as the face or an arm. The objective, step-by-step, sensory approach of the Jacobson procedure associated with the differential relaxation feature has caused progressive relaxation to be widely used in speech-language pathology. Circumlaryngeal massage, laryngeal reposturing technique, was first introduced by Aronson (1990) and has been further studied by Leeper (1993) and Roy, Ford, and Bless (1996). This procedure involves applying manual tension reduction techniques using the hands of the speech-language pathologist or patient. The pressure is applied in a circular and downward motion. Roy and Leeper (1993) demonstrated a significant improvement in voice quality with this technique for patients with muscle tension dysponia and spasmodic dysphonia (Roy et al., 1996; Roy, Mauszycki, Merrill, Gouse, & Smith, 2007).

Voice Training

The six procedures of the direct approach we have discussed so far have not included much discussion of the voice itself and what can be done to rehabilitate or improve it. Vocal training is designed to improve the voice to the maximum extent possible. Some of the rehabilitative procedures that are used most commonly include eliminating factors that are harmful to the voice, finding the best sounds, reducing excessively tense phonation, increasing phonatory efficiency, modifying vocal pitch, increasing vocal loudness, and altering vocal resonance.

Eliminating Factors Harmful to the Voice   Factors that are harmful to the voice must be eliminated or else voice therapy approaches attempting to remediate the dysfunction will not be as effective. The first step is a careful analysis of the amount of loudness in the individual's typical speech and singing. Subsequently, a prescription for the reduction of both the quantity of vocal use and the loudness level is developed. The plan is often implemented through the application of behavior modification techniques.

Finding the Best Sounds   Everyone (except someone who is mute) has a repertoire of vocal sounds. Some sounds will be produced more easily and with better quality than others. The best sounds can be located by asking the child or adult to produce a variety of vowel sounds at low, medium, and high pitches and with different loudness levels. The most pleasant or most effortless phonation is selected as a guide, or target, voice (Boone & McFarlane, 1994). The person is taught to feel and hear the best production, and an effort is made to produce other sounds equally well. Finding the best voice is closely related to the listening training we have described.

Reducing Excessively Tense Phonation   Tense phonation signals overly tight glottal closure or excessive effort to close the glottis when an organic problem interferes. This pattern can usually be relieved by the combination of general relaxation and phonation drills that stress excessively breathy sounds. Sentences such as *Hold hope high, How high is his house?* and *He hid Harry's hat* can be used to open the glottis and relieve excess tension. Many available textbooks contain stimuli with these speech sounds, so that you can easily incorporate them into the therapy program.

Increasing Phonatory Efficiency   Phonatory efficiency implies maximum balance between air supply and adjustment of the laryngeal mechanism. Stated negatively, if there is air waste or the vocal folds are adjusted with too much or too little glottal opening, phonatory efficiency is reduced. When excessive air escapes during phonation or, in contrast, when the inefficiency of phonation reflects a glottal closure that is too tight, efficiency may be increased by tone prolongation. In this type of drill, the individual practices vocalizing as long as possible on each breath, at various pitch and loudness levels, and while as relaxed as possible. The tonal drills can be extended into phrases and sentences in which the number of words on one breath can be gradually increased.

Modifying Vocal Pitch   Vocal pitch is abnormal when it is either higher or lower than the voice expected in most persons of the same age and sex as the speaker or when it is monotonous. The high-pitch, effeminate voice in men and low-pitch, masculine voice in women can be serious social and economic handicaps. If medical examination reveals a normal larynx in the male, vocal retraining that includes intentionally lowering the pitch, changing the head position (such as tilting the head backward), prolonging throat-clearing sounds, and sometimes manually manipulating the larynx usually produces improvement if the person really wants to change (Fawcus, 1986). When the pitch of a woman's voice becomes low enough to cause her to be falsely identified as a male in telephone conversations, the basic problem may be related to hormonal imbalance or a mass lesion of the vocal folds. Medical treatment may arrest the change, but does not reverse it. Voice therapy emphasizes forward articulatory adjustments of the tongue and female prosodic patterns, such as upward pitch changes in word stress. When an individual speaks with little pitch variation, the voice may reflect an identity problem such as that of men who wish to sound "more masculine" by speaking monotonously at the bottom end of the pitch range. If these individuals want to change their voices, they usually can do so through ear training, self-monitoring, and pitch-flexibility drills of the type mentioned previously. Obviously, combinations of mental hygiene and pitch drills are needed. Finally, inability to vary pitch could be due to an organic or neurological condition.

Increasing Vocal Loudness   People who do not speak loudly enough for their needs do so for one or a combination of four reasons: (1) There is an organic or neurologic problem that impairs normal function, (2) the person is shy and reticent about speaking,

(3) there is a hearing loss, or (4) the person does not know how to use a big voice without damaging the mechanism. When an individual has an organic problem such as paralysis, a postsurgical condition, or some other disability that prevents glottal closure during vocal fold vibration, the voice may never be loud enough; however, we do have a few procedures that often prove helpful. One is greater airflow, which improves the approximation of the vocal folds by increasing the amplitude of their vibration. A mechanical aid, through the use of various portable amplification devices, can also be a useful solution for inadequate loudness. Finally, surgical procedures are also an option. These procedures medialize the paralyzed vocal fold so that glottal closure can be obtained. Of further assistance to the person with a continuously weak voice is improvement in articulatory precision. When words are spoken with precise movements of the tongue, lips, and soft palate, the speech is easier to understand, and there is less demand on the phonatory mechanism. The person who is capable of producing adequately loud sound, but who is reluctant to speak with sufficient voice, usually needs help with personality adjustment and the development of more self-confidence. In addition to mental hygiene methods, there are some procedures that reduce the voice problem and contribute to self-confidence. One is supplying masking noise through headphones while the person reads aloud. This technique causes the speaker to use a louder voice unknowingly, which can be recorded and played back to the client to demonstrate that an adequate voice can be produced. Another approach is role playing with a play script or hand puppets to facilitate imitation of other characters and their voices. The person who must be able to use a loud voice, such as a minister, lawyer, athletic coach, or actor, but who is unable to do so for more than a few minutes without feeling discomfort or becoming hoarse needs help in building a voice. Those who have this problem usually come to the speech-language pathologist with hypertense muscle adjustments in the larynx and also in the tongue, soft palate, and jaw. These adjustments are often accompanied by generalized, excessive muscular tension, poor posture, and respiratory habits that are inadequate for sustained loud speaking. These people also often have vocal nodules or chronic laryngitis.

Remediation is a long-term process. This fact often surprises or even irritates people with a problem; they want something done to them or for them immediately. They frequently find it difficult to accept the concept that whatever is done is done *with* them, not *to* them; remediation is a collaboration among patient, speech-language pathologist, and other professionals. Many patients fail to realize that the coordination needed for effective voice production is probably subtler and less easily modified than movements of arms, legs, and torso.

The specific procedures to be instituted—in addition to explanation, relaxation, respiration, and posture—include drills for easy phonation, unvoiced-voiced fricative production at minimum and maximum intensities, and the drills for prolongation to increase the efficiency of breath usage. In addition to these exercises, practice should be gradually carried over into an environment in which the person needs to be functional. For those needing a big/loud voice, practicing exercises in a large hall would be advocated. At first, the voice should be produced gently as though attempting to reach only the first few rows of seats. Gradually, over a period of weeks, as each loudness level becomes established, the loudness should be increased to reach successive rows. An efficient, relatively relaxed, loud voice for long periods of time is the ultimate objective. The Lee Silverman Voice Treatment (LSVT) program developed by Dr. Lorraine Ramig incorporates many of the strategies listed above in an intensive, programmatic model of therapy. The LSVT program promotes models of exercise-based theories and is a proven, effective speech treatment for individuals with Parkinson's disease or other hypofunctional voice disorders (Ramig, Countryman, O'Brien, Hochn, & Thompson, 1996; Ramig et al., 2001; Ramig, Sopir, Fox, & Countryman, 2001). It uses vocal loudness as a "trigger" for stimulating increased effort and coordination during speech production (www.lsvt.org/main_site.html). Other symptoms targeted by the program include breathiness, pitch, reduced articulatory movements, and respiration.

Altering Vocal Resonance   As discussed, the resonance characteristics of the vocal tract have a marked influence on voice quality. When organic variations do not interfere, resonance is modified primarily by moving the tongue, positioning the lips, opening or closing of the velopharyngeal valve, and changing the size of the pharynx. When the tongue is carried forward in the mouth, the voice has a "thin" quality. Frequently, this quality is accompanied by broad-smile or slit-shaped lip positions during the articulation of the back, lip-rounded vowels. A thin voice especially can generate many impressions in a listener, ranging from immaturity (Fisher, 1966), through helplessness, to femininity. Of course, the listener should realize that these vocal perceptions might depend as much on the attitudes of the listener as on the properties of the voice. In contrast to the forward carriage of the tongue, when the tongue is retracted, the voice tends to sound "throaty." This quality is heard most frequently in men, particularly those who attempt to speak at the low end of their pitch range. Direct drills that stress front vowels are beneficial, particularly when used with the bilabial and lingua-alveolar consonants (Andrews, 1994).

Many of these resonance problems can be relieved with exercises in which the person is taught to sense the tongue positions and hear the deviant sounds by exaggerating the malpositions and distorted sounds. However, serious emotional problems may arise for these speakers when specific voice qualities do not match the gender expectations of our culture. Two current and popular voice therapy programs that are considered to be physiologically based and that address resonance are Vocal Function Exercises (VFE), developed by Dr. Joseph Stemple, and Lessac-Madsen Resonant Voice Therapy (LMRVT), developed by Dr. Katherine Verdolini. Both are well suited for use with patients that have hyper- and hypofunctional voice disorders. VFE can be used with all age groups. Steps to the VFE program include vocal warm-up, pitch glides, and prolonged phonation of /o/ at selected pitches. VFE outcome was tested on a randomized group of subjects with normal voice who were placed into experimental, placebo, and control groups. After 4 weeks of VFE, the experimental group produced improved phonation volumes, phonation times, and frequency range compared to the placebo and control groups (Stemple, Lee, D'Amico, & Pickup, 1994). A study by Roy et al. (2001) examined the functional effects of two voice therapy programs, one being VFE and the other a vocal hygiene program, on a group of nearly fourty teachers with voice disorders. A control group of 20 teachers who went untreated was also included. Findings indicated that the VFE group had an overall greater improvement in ease and clarity of their voice production. The LMRVT program augments introductory approaches to "resonant voice" with early training centered on humming and production of resonant words and phrases following a prescribed sequence and hierarchy. The basic premise of LMRVT is that a target laryngeal configuration produces the strongest voice, while using the least amount of respiratory effort and placing the least amount of impact stress on the vocal folds, thereby reducing laryngeal injury (Verdolini Abbott, 2000). Currently, clinical trials are ongoing with the intent to provide evidence of LMRVT outcome. Students should stay abreast of emerging literature on treatment outcomes.

The most obvious resonance disorders are hyper- and hyponasality. When hypernasality is present without an apparent organic cause, the speech usually responds to voice treatment. The basic objective, of course, is to achieve closure of the velopharyngeal port at the proper time in conjunction with adequate mouth opening. Individuals with communication problems usually do not fit into neat categories. Their complex problems often require interdisciplinary management.

Speech Without a Larynx

Approximately 12,000 new cases of laryngeal cancer are diagnosed each year in the United States (Casper & Colton, 1998). Many of these cases have to undergo a total laryngectomy, which results in complete loss of the larynx and some associated structures. The result is an absolute loss of voice. Speech pathologists and surgeons have been searching for an effective technique of vocal rehabilitation since the first laryngectomy was performed in 1873. Artificial larynges and esophageal speech (see discussion below) have been used as alternative voicing methods. The more effective method, however, appears to be the tracheoesophogeal puncture (TEP) and the voice prosthesis introduced by Singer and Blom in 1980. The unique speech problems of the laryngectomized justify extra study; see the books by Blom, Singer, and Hamaker (1998), Casper and Colton (1998) P.C. Doyle (1994), and Graham (1997). Earlier in this chapter, in the review of the relationship between phonation and resonance, the larynx was described as the generator of linguistically undifferentiated sound that is modified into meaningful speech by the movements and positions of the articulators. In other words, any complex sound could substitute for the laryngeal sound if it were put into the upper airway. Loss of the larynx occurs usually as the result of surgical treatment for cancer or, occasionally, from injury that requires laryngectomy as a life-preserving measure. Removal of the larynx alters the structures in the anterior part of the neck. The removal of the total larynx occurs. A stoma, or opening, is created in the lower front of the neck. The trachea is attached to this stoma, and the person breathes through it. There is complete separation between the airway to the lungs and the alimentary tract. After the larynx has been removed, the laryngectomized person has three possible substitute sound sources as mentioned above: artificial larynges, esophageal speech, or a voice prosthesis available through a TEP.

Artificial Larynges

Artificial larynges can be classified according to their source of power: pneumatic or electronic. The pneumatic instruments use pulmonary air, are hand held, and have an air supply tube, sound source, and sound-conducting tube. When a laryngectomee speaks with one of these instruments, the air supply tube is held against the stoma to conduct the exhaled air to the sound source, which is located in the capsule displayed in the figure. The capsule contains a vibrator, either a reed or a broad rubber band that is activated by the airflow. The sound that is generated is conducted into the mouth through a small tube that passes between the lips and opens above the tongue in the vault of the mouth. Articulating in the usual manner produces intelligible speech.

The electronic artificial larynges are more common than the pneumatic instruments, primarily because they are easier to use and maintain. These units take several forms according to the manufacturers' designs, but their function in speaking is similar. A battery and associated circuit, which are located in the handle, vibrate a small disc at one end. This generates a buzzing sound that can be turned on and off with a thumb switch. Some models have variable controls for both pitch and volume. When a laryngectomized person speaks with this type of instrument, the sound-producing end is placed firmly against the upper part of the neck at a location that has been experimentally determined to produce the loudest speech. The sound passes through the skin and other tissues of the neck into the pharynx and mouth, where it is available for speech. Electrolaryngeal devices are the most frequently used means of communication by laryngectomees (Culton & Gerwin, 1998). Another device conducts the sound from an earphone-type sounder through a tube into the mouth. The speaker unit is held in the user's hand and can be turned on and off with a push-button switch. The power for the unit comes from a battery carried in a pocket or other convenient container. A variant of this concept has a speaker unit mounted in the bowl of a tobacco pipe or cigarette holder and uses the stem to transmit the sound into the mouth. These units have not been widely used; they are mentioned here to suggest the range of aids developed to help the laryngectomee.

A major advantage of artificial larynges is that laryngectomees are able to use them effectively with very little training. However, the quality of speech produced by artificial larynges is generally monotone, and in the case of the electrolarynx, the speech has a mechanical sound. Also, these devices require the use of one hand, which hinders laryngectomees from completing two-handed tasks while simultaneously communicating.

Esophageal Speech

A natural sound source is present in the neck area of almost everyone. This voice generator is usually located at the junction between the pharynx and esophagus, an area sometimes called the pharyngeoesophageal (P-E) segment. The sound is produced when air in the esophagus is forced through the constriction at the P-E segment, causing it to vibrate (see Figure 8.11). The sound is in the form of a belch, burp, or eructation. The air is released in a sequence of puffs that create sound pressure waves similar to those produced at the vocal folds. The esophageal sound can be used in speaking if it is prolonged and available when needed. The requirement, then, is to learn to take air into the esophagus and return it with sound when desired. Reported success rates for individuals who are able to use esophageal speech as a means of effective communication vary greatly, from 30 percent (Gates, Ryan, Cantu, & Hearne, 1982) to 63 percent (Natvig, 1983). The use of esophageal speech is appealing to some laryngectomees because it does not require the use of any external devices or any additional surgical procedures. However, one major disadvantage of esophageal speech is the limited duration of speech utterances due to the restricted amount of air that is inhaled.

Surgical Procedures

Many surgical procedures to aid voice production have been developed with varying degrees of success. Some reconstruct a vibrator, a pseudoglottis at the laryngeal site from the remaining tissue, and the pulmonary air activates this. Others incorporate an external device with a reed-type vibrator through which the pulmonary air flows to create a sound that is carried back into the pharynx through a small tube passing through a surgically created opening in the neck.

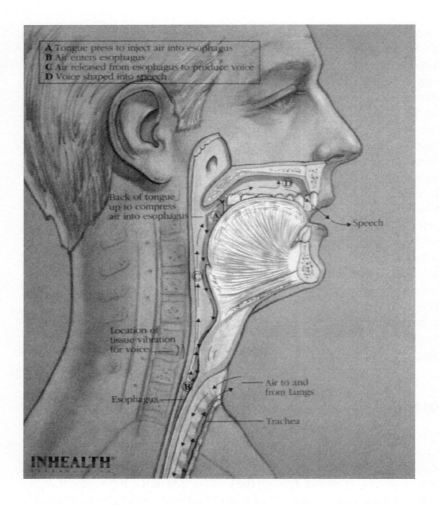

A third surgical procedure, and the most widely used, employs a shunt (fistula), a tunnel that connects the trachea with the esophagus. This channel allows the pulmonary air to pass from the trachea into the esophagus and up through the P-E constriction, where vibration occurs to create sound (M.I. Singer & Blom, 1980) (see Figure 8.12). The TEP is frequently performed as a primary procedure at the time of the laryngectomy. However, the TEP may be performed as a secondary procedure 6 to 8 weeks after the initial surgery or radiation treatment (Kao, Mohr, Kimmel, Getch, & Silverman, 1994).

Shunts tend to close; consequently, they are kept open by the insertion of a plastic tube that permits relatively easy flow of the breath when the tracheal stoma is closed. Figure 8.12 indicates the route of the air when the thumb or a special valve intentionally closes the stoma. These are one-way valves that allow the exhaled air to pass into the esophagus and prevent food and liquids from going the other way into the trachea. Since air from the lungs activates the vibrator, the length of sentences and fluency can be similar to speaking with a normal larynx. A "tracheostoma" valve may be placed at the stoma, instead of a thumb, to direct the air through the fistula for speaking. The valve allows inhalation and exhalation for ordinary respiration, but a sudden slight increase in airflow to initiate speech closes the valve, thereby causing the breath to flow through the fistula. The valve will also open completely to accommodate a cough. The shunt procedure helps many laryngectomized persons to speak well, and it frees both

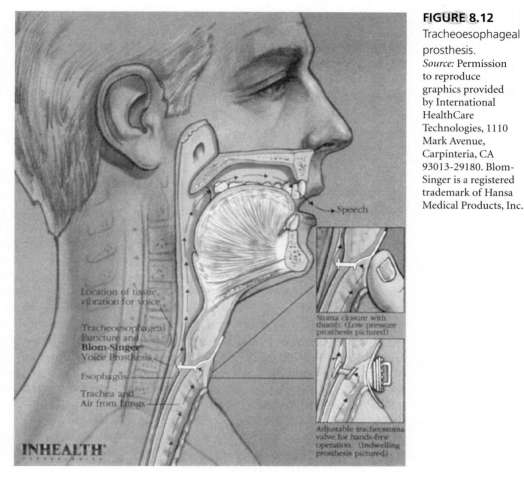

FIGURE 8.12
Tracheoesophageal prosthesis.
Source: Permission to reproduce graphics provided by International HealthCare Technologies, 1110 Mark Avenue, Carpinteria, CA 93013-29180. Blom-Singer is a registered trademark of Hansa Medical Products, Inc.

hands for ordinary activities, but it is not for everyone. The Blom-Singer Adjustable Tracheostoma Valve is a commonly used device with a reported success rate among users of 66 percent (Grolman et al., 1995). Postsurgical structural conditions may prevent the use of tracheoesophageal puncture techniques. Also, removing, cleaning, and reinserting the prosthesis requires dexterity and personal management that may be beyond the capacity of some patients, so that not all laryngectomees are candidates for this procedure. Recently, a long-term indwelling voice prosthesis was developed that reduces routine maintenance of the device (Blom, 1995). It can be left in place for approximately 6 months. And the most current indwelling device being experimented with may be able to stay in for as long as a year.

Limitations

No alaryngeal form of speaking is as desirable as normal speech, but any of the forms, when used well, can be extremely serviceable. Of the available options for alaryngeal speech, tracheoesophageal speech seems to be the most natural sounding. High rates of success have been associated with tracheoesophageal speech. Geraghty, Wenig, Smith, and Portugal (1996) report a 66 percent success rate for the long-term effectiveness of tracheoesophageal speech. Slightly higher rates for effective communication have been reported for individuals who have TEP as a primary procedure (93%) compared to those who have TEP as a secondary procedure (83%) in regard to short-term usage (Kao et al., 1994). In a survey of perceptions of speech-language pathologists toward the different types of alaryngeal speech, TEP was ranked as the most preferred method of laryngectomy rehabilitation. The artificial larynx was ranked as the least preferred (Culton & Gerwin, 1998).

Treatment Accountability

Professionals working in the area of voice are very sensitive about the issues surrounding evidence-based outcomes. There have been numerous national initiatives focused on strengthening our position as rehabilitation specialists. Working in teams, professionals in the area of voice and voice disorders have developed evidence-based outcome tools that will help define the success or failure of particular treatment modalities. Evidence-based outcome research places emphasis on the dissemination of information, as well as its collection, so that the evidence can reach clinical practice. Outcomes are assessed by the therapist and by the patient so that treatment tools can be validated as well as refined in practice. One such tool that has been recently developed in the CAPE-V, which stands for the Consensus of Auditory Perceptual Evaluation of Voice. This tool is being tested as a potential standardized method for evaluating the voice quality of a disordered voice and documenting its response to treatment. More information about the CAPE-V can be found at www.asha.org. There are other tools that have focused on defining functional outcomes from the patient's perspective. These are termed quality-of-life indices. Two such indices that are commonly used are the Voice Handicap Index (B.H. Jacobson et al., 1997) and the Voice-Related Quality of Life Scale (Hogikyan & Sethurman, 1999). These scales allow the clinician to assess the impact a voice disorder has on physical, social, and emotional factors as perceived by the patient as well as to determine how the impact of the voice disorder changes following intervention. Like all work in the area of rehabilitation, it is the role of the researcher to define which treatments are efficacious and effective by comparing and contrasting the many available techniques.

case study KEITH

Keith, a 27-year-old high school football coach and teacher in excellent physical condition, referred himself to a speech and hearing clinic with a moderately severe breathy, hoarse voice with intermittent moments of total voice loss. His pitch range was limited to the low notes in his potential range. He had lost the higher notes as the voice disorder progressed. The coach reported to the speech-language pathologist that he talked a lot, which was confirmed during the evaluation.

Keith reported a long history of hoarseness. He had always been active physically and vocally and noted that the hoarseness had recently become worse. An older friend and coach also had a laryngeal tumor of some sort that required surgery. This experience frightened Keith into attending to his own voice.

His typical daily routine began at 5:00 A.M. with 7 miles of jogging. At 6:30 A.M., he conducted football practice, which continued until the start of the regular school schedule. He taught five classes each day in which he lectured most of the time. After school, there was more football practice, and sometimes he held private classes in gymnastics. He arrived home around 8:00 P.M.; after dinner, he often read bedtime stories to his 3-year-old son. During those evenings when his team had a football game, he shouted and yelled almost continuously throughout the game. His voice was always extremely hoarse following a game.

A medical examination showed bilateral vocal nodules of moderate size. Both vocal folds were slightly inflamed. A diagnosis of moderately severe breathy-hoarseness with intermittent loss of voice resulting from the medium-size, bilateral vocal nodules was made. These lesions were caused by excessive vocal use and abuse in his occupation as coach and teacher.

Unfortunately, Keith lived in a region where he could not obtain direct aid from a speech-language pathologist. Consequently, a program was planned for him that contained the following: (1) He received a detailed description of vocal nodules—this information was presented at the time of the voice evaluation with the aid of photographs of vocal nodules and the playing of his voice recording; the need to eliminate vocal abuse and reduce speaking to a minimum was stressed. (2) We reviewed the work situation to identify places where vocal abuse could be reduced—this discussion resulted in the following actions: elimination of all but essential speaking (he put himself on almost complete silence for 10 days), introduction of a whistle and bullhorn for signaling and giving instructions on the football field, alteration of his classroom methods (use students in instruction, more written work, and the like), and restraint of vocal output during games.

After 1 month, Keith returned to the voice clinic for reevaluation. His voice had improved substantially, and although the nodules were still present, the general inflammation had subsided and the nodules were somewhat smaller. A continuation of the same therapy regimen was recommended. Subsequent evaluations over the next several months revealed continued improvement except for temporary setbacks following games during which he had yelled.

One of the most important changes affecting the ultimate management of this voice problem was in Keith's perception of his role as coach. He came to realize that his excessive yelling was an extension of his own participation in the sport. During the games and practice sessions, he partially reverted to his playing days through his shouting and excessive verbal output. When his thinking became more mature, Keith was able to exert appropriate control of his voice.

Have you ever heard a voice with any intermittent aphonia, hoarseness, nasality, or breathiness? What would you, as a speech-language pathologist, do with and for the man whose case summary was presented? Discovering answers to questions about voice problems is the goal for this chapter.

Prevention

Preventing voice disorders relies on awareness and education. Voice disorders can be caused by physical, social, emotional, and environmental factors. Educating individuals who use their voice occupationally and developing awareness of good vocal hygiene strategies should be done in a proactive manner rather than reactive manner. While it is obvious that some disorders are not preventable, the majority of them are. It is the role and responsibility of the speech-language pathologist to be the educator and provide appropriate and up-to-date material to individuals who use their voices in the workforce.

Remedial programs for voice disorders must recognize the causes in each individual case and attempt to modify those causes where possible. Therapy programs must also incorporate the means for increasing function to maximum efficiency. The full restoration or development of normal voice is not always possible, but usually we have remedial techniques available that can at least facilitate more intelligible speech, more normal vocal sound, and more efficient, trauma-free voice production. In a society such as ours, which depends heavily on spoken communication, every step toward better communication is a valuable contribution.

STUDY QUESTIONS

1. What kinds of vocal use can be classified as phonotraumatic?

2. How can the laryngeal structures be seen and laryngeal function be evaluated?

3. Many untrained young singers of popular music destroy their voices within a period of 2 or 3 years. Can you trace the probable sequence of events and changes that might occur in a hypothetical singer who develops hoarseness?

4. Why do voice deviations tend to be of less concern within the general population than other communication problems such as stuttering and articulation disorders?

SELECTED READINGS

American Speech-Language-Hearing Association. Accessed August 15, 2009, from www.asha.org.

Andrews, M. L. (1994). *Manual of voice treatment: Pediatrics to geriatrics.* Florence: Thomson Learning.

Colton, R. H., Casper, J. K., & Leonard, R. (2006). *Understanding voice problems: A physiological perspective for diagnosis and treatment* (3rd ed.). Baltimore, MD: Williams & Wilkins.

Doyle, P. C. (1994). *Foundations of voice and speech rehabilitation following laryngeal cancer.* Florence, KY: Thomson Learning.

Doyle, P. C,, & Keith, R. (Eds.). (2005). *Contemporary considerations in the treatment and rehabilitation of head and neck cancer: Voice, speech, and swallowing.* Austin, TX: Pro-Ed.

Hogikyan, N. D., & Sethurman, G. (1999). Validation of an instrument to measure voice-related quality of life (V-RQOL). *Journal of Voice, 13*(4), 555–569.

Roy, N., & Leeper, H. A. (1993). Effects of the manual laryngeal: Musculoskeletal tension reduction technique as a treatment for functional voice disorders–perceptual and acoustic measures. *Journal of Voice, 7,* 242–249.

Roy, N., Merrill, R. N., Gray, S. D., & Smith, E. M. (2005). Voice disorders in the general population: Prevalence, risk factors, and occupational impact. *Laryngocope, 115*(11). 1988–1995.

Sapeinza, C., & Hoffman Ruddy, B. (2008). *Voice disorders.* San Diego, CA: Plural.

Stemple, J. C. (Ed.). (2000). Voice therapy and clinical studies (2nd ed.). San Diego, CA: Singular Publishing Group.

Stemple, J. C., Glaze, L., & Gerdeman, B. (2000). Clinical voice pathology: Theory and management (3rd ed.). San Diego, CA: Singular Publishing Group.

Titze, I. R. (1994). *Principles of voice production.* Englewood Cliffs, NJ: Prentice-Hall.

Wilson, D. K. (1987). Voice problems of children (3rd ed.). Baltimore, MD: Williams & Wilkins.

WEBSITES OF INTEREST

American Cancer Society
www.cancer.org
American Speech-Language-Hearing Association, Division 3, Voice and Voice Disorders
www.asha.org/members/divs/div_3.htm
American Speech-Language-Hearing Association. Voice Disorders
www.asha.org/public/speech/disorders/voice.htm
Glottal Enterprises
www.glottal.com
InHealth Technologies
www.inhealth.com
KayPentax
www.kaypentax.com

National Cancer Institute
www.nci.gov
National Center for Voice and Speech
www.ncvs.org
National Institutes of Health, Voice Disorders
health.nih.gov/topic/VoiceDisorders
Sensimetrics Corporation
www.sens.com
Tucker Davis Technologies
www.tdt.com
Voice Foundation
www.voicefoundation.org
Voiceproblem.org
www.voiceproblem.org

Chapter NINE

Cleft Lip and Palate and Other Craniofacial Disorders

Ann W. Kummer
Cincinnati Children's Hospital Medical Center and
University of Cincinnati Medical Center

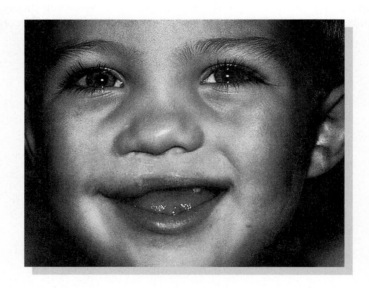

personal **PERSPECTIVE**

ANN W. KUMMER

If we define "success" as obtaining ultimate professional satisfaction, I am one of the most successful speech-language pathologists in the world today! This is because my career has been defined by helping children with clefts and craniofacial anomalies achieve normal speech, despite sometimes significant obstacles. This has been immensely gratifying because communication is such an important human skill. It keeps us connected with others and enhances our relationships. As with facial appearance, the quality of our speech is important because it leaves a first and lasting impression on others.

My first job as a speech-language pathologist was working in the public schools of North Carolina. In that position, I had a child named Justin on my caseload. Justin had perfect articulation, but terrible speech due to a loud nasal distortion on consonants. I referred Justin to an otolaryngologist who looked in his mouth and said all was fine. He recommended speech therapy, which I did for another 3 years. At the end of my time in that school, Justin had made no progress with speech therapy.

What I didn't know then, but what I do know now, is that Justin had a nasal rustle during consonant production, which is typically due to a small velopharyngeal opening. There was probably a defect on the nasal surface of the velum, so it would not have been detected from an intra-oral examination alone. Because this is a structural problem, it requires surgery for correction—not speech therapy. I also now understand that most otolaryngologists are unfamiliar with velopharyngeal dysfunction unless they specialize in this area. I should have referred Justin to a craniofacial team, where there are specialists who can evaluate and treat this disorder appropriately. I think of that child periodically and just wish I had had the right information then in order to help him and make a positive difference in his life.

After 3 years in North Carolina, I began working at Cincinnati Children's Hospital Medical Center. There, I was fortunate to be assigned to the Craniofacial Team, where I found my passion. For many years now, I have been able to work with an interdisciplinary group of professionals who are experts in the evaluation and treatment of children with clefts and complex craniofacial syndromes. Although not all outcomes are good, for the most part we are able to make a very positive impact on the lives and futures of these children. This is very rewarding and therefore, that is what I call success!

case study

Angela was born with a unilateral complete cleft lip and palate. The lip was repaired at 3 months of age and the palate was repaired at 10 months. Angela was initially followed by a craniofacial team near her home. However, the parents got divorced and the family moved. Therefore, she was lost to follow-up.

When Angela was 9 years old and just starting fourth grade, the school speech-language pathologist called me to ask for advice. Angela had been receiving speech therapy at that school since she was in kindergarten. According to the records, the previous speech-pathologist used blowing, sucking, and oral motor exercises (all of which are very inappropriate!) and articulation therapy. Angela made virtually no progress with the 4 years of speech therapy.

I recommended bringing Angela in to our craniofacial team for a comprehensive evaluation. In the evaluation, it was determined that Angela's speech consisted of hypernasality, nasal air emission, and compensatory articulation productions. As a result, intelligibility of speech was poor. Angela expressed embarrassment about her speech, and as a result, she was very shy and had few friends. A nasopharyngoscopy evaluation showed a moderate-sized velopharyngeal opening. Therefore, a pharyngeal flap was done to correct the velopharyngeal insufficiency.

Angela received about 6 months of postoperative speech therapy for correction of the compensatory speech productions. This was done though a coordinated effort of the speech pathologists at Cincinnati Children's Hospital and in her school. Her mother also worked with Angela on speech practice every day at home. As a result of these efforts, Angela was finally discharged from speech therapy at the end of fourth grade. At that time, she had normal speech and resonance and much more social confidence. Incidentally, she also had a bone graft to the alveolus and a lip revision and began dental/orthodontic treatment with the team specialists during that year.

The lessons learned from this case are many. First, about 25–30 percentage of children with a history of cleft palate will have velopharyngeal insufficiency (VPI), which causes hypernasality, nasal air emission, and articulation errors. VPI is a structural problem that cannot be corrected with speech therapy (which only changes function). Instead, VPI requires surgical correction. Ideally, Angela should have had the pharyngeal flap between the ages of 3 and 4. Another point is that blowing, sucking, and oral motor exercises are totally inappropriate as a treatment for VPI in all cases. They simply don't work, even when there is motor involvement. Although articulation therapy is appropriate for correction of the compensatory errors, it is not very effective until the abnormal structure is corrected. Therefore, the years of speech therapy were very ineffective and only served to negatively affect Angela's self-esteem. Finally, children with a history of cleft lip and palate require coordinated services from a variety of medical, surgical, dental, psychological, and allied health professionals throughout childhood. Therefore, team care and follow-up are essential for optimal outcomes.

Most speech pathologists, particularly those who work with children, are likely to encounter clients on their caseload with speech problems secondary to cleft lip and/or palate. Unfortunately, due to the depth of the field, courses on clefts and craniofacial anomalies are usually not required in speech pathology or communication sciences training programs. As a result, many practicing speech-language pathologists have little education or experience in this area. This is a particular problem because children with a history of cleft present speech disorders that are unique—and very different than other types of speech disorders. However, the speech-language pathologist is often the person who is best able to determine if the speech disorder can be corrected by speech therapy or needs correction through surgical intervention.

The purpose of this chapter is to provide basic information about craniofacial anomalies, particularly cleft lip and palate, and to discuss how these anomalies can affect speech, language, voice, and resonance. The reader will learn how to evaluate speech and resonance and when to refer for a specialty evaluation of velopharyngeal function. Finally, specific treatment techniques will be provided. It is hoped that with this information, the reader will be able to make appropriate decisions to ensure the best outcome for children with clefts or craniofacial syndromes.

Structures of the Lip and Palate

Before discussing cleft lip and palate, it is important to point out various structures and embryological suture lines. An examination of the upper lip (Figure 9.1) will reveal the *philtrum*, which is a long dimple or indentation that courses from the nose down to the upper lip. On either side of the philtrum are *philtral ridges*. These ridges are actually embryological suture lines that are formed as the segments of the upper lip fuse. If there is a cleft lip, the cleft (opening) will be along one or both of those lines.

An intra-oral examination (Figure 9.2) will reveal the *maxillary teeth* and *alveolar ridge* just behind the teeth. One can first see the *hard palate*, which is a

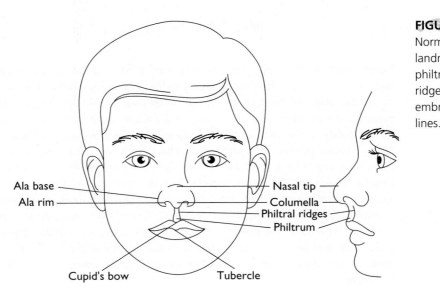

FIGURE 9.1

Normal facial landmarks. Note the philtrum and philtral ridges, which are embryological suture lines.

Ala base —
Ala rim —
Nasal tip —
Columella —
Philtral ridges —
Philtrum —
Cupid's bow   Tubercle

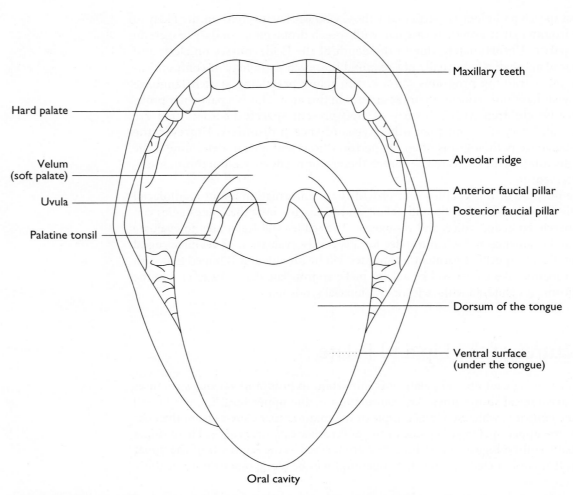

Hard palate

Velum
(soft palate)

Uvula

Palatine tonsil

Maxillary teeth

Alveolar ridge

Anterior faucial pillar

Posterior faucial pillar

Dorsum of the tongue

Ventral surface
(under the tongue)

Oral cavity

FIGURE 9.2   The structures of the oral cavity as viewed through an intra-oral
examination.

bony structure that separates the oral cavity from the nasal cavity. Posterior to the
hard palate is the *velum* (frequently called the soft palate). The velum is soft and
muscular and can be seen to elevate with phonation. At the posterior edge of the
velum is the pendulous *uvula*. Two *faucial pillars* (curtainlike structures) can be seen
on each side of the oral cavity. The *tonsils* (when present) are located between each
set of faucial pillars. The *pharynx* is the throat area that also serves as part of the
upper airway. The lateral and posterior pharyngeal walls surround the pharynx.
Finally, looking at the bony structure of the hard palate (Figure 9.3), there are two
incisive suture lines. These are embryological suture lines that course through the
alveolar ridge to the *incisive foramen*. These lines border the triangle-shaped
premaxilla, which will contain the maxillary incisors. Finally, there is the *median
palatine suture line* that courses through the middle of the hard palate. If any of these
sutures lines do not completely close during embryological development, a cleft will
be the result.

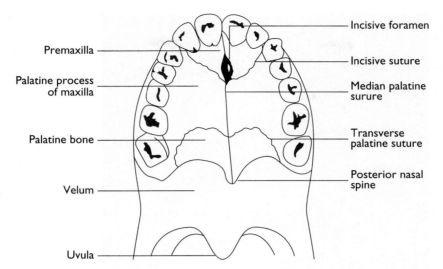

FIGURE 9.3 Bony structures of the hard palate and the soft tissue of the velum and uvula.

Labels on figure:
- Premaxilla
- Palatine process of maxilla
- Palatine bone
- Velum
- Uvula
- Incisive foramen
- Incisive suture
- Median palatine surure
- Transverse palatine suture
- Posterior nasal spine

Cleft Lip and Palate

Overt Cleft Lip and Palate

In normal embryological development, sections of the embryonic facial tissue and palate move toward each other to fuse. The lip usually fuses around 7 weeks of gestation, and the palate fuses at 9 weeks of gestation. Cleft lip and/or palate is the result of a disruption in the embryological fusion during the first trimester of pregnancy. If fusion fails to occur, a cleft (opening) is the result. Clefts can occur in the lip and alveolus without a cleft palate or in the palate without a cleft lip. Clefts of the lip and alveolus can be unilateral (Figure 9.4) or bilateral (Figure 9.5). Note that with a bilateral cleft, the premaxilla is separated from the rest of the palate due to the clefts through the incisive suture lines.

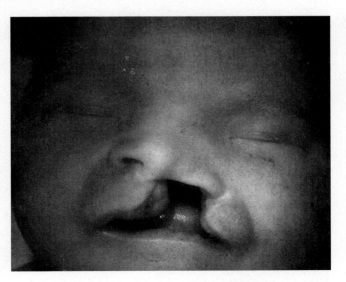

FIGURE 9.4
Patient with a wide unilateral complete cleft of the primary palate (lip and alveolus).

Note: Figures 9.4, 9.5, 9.6, 9.7, 9.8, 9.9, 9.10, 9.11, 9.12, 9.13, 9.14, 9.21, 9.22, 9.24, 9.25, 9.26, 9.27, 9.28 (left), and 9.29 from Kummer, *Cleft Palate and Craniofacial Anomalies*, 2E. © 2008 Delmar Learning, a part of Cengage Learning, Inc. Reproduced by permission. www.cengage.com/permissions

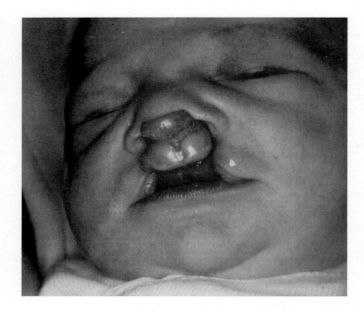

Clefts vary in the extent (or severity) of the defect. For example, an incomplete cleft lip could be as minor as a small notch in the upper lip. On the other hand, a complete cleft of the lip will extend through the entire lip, through the base of the nostril, and through the alveolar ridge (following the incisive sutures lines) to the area of the incisive foramen. An incomplete cleft palate may be as slight as a bifid (split) uvula, or it may include only the velum (not the hard palate). However, a complete cleft of the palate extends from the uvula to the incisive foramen, which is right behind the alveolar ridge (Figure 9.6). A bilateral complete cleft lip and palate includes the lip, alveolus and palate. (Figure 9.6).

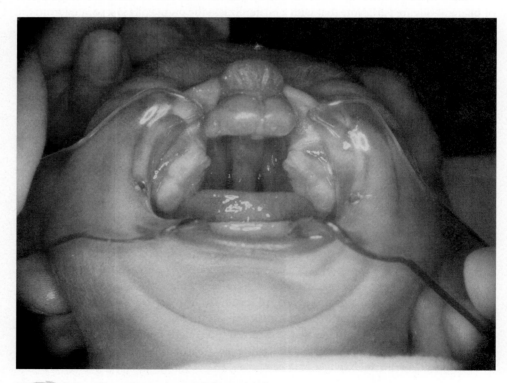

FIGURE 9.6   Bilateral complete cleft lip and palate.

Submucous Cleft

A submucous cleft palate is a congenital defect that affects the underlying structure of the palate, while the oral surface mucosa is intact (K. T. Chen, Wu, & Noordhoff, 1994; Garcia Velasco, Ysunza, Hernandez, & Marquez, 1988). This defect often involves the muscles and nasal surface of the velum. An *overt* submucous cleft is one that can be identified through an intra-oral examination (Figure 9.7a and 9.7b). The most common characteristic of an overt submucous cleft is a bifid or hypoplastic uvula. In some cases, a zona pellucida (thin zone) is noted in the velum as a dark or bluish area. The zona pellucida is due to diastasis (separation) of the muscles. If the submucous cleft extends to the hard palate, a notch can often be seen or felt in the posterior border of the hard palate.

An *occult* (which means hidden) submucous cleft is a defect in the velum that is not apparent on the oral surface (Gosain, Conley, Marks, & Larson, 1996; Gosain, Conley, Santoro, & Denny, 1999; Kaplan, 1975). In fact, it can be appreciated only by viewing the nasal surface of the velum through nasopharyngoscopy (Croft, Shprintzen, & Ruben, 1981; Shprintzen, 2000a) or through surgical dissection. Unless there is hypernasal speech and a nasopharyngoscopy evaluation is done, an occult submucous cleft will go undetected.

Prevalence

It is estimated that 1 in 700 children is born with cleft lip (with or without cleft palate) and 1 in 2,000 children is born with cleft palate (Edmonds & James, 1990; Gorlin, Cohen, & Hennekam, 2001; K. L. Jones, 2006; Wyszynski, Beaty, & Maestri, 1996). However, the prevalence of clefts varies by racial background. Individuals of Native American descent have the highest rate of clefts, followed by those of Asian descent.

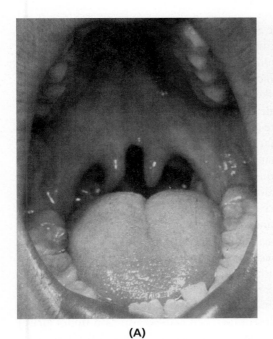

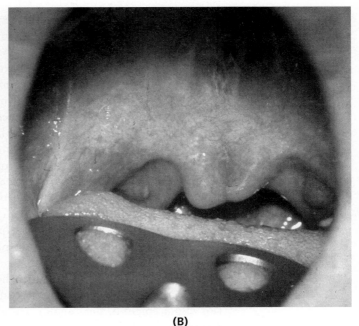

(A)   (B)

FIGURE 9.7 **(A)** A submucous cleft palate with bifid uvula and zona pellucida; **(B)** A submucous cleft with a zona pellucida and hypoplastic uvula with a faint line in the middle.

Caucasians have the third highest rate, and those of African descent have the lowest rate of clefts.

Cleft lip and palate occurs more often in boys. However, cleft palate alone occurs more commonly in girls. Cleft lip alone occurs about 25 percentage of the time, cleft palate alone occurs about 25 percentage of the time, and cleft lip and palate occurs about 50 percentage of the time. A unilateral cleft lip and palate is more common than a bilateral cleft lip and palate, and it is more common on the left side than the right.

Causes of Clefts

The cause of clefts is considered to be multifactorial (Gorlin et al., 2001; M. C. Jones, 1988; Lidral & Moreno, 2005; Wyszynski et al., 1996). Therefore, in most cases, there is both a genetic predisposition and additional environmental factors during embryological development that come together to cause the cleft. Environmental factors associated with clefts include maternal nutritional deficiencies, metabolic imbalance, disease or infection (rubella or cytomegalovirus), drugs (valium, dilantin), alcohol, chemicals, and radiation (M. C. Jones, 1988; Murray, 2002).

Many children born with clefts also have other anomalies as part of an identifiable genetic syndrome. These other anomalies further complicate treatment and can affect the overall prognosis for normal speech, language, and cognition. This is particularly true of children born with cleft palate only (Persson, Elander, Lohmander-Agerskov, & Soderpalm, 2002). Children born with cleft lip (with or without cleft palate) are far less likely to have a syndrome or other birth defects. Because many syndromes are autosomal dominant, the risk of another offspring with this syndrome can be as high as 50 percentage.

Other Craniofacial Anomalies

In addition to cleft lip and palate, there are numerous other congenital craniofacial anomalies. When multiple anomalies commonly occur together and are pathogenically related, they are identified as a *syndrome* (M. Cummings, 1997; K. L. Jones, 2006; Mange & Mange, 1999). Because craniofacial syndromes affect the facial features, they can cause affected individuals to look alike, even when there is no family relationship. A good example of this is Down syndrome. Many children with craniofacial conditions have underlying syndromes. In fact, there are over 400 craniofacial syndromes that are associated with cleft palate and velopharyngeal insufficiency. Recognizing the syndrome can be important for medical management. Because there is usually a genetic component to most craniofacial syndromes, the affected child should have a complete genetic evaluation and follow-up evaluations over time.

In contrast to a syndrome, a *sequence* is a pattern of multiple anomalies that arise consecutively from a single initiating cause (M. Cummings, 1997). Perhaps the best understood example is Pierre Robin sequence. This sequence begins with lack of development of the mandible in the first trimester. The small mandible prevents the tongue from moving down and forward in the oral cavity. Because the tongue remains high, it interferes with closure of the velum. Therefore, when the baby is born, there is usually a wide, U-shaped cleft palate; micrognathia (small lower jaw); and glossoptosis (posterior displacement of the tongue). The glossoptosis can cause significant upper airway obstruction and, in some cases, life-threatening respiratory distress. Although Pierre Robin sequence is not a syndrome by itself, it is part of many inherited craniofacial syndromes that include micrognathia as part of the syndrome's phenotype.

It is impossible to address all craniofacial syndromes in the chapter. However, the most common are velocardiofacial syndrome (Figure 9.8), Stickler syndrome (Figure 9.9), hemifacial microsomia (Figure 9.10), Crouzon syndrome (Figure 9.11), Apert syndrome (Figure 9.12), and Treacher Collins syndrome (Figure 9.13) (Shprintzen, 2000a). The phenotypic features of these syndromes are listed in Table 9.1.

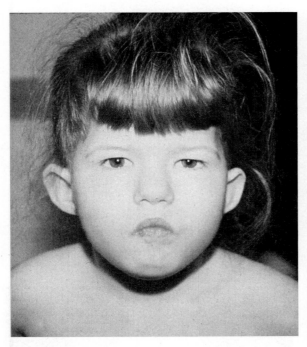

FIGURE 9.8   Patient with velocardiofacial syndrome. She has a long oval face, broad nasal tip, and small mouth.

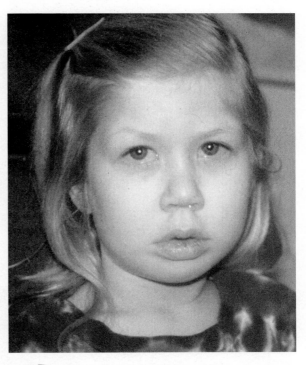

FIGURE 9.9   A child with Stickler syndrome.

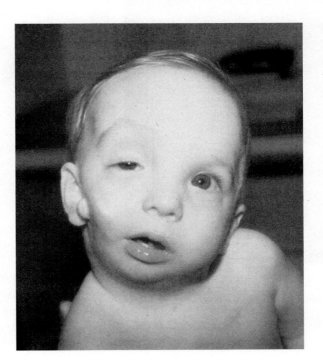

FIGURE 9.10
Patient with hemifacial microsomia. Note the facial dysplasia on the right side.

FIGURE 9.11
Sisters with Crouzon syndrome. Note the midface deficiency, which causes exopthalmus.

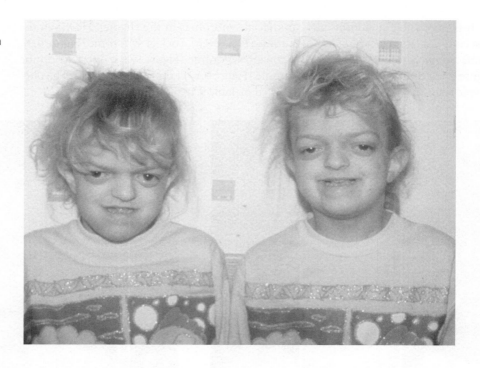

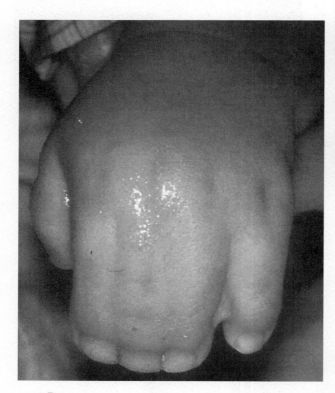

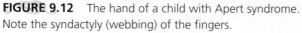

FIGURE 9.12   The hand of a child with Apert syndrome. Note the syndactyly (webbing) of the fingers.

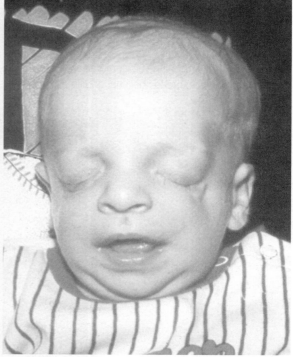

FIGURE 9.13   Patient with Treacher Collins syndrome. He has micrognathia, severe hypoplasia of the zygomatic arches, secondary low-set ears, and downslanting palpebral fissures.

TABLE 9.1   Common Craniofacial Syndromes

Velocardiofacial Syndrome (Figure 9.8)

Velocardiofacial syndrome (VCFS), also known as De George syndrome and 22q11.2 syndrome, is now recognized as the second most common genetic syndrome, following Down syndrome (Trisomy 21) as most common (Shprintzen, 2000a). VCFS is commonly identified in patients with hypernasality often of unknown etiology. In addition to the characteristic hypernasality, the individual often demonstrates language and learning problems, an articulation disorder, and hearing loss. Therefore, it is the speech pathologist that may be the first to detect the problem and refer the patient for further medical assessment and intervention.

- **Velo:** velopharyngeal dysfunction causing hypernasality, usually secondary to an occult submucous cleft or pharyngeal hypotonia.

- **Cardio:**   minor cardiac and vascular anomalies, including ventriculoseptal deviation (VSD), atrial septal defect (ASD), patent ductus arteriosis (PDA), pulmonary stenosis, tetralogy of Fallot, right-sided aortic arch, medially displaced internal carotid arteries, and tortuosity of the retinal arteries. Parents often report a history of heart murmur at birth.

- **Facial:**   microcephaly; long face with vertical maxillary excess; micrognathia (small jaw) or retruded mandible, often with a Class II malocclusion; nasal anomalies, including wide nasal bridge, narrow alar base, and bulbous nasal tip; narrow palpebral fissures (slitlike eyes); malar flatness; thin upper lip; minor auricular anomalies; abundant scalp hair; and others.

- **Learning and cognitive problems:**   learning disabilities; mild to moderate mental retardation in about 40% of the cases; concrete thinking; language disorders.

- **Communication problems:**   hypernasality due to velopharyngeal insufficiency and pharyngeal hypotonia; misarticulations, often due to verbal apraxia; conductive and/or sensorineural hearing loss; language disorders with learning problems; and high-pitched voice. Abnormal speech is the most common characteristic.

- **Other common physical and medical characteristics:**   long slender digits; hyperextensibility of the joints; short stature, usually below the 10th percentile; Robin malformation sequence (cleft palate, micrognathia, glossoptosis with airway obstruction); umbilical and inguinal hernias; and laryngeal web.

Other common functional problems: early feeding problems, gross and fine motor delays, social disinhibition, and risk of onset of psychosis in adolescence.

Stickler Syndrome   (Figure 9.9)

Stickler syndrome is an autosomal dominant condition that includes Pierre Robin sequence with the characteristic cleft palate, micrognathia, and glossoptosis. In addition, it includes sensorineural hearing loss, myopia (nearsightedness), and early onset of osteoarthritis.

Hemifacial Microsomia   (Figure 9.10)

Hemifacial microsomia (HFM) is also known as facio-auriculo-vertebral spectrum (FAV) and Goldenhar syndrome. This is a relatively common multiple anomaly disorder with a birth incidence of 1 in 3,000 to 5,000 live births (K. L. Jones, 2006). Features include unilateral lack of development (hypoplasia) of face; hypoplasia of malar, maxillary, and mandibular processes; cleftlike extension of the corner of the mouth; microtia/anotia (small or absent external ear or middle-ear anomalies); preauricular tags or pits; and hearing loss. Some affected individuals have unilateral velar paresis or paralysis, which causes velopharyngeal incompetence.

(Continued)

TABLE 9.1 *(Continued)*

Crouzon Syndrome (Figure 9.11)

Crouzon syndrome is due to premature closure of the coronal sutures of the skull. As a result, the skull grows laterally, but is restricted in the anterior-posterior dimension. This usually results in shallow orbits, causing exophthalmos (protrusion of the eyeballs), hypertelorism (wide space between the eyes), strabismus, and midface hypoplasia. Development is usually normal, although there can be developmental disabilities related to brain anomalies, including hydrocephalus and agenesis of the corpus callosum. Cleft palate and submucous cleft palate are occasionally seen in these patients (K. L. Jones, 2006).

Apert Syndrome (Figure 9.12)

Apert syndrome is similar to Crouzon syndrome. However, individuals with Apert syndrome are more likely to have cleft palate and developmental disabilities. The upper nasal and pharyngeal airway may be narrowed, causing respiratory obstruction and hyponasality in some patients. The main distinguishing feature of this syndrome, however, is that individuals with Apert syndrome have syndactyly (mittenlike webbing of the fingers and toes).

Treacher Collins Syndrome (Figure 9.13)

Treacher Collins syndrome includes downward slanting of the palpebral fissures (eye openings), colobomas (notching) of the lower eyelids, microtia or small dysplastic ears, hypoplastic zygomatic arches, and macrostomia or microstomia (large or small mouth). Treacher Collins syndrome usually includes Pierre Robin sequence, although most individuals with this condition do not have clefts, despite having pronounced micrognathia.

Effect of Clefts on Feeding

All babies feed by latching on to a nipple and then sucking. Babies with only a cleft lip may have some initial difficulty latching on to the nipple, but they do not have major problems with feeding and are usually able to breast-feed. Babies with a small cleft of the soft palate may also be able to feed without significant difficulty. However, babies with a complete cleft palate have feeding problems because the opening of the cleft makes sucking virtually impossible. It can take a long time for them to feed, which burns more calories and makes weight gain a problem. Other problems include nasal regurgitation of the milk, choking, gagging, and the swallowing of too much air.

Breast-feeding a baby with a cleft palate is not possible due to the sucking issues. However, these babies can be successfully bottle-fed with simple modifications. For example, it is important to put the nipple under a hard bone in the baby's mouth (not in the cleft area) so that the baby can compress the nipple against the bone. Also, there are special nipples that can help a baby get the most out of feeding. When a soft nipple is used or the nipple opening is enlarged, the baby can express the milk with less need for sucking. A special squeeze bottle can allow the caregiver to assist the baby in getting the milk out of the nipple. Finally, nasal regurgitation and choking can be reduced by feeding the baby in a semi-upright position. Once the palate is repaired and the baby is no longer bottle-fed, feeding is no longer an issue.

Causes of Speech Disorders Secondary to Clefts

A history of clefts or other craniofacial anomalies can have a negative effect on various aspects of communication, including speech, resonance, voice, and even language development (Kummer, 2008). Some of the reasons are as follows:

Nasal Obstruction

Depending on the type and severity of the cleft, it may result in additional anomalies of the inside of the nose and the septum. In addition, surgical correction of the lip and nose can result in a narrowing of the nares (nostrils). As the individual with a cleft grows, the maxilla and entire midface may be retrusive (too far back). This can compromise the pharyngeal airway. All of these conditions can cause hyponasality or cul de sac resonance. In addition, children with clefts often have airway issues and sleep apnea.

Short Upper Lip

Children with a history of cleft lip may present with a relatively short upper lip and bilabial incompetence. This may be due to too much scar contraction after the lip repair or a protrusive premaxilla despite surgical repair, or it may be secondary to the underlying dysmorphology. The lip incompetence is a cosmetic issue, but can also affect the production of bilabial sounds (p, b, m). Typically, the child will compensate by using a labiodental placement.

Dental and Occlusal Abnormalities

Dental anomalies, including missing, malpositioned, or supernumerary (extra) teeth, are commonly seen in the line of the cleft as it goes though the alveolar ridge. These usually do not affect speech unless there is interference with tongue tip movement. On the other hand, malocclusion (abnormal closure of the jaws) can have a significant effect on articulation. The biggest issue is with Class III malocclusion (Figure 9.14), where the top jaw (maxilla) is relatively retrusive and/or the bottom jaw (mandible) is relatively protrusive. This is very common with a history of cleft lip and palate. Because the tongue goes with the mandible, this relationship leaves the tongue tip in front of

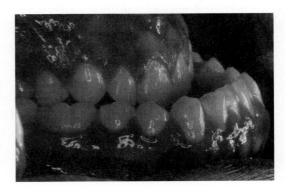

FIGURE 9.14 A dental and skeletal Class III malocclusion with underbite and underjet. These are manifestations of the lack of midfacial growth often seen in patients with cleft lip and palate.

the alveolar ridge and even the teeth. Therefore, tongue tip (lingual alveolar) sounds (t, d, n, l, s, z, sh, ch, j) may not be produced normally. Some of the same sounds can be affected with an anterior crossbite, where the jaws are normal, but the maxillary teeth are inside the mandibular teeth. Tongue-tip sounds can even be affected if the alveolar ridge is too far forward, as in a protrusive premaxilla.

Speech errors due to structural abnormalities, including abnormal occlusion, may be obligatory or compensatory. *Obligatory distortions* occur when the function is normal, but the abnormal structure results in speech distortion. For example, if the speaker has a Class III malocclusion and the tongue is in the right place in the mandible during speech, the maxillary teeth will come down on top of the tongue, causing a frontal lisp distortion on sibilant sounds (s, z, sh, ch, j). *Compensatory errors* are those that occur when the function (articulation) is changed because of the abnormal structure. If that same individual with a Class III malocclusion tries to compensate for the fact that the tongue tip is in front of the maxillary teeth and not under the alveolar ridge, he might use the dorsum of the tongue for articulation instead. This would result in several distorted speech sounds, including a lateral lisp on sibilants. See Table 9.2 for common obligatory distortions and compensatory errors.

Oronasal (Palatal) Fistula

A fistula (opening) in the palate is always a risk after palate repair (Figure 9.15). Fistulas can be related to the preoperative size of the cleft, the surgical procedure, or even the skill of the surgeon. They can also be due to postoperative infection. When maxillary expansion is needed, the opening of a fistula is always a risk.

The effect of a fistula on speech depends on its size and location. A small opening may not be symptomatic for speech because typically the airflow in the oral cavity is horizontal to the opening. A fistula the size of a dime will cause nasal emission during speech. If it is even larger, it will cause hypernasality. A fistula will be particularly symptomatic if it is located above the tongue tip. This is because, as the tongue moves upward for speech sounds, it directs the airflow into the fistula.

TABLE 9.2   Common Obligatory Distortions and Compensatory Speech Productions in Individuals with History of Cleft Lip and Palate and/or VPI

	Anterior Crossbite/Class III	*VPI*
Obligatory Distortions	■ Frontal lisp	■ Nasalized phonemes
		■ Hypernasality
		■ Nasal emission (on all pressure sounds)
Compensatory Productions	■ Reverse labiodentals	■ Generalized backing
	■ Palatal-dorsal production of lingual alveolars (t, d, n)	■ Posterior nasal fricative
	■ Lateral lisp	■ Pharyngeal plosive
		■ Pharyngeal fricative/affricate
		■ Glottal stop

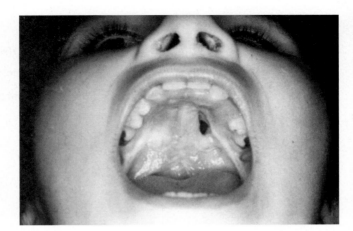

FIGURE 9.15 An oronasal fistula. *Source:* Photo by Ann Kummer.

Hearing Loss

The eustachian tube connects the middle ear with the back of the pharynx. Its role is to open during swallowing (and yawning), which allows fluids to drain out of the middle ear. It also helps to equalize air pressure between the middle ear and the environment. (You can feel it work when your ears pop on an airplane.) Unfortunately, children under the age of 5 or 6 have poor eustachian tube function, and therefore, they are prone to middle-ear effusion and ear infections. This is because the eustachian tube is in a horizontal position at this age, resulting in poor drainage. As the child grows, the relative position of the tube changes to a 45 degree angle. This results in better drainage of the middle ear and a significant decrease in middle-ear dysfunction.

Children with a history of cleft palate (not cleft lip only) or velopharyngeal insufficiency are at even greater risk for middle-ear disease (Sheahan, Miller, Earley, Sheahan, & Blayney, 2004). This is because the tensor veli palatini muscle, which opens the eustachian tube during swallowing and yawning, originates in the velum. If there is or has been a cleft in that area, the muscle may not function properly. If this is the case, the eustachian tube does not open, negative pressure is not released, and there is an accumulation of fluids (middle-ear effusion) that can't drain. Infection can occur, resulting in otitis media. Chronic middle-ear effusion and otitis media can cause a conductive hearing loss and delay speech and language development. Because this is a known issue in children with cleft palate, it is treated prophylactically with the insertion of pressure-equalizing (PE) tubes at the time of the first surgery (lip or palate repair). In order to avoid conductive hearing loss and its detrimental effect on speech and language development, aggressive monitoring of hearing and middle-ear function is important, especially in the preschool years. PE tubes may be required several times before eustachian tube function normalizes in the late childhood–early adolescent years.

Tonsils and Adenoids

The tonsils and adenoids are most prominent in young children until they reach puberty. Although adenoids play a role in the immune system, they also have a role in speech. As will be discussed below, velopharyngeal closure is important in closing off the nasal cavity from the oral cavity during speech. However, young children actually have velo-adenoidal closure until the pharynx and facial bones change with growth

FIGURE 9.16

Position of the adenoid in the pharynx. The adenoid pad can help with closure in many cases. In many young children, there is velo-adenoidal closure rather than velopharyngeal closure.

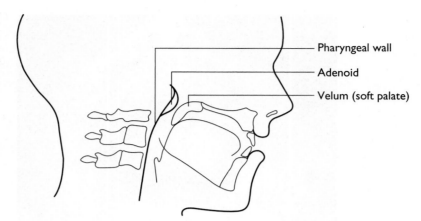

Pharyngeal wall

Adenoid

Velum (soft palate)

(Figure 9.16). Therefore, adenoidectomy carries a risk of hypernasality because it increases the space in the pharynx and may result in a velopharyngeal opening during speech (Andreassen, Leeper, & McRae, 1991; Croft, Shprintzen, & Ruben, 1981; Donnelly, 1994; Fernandes, Grobbelaar, Hudson, & Lentin, 1996; Kummer, Myer, Smith, & Shott, 1993; Ren, Isberg, & Henningsson, 1995; Saunders, Hartley, Sell, & Sommerlad, 2004). This is a particular risk for children with a history of cleft palate or submucous cleft.

Adenoid involution typically occurs around puberty. The process is gradual and occurs with changes in the skeletal and soft tissue relationships that result in more velopharyngeal closure. Therefore, the gradual atrophy of the adenoid usually has no negative effect on speech. In children with tenuous velopharyngeal closure due to a history of cleft palate or submucous cleft, there can be a gradual onset of hypernasality with this involution. This is rare, but it does occur. Usually, parents begin to complain that the child has begun to "mumble."

There is a very big misconception that tonsillectomy can also have a negative effect on speech. This is not true because the tonsils are in the oral cavity and do not contribute to velopharyngeal closure. Therefore, tonsillectomy is never a risk for speech. In fact, tonsillectomy is more likely to improve speech. This is because large tonsils or adenoids can cause hyponasality or cul-de-sac resonance. When this is the case, removal can improve the resonance and eliminate airway obstruction.

Velopharyngeal Dysfunction

For children with cleft palate, the biggest potential risk for speech is velopharyngeal dysfunction—specifically velopharyngeal insufficiency. Because this is a complex disorder, it is addressed in the following sections.

Normal Velopharyngeal Function and Velopharyngeal Dysfunction

It is important to understand normal velopharyngeal function before one can appreciate velopharyngeal dysfunction. Normal velopharyngeal closure is accomplished by the coordinated action of the velum (soft palate), the lateral pharyngeal walls, and the posterior pharyngeal wall (J. B. Moon & Kuehn, 1996, 2004). These structures function as a valve that closes off the nasal cavity from the oral cavity during speech.

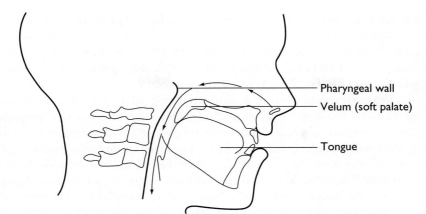

FIGURE 9.17
Lateral view of the velum and posterior pharyngeal wall during normal nasal breathing. The velum rests against the base of the tongue, resulting in a patent airway.

The velopharyngeal valve is a dynamic mechanism. During normal nasal breathing, the velum is down and rests against the base of the tongue (Figure 9.17). The pharyngeal walls are also at rest. This results in a patent airway for unobstructed nasal breathing. During speech, however, the velum moves up and back to close tightly against the posterior pharyngeal wall (back wall of the throat) (Figure 9.18). At the same time, the lateral pharyngeal walls (side walls of the throat) move medially to close against or behind the velum. The posterior pharyngeal wall moves forward to close against the velum. These actions close the velopharyngeal valve, which effectively closes off the nasal cavity from the oral cavity (Moon & Kuehn, 1996, 2004).

Velopharyngeal closure is important for speech and also for other pneumatic activities, such as blowing, whistling, sucking, and even kissing. It is also important for certain nonpneumatic activities, such as swallowing and vomiting. It should be kept in mind, however, that the locus and type of closure are different for speech than for these other activities. (This is one reason that working on blowing and sucking will not improve velopharyngeal closure for speech.)

During speech, air from the lungs provides the airflow and air pressure needed for the production of consonants. At the same time, sound from the vocal cords provides

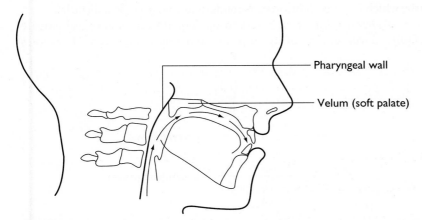

FIGURE 9.18   Lateral view of the velum and posterior pharyngeal wall during speech. The velum elevates and closes against the posterior pharyngeal wall. This allows the air from the lungs and the sound from the larynx to be redirected from a superior direction to an anterior direction to enter the oral cavity for speech.

the acoustic energy that resonates (vibrates) for the production of vowels and voiced consonants. As we speak, the air and sound travel upward through the vocal tract. If it weren't for the closed velopharyngeal valve, all the air and sound would continue to travel upward and out through the nose. With the valve closed, however, the air and sound are redirected into the mouth for speech.

Velopharyngeal closure is important for all vowels and most consonants—particularly plosives, fricatives, and affricates, which require oral pressure. The only sounds that do not require velopharyngeal closure are nasal sounds (m, n, ng) because, as their name implies, these sounds are produced through the nose with the velopharyngeal valve open. To prove this, produce the syllable "ba" repetitively and then close your nose. There should be no difference in the sound because the nasal cavity is already closed by the velopharyngeal valve. Now produce the syllable "ma" repetitively and close your nose again. With the nose closed, there is a definite difference in the sound. This is because the velopharyngeal valve is open during production of nasal sounds, allowing the sound to resonate in the nasal cavity and pass out through the nose.

Velopharyngeal dysfunction (VPD) is a condition where the velopharyngeal valve does not close completely during speech for some reason. *Velopharyngeal insufficiency* (VPI) (Figure 9.19) is typically used to describe an anatomical or structural defect that prevents adequate velopharyngeal closure. Velopharyngeal insufficiency is the most common type of VPD because it includes a short or defective velum, which is common in individuals with a history of cleft palate (despite palate repair) or submucous cleft (Moon & Kuehn, 1996, 2004). Other causes of velopharyngeal insufficiency include cranial base anomalies that can result in a very deep pharynx and irregular adenoids that can prevent a tight velo-adenoidal seal. Velopharyngeal insufficiency can even occur after certain surgeries, such as adenoidectomy (not tonsillectomy) or LeFort I maxillary advancement, which brings the maxilla (hard palate) and soft palate forward.

Velopharyngeal incompetence (VPI) (Figure 9.20) is used to refer to a neuromotor (physiological) disorder that results in poor movement of the velopharyngeal structures. Causes of velopharyngeal incompetence include velar or pharyngeal hypotonia, velar paralysis or paresis due to a brain stem injury, neuromuscular disorders (i.e., myasthenia gravis), and neurological injuries. Velopharyngeal incompetence is a common characteristic of dysarthria, which is a speech disorder secondary to a neurological disorder.

Finally, *velopharyngeal mislearning* refers to inadequate velopharyngeal closure secondary to faulty development of appropriate articulation patterns. Examples

FIGURE 9.19
Velopharyngeal insufficiency. The velum is too short to achieve velopharyngeal closure during speech.

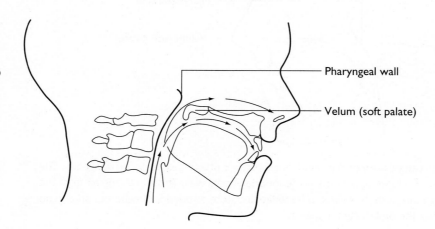

Pharyngeal wall

Velum (soft palate)

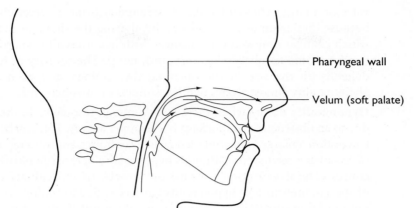

Pharyngeal wall

Velum (soft palate)

include the mislearned substitution of nasal sounds for oral sounds (i.e., ng/l or ng/final /r/) or the use of pharyngeal or nasal fricatives for oral sibilants (s, z, sh, ch, j). Because of the way these sounds are produced, these misarticulations result in abnormal nasal resonance or nasal emission. It should be noted that these types of misarticulations can be found in individuals with no history of cleft palate or VPI. They are also found in individuals who have VPI (or a history of VPI) and have learned these articulation productions as a way to compensate for inadequate intra-oral air pressure. Even if the VPI is corrected surgically, these misarticulations (and their associated nasal emission or hypernasality) will remain until they are treated with speech therapy.

A differential diagnosis of the cause of the velopharyngeal dysfunction is very important because it has implications for treatment. Velopharyngeal insufficiency and incompetence almost always require physical management through surgery or a prosthesis. On the other hand, velopharyngeal mislearning always requires speech therapy.

Effect of Clefts and Velopharyngeal Dysfunction on Speech

The structural abnormalities associated with cleft lip and/or palate and velopharyngeal dysfunction can cause problems with resonance, air pressure and airflow, articulation, and phonation (Harding & Grunwell, 1996; D. L. Jones, 2005; Kummer, 2008).

Abnormal Resonance

Resonance, as it relates to voiced speech, is the modification of the sound that is generated by the larynx as it vibrates and travels through the vocal tract. Resonance is partly determined by the size and shape of the cavities of the vocal tract (pharynx, oral cavity, and nasal cavity) because they selectively enhance certain frequencies. Resonance is also determined by the function of the velopharyngeal valve. Abnormal resonance is due to either obstruction in any of these cavities or velopharyngeal dysfunction. The following are the types of abnormal resonance:

- **Hypernasality** occurs when there is too much sound resonating in the nasal cavity during speech. This is usually due to incomplete closure of the velopharyngeal valve or a large oronasal fistula. Hypernasality is most perceptible on vowels because these sounds are produced by altering the shape of the oral cavity, which changes oral sound resonance. With hypernasality, voiced oral consonants become nasalized (i.e., m/b, n/d, ng/g). The severity of hypernasality depends on the size of the opening, the etiology, and even articulation. Hypernasality almost always requires surgical or prosthetic management.

- **Hyponasality** occurs when there is not enough resonance in the nasal cavity due to an obstruction or blockage in the upper airway. This can be due to nasal congestion, enlarged adenoids, a deviated septum, stenotic nares, nasal polyps, or maxillary retrusion. Although hyponasality is most perceptible on nasal consonants, it can also be heard on vowels. In individuals with apraxia of speech, intermittent hyponasality can occur due to timing errors in lowering the velum for the production of nasal sounds. Unless it is due to faulty articulation or timing, hyponasality is treated through medical or surgical management.

- **Cul-de-sac resonance** occurs when the sound resonates in the pharynx or nasal cavity, but it is not released due to an obstruction. This can occur when there is velopharyngeal insufficiency and anterior nasal blockage. It occurs commonly with very large tonsils, which can block the sound from entering into the oral cavity. The sound remains in the pharynx and is absorbed by the tissues. Cul-de-sac resonance sounds muffled and low in volume. As with hypernasality, parents may describe it as "mumbling."

- **Mixed nasality** occurs when there is hypernasality or nasal air emission on oral consonants and hyponasality on nasal consonants. This can occur if there is any form of nasopharyngeal obstruction (such as enlarged adenoids) and also incomplete velopharyngeal closure on oral sounds. It can also occur with apraxia of speech due to poor motor coordination of the velopharyngeal valve.

Abnormal Airflow and Air Pressure

Nasal air emission is abnormal nasal airflow (in contrast to hypernasality, which is abnormal resonance of sound). It occurs when there is an attempt to build up oral air pressure for consonants, but there is a leak in the velopharyngeal valve. Unlike hypernasality, which occurs on vowels and voiced consonants, nasal emission occurs only on pressure-sensitive consonants (plosives, fricatives, and affricates), particularly those that are voiceless.

Depending on the size of the opening, nasal emission can be very loud and distracting, or it can be totally inaudible. When there is a large opening, there is a significant loss of air pressure through the nose during speech. However, nasal emission will not be very audible. This is because there is little resistance to the flow, and therefore, minimal friction is produced. In addition, there is a co-occurrence of hypernasality, which is louder. When there is a smaller velopharyngeal opening, there is greater resistance to the flow, causing the nasal emission to be more audible. When the opening is very small, the airflow passes through the valve with a great deal of pressure. As it is released, the air pressure causes bubbling of the nasal secretions. The bubbling causes a loud and distracting *nasal rustle* (also called nasal turbulence), which is not too different than the sound that occurs when blowing the nose.

When there is a large velopharyngeal opening and a great loss of air pressure through the nose, this reduces the amount of air pressure in the oral cavity for the production of consonants. As a result, oral consonants, particularly the pressure-sensitive consonants, become weak in intensity and pressure. The loss of air through the nose also compromises breath support. This causes a need to increase respiratory effort and take more frequent breaths during speech to compensate. As a result, utterance length may be short, and connected speech can sound choppy. Finally, a nasal grimace is often observed to accompany nasal emission. A nasal grimace is a muscle contraction that occurs above the nasal bridge or at the side of the nares. It is actually an overflow muscle reaction that occurs with extreme effort to achieve velopharyngeal closure. Once velopharyngeal function is corrected, nasal grimace during speech usually disappears spontaneously.

Abnormal Articulation

As with dental and occlusal anomalies, VPI can cause obligatory distortions and compensatory errors. For example, if articulation placement is normal, but there is a large velopharyngeal opening during speech, plosives will be nasalized—in other words, substituted by their nasal cognates (i.e., m/b, n/d, ng/g). This is an obligatory speech distortion that cannot be corrected with speech therapy.

Compensatory articulation productions often occur when there is inadequate intra-oral air pressure for the production of consonant sounds. Compensatory productions secondary to VPI typically maintain the manner of production (plosive, fricative, or affricate), but sacrifice the placement of articulation. The speaker compensates by moving the placement of sounds posteriorly in the vocal tract where there is air pressure. As a result, common compensatory productions for VPI include glottal stops (plosives), pharyngeal fricatives, posterior nasal fricatives, and so on. For a description of common obligatory distortions and compensatory errors, see Table 9.2.

Abnormal Phonation

Dysphonia is characterized by hoarseness, breathiness, low intensity, and/or glottal fry. Children with a history of congenital anomalies or VPI have an increased risk for dysphonia for several reasons (Hamming, Finkelstein, & Sidman, 2009). Vocal cord nodules are common in this population due to the use of glottal stops during articulation and the hyperfunction that develops in the vocal tract with attempts to achieve velopharyngeal closure. In addition, individuals with craniofacial anomalies often have other congenital abnormalities of the vocal cords or larynx. Finally, breathiness is used by some individuals with VPI as a compensatory strategy because it masks the sound of hypernasality and nasal emission.

Perceptual and Intraoral Assessment

The perceptual assessment of speech should include evaluation of the following speech components:

- **Resonance:**   Resonance as noted on the vowel sounds and in connected speech should be assessed. A determination should be made as to whether the resonance is normal, hypernasal, hyponasal, cul-de-sac, or mixed. Although many clinicians assign a severity rating to abnormal resonance (i.e., mild, moderate, or severe), in reality it doesn't matter. This is because it is the type of resonance, not the severity, that determines treatment.

■ **Airflow and air pressure:**   The examiner should listen for nasal emission on consonant sounds. If there is nasal emission, the examiner should note if it is soft and barely audible or loud and distracting. This information can indicate the approximate size of the opening. In addition, the examiner should determine if the nasal emission occurs on all pressure-sensitive sounds or only on certain sounds. If it occurs on all pressure sounds, it is due to a structural defect in the valve that will require surgery. If it occurs only on certain sounds (i.e., sibilants) consistently, this may be due to mislearning and could be corrected with speech therapy alone. The examiner should also note whether the consonants are weak in intensity and pressure due to inadequate air pressure. Finally, the examiner should determine whether breath support is compromised by the leak of nasal air. This can be done by having the individual count to 20 and noting if breaths have to be taken before reaching the end.

■ **Articulation:**   All speech sounds should be assessed and errors noted. In children, it is important to determine the errors that are developmental in nature versus those that are misarticulations due to mislearning. When there are structural anomalies, it is also important to determine which distortions are obligatory and which are due to compensatory articulation productions.

■ **Voice (phonation):**   The quality of phonation should be determined. The presence of dysphonic features (hoarseness, breathiness, abnormal pitch, or glottal fry) should be noted.

When assessing speech characteristics and velopharyngeal function, it is important to select an appropriate speech sample to obtain the information that is needed for a definitive diagnosis (Kummer, 2008). The following speech samples should be considered:

■ **Formal articulation tests:**   Although a formal articulation test with single articulatory targets is usually easiest for the novice clinician, normal speech does not usually consist of single words. In addition, velopharyngeal function (and even articulation) may be normal in single-word productions, but abnormal in connected speech, which increases the demands on the oral motor system. Therefore, it is far better to assess articulation in connected speech, or at least with repetitive syllables.

■ **Syllable repetition:**   The syllable repetition test is powerful because it isolates individual phonemes, eliminates the effects of other speech sounds, and simulates connected speech. The examiner should ask the individual to produce consonants (particularly plosives, fricatives, and affricates) in a repetitive manner ("pah, pah, pah; pee, pee, pee; tah, tah, tah; tee, tee, tee," etc.). Each of the pressure-sensitive phonemes should be tested with a low vowel (i.e., "ah") and then again with a high vowel (i.e., "ee").

■ **Sentence repetition:**   Both articulation and velopharyngeal function can be tested by having the child repeat a battery of sentences, as can be found in Table 9.3. It is preferable to use sentences that contain phonemes that are similar in articulatory placement (such as "Take Teddy to town."). This is much faster than a single-word articulation test and less expensive because there is nothing to buy, and it is actually a more valid test of normal speech production than a formal articulation test.

TABLE 9.3   Sample Sentences for Assessment of Articulation, Nasal Emission, and Resonance

Have the child repeat the following sentences:

p	Popeye plays in the pool.
b	Buy baby a bib.
m	My mommy made lemonade.
w	Wade in the water.
y	You have a yellow yo-yo.
h	He has a big horse.
t	Take Teddy to town.
d	Do it for Daddy.
n	Nancy is not here.
k	I like cookies and cake.
g	Go get the wagon.
ng	Put the ring on her finger.
f	I have five fingers.
v	Drive a van.
l	I like yellow lollipops.
s	I see the sun in the sky.
z	Zip up your zipper.
sh	She went shopping.
ch	I ride a choo-choo train.
j	John told a joke to Jim.
r	Randy has a red fire truck.
er	The teacher and doctor are here.
th	Thank you for the toothbrush.
blends	splash, sprinkle, street

Source: From Kummer, *Cleft Palate and Craniofacial Anomalies,* 2E. © 2008 Delmar Learning, a part of Cengage Learning, Inc. Reproduced by permission. www.cengage.com/permissions.

- **Counting:**   To test velopharyngeal function, the clinician should ask the child to count from 60 to 70 or simply repeat "60, 60, 60, 60" or "66, 66, 66." The word *sixty-six* is a great screening word because it contains several /s/ sounds and a high vowel ("ee"), both of which are particularly sensitive to velopharyngeal dysfunction. In addition, it contains several /s/ blends ("kst" and "ks"), which further tax the velopharyngeal mechanism. If there are concerns regarding possible hyponasality, counting from 90 to 99 allows the examiner to assess the production of the nasal /n/ in connected speech.

- **Spontaneous connected speech:**   In addition to the syllable and sentence repetition tests, the examiner should listen to spontaneous speech. Connected speech increases the demands on the velopharyngeal valving system to achieve and maintain closure.

If the examiner is unsure about the resonance or nasal emission, there is a very simple test that can be done using a straw, preferably a bending straw. The examiner

FIGURE 9.21
Straw test. A straw can be used to test for nasal air emission and hypernasality. The straw is placed in the child's nostril as he produces pressure-sensitive sounds. If there is nasal air emission or hypernasality, this can be heard through the straw.

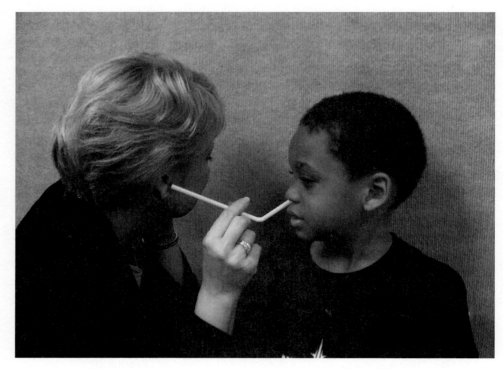

should place one end of the straw at the entrance to the child's nose and the other end at the examiner's ear (Figure 9.21). The child is then asked to produce speech samples containing only oral sounds (e.g., sa, sa, sa, sa; or prolongation of vowels) and then speech samples with nasal phonemes (e.g., ma, ma, ma, ma). If speech is normal, there should be no sound coming through the straw during production of oral sounds, but loud sound coming through the straw during production of nasal sounds. Therefore, if sound is heard through the straw on vowel sounds or voiced plosives, this indicates hypernasality. If air is heard through the straw on oral consonants, this indicates nasal emission. If there is not much sound coming through the straw on nasal consonants, this may indicate hyponasality or even nasal cul-de-sac resonance.

An intra-oral exam should be done to determine if there are large tonsils (which can cause hyponasality or cul-de-sac resonance), a submucous cleft, or a fistula (if the child has a history of cleft). The examiner should ask the child to open his mouth and say "aaah" instead of "ahhh" and to stick out his tongue as far as possible. The "aaah" sound is best because it brings the back of the tongue down and forward for a better view of the velum, uvula, and tonsils. Using this sound, the exam can usually be done without a tongue blade. If there is a bifid or hypoplastic uvula, if there is a bluish color in the velum, or if the velum appears like an inverted "V" during phonation, a submucous cleft should be suspected. Unfortunately, you cannot assess velopharyngeal function through an oral exam because the velopharyngeal valve is above your level of view and behind the velum.

Instrumental Assessment

Although a perceptual assessment of the speech characteristics of velopharyngeal dysfunction is the gold standard, it is also important to use instrumental procedures for the assessment of velopharyngeal function. There are two types of instrumental procedures that are typically used—direct measures and indirect measures (Kummer, 2008). *Direct measures* include videofluoroscopy and nasopharyngoscopy. These procedures allow the examiner to view the valve and determine the approximate size and location of the opening. This information is particularly helpful preoperatively because it guides the surgeon in choosing the best procedure for that child. The disadvantage is that these procedures are interpreted subjectively. *Indirect measures* include aerodynamic instrumentation and nasometry. These instruments allow the examiner to obtain objective data regarding the opening. This can be helpful in determining changes in velopharyngeal function as a result of surgery. The disadvantage of indirect measures is that the examiner cannot see the valve or determine the location (or even the cause) of the opening.

A brief description of instrumental procedures follows:

- **Videofluoroscopy:** A videofluoroscopic speech study is a radiographic technique that consists of multiple views of the velopharyngeal sphincter during speech. The lateral view documents the length of the soft palate, the depth of the pharynx, the elevation and elongation of the soft palate with speech, and the anterior motion of the posterior pharyngeal wall, which may contribute to closure (Figure 9.22). The frontal view allows assessment of lateral pharyngeal wall motion and its contribution to velopharyngeal closure. The base view permits an enface view of the entire sphincter. Videofluoroscopy is particularly helpful in assessing the relative elevation of the velum during speech and the entire length of the posterior pharyngeal wall. However, the visualization of the velopharyngeal opening is limited, and there is the risk of radiation exposure, although minimal, with this procedure. Also, small openings cannot be seen with this procedure.

- **Nasopharyngoscopy:** Nasopharyngoscopy is a minimally invasive endoscopic procedure that allows direct assessment of the velopharyngeal mechanism during speech. To open up the nasal cavity and numb it at the same time, a nasal spray is used that contains a mixture of neosynephrine and pontocaine. Then the endoscope is passed through the middle meatus of the nose to the back of the pharynx (Figure 9.23). It is then turned down in order to view the velopharyngeal port from above. With the endoscope in place in the nasopharynx, the function of the velopharyngeal valve can be clearly visualized during connected speech (Figure 9.24). Even a very small velopharyngeal opening can be clearly seen with

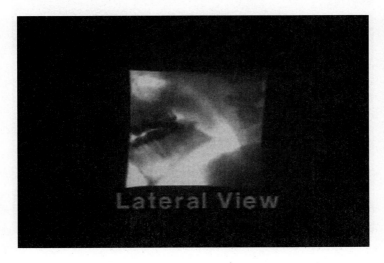

FIGURE 9.22
Videofluoroscopy. This lateral view shows a short velum relative to the posterior pharyngeal wall, resulting in velopharyngeal insufficiency.

FIGURE 9.23
Nasopharyngoscopy. For evaluation of velopharyngeal function, the scope is guided into the middle nasal meatus and then back to the nasopharynx, where it periscopes down to view the velum.

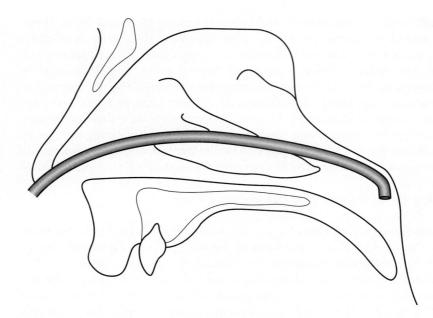

this procedure. In addition, the nasal surface of the soft palate can be assessed for signs of a submucous cleft palate (Figure 9.25). Finally, the vocal folds can be viewed, which is important because of the high incidence of vocal fold nodules and laryngeal anomalies in patients with VPI or craniofacial syndromes.

- **Aerodynamic instrumentation:**   Because speech production requires a buildup and release of air pressure at the various valving points in the vocal tract, a pressure-flow procedure can be used to evaluate velopharyngeal function (Figure 9.26). The instrumentation includes catheters that are placed in both the mouth and one nostril. These catheters are connected to a pressure

FIGURE 9.24   A nasopharyngoscopy view of normal velopharyngeal structures. The nasal surface of the velum is always at the bottom of the screen, and the posterior pharyngeal wall is always at the top of the screen. The opening to the eustachian tube can be seen on the left side of this picture.

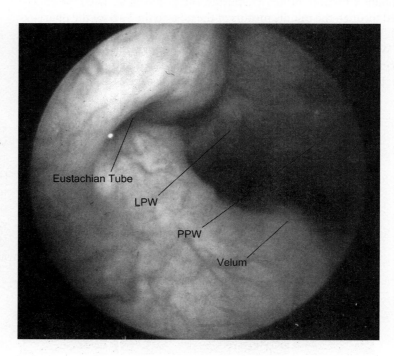

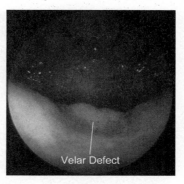

Velar Defect

FIGURE 9.25
A nasopharyngoscopy view of a submucous cleft. Note the notch in midline and the depression on the top of the velum where there should be a bulge from the musculus uvulae muscles.

transducer. A flow tube is placed in the other nostril and connected to a heated pneumotachograph. The child produces a single word, usually "hamper." Using a special formula, an estimate of the cross-sectional area of the velopharyngeal orifice can be calculated because the differential pressure and rate of airflow are measured simultaneously.

■ **Nasometry:**   The Nasometer (KayPentax, Pine Brook, NJ) is a computer-based instrument that measures the acoustic correlates of resonance and velopharyngeal function. The child wears a headset with a sound separator plate that rests on the upper lip (Figure 9.27). There is a microphone on the top of the plate to measure nasal acoustic energy during speech and a microphone below the plate to measure oral acoustic energy. Nasometry testing gives the examiner a *nasalance score*, which is the percentage of nasal acoustic energy of the total (nasal plus oral) energy. When standardized passages are used, this score can be compared to normative data. In addition, by testing certain speech phonemes in syllables, the Nasometer can provide important differential diagnostic information (MacKay-Kummer SNAP Test–R; Kummer, 2005).

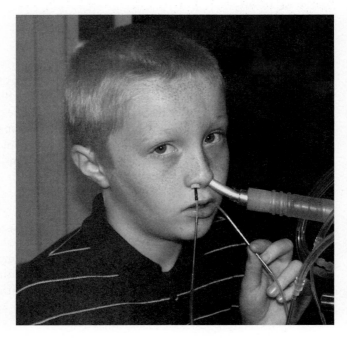

FIGURE 9.26
Aerodynamic instrumentation. The pressure-flow technique using aerodynamic instrumentation can help to estimate velopharyngeal orifice areas during the production of a few speech sounds. This figure illustrates the catheters that are placed in both the mouth and one nostril and the flow tube that is placed in the other nostril.

FIGURE 9.27
Nasometry. The headset is positioned on the child so that the sound separator plate is perpendicular to the face or in a horizontal position. The microphones should be directly in front of the mouth and the nose.

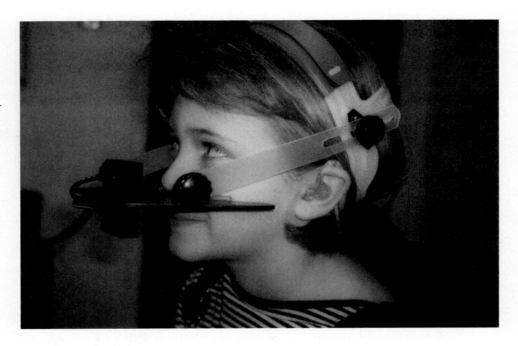

Treatment of Speech Disorders Secondary to Clefts

The treatment of abnormal speech and resonance involves physical management for the abnormal structure and behavioral management for the abnormal function. Physical management includes dental and orthodontic treatment, surgery, and prosthetics. Behavioral management involves speech therapy. These treatment options are discussed below.

Dental and Orthodontic Treatment

Because dentition and occlusion are affected by clefts and other craniofacial anomalies, early and consistent dental care is important. A child with a cleft lip and palate may require a maxillary expansion device in preschool, a bone graft to the alveolus around age 7, and orthodontic treatment during adolescence after all permanent dentition has erupted. The expansion devices and orthodontic treatment rarely interfere with speech or speech therapy. Certainly, normalizing the dentition and occlusion always has a positive effect on speech.

Many children with cleft lip/palate will develop maxillary retrusion with Class III malocclusion as they grow older. Because this is a skeletal problem, rather than dental problem, it cannot be corrected with orthodontics alone. Instead, correction of the occlusion has to be done with a combination of orthodontia and surgery. The surgery may involve a LeFort I maxillary advancement or distraction osteogenesis, where the bone is cut and gradually moved through a distraction device to allow a natural fill-in of new bone. Unfortunately, neither procedure can be done until after facial growth is complete. This is around age 14–15 in girls and age 18–19 in boys.

Surgery

Children born with cleft lip and palate often undergo several surgeries during child-hood. The lip repair is usually done around 3 months of age. Its purpose is solely aesthetic. The surgeon attempts to provide an upper lip with a symmetrical "cupid's bow" and a nose with adequate nasal tip projection and symmetrical nostrils. A lip revision is often needed at a later date. The palate is repaired around 10 months. The goal of the palate repair is purely functional. The repair is done to provide appropriate structure and function for speech and, to a lesser extent, for feeding.

Despite the palate repair, about 25 percentage of children with a history of cleft palate will have velopharyngeal insufficiency. This requires a secondary surgical procedure. Although ideally we would want normal structure before the child begins speaking, the secondary procedure for speech is usually not done until the age of 3 or 4. One reason for this is that the child has to be old enough to be talking in at least short utterances and to be cooperative for a speech and instrumental evaluation. Another reason for the delay is that all secondary procedures compromise the upper airway to some extent. This is particu-larly a concern in children with cleft palate secondary to Pierre Robin sequence. Therefore, most surgeons prefer to wait until the child's airway is big enough (between the ages of 3 and 4) to reduce the risk of postoperative airway obstruction and sleep apnea.

The following are common secondary procedures for VPI:

- **Pharyngeal augmentation:**   A filler substance (i.e., collagen or hydroxyl apetit) is injected in the posterior pharyngeal wall in the area of the opening. This helps to fill small, localized gaps or irregularities on the posterior pharyn-geal wall.

- **Furlow Z plasty:**   This procedure can be used as the primary palate repair or as a secondary procedure. Its purpose is to lengthen the velum. It works best with narrow coronal gaps.

- **Pharyngeal flap:**   A flap is elevated from the posterior pharyngeal wall and sutured into the velum to partially close the nasopharynx through this tissue bridge in midline. Lateral ports are left on either side for nasal breathing. This procedure is appropriate for large openings and midline gaps, which are most common with a history of cleft palate.

- **Sphincter pharyngoplasty:**   The posterior faucial pillars, including their internal muscles, are released at the base and rotated back to be sutured together on the posterior pharyngeal wall. This forms a type of sphincter. This procedure is best for lateral gaps or narrow coronal gaps.

In performing these procedures, the surgeon needs to balance the need to close down the velopharyngeal port for speech with that of keeping it open enough for nasal breathing (Liao, Chuang, Chen, Chen, Yun, & Huang, 2002; Yamashita & Trindade 2008). This can be a tricky balance. Therefore, these procedures often require revisions to either close the port more for speech or open it more for the airway.

Prosthetics

Prosthetic devices for speech are typically used when surgery is not an option or when it is being delayed due to airway or other concerns. These devices are made of either acrylic or metal and are similar to a dental retainer. As with a dental retainer, they hook onto the teeth for stabilization and are removable. There are three types of prosthetic devices for speech: palatal lift, palatal obturator, and speech bulb obturator.

- **Palatal lift:**   The palatal lift serves to raise the velum when velar mobility is poor, as would be seen in velopharyngeal incompetence. It is a great option for hypernasality secondary to dysarthria.
- **Palatal obturator:**   An obturator is used to occlude an open cleft or oronasal fistula for speech.
- **Speech bulb obturator (speech aid):**   The speech bulb goes behind the velum and up in the pharynx to occlude the nasopharynx. It is used when the velum is too short to achieve closure, as in velopharyngeal insufficiency. It can be combined with a palatal obturator. This is commonly done for individuals who have undergone a maxillectomy for treatment of cancer.

With the right individuals, prosthetic devices can be very helpful. However, they have some distinct disadvantages. They are expensive, yet they have to be remade periodically for children due to growth. They require manual dexterity for insertion and removal. They can be lost or damaged, and compliance is often poor because they can be uncomfortable. The biggest limitation is that they don't permanently correct the problem. Therefore, surgical correction is usually preferable whenever it is possible.

Speech Therapy

Speech therapy is usually not necessary for children under the age of 3 years. At this time, the primary focus of intervention for communication should be *quantity* (language). In other words, the goal should be to constantly increase the number of words that the child can understand, say, and then put together in sentences. Parents should be counseled on language and speech-sound stimulation techniques. If language development is not normal, language therapy should be started right away.

Between the ages of 3 and 4, the focus should shift to *quality* (articulation and resonance). It is at this time that speech and velopharyngeal function should be evaluated and that treatment (surgery and/or speech therapy) should be initiated. It should be kept in mind that speech therapy cannot change hypernasality or nasal emission due to abnormal structure— even if there is only a small gap! Also, speech therapy is usually not effective in improving nasality due to abnormal physiology. When there is VPI, surgery (or a prosthetic device) is required for correction.

Therapy *is* effective and appropriate for the following:

- Compensatory articulation productions secondary to VPI that cause nasal emission,
- Misarticulations that cause nasal air emission or hypernasality that is phoneme specific,
- Hypernasality or variable resonance due to apraxia, and
- Hypernasality or nasal emission following surgical correction. This is because changing structure does not change function. The child may need to learn to use the corrected velopharyngeal valve through auditory feedback.

If the child has VPI, but surgical correction is being delayed due to airway concerns, work can still be done on articulation placement. However, articulation placement is very difficult to learn without adequate oral air pressure. Therefore, the nose should be closed during therapy with a nose clip. The nose clip should also be worn at home during practice and whenever possible.

When therapy is appropriate, there are some simple techniques that are usually effective (Kummer, 2008). For example, if there is nasal emission on sibilants only due to the use of a pharyngeal or nasal fricative, it is helpful to have the child produce a /t/ sound with the teeth closed. Next, the child should be instructed to prolong that sound. If the child has a normal velopharyngeal valve, this should result in a normal /s/ without nasal emission. This skill can then be transferred to the other sibilant sounds.

If the child co-articulates /ng/ for /l/, it is often helpful to have the child co-articulate a yawn with the sounds. With a yawn, the back of the tongue goes down, and the velum goes up.

If the child produces glottal stops for plosives, these can be eliminated by starting with a voiceless plosive (i.e., /p/). The child should be instructed to first produce the sound without the vowel. Then the child should be shown how to produce the vowel preceded by an /h/ (i.e., ha). Finally, the child should be told to combine the consonant and the /h/ plus vowel. For example, the child should say "p . . . ha." Inserting the /h/ makes it impossible to produce a glottal stop.

When working on eliminating hypernasality or nasal emission by changing articulation placement or after surgery, auditory feedback is very important. This is best done by using a "listening tube" or stethoscope. One end of the tube is placed in the entrance of a nostril and the other end near the child's ear. If there is any nasality, the child will hear it loudly through the tube. To allow the speech pathologist (or parent) to receive the same auditory feedback, the Oral & Nasal Listener (Super Duper Publications, www.superduperinc.com) (Figure 9.28) is particularly helpful.

In speech therapy, *never* use blowing, sucking, velar, or oral motor exercises! The problem is rarely muscle weakness, and these exercises do not work! Also, do not pinch

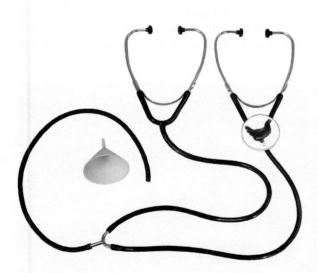 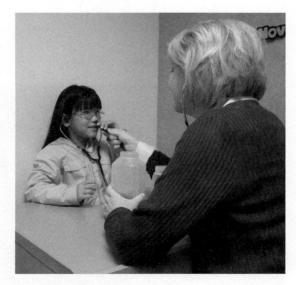

FIGURE 9.28   The Oral & Nasal Listener (ONL). The ONL is designed to allow the speech-language pathologist (or parent) and the child to hear the nasality (hypernasality or nasal emission) at the same time. This allows the adult to give appropriate feedback.
Note: The Oral & Nasal Listener is available through Super Duper Publications [superduperinc.com]. It was developed by Jonathan Cross, Jessica Link, and Ann Kummer at Cincinnati Children's Hospital Medical Center and is patented under the name Nanoscope, 12/2/03, patent number: 6656128.
Source: Photo on the right supplied by Ann Kummer.

the nose to try to improve velopharyngeal function. Closing the nose actually makes it impossible for the velum to go up. Instead, use general articulation procedures to establish correct articulation placement. In some cases, this may result in the establishment of correct oral airflow. As with other children in therapy, it is important to make sure that the child practices frequently at home. Speech therapy is like taking piano lessons. The success depends on the frequency and consistency of practice between sessions!

If the child continues to demonstrate hypernasality or nasal emission after a short period of therapy, he should be referred to a specialist for further assessment and consideration of physical management. No child should be kept in therapy and continually asked to perform a speech task that is physically impossible to do! It is best to refer the child to a *craniofacial team* (not a general otolaryngologist) for further evaluation of velopharyngeal function. Surgical intervention or surgical revision may be necessary. With appropriate management, the child should achieve the ultimate goal of normal (not just "acceptable") speech and resonance.

Importance of Team Care

As noted above, children with craniofacial anomalies, including cleft lip and palate, often demonstrate multiple complex issues, including early feeding and nutritional problems, developmental delay, hearing loss, abnormal speech and/or resonance, dentofacial and orthodontic abnormalities, aesthetic issues, and possible psychosocial problems (American Cleft Palate–Craniofacial Association, 1993). It is not possible for one professional to deal with all of these areas of concern. In fact, these children often have the need for medical, surgical, dental, speech pathology, and psychological treatment. The American Cleft Palate–Craniofacial Association recommends that cleft palate/craniofacial teams have at least a plastic surgeon, dental professional, and speech-language pathologist. However, most teams also include other professionals, such an oral surgeon, otolaryngologist, pediatrician, geneticist, dentist, orthodontist, psychologist, and audiologist (Figure 9.29). Patients with craniofacial anomalies not only require evaluation and

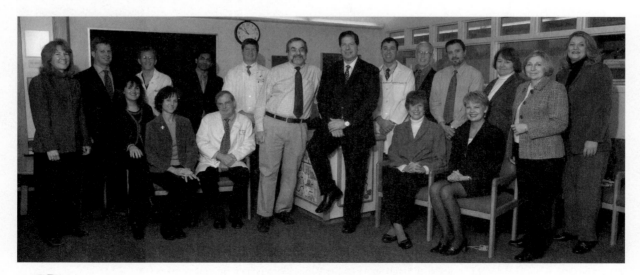

FIGURE 9.29   Team members of the Craniofacial Center at Cincinnati Children's Hospital Medical Center, 2006.

treatment from a variety of professionals, but also need follow-up over a long period of time. The entire habilitative process can last from infancy into adulthood. Even the most knowledgeable of families prefer a coordinated team approach of appointments and procedures. However, the most important reason for team care is to provide coordinated treatment by a group of specialists in order to achieve the best possible outcomes.

Summary

Cleft lip and palate and other craniofacial disorders affect the two ways that we interact with others—our facial appearance and our speech. Fortunately, with the coordinated effort of craniofacial team specialists, including the speech-language pathologist, the prognosis for children affected by these anomalies is excellent. It is truly a joy to be a part of the process of making a difference in the lives of these children!

STUDY QUESTIONS

1. Why is it important to repair a cleft palate before the onset of first words?

2. What are the possible causes of speech disorders secondary to cleft lip and palate? Explain how each can affect speech or resonance.

3. What is the difference between an obligatory speech distortion and a compensatory speech error? Which is treated with physical management only?

4. Why is adenoidectomy a potential cause of velopharyngeal insufficiency? Why is tonsillectomy never a risk factor for speech?

5. What are the speech characteristics that are secondary to velopharyngeal insufficiency?

6. Name two indirect and two direct instrumental procedures. What are the advantages and disadvantages of each?

7. What surgical procedures can be considered for velopharyngeal insufficiency?

8. Why is speech therapy ineffective and inappropriate as a means to correct velopharyngeal insufficiency?

9. In what cases is speech therapy appropriate for correction of nasal emission?

10. Why is team management so important for individuals with a history of cleft lip and palate?

SELECTED READINGS AND RESOURCES

American Cleft Palate–Craniofacial Association (ACPA). www.acpa-cpf.org.

Golding-Kushner, K. J. (2001). *Therapy techniques for cleft palate speech and related disorders*. San Diego, CA: Singular Publishing Group.

Kummer, A. W. (2007). *Oral & Nasal Listener*. Greenville, SC: Super Duper Publications.

Kummer, A. W. (2007). *Resonance disorders and velopharyngeal dysfunction: Evaluation and treatment* (a 4-hour self-study course on DVD with manual). Rockville, MD: American Speech-Language-Hearing Association.

Kummer, A. W. (2008). *Cleft palate and craniofacial anomalies: The effects on speech and resonance* (2nd edn.). New Albany, NY: Delmar Cengage Learning.

Kummer, A. W., & Marsh, J. H. (1998). Pediatric voice and resonance disorders. In A. F. Johnson & B. H. Jacobson (Eds.), *Medical speech-language pathology: A practitioner's guide*. New York, NY: Thieme.

Nasometer. Information available at: www.kaypentax.com/snaptestr.htm.

Shprintzen, R. J. (1997). *Genetics, syndromes, and communication disorders*. San Diego, CA: Singular Publishing Group.

Chapter TEN

Neurogenic Disorders of Speech in Children and Adults

Bruce E. Murdoch
The University of Queensland

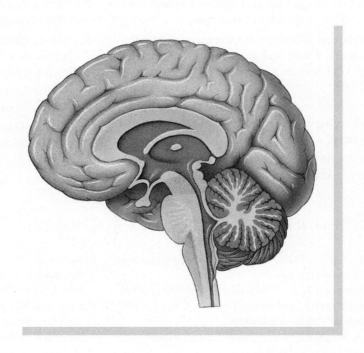

personal PERSPECTIVE

BRUCE E. MURDOCH

The functioning of biological organisms always fascinated me from an early age. This fascination in my later teens focused in particular in the area of the functioning of the nervous system. How did the brain work? In an attempt to gain at least a rudimentary understanding of the answer to this question, I initially undertook a science degree with a major in human physiology and eventually completed a Ph.D. in the field of neurophysiology. In the mid-1970s, my work in neurophysiology collided with an area that previously had been unknown to me—namely, speech-language pathology. This collision occurred as a consequence of a lecture course in neuroanatomy that I agreed to give to a group of speech-language pathology students as part of their degree program. My readings in aphasia, dysarthria, and other associated neurogenic communication disorders, as part of my preparing for this course, ignited my interest in the field. Here was an area where my knowledge of neuroanatomy and neurophysiology could be applied to answer real and important clinical questions and hopefully have some benefit for individuals with communication impairments. A subsequent period of study under the direction of Dr. Malcolm McNeil at the University of Wisconsin–Madison provided the necessary impetus and background for me to change my research direction and focus my efforts on further exploration of the brain mechanisms involved in speech and language. Since the early 1980s, this research has been my passion, and my interest in discovering new aspects of the workings of the brain is greater today then ever.

Speech is one of the most complex activities regulated by the nervous system and involves the coordinated contraction of a large number of muscles for its production. Contraction of the muscles of the speech mechanism is controlled by nerve impulses that originate in the cerebral cortex of the brain and then pass to the muscles by way of the motor pathways that run within the central and peripheral nervous systems. Overall, the control of muscular activity, including the muscles of the speech production mechanism, can be thought of as a series of levels of functional activity involving the nervous system.

The lowest level of muscle control is provided by **neurons** (nerve cells) that connect the **central nervous system** (brain and spinal cord) to the muscle fibers. These neurons, referred to as lower motor neurons, form the only route by which nerve impulses can travel from the central nervous system to cause contraction of the muscle fibers and, for this reason, are also known as the final common pathway. In regard to the muscles of the speech production mechanism, which includes the face, lips, jaw, tongue, soft palate, larynx, and respiratory system, the majority of the lower motor neurons reach the muscles via nerves arising from the base of the brain, the so-called cranial nerves (e.g., the muscles of the tongue, face, larynx, and soft palate), while others extend to the muscles via spinal nerves that originate from the spinal cord (e.g., the muscles of respiration).

The areas of the cerebral cortex responsible for the initiation of voluntary muscle activity, called the motor areas, constitute the highest level of muscle control. These areas can dominate the lower motor neurons arising from the base of the brain and spinal cord, via either direct pathways or indirect pathways. The neurons that make up the direct and indirect pathways run within the central nervous system and are collectively referred to as upper motor neurons. Coordination of muscular contraction is a function of the cerebellum.

Damage to the nervous system causing disruption to any level of the motor system involved in the regulation of the speech mechanism can lead to a disturbance in speech production. The type of neurogenic (arising from the nervous system) speech disorder that results from damage to the neuromuscular system depends very much on where in the neuromuscular system that damage is located. The present chapter will focus on the two commonly recognized motor speech disorders resulting from damage to the neuromuscular system: apraxia of speech and the dysarthrias. In adults, these conditions are acquired disorders, meaning that they result from some sort of damage or trauma to the neuromuscular system (e.g., stroke, head trauma, Parkinson's disease) that occurs after birth. In children, both acquired and developmental forms of apraxia of speech and dysarthria occur, the latter being associated with conditions present before or shortly after birth that affect the functioning of the neuromuscular system (e.g., cerebral palsy). For a detailed account of the clinical characteristics and neuropathological basis of acquired neurogenic speech disorders, the reader is referred to Murdoch (2009).

Definitions

Darley (1982, p. 10) described **apraxia of speech** (also called verbal apraxia) as "a disorder in which the patient has trouble speaking because of a cerebral lesion that prevents his executing voluntarily and on command the complex motor activities involved in speaking, despite the fact that muscle strength is undiminished." The pattern of deviant speech cannot be explained by the loss or impairment of the phonologic rules of the native language or by the weakening or paralysis of the muscles of the speech mechanism. Articulation errors are the primary feature of apraxia of speech, with alterations of prosody (i.e., changes in speech stress, intonation, or rhythm) also occurring either as a primary part of the condition or, as many researchers believe, in compensation for it.

Dysarthria has been defined as "a collective name for a group of related speech disorders that are due to disturbances in muscular control of the speech mechanism resulting from impairment of any of the basic motor processes involved in the execution of speech" (Darley, Aronson, & Brown, 1975). According to this definition, the term *dysarthria* is restricted to those speech disorders that have a neurogenic origin (i.e., those speech disorders that result from damage to the central or peripheral nervous system) and does not include those speech disorders associated with either somatic structural defects (e.g., cleft palate, congenitally enlarged pharynx, congenitally short palate, and malocclusion) or psychological disorders.

Classification, Causes, and Characteristic Features of Neurogenic Speech Disorders

Dysarthria

According to the definition provided above, dysarthria is the outcome of a motoric impairment, or a fundamental disturbance of movement, of the muscles of the speech production mechanism. The specific muscles affected may include the muscles of respiration and the muscles of the larynx, pharynx, soft palate, or articulators (lip, tongue). The features of movement that may be compromised include muscle strength, speed, range, accuracy, steadiness, and muscle tone.

According to which level(s) of the motor system is affected, a number of different types of dysarthria may be recognized, each of which is characterized by its own set of auditory perceptual features. The system of classification most universally accepted by speech pathologists and neurologists, and, therefore, the system most used clinically, is the perceptually based classification scheme devised by Darley and colleagues (1975). This system is based on classifying the neuromuscular status of the muscles whose dysfunction causes the dysarthria. The six types of dysarthria identified by the Darley and colleagues (1975) system, together with their localization, are listed in Table 10.1.

Each of these different types of dysarthria is described below.

Flaccid Dysarthria   *Flaccid dysarthria* is a collective name for the group of speech disorders arising from damage to the lower motor neurons supplying the muscles of the speech mechanism and/or to the muscles of the speech mechanism itself. The term *flaccid dysarthria* is derived from the major symptom of lower motor neuron damage—namely, flaccid paralysis. Lower motor neurons form the ultimate pathway (i.e., the final common pathway) through which nerve impulses are conveyed from the central nervous system to the skeletal muscles, including the muscles of the speech mechanism. Lesions of the motor cranial nerves and spinal nerves represent lower motor neuron lesions and interrupt the conduction of the nerve impulses from the central nervous system to the muscles. Consequently, voluntary control of the affected muscles is lost. Simultaneously, in that the nerve impulses necessary for the maintenance of

TABLE 10.1 Clinically Recognized Types of Dysarthria Together with Their Lesion Sites

Dysarthria Type	Lesion Site
Flaccid dysarthria	Lower motor neurons
Spastic dysarthria	Upper motor neurons
Ataxic dysarthria	Cerebellum and/or its connections
Hypokinetic dysarthria	Basal ganglia and associated brain stem nuclei
Hyperkinetic dysarthria	Basal ganglia and associated brain stem nuclei
Mixed dysarthria e.g. Mixed flaccid-spastic dysarthria	Both lower and upper motor neurons (e.g., amyotrophic lateral sclerosis)
Mixed ataxic-spastic-flaccid dysarthria	Cerebellum/cerebellar connections, upper motor neurons and lower motor neurons (e.g., Wilson's disease)

muscle tone are also lost, the muscles involved become flaccid (hypotonic). Muscle weakness, a loss or reduction of muscle reflexes, atrophy of the muscles involved, and fasciculation (spontaneous twitches of individual muscle bundles—fascicles) are further characteristics of lower motor neuron lesions. All or some of these characteristics may be manifest in the muscles of the speech mechanism of persons with flaccid dysarthria with hypotonia—with weakness and reduced reflex activity being the primary characteristics of flaccid paralysis. The actual lower motor neurons that, if damaged, may be associated with flaccid dysarthria are listed in Table 10.2.

Neurological Disorders Associated with Flaccid Dysarthria. With the exception of the muscles of respiration, the motor cranial nerves that arise from the bulbar region (pons and medulla oblongata) of the brain (i.e., cranial nerves V, VII, IX, X, XI, and XII) innervate the muscles of the speech mechanism. Bulbar palsy, the name

TABLE 10.2 Lower Motor Neurons Associated with Flaccid Dysarthria

Speech Process	Muscle	Site of Cell Body	Nerves Through Which Axons Pass
Respiration	Diaphragm	3rd–5th cervical segments of spinal cord	Phrenic nerves
Phonation	Laryngeal muscles	Nucleus ambiguus in medulla oblongata	Vagus nerves (X)
Articulation	Pterygoids, masseter, temporalis, etc.	Motor nucleus of trigeminal in pons	Trigeminal nerves (V)
	Facial expression, e.g., orbicularis oris	Facial nucleus in pons	Facial nerves (VII)
	Tongue muscles	Hypoglossal nucleus in medulla oblongata	Hypoglossal nerves (XII)
Resonation	Levator veli palatini	Nucleus ambiguus in medulla oblongata	Vagus nerves (X)
	Tensor veli palatini	Motor nucleus of trigeminal in pons	Trigeminal nerves (V)

commonly given to flaccid paralysis of the muscles supplied by the cranial nerves arising from the bulbar region of the brain stem, can be caused by a variety of conditions that may affect either the cell bodies or the axons of the lower motor neurons as they course through the peripheral nerves.

Flaccid dysarthria can also be caused by conditions that impair nerve impulse transmission across the neuromuscular junction (e.g., myasthenia gravis) or by disorders that involve the muscles of the speech mechanism directly (e.g., muscular dystrophy).

Clinical Characteristics of Flaccid Dysarthria.   The specific characteristics of the speech disorder manifest in patients with flaccid dysarthria vary from case to case depending upon which particular nerves are affected and the relative degree of weakness resulting from the damage. A number of subtypes of flaccid dysarthria are therefore recognized, each with its own speech characteristics determined by the specific nerve or combination of nerves involved.

Trigeminal, facial, and hypoglossal nerve lesions.   The functioning of the articulators (i.e., tongue, lips, jaw) are regulated by the Vth (trigeminal), VIIth (facial), and XIIth (hypoglossal) nerves. The trigeminal nerves are the largest of the cranial nerves and emerge from the brain stem on the lateral side of the pons. The motor fibers of the trigeminal nerve innervate the muscles of mastication, which include, among others, the temporalis, masseter, and medial and lateral pterygoid muscles. Bilateral trigeminal lesions may leave the elevators of the mandible (e.g., masseter and temporalis muscles) too weak to approximate the mandible and maxilla. This in turn may prevent the tongue and lips from making the contacts with oral structures required for the production of labial and lingual consonants and vowels, with devastating consequences for speech intelligibility. In contrast, unilateral trigeminal lesions cause only minor impairment to the patient's ability to elevate the mandible and consequently are associated with only a minor effect on speech intelligibility. In most cases, lesions to the trigeminal nerves occur in combination with other cranial lesions, with isolated trigeminal lesions occurring only rarely.

The facial nerves emerge from the lateral aspects of the brain stem and innervate the muscles of facial expression (including the occipito-frontalis, orbicularis oris, and buccinator). Lesions in one of the facial nerves leads to unilateral flaccid paralysis on the ipsilateral side (same side) of the face, causing distortion of bilabial and labiodental consonants. Due to the weakness of the lips on the affected side, patients with unilateral facial paralysis are unable to seal their lips sufficiently to prevent air escape from the mouth during the buildup of intra-oral pressure. Consequently, the production of plosives, in particular, is defective. These symptoms are more extreme in patients with bilateral facial paralysis (as occurs, e.g., in Mobius syndrome), with the bilateral weakness leading to speech impairments ranging from distortion to complete obliteration of bilabial and labiodental consonants. Vowel distortion may also be evident in severe cases due to problems with either lip rounding or lip spreading. Lesions involving the VIIth nerves can occur in isolation or in combination with lesions to other cranial nerves.

The hypoglossal nerves emerge from the brain stem and innervate the muscles of the tongue. By interfering with normal tongue movements, lesions of the hypoglossal nerves cause disturbances in articulation. Unilateral hypoglossal lesions cause ipsilateral paralysis of the tongue and may result from either brain stem conditions such as medial medullary syndrome or peripheral nerve lesions such as submaxillary tumors compressing one of the hypoglossal nerves. Although this may be associated with mild, temporary articulatory imprecision, especially during production of linguo-dental and linguo-palatal consonants, in most cases the patient learns to compensate rapidly for the unilateral tongue weakness or paralysis. Bilateral hypoglossal lesions, however, are associated with more severe articulatory disturbances. In such cases, tongue movement may be severely restricted, and speech sounds such as high front vowels and consonants that require elevation of the tip of the tongue to the upper alveolar ridge or hard palate (e.g., /t/, /d/, /n/, /l/) may be grossly distorted.

Vagus nerve lesions.   Each vagus nerve arises from the brain stem and supplies the muscles of the pharynx and larynx and the levator muscles of the soft palate.

Lesions that involve the brain stem (as occurs in lateral medullary syndrome) or the vagus nerve near to the brain stem cause paralysis of all muscles that are supplied by the vagus. In such cases, the vocal cord on the affected side is paralyzed, leading to flaccid dysphonia characterized by moderate breathiness, harshness, and reduced volume. Additional voice characteristics that may also be present include diplophonia, short phrases, and inhalatory stridor. Further, the soft palate on the same side is also paralyzed, causing hypernasality in the patient's speech. If the lesion is bilateral, the vocal cords on both sides are paralyzed, and elevation of the soft palate is also impaired bilaterally, causing more severe breathiness and hypernasality. The major clinical signs of bilateral flaccid vocal cord paralysis include breathy voice (reflecting incomplete adduction of the vocal cords that results in excessive air escape), audible inhalation (inspiratory stridor, reflecting inadequate abduction of the vocal cords during inspiration), and abnormally short phrases during contextual speech (possibly as a consequence of excessive air loss during speech as a result of inefficient laryngeal valving). Other signs seen in some patients include monotony of pitch and monotony of loudness. Bilateral weakness of the soft palate is associated with hyernasality, audible nasal emission, reduced sharpness of consonant production (as a consequence of reduced intra-oral pressure due to nasal escape), and short phrases (reflecting the premature exhaustion of expiratory air supply as a result of nasal escape). Lesions to the vagus nerve below the branch that supplies the soft palate (the pharyngeal branch) have the same effect on phonation as brain stem lesions. However, such lesions do not produce hypernasality, since functioning of the levator veli palatini is not compromised.

Phrenic and intercostal nerve lesions.   The muscles of respiration are important for the motor production of speech in that the exhaled breath provides the power source for speech. It follows, therefore, that interruption of the nerve supply to the respiratory muscles would interfere with normal speech production.

Lesions involving either the phrenic or the intercostal nerves may lead to respiratory hypofunction in the form of reduced tidal volume and vital capacity and impaired control of expiration. In general, diffuse impairment of the intercostal nerves is required to have any major effect on respiration. Spinal injuries that damage the 3rd to 5th segments of the cervical spinal cord (i.e., the origin of the phrenic nerves) can paralyze the diaphragm bilaterally, thereby leading to significant impairment of respiration. Respiratory hypofunction may in turn affect the patient's speech, resulting in speech abnormalities such as short phrases due to more rapid exhaustion of breath during speech.

Multiple cranial nerve lesions.   Multiple cranial nerve lesions are most commonly caused by intracranial (within the skull) conditions affecting the brain stem. In that the functioning of several cranial nerves is compromised simultaneously, the resulting flaccid dysarthria is usually severe. For example, in bulbar palsy the muscles supplied by cranial nerves V, VII, IX, X, XI, and XII may dysfunction simultaneously. As a result, functioning of the muscles of the lips, tongue, jaw, palate, and larynx are affected in varying combinations and with varying degrees of weakness. Disorders evident in the affected person's speech may include hypernasality with nasal emission due to disruption of the palatopharyngeal valve; breathiness, harsh voice, audible inspiration, monopitch, and monoloudness associated with laryngeal dysfunction; and distortion of consonant production due to impairment of the articulators.

Myasthenia gravis.   Myasthenia gravis is a condition characterized by muscle weakness that progressively worsens as the muscle is used (fatigability) and rapidly recovers when the muscle is at rest. The condition represents a disorder of neuromuscular transmission. As these patients speak, fatigue of the muscles supplied by the bulbar cranial nerves becomes more and more evident, resulting in increasing levels of hypernasality, deterioration of articulation, onset and increase of dysphonia, and a reduction in loudness levels. Eventually, speech becomes unintelligible.

Spastic Dysarthria   The term *spastic dysarthria* is used to describe the speech disturbance seen in association with damage to the upper motor neurons (i.e., the neurons that convey nerve impulses from the motor areas of the cerebral cortex to the lower motor neurons). The reference to **spastic** in the term *spastic dysarthria* is, therefore, a reflection of the clinical signs of upper motor neuron damage present in the bulbar musculature of these patients, which includes spastic paralysis or paresis (weakness) of the involved muscles, hyperreflexia (e.g., hyperactive jaw-jerk), little or no muscle atrophy, and the presence of pathological reflexes (e.g., sucking reflex). Lesions that disrupt the upper motor neurons causing spastic dysarthria can be located in the cerebral cortex, the internal capsule, the cerebral peduncles, or the brain stem.

Neurological Disorders Associated with Spastic Dysarthria.   Damage to the upper motor neurons is associated with two major syndromes: pseudobulbar palsy (also called supranuclear bulbar palsy) and spastic hemiplegia. Both of these conditions are characterized by spasticity and impairment or loss of voluntary movements.

Pseudobulbar palsy takes its name from its clinical resemblance to bulbar palsy (*pseudo* = false) and is associated with a variety of neurological disorders that bilaterally disrupt the upper motor neuron connections to the bulbar cranial nerves (e.g., bilateral cerebrovascular accidents, traumatic brain injury, extensive brain tumors, degenerative neurological conditions such as motor neuron disease). In this condition, the bulbar muscles, including the muscles of articulation, the velopharynx, and the larynx are hypertonic and exhibit hyperreflexia. In addition, there is a reduction in the range and force of movement of the bulbar muscles as well as slowness of individual and repetitive movements. The rhythm of repetitive movements, however, is regular and the direction of movement normal. Symptoms of pseudobulbar palsy include bilateral facial paralysis, dysarthria, dysphonia, bilateral hemiparesis, incontinence, and bradykinesia. Drooling from the corners of the mouth is common, and many of these patients exhibit lability. A hyperactive jaw reflex and positive sucking reflex are also evident, and swallowing problems are a common feature.

In contrast, unilateral upper motor neuron lesions produce spastic hemiplegia, a condition in which the muscles of the lower face and extremities on the opposite side of the body are primarily affected. The bulbar muscles are not greatly affected, with weakness being confined to the contralateral lips, lower half of the face, and tongue. In addition, the forehead, palate, pharynx, and larynx are largely unaffected. Consequently, unlike pseudobulbar palsy, spastic hemiplegia is not associated with problems in mastication, swallowing, velopharyngeal function, or laryngeal activity. The tongue appears normal in the mouth, but deviates to the weaker side on protrusion. Only a transitory dysarthria comprised of a mild articulatory imprecision, rather than a persistent spastic dysarthria, is present.

Clinical Characteristics of Spastic Dysarthria.   All aspects of speech production including articulation, resonance, phonation, and respiration are affected in spastic dysarthria, but to varying degrees. The condition is characterized by slow and labored speech produced only with considerable effort. Perceptually, the deviant speech characteristics of spastic dysarthria are reported to cluster primarily in the areas of articulatory incompetence, phonatory stenosis (narrowing), and prosodic insufficiency and include imprecise consonants, monopitch, reduced stress, harsh voice quality, monoloudness, low pitch, slow rate, hypernasality, strained strangled voice quality, short phrases, distorted vowels, pitch breaks, continuous breathy voice, and excess and equal stress.

Ataxic Dysarthria   Damage to the cerebellum or its connections leads to a condition called *ataxia* in which movements become uncoordinated. If the ataxia affects the muscles of the speech mechanism, the production of speech may become abnormal, leading to a cluster of deviant speech dimensions collectively referred to as *ataxic dysarthria.*

Although even simple movements are affected by cerebellar damage, the movements most disrupted by cerebellar disorders are the more complex, multicomponent sequential movements. Following damage to the cerebellum, complex movements tend to be broken down or decomposed into their individual sequential components, each of which may be executed with errors of force, amplitude, and timing, leading to uncoordinated movements. As speech production requires the coordinated and simultaneous contraction of a large number of muscle groups, it is easy to understand how cerebellar disorders could disrupt speech production and cause ataxic dysarthria.

Diseases of the Cerebellum.   Functioning of the cerebellum can be adversely affected by a number of conditions, including chromosomal disorders, demyelinating disorders (e.g., multiple sclerosis), hereditary ataxias (e.g., Friedreich's ataxia), infections (e.g., cerebellar abscess), toxic/metabolic disorders (e.g., heavy metal poisoning), trauma, tumors, or cerebrovascular accidents. The signs and symptoms of cerebellar dysfunction are generally the same, regardless of etiology. In those disorders where the lesion is slowly progressive (e.g., cerebellar tumor), however, symptoms of cerebellar disease tend to be much less severe than in conditions where the lesion develops acutely (e.g., traumatic brain injury, cerebrovascular accident). In addition, considerable recovery from the effects of an acute lesion can usually be expected.

Clinical Characteristics of Ataxic Dysarthria.   Inaccuracy of movement, irregular movements, and hypotonia of affected muscles appear to be the principal neuromuscular deficits associated with cerebellar damage that underlie ataxic dysarthria.

The most predominant features of ataxic dysarthria include a breakdown in the articulatory and prosodic aspects of speech. The 10 deviant speech dimensions most characteristic of ataxic dysarthria can be divided into three clusters: articulatory inaccuracy, characterized by imprecision of consonant production, irregular articulatory breakdowns, and distorted vowels; prosodic excess, characterized by excess and equal stress, prolonged phonemes, prolonged intervals, and slow rate; and phonatory-prosodic insufficiency, characterized by harshness, monopitch, and monoloudness. It has been suggested that the articulatory problems are the product of ataxia of the respiratory and oral-buccal-lingual musculature, while prosodic excess is thought by some authors to result from slow movements. The occurrence of phonatory-prosodic insufficiencies has been attributed to the presence of hypotonia.

Hypokinetic Dysarthria   Darley, Aronson, and Brown (1969a) first used the term *hypokinetic dysarthria* to describe the speech disorder associated with Parkinson's disease, a progressive, degenerative, neurological disease associated with selective loss of dopaminergic neurons in the brain. It has been estimated that 60 to 80 percent of patients with Parkinson's disease exhibit a hypokinetic dysarthria, with the prevalence increasing as the disease advances. Some authors have suggested that more than 75 percent of people with Parkinsonism eventually develop speech and voice deficits that decrease their ability to communicate with family and friends and limit their employment opportunities.

Clinical Characteristics of Hypokinetic Dysarthria.   Features of the speech disorder seen in association with Parkinson's disease are frequently described as including a monotony of pitch and loudness, decreased use of all vocal parameters for effecting stress and emphasis, breathy and harsh vocal quality, reduced vocal intensity, variable rate including short rushes of speech or accelerated speech, consonant imprecision, impaired breath support for speech, reduction in phonation time, difficulty in the initiation of speech activities, and inappropriate silences.

The hypokinetic dysarthria resulting from Parkinson's disease has been the subject of extensive perceptual, acoustic, and physiological analyses in order to produce a definitive description of the speech disorder and provide a basis for treatment programming. Although various studies have identified impairment in all aspects of speech production (respiration, phonation, resonance, articulation, and prosody) involving the various subsystems of the speech production mechanism, the individual with Parkinson's disease is most likely to exhibit disturbances of prosody, phonation, and articulation.

Hyperkinetic Dysarthria   Hyperkinetic dysarthria occurs in association with a variety of neurological disorders in which the deviant speech characteristics are the product of abnormal involuntary movements that disturb the rhythm and rate of motor activities. Although known to be associated with dysfunction of the basal ganglia (large nuclei within the cerebral hemispheres), the underlying neural mechanisms by which these abnormal involuntary movements are produced are poorly understood.

Neurological Disorders Associated with Hyperkinetic Dysarthria.   Any process that damages the basal ganglia or related brain structures has the potential to cause hyperkinetic dysarthria, including degenerative, vascular, traumatic, inflammatory, toxic, and metabolic disorders. In some cases, the cause of hyperkinetic dysarthria is idiopathic. The major types of hyperkinetic disorders are outlined in Table 10.3.

Mixed Dysarthria   A number of disorders of the nervous system affect more than one level of the motor system. Consequently, although pure forms of dysarthria do occur, mixed dysarthria, involving a combination of two or more types of dysarthria, are often exhibited by neurological cases referred to speech pathology clinics. A variety of neurological disorders can cause mixed dysarthria, including central nervous system

TABLE 10.3   Major Types of Hyperkinetic Disorders

Disorder	Symptoms	Effect on Speech
Myoclonic Jerks	Characterized by abrupt, sudden, unsustained muscle contractions that occur irregularly. Involuntary contractions may occur as single jerks of the body or may be repetitive. Two forms—palatal myoclonus and action myoclonus—may affect speech.	Speech disorder in palatal myoclonus usually characterized by phonatory, resonatory, and prosodic abnormalities (e.g., vocal tremor, rhythmic phonatory arrests, intermittent hypernasality, prolonged intervals, and inappropriate silences). With action myoclonus, speech is disrupted as a result of fine, arrhythmic, erratic muscle jerks, triggered by activity of the speech musculature.
Tics	Brief, unsustained, recurrent, compulsive movements. Usually involve a small part of the body (e.g., facial grimace).	Gilles de la Tourette's syndrome characterized by development of motor and vocal tics plus behavioral disorders. Vocal tics include simple vocal tics (e.g., grunting, coughing, barking, hissing) and complex vocal tics (e.g., stuttering-like repetitions, palilalia, echolalia, and corprolalia).
Chorea	A choreic movement consists of a single, involuntary, unsustained, isolated muscle action producing a short, rapid, uncoordinated jerk of the trunk, limb, face, tongue, diaphragm, or the like. Contractions are random in distribution and timing is irregular. Two major forms are Sydenham's and Huntington's chore.	A perceptual study of 30 patients with chorea demonstrated deficits in all aspects of speech production (Darley et al., 1969a). Physiological studies of the speech disturbance in chorea are as yet unreported.
Ballism	Rare hyperkinetic disorder characterized by involuntary, wide-amplitude, vigorous, flailing movements of the limbs. Facial muscles may also be affected.	Least important hyperkinetic disorders with regard to occurrence of hyperkinetic dysarthria.
Athetosis	Slow hyperkinetic disorder characterized by continuous, arrhythmic, purposeless, slow, writhing-type movements that tend to flow one into another. Facial grimacing, protrusion and writhing of the tongue, and problems with speaking and swallowing result when muscles of the face, neck, and tongue are affected.	Descriptions of the speech disturbance in athetosis largely related to athetoid cerebral palsy rather than hyperkinetic dysarthria in adults.
Dyskinesia	Two dyskinetic disorders—tardive dyskinesia and levodopa-induced dyskinesia—are included under this heading. Basic pattern of abnormal involuntary movement in both of these conditions is one of slow, repetitive, writhing, twisting, flexing, and extending movements, often with a mixture of tremor. Muscles of the tongue, face, and oral cavity most often affected.	Accurate placement of the articulators of speech may be severely hampered by the presence of choreoathetoid movements of the tongue, lip pursing and smacking, tongue protrusion and sucking, and chewing behaviors.
Dystonia	Characterized by abnormal involuntary movements that are slow and sustained for prolonged periods of time. Involuntary movements tend to have an undulant, sinuous character that may produce grotesque posturing and bizarre writhing, twisting movements.	Dystonias affecting the speech mechanism may result in respiratory irregularities and/or abnormal movement and bizarre posturing of the jaw, lips, tongue, face, and neck. In particular, focal cranial/orolingual-mandibular dystonia and spasmodic torticollis have the most direct effect on speech function.

degenerative diseases (e.g., amyotrophic lateral sclerosis, Wilson's disease), cerebrovascular accidents, traumatic brain injury, demyelinating disorders, brain tumors, and toxic, metabolic, and inflammatory disorders.

Acquired Dysarthria in Childhood   Although traditionally acquired childhood dysarthria has been described and classified according to criteria pertaining to the adult dysarthric population, it must be remembered that children, depending on age, are either beginning to develop or are still developing speech concurrent with damage to the nervous system. Consequently, unlike adults, motor speech disorders in children are complicated by the interaction between the acquired and developmental components of the disorder. The impact of a congenital or acquired central nervous system lesion on the developmental continuum of speech is, however, unclear, as is the contribution of developmental speech patterns to the perceived congenital or acquired dysarthria and to its resolution or progression.

Another difference between acquired dysarthria in children and acquired adult dysarthria is the difference in recovery potential between the two populations. The potential of the central nervous system to recover from brain trauma sustained at a young age has often been reported as favorable relative to recovery expected following brain damage in adults. It is also possible that the relationship between the site of the lesion and the type of dysarthria determined in adults will not be readily applicable to the developing central nervous system.

The impact of a central nervous system lesion on a child who is still developing adult speech is clearly influenced by a number of variables that are unique to that population. Unfortunately, descriptions of the nature and course of specific forms of acquired childhood dysarthria have only rarely been reported. Consequently, the literature on dysarthria in children has little to offer the clinician in either the diagnosis or the treatment of these children. While the difficulty of applying terminology, classification systems, and theories developed for adult dysarthria to children, particularly those still developing speech, is acknowledged, until further studies of childhood dysarthria are completed it appears such terminology, classification systems, and models are all that are currently available to help clinicians in the assessment and treatment of children with acquired dysarthria.

Developmental Dysarthria in Childhood   A number of neurological conditions in the developmental population primarily consisting of neuromotor dysfunction are also associated with the presence of developmental dysarthria. These conditions are largely caused by damage to specific areas of the brain, either during fetal development or during or shortly after birth. However, developmental dysarthria, where it occurs, is most commonly associated with cerebral palsy. Consequently, discussion of developmental dysarthria will focus on the population of children with cerebral palsy.

Cerebral Palsy.   Cerebral palsy is characterized by an inability to fully control motor function, particularly muscle control and coordination. The term **cerebral palsy** refers to a group of disorders with similar disturbances to movement control. Damage to the motor areas of the brain disrupt its ability to adequately control movement and posture. Depending on which areas of the brain have been damaged, one or more of the following symptoms may manifest in this population: muscle tightness or spasticity, involuntary movement, disturbance in gait or mobility, difficulty swallowing, and speech disturbances. Other issues may consist of abnormal sensation and perception, impairment of sight or hearing, seizures, intellectual disturbances, and learning disorders.

The types of cerebral palsy can be classified into three categories based on the type of movement disorder exhibited: spastic, athetoid, and ataxic. A fourth category may also be represented by various combinations of these types.

1. *Spastic cerebral palsy* (stiff and difficult movement)—This form of cerebral palsy accounts for 70 to 80 percent of the overall incidence in children. Muscles are stiff and permanently contracted. The type of spastic cerebral palsy diagnosed is described according to the limb involvement (e.g., spastic diplegia—both legs; left hemiparesis—the left side of the body).

2. *Athetoid (or dyskinetic) cerebral palsy* (involuntary and uncontrolled movement)—This category is characterized by uncontrolled, slow, writhing movements, which usually affect the hands, feet, arms, or legs. Often the muscles of the face and articulators are also involved (developmental dysarthria), which also results in distorted facial patterning and/or drooling. Such movements often increase during times of excitement or distress and are reduced during rest.

3. *Ataxic cerebral palsy* (disturbed sense of balance and depth perception)— This form of cerebral palsy is the least common at an incidence of 5 to 10 percent of patients diagnosed. It involves disturbances to balance and depth perception. Characteristics include poor coordination, unsteady gait patterns, and difficulty in attempting fast, precise movements such as writing or buttoning a shirt. An intention tremor has also been noted in these patients.

4. *Mixed cerebral palsy*—It is not uncommon for individuals to have symptoms of more than one of the above three varieties of cerebral palsy. The most common mixed form includes spasticity and athetoid movements, with other combinations possible.

Given that the primary feature of cerebral palsy is the presence of a developmental neuromotor disorder, the pervading communication deficit and the most distinctive feature of this population is developmental dysarthria. Developmental dysarthria is characterized by a disruption in the development of the ability to generate motor speech function due to the dysfunction of the speech subsystems. The main difference between the acquired and developmental dysarthrias is that individuals with acquired dysarthria experience an impairment of the speech production skills that had previously been developed prior to an insult to the nervous system, whereas individuals with developmental dysarthria require treatment to modify motor patterns to develop a skill that they have not yet acquired.

The most commonly involved subsystems in children with developmental dysarthria consist of respiration, phonation, and articulation. Although these speech systems will be considered individually, it is important to note that all features of speech production are closely related and do not operate in an independent manner in children with cerebral palsy. Therefore, a breakdown in one of the following areas is likely to impact others and may contribute overall to the characteristics of the speech production mechanism.

Respiration.   Respiration is reportedly affected in a variety of ways in individuals with cerebral palsy, which subsequently impacts speech production related to developmental dysarthria. While a speech breathing pattern consisting of a brief inhalation followed by a prolonged and controlled exhalation is present in normal individuals, this population commonly attempts to speak on the expiratory component of the rest breathing cycle. This aspect of the cycle may be too short to support speech production, as it is often difficult for these children to hold their breath momentarily or exhale slowly.

It is poor neuromuscular control, however, that accounts for reduced prolongation of exhalation in this population, which subsequently impacts communication by preventing inadequate levels of air pressure to be achieved for connected speech. Children with cerebral palsy often expire more air per unit of speech than do those with normally functioning mechanisms. Thus, they also deplete the air supply used to generate speech very quickly, with body effort and exertion at the end of phrases often seen as they attempt to continue speech production.

A phenomenon termed *reversed breathing* is also characteristic of the respiration patterns in children with cerebral palsy. While breathing in normal individuals consists of a simultaneous increase in volume in both the thoracic and the abdominal areas, children with cerebral palsy are often unable to develop or maintain coordinated thoracic and diaphragmatic activity.

In such instances of impaired respiratory control in children with cerebral palsy, speech output is characterized by poor prosody and particularly inappropriate variations in loudness. Short utterances with inhalations between each, as well as an overall appearance of increased effort for speech, a slowing of speech, and a strained vocal quality at the end of phrases, are notably also characteristic. Speech rate is, therefore, also commonly affected.

Phonation.　Some individuals with developmental dysarthria experience difficulty coordinating phonation with exhalation. Often the vocal folds open during exhalation, making phonation impossible. Even if the vocal folds are open during the initial stage of phonation, air will escape easily and leave little for speech when the folds do adduct. This is especially crucial in the event of short or poorly controlled expirations.

An additional feature noted in individuals with cerebral palsy involves excessively strong adduction of the vocal folds, where the subglottal pressure is inadequate to separate the vocal folds and initiate phonation. Irregulation of vocal fold tension may also impact phonation in this population. Whereas an inability to vary tension may result in a monotone pitch, an inability to control tension changes is likely to cause inappropriate pitch variations. Inappropriate timing of phonation, including extraneous phonations unrelated to utterance, may also present.

Resonance.　Altered posture often seen in children with cerebral palsy can greatly impact resonatory function involved in speech production. Hyperextension of the head and neck, as well as severe depression of the jaw, is often seen as a contributing factor in altering the size of the oral and pharyngeal cavities. In turn, abnormal resonatory characteristics result. When the jaw is depressed, the back of the tongue is pulled downward. Connections with the soft palate are subsequently disrupted, which in turn interrupts palatal movement required to close the nasopharyngeal cavity. Underdeveloped velopharyngeal musculature may also impact speech production in these speakers. Severity of resonatory dysfunction ranges from slight nasalization to an involvement of all sounds and severely reduced intelligibility.

Articulation.　When the jaw is depressed, the lips may be drawn apart and stretched, which often makes it extremely difficult to approximate, protrude, or retract the articulators for specific sound production. Lip function may also be impaired in the presence of jaw movement that is minimally impacted, as with general lip immobility and reduced lip gesture and protrusion. Additionally, the tongue may be pulled downward, preventing approximation of target placements. Abnormal lingual movements may also be seen in children with cerebral palsy, causing various effects that range from misarticulation through to an inability to shape or approach the target area for speech sound production. Due to difficulty with oral motor control, children with cerebral palsy also experience difficulty combining sounds to create consonant–vowel combinations.

Prosody.   Prosodic disturbances and suprasegmental dysfunction may be seen in this population for a variety of reasons. As mentioned above, poor respiratory control commonly contributes to prosodic disturbances in children with cerebral palsy due to reduced support for speech and, among other things, may result in shortened utterance length, inappropriate stress patterning, reduced rate, and increased loudness. Poor control of laryngeal musculature may result in pitch variation, as outlined above, which results in abnormal intonation patterns as well as contributing to inappropriate volume levels. Stress patterning may also be poor due to a reduced ability to produce accurate and precise articulatory movements and target approximations.

Apraxia of Speech

Acquired Apraxia of Speech   **Apraxia of speech** (acquired verbal apraxia) is a motor speech programming disorder characterized primarily by errors in articulation and secondarily by what are thought by many to be compensatory alterations of prosody (e.g., pauses, slow rate of speech, equalization of stress). Articulation errors, therefore, are the primary features of this motor speech disorder. As they speak, individuals with apraxia of speech struggle to correctly position their articulators. As they struggle, affected individuals appear to visibly and audibly grope to achieve the correct individual articulatory postures and sequences of articulatory postures to produce sounds as well as words. The resulting articulation, however, is frequently off-target. As persons with apraxia of speech are aware of their articulatory mistakes, however, they usually attempt to correct them. Often these attempted corrections are also erroneous, but importantly are not always the same as the original error in articulation. In fact, in a series of trials, the articulatory errors exhibited by individuals with apraxia of speech were highly variable. Further, the number of articulatory errors exhibited by individuals with apraxia of speech was greater during repetition than during conversational speech. Consequently, apraxia of speech is most clearly illustrated when the individual is asked to repeat spoken language.

The number of articulatory errors produced by individuals with apraxia of speech also increases as the complexity of the articulatory exercise increases. Repetitions of a single consonant such as "puh," "tuh," or "kuh" is ordinarily more easily accomplished than repetition of the sequence "puh-tuh-kuh." The number of articulatory errors produced by these individuals has also been found to increase as the length of the word increases. For example, as these individuals produce a series of words with an increasing number of syllables (e.g., door, doorknob, doorkeeper, dormitory), more errors occur during production of the longer words.

In addition to the impairment in articulation, the prosodic features of the speech of individuals with apraxia of speech are disturbed. The prosodic deficits occur as a result of the fact that, as these patients speak, they slow down their rate of speech, space their words and syllables more evenly, and stress each of them more equally in an attempt to avoid articulatory errors. Individuals with apraxia of speech also display a marked discrepancy between their relatively good performance at automatic and reactive speech productions and their relatively poor volitional-purposive speech performance. These individuals may sound normal when producing words and phrases that are well known to them through practice or usage (e.g., repeating rhymes or jingles, reacting to a sudden stimulus, counting). In contrast, these same individuals exhibit effortful and off-target groping in spontaneous speech or when they are required to select a particular target word.

Although most of what we know about apraxia of speech comes from studies of adults, it has been speculated that acquired apraxia of speech can also occur in children with brain injuries. Unfortunately, only scant information regarding the nature and occurrence of this disorder in childhood is available in the literature, with the presence of this condition occasionally being noted by authors as one of the speech-language disorders to occur following brain injury, but with few details being provided.

Developmental Apraxia of Speech   **Developmental apraxia of speech** (also known as **developmental verbal dyspraxia** or DVD) is an impairment of speech production at the motor level that largely impacts the phonological development of children. Whereas the term *apraxia* has historically been used to describe the characteristics of this variety of acquired speech disorder in adults, it has also been adopted to describe similar symptoms in children's speech.

While this disorder has created extensive debate regarding the commonly presenting features in childhood, a diagnosis is based on the presence of a number of co-occurring clinical symptoms rather than being based on a single symptom. Specific characteristics may include difficulty in planning volitional oral motor movements, deviant speech development (compared to delayed development), vowel errors, inconsistent patterns of speech-sound errors, reduced phoneme repertoire, difficulty in producing individual phonemes or sequences of phonemes volitionally with possible groping of articulators, voicing errors, reduced prosody, increased errors with increased performance load, and reduced diadokokinetic rates (particularly with alternating sounds or syllables). Potential linguistic involvement has also been reported.

The pattern of presenting symptoms may vary considerably between children, with numerous combinations possible. Varying degrees of severity also play a part in the presentation of this collection of features, ranging from mild unintelligibility (such as within multisyllabic words or connected speech) to a complete absence of intelligible speech or a nonverbal presentation. Children diagnosed with developmental apraxia of speech have an overall reduced capacity to develop adequate mechanisms of speech production and, while having adequate range and rate of movement of the articulators, display inappropriate movements during speech.

Differentiation of Apraxia of Speech from Dysarthria

Although apraxia of speech and dysarthria are both motor speech disorders, each represents a breakdown at a different level of speech production. Individuals with apraxia, on neurological examination, show no significant evidence of slowness, weakness, incoordination, paralysis, or alteration of tone of the muscles of the speech production mechanisms that can account for the associated speech disturbance. Individuals with dysarthria, on the other hand, dependent on the type of dysarthria present, may exhibit either hyper- or hypotonus of the speech muscles, a restricted range of movement, and so on. Whereas individuals with dysarthria often show variable disturbances in all of the basic motor processes that underlie speech production—including respiration, phonation, resonation, articulation, and prosody—in apraxia of speech the continuing impairment is specifically articulatory, with prosodic alterations occurring as compensatory phenomena. Further, the nature of the articulatory disturbance differs between the two conditions. In dysarthria, the errors of articulation are characteristically errors of simplification (e.g., distortions or omissions), whereas in apraxia of speech, the articulatory errors largely take the form of complications of speech (e.g., substitution of one phoneme for another, addition of phonemes, repetition of phonemes).

Assessment of Neurogenic Speech Disorders

Appropriate assessment of neurogenic speech disorders is essential to aid clinicians in their formulation of a diagnosis and their determination of specific treatment priorities. A comprehensive assessment of persons affected by neurological speech impairments usually includes the following components: a detailed case history, an oro-motor examination, and a determination of the clinical characteristics of the speech disorder and an identification of their neurological substrates.

A detailed case history can inform the clinician of the salient features of the speech disorder from the perspective of the client and should be taken prior to administration of any formal tests. Essential background information to be collected as part of the case history should include the following client details: age, education level, occupation, marital and family status, prior history of speech-language impairment (including developmental conditions experienced in childhood), onset and course of the disorder, associated deficits (e.g., drooling, hemiplegia, swallowing impairments), emotional disturbances, prior treatment and management regimens, client's awareness and understanding of the disorder, and consequences of the disorder for the client (e.g., disruption to work, school, social activities). An oro-motor examination primarily involves visual and tactual observation of the speech production mechanism during performance of a range of nonspeech activities and provides important information about the size, strength, symmetry, range, tone, steadiness, speed, and accuracy of movements of the face, jaw, tongue, and soft palate (velum).

Techniques available for determination of the key features of the speech disorder and identification of their neurological substrates for the purposes of differential diagnosis and determination of treatment priorities can be broadly divided into three major categories: perceptual techniques—these assessments are based on the clinicians' impressions of the auditory-perceptual attributes of the speech; acoustic techniques—assessments in this category are based on the study of the generation, transmission, and modification of sound waves emitted from the vocal tract; and physiological techniques—these methods are based on instrumental assessment of the functioning of the various subsystems of the speech production apparatus in terms of their movements, muscular contractions, biomechanical activities, and such.

Perceptual Assessment

In the past years, perceptual analysis of dysarthric speech has been the "gold standard" and preferred method by which clinicians make differential diagnoses and define treatment programs for their clients with motor speech disorders. In fact, many clinicians have relied almost exclusively on auditory-perceptual judgments of speech intelligibility, articulatory accuracy, or subjective ratings of various speech dimensions to diagnose dysarthric speech and plan their interventions. The use of auditory perceptual assessment to characterize the different types of dysarthria and to identify the spectrum of deviant speech characteristics associated with each was pioneered by Darley and colleagues (1969a, 1969b, 1975). As indicated earlier, it was from the findings of their auditory-perceptual studies of dysarthria that the system of classification of dysarthria used most frequently in clinical settings and used throughout the present chapter was developed. Darley and colleagues (1969a, 1969b) assessed speech samples taken from 212 dysarthric speakers with a variety of neurological conditions on 38 speech dimensions that fell into six categories: pitch, loudness, voice quality (including both laryngeal and resonatory dysfunction), respiration, prosody, articulation, and two summary dimensions relating to intelligibility and bizarreness. A key component of their research was the application of the "equal-appearing intervals scale of severity," which utilized a seven-part scale of severity. In addition to rating scales, other perceptual assessments used to investigate dysarthric speech include application of intelligibility measures, phonetic transcription studies, and articulation inventories. A full description of these methods is beyond the scope of the present chapter; however, the reader is referred to an excellent review of perceptual techniques by Kent (2009).

The major advantages of perceptual assessment are those that have led to its preferred use as the tool for characterizing and diagnosing dysarthric speech. Perceptual assessments are readily available and require only limited financial outlay. In addition, all students of speech-language pathology are taught how to test for and identify perceptual symptoms. Finally, perceptual assessments are useful for monitoring the effects of treatment on speech intelligibility and the adequacy of communication.

Clinicians need to be aware, however, that there are a number of inherent inadequacies with perceptual assessment that may limit their use in determining treatment priorities. First, accurate, reliable perceptual judgments are often difficult to achieve, as they can be influenced by a number of factors, including the skill and experience of the clinician and the sensitivity of the assessment. In particular, raters must have extensive structured experience in listening prior to performing perceptual ratings.

Second, perceptual assessments are difficult to standardize in relation to both the patient being rated and the environment in which the speech samples are recorded. Patient variability over time and across different settings prevents maintenance of adequate intra- and interrater reliability. Further, the symptoms may be present in certain conditions and not others. This variability is also found in the patients themselves such that characteristics of the person being rated (e.g., age, premorbid medical history, and social history) may influence speech as well as the neurological problem itself.

A third factor that limits reliance on perceptual assessments is that certain speech symptoms may influence the perception of others. This confound has been well reported in relation to the perception of resonatory disorders, articulatory deficits, and prosodic disturbances.

Probably the major concern of perceptual assessments, particularly as they relate to treatment planning, is that they have restricted power for determining which subsystems of the speech motor system are affected. In other words, perceptual assessments are unable to accurately identify the pathophysiological basis of the speech disorder manifest in various types of dysarthria. It is possible that a number of different physiological deficits can form the basis of perceptually identified features and that different patterns of interaction within a patient's overall symptom complex can result in a similar perceptual deviation (e.g., distorted consonants can result from reduced respiratory support for speech, from inadequate velopharyngeal functioning, or from weak tongue musculature). When crucial decisions are required in relation to optimum therapeutic planning, an overreliance on only perceptual assessment may lead to a number of questionable therapy directions.

Acoustic Assessment

Acoustic analyses can be used in conjunction with perceptual assessments to provide a more complete understanding of the nature of the disturbance in dysarthric speech. In particular, acoustic assessment can highlight aspects of the speech signal that may be contributing to the perception of deviant speech production and can provide confirmatory support for perceptual judgments. For example, acoustic assessment may confirm the perception that speech is slow and demonstrate that the reduced rate of speech may be the result of increased interword durations and prolonged vowel and consonant production. As a further example, an acoustic analysis might be used to confirm the perception of imprecise consonant production and to show that such imprecision is the result of spirantization of consonants and reduction of consonant clusters. In addition to altered speech rate and consonant imprecision, other perceived deviant speech dimensions that can be confirmed by way of acoustic analysis include, among others, breathy voice, voice tremor, and reduced variability of pitch and loudness. Acoustic analysis is also useful for providing objective documentation of the effects of treatment and disease progression on speech production.

Acoustic measurements can be taken primarily from two different types of acoustic displays: oscillographic displays and spectrographic displays. An oscillographic display is a two-dimensional waveform display of amplitude (on the y-axis) as a function of time (x-axis). Oscillographic displays are easy to generate and can provide information on a variety of acoustic parameters such as segment duration (e.g., vowel duration, word duration), amplitude, fundamental frequency, and the presence of some acoustic cues of articulatory adequacy such as voice onset time, spirantization, and voiced–voiceless distinctions. Measurements from oscillographic displays can be made either manually or by using computer-controlled acoustic analysis software.

In contrast to the two-dimensional oscillographic display, a spectrographic display is actually a three-dimensional display, with both frequency and amplitude as a function of time, where time is on the x-axis and frequency is displayed on the y-axis. There are two different types of spectrographic displays: wide-band displays (also called broad-band displays) and narrow-band displays. Wide-band spectrographic displays are used to determine accurate temporal measurements, while narrow-band spectrograms are useful for making measurements of fundamental frequency and the prosodic aspects of speech.

While there is no "standard" set of parameters included in all acoustic analyses, there are a number of different acoustic measures that can provide important information about the acoustic features of dysarthric speech. These parameters can be loosely arranged into groups of measures, including fundamental frequency measures, amplitude measures, perturbation measures, noise-related measures, formant measures, temporal measures, measures of articulatory capability, and evaluations of manner of voicing.

Physiological Assessment

Traditional therapeutic approaches to the rehabilitation of dysarthric speech are based primarily on subjective, perceptual assessments and techniques. Some clinicians believe that such methods lack the objectivity and specificity required to ensure the most effective rehabilitation, especially given the acknowledged inability of perceptual assessment to provide information regarding the pathophysiological basis of the speech disorder. What is needed is a more objective, physiological approach to dysarthria therapy—one that is based on a comprehensive instrumental assessment of the functioning of the subsystems of the speech production apparatus. Such an approach, often referred to as the physiological approach, has been advocated by several researchers.

The physiological approach to dysarthria rehabilitation is based on the concept that assessment of the individual motor subsystems of the speech mechanism (i.e., respiratory, laryngeal, velopharyngeal, and articulatory subsystems) is crucial in defining the underlying speech motor pathophysiology necessary for the development of optimal treatment programs. Therefore, in this approach the initial step is to undertake a comprehensive physiological assessment of the various components of the speech production mechanism of the dysarthric speaker to determine, first, those components that are malfunctioning and, second, the physiological nature and severity of the malfunction. Essentially, the goal of the physiological assessment is to evaluate the integrity of the speech components (lips, tongue, jaw, velopharynx, larynx, etc.) and systems (articulation, phonation, respiration, etc.) that generate or valve the expiratory airstream and subsequently to relate this information to the perceived dysarthric symptom. Whereas perceptual and acoustic assessments focus on the signal emitted from the vocal tract, physiological assessments analyze muscle contractions and movements within the speech mechanism and address whether specific deviant speech dimensions are the outcome of factors such as muscle weakness or spasticity.

A wide variety of different types of instrumentation has been described in the literature for use in the assessment of the functioning of the various components of the speech production apparatus. Physiological instruments most commonly used to assess the functioning of the speech mechanism include electromyography, kinematic measures, and aerodynamic measures. Each of these instruments has been designed to provide information on a specific aspect of speech production, including muscular activity, structural movements, airflows, and air pressures generated in the various parts of the speech mechanism. It is, however, beyond the scope of the present chapter to review all of the types of instrumentation available or to go into the specific details of the instrumental techniques. For a comprehensive set of reviews of instrumental assessment of the speech mechanism, the reader is referred to Barlow, Finan, Andreatta, and Boliek (2009), Luschei and Finnegan (2009), and Zajac, Warren, and Hinton (2009).

In summary, although instrumentation has opened a whole new range of assessment techniques, physiological data should be integrated with data from other appraisal procedures (i.e., perceptual, acoustic, and physiological information should be combined) to ensure than an accurate diagnosis is made and that the subsequent remediation techniques are appropriate. In particular, the limitations of each instrumental procedure should be kept in mind when making clinical decisions based on its findings. It also must be remembered that, despite the wide variety of objective instrumental measures available for documenting the physiology of speech production, to date the clinical application of these techniques has been limited. Increasing the use of instrumentation in the clinical setting, for the purposes of both assessment and treatment, will require the implementation of training programs for the clinicians as well as an increase in clinical research projects designed to demonstrate the clinical utility of instrumental techniques and to validate the role of instrumentation in dysarthria management.

Treatment of Acquired Neurogenic Speech Disorders

A range of treatment options exists in the management of dysarthria and apraxia of speech. However, the overall goal in treatment programs for individuals with neurogenic speech disorders is to improve intelligibility by enhancing physiological support for speech and by teaching compensatory speech behaviors. Occasionally, the speech pathologist may also be required to work in collaboration with medical professionals and specialists in order to explore surgical or prosthetic approaches to management.

Regardless of the best applicable treatment technique, the following five principles are considered practical strategies that promote greater success in the treatment of neurogenic motor speech disorders in both adult and child populations (Darley et al., 1975; Murdoch, Ozanne, & Cross, 1990).

1. *Compensatory strategies.*   Helping the patient to utilize his remaining strengths and potential is an important strategy. Children in particular often have more of a tendency to compensate due to their ongoing development, as speech patterns prior to an acquired disturbance such as brain injury tend to be less well established than in adults.

2. *Purposeful activity.*   As the individual becomes aware of how her articulators work and interact, she is able to more effectively learn a range of strategies designed to increase the intelligibility of her speech. What was once an automatic response now needs to be learned as a purposeful behavior.

3. *Early treatment.*   It is essential to begin rehabilitation early. The sooner the patient becomes aware of how his speech system works, the greater the chance that effective self-monitoring skills will be established.

4. *Monitoring.*   Self-monitoring of behaviors and behavioral change is a key strategy in effectively treating neurogenic speech deficits in adults and children and generalizing. Children may find this skill more difficult to learn, but it may be taught as a set strategy with steps that can be followed in contextual situations.

5. *Motivation.*   This ingredient will ensure much greater success and better outcomes in treating the individual's speech deficit and in reducing unintelligibility.

Treatment in the Acute Period

Treatment in the early phase of recovery for motor speech disorders across both adult and pediatric populations may initially consist of feeding and dysphagia treatment and oral/facial stimulation until the patient is sufficiently responsive and medically stable to actively participate in learning treatment techniques for improving communication and intelligibility. Often a period of mutism is described in the early recovery period associated with dysarthria and dyspraxia. During this phase of recovery, it is of utmost importance to establish a form of communication aside from verbal output until speech becomes more functional. This may include signals, gesture, or more formal signing, to be introduced as one of the earliest treatment goals. All gesture and attempts at communication by the patient should be encouraged. Symbol systems such as Compic and the Picture Exchange Communication System (PECS) or self-made photograph communication boards may be appropriate methods of communication, particularly if physical abilities are also restricted and limit the use of sign. The communication system selected, however, should rely on the patient's cognitive level, receptive language skills, perceptual and motor abilities, and level of desire to interact and communicate.

In some cases, the use of an augmentative communication system may facilitate the return of verbal communication. Some patients may, however, have more severe motor involvement or apraxia of phonation, in which case recovery may either occur spontaneously or require specific treatment. Many of these individuals, particularly children, may vocalize spontaneously in emotional situations (laughing, etc.), in play settings, or in other active therapy sessions. The speech-language clinician may, therefore, find it beneficial to be present and participate in team therapy sessions in order to shape and build on these vocalizations. Patients with severe involvement and poorer prognosis for recovery may require a more advanced communication device such as a voice output device or a computer-based system with context-based control options.

Treatment Approaches

Several key therapy goals can be achieved through a combination of different approaches and techniques, and largely include the strategies outlined below.

Behavioral approach.   The focus of this approach is to teach patients new skills or compensatory techniques that utilize traditional techniques that involve the presentation of stimulus and patient response. Due to the portability, flexibility, and low-cost nature of this approach, it is the technique most widely used in clinical situations.

Biofeedback/instrumental approach.   The use of biofeedback or instrumentation is based on the principle that effective motor speech learning is dependent on the patient receiving immediate and specific feedback regarding his performance across each component of the speech production mechanism. Therefore, instruments are used to determine the exact level of functioning of the tongue, lip, and jaw and to ascertain the presence and nature of facial weakness, respiratory dysfunction, velopharyngeal incompetence, and prosodic impairment. The information is then presented in a way that facilitates the patient's control of the variable, in turn providing a large range of possible treatment strategies.

Surgical and prosthetic approaches.   As an alternative to traditional or biofeedback therapy techniques, surgical procedures or prosthetic involvement may be used in the management of severe cases of dysarthria. Techniques such as amplification devices, palatal lifts, or bite blocks may be used to assist the patient in compensating for reduced or impaired functioning of a specific aspect of the speech mechanism where other approaches are not feasible. Surgical procedures such as Teflon injections, laser surgery, and pharyngeal flap surgery are often utilized in patients who have severe impairments and are unresponsive to other therapeutic approaches.

Pragmatic approach.   Rather than focusing on improving the actual physiological aspects of the speech mechanism, this approach aims to assist the patient in providing strategies that maximize communication within the context of daily life situations. Such methods may include altering the communicative environment (e.g., avoiding communication in dark or noisy situations, reducing distance between communicative partners), modifying utterance/sentence length, teaching repair strategies, and providing attention and topic orientation.

Specific Treatment Methods

Specific treatment techniques are designed to target each of the subsystems that make up the speech production mechanism, in combination with associated prosodic features. A range of techniques for the common features associated with dysarthria and apraxia of speech is explored below, covering treatment approaches for disorders that present in speech breathing, phonation, resonance, articulation, and prosody. Often techniques that focus on one specific characteristic may have beneficial effects for other areas of concern.

Treatment of Speech Breathing Disorders   The remediation of respiratory deficits in individuals with dysarthria usually involves a combination of strategies to improve physiological support and guide compensatory behaviors that will enable optimal available respiratory support for speech. A primary and commonly used behavioral strategy for this physiological component of the speech mechanism consists of training the patient to maintain adequate posture for respiration. Instrumental techniques range from simple homemade devices to complex instrumentation to provide biofeedback on respiratory function and are extremely useful for promoting controlled exhalation—for example, using a straw to blow bubbles in a glass of water or using a U-shaped manometer where a patient blows into one end of plastic tubing to maintain a consistent water level. In those patients with more severe respiratory impairment, prosthetic approaches such as supporting the abdominal muscle with an elastic bandage for short periods have been tried and have appeared to provide the patient more control over expiratory breath.

Treatment of Phonation Disorders   Techniques addressing disturbances to laryngeal function and phonation in individuals with dysarthria will vary depending on the underlying neuromuscular issue and the actual motor speech disorder. Treatment of this collection of phonation disorders in dysarthria often incorporates mostly behavioral and instrumental techniques, with possible use of prosthetic compensatory devices. Surgical intervention may be required in such cases to maximize the effectiveness of the other treatment approaches. However, it is important to identify the underlying pathophysiology and the impact of other speech subsystems on phonatory disturbances that exist prior to treatment planning.

Excessive vocal fold adduction, or hyperadduction, produces varying degrees of low-pitched, strained-strangled, harsh vocal quality that ranges from an inability to phonate at all to a more mild form of hyperadduction that presents as pitch breaks, mild vocal strain, and harshness. Intervention involves overall body and specific head and neck relaxation and exercises to decrease tension in the vocal cords. These include the chewing method, the yawn–sigh approach, and gentle voice onsets.

Hypoadduction of the vocal folds involves inadequate adduction of the vocal folds for phonation and presents as increased airflow through the glottis due to a decrease in laryngeal resistance, reduced loudness level, breathiness, hoarseness, and short phonation time. Treatment techniques to facilitate adduction of the vocal folds include pushing, pulling, and lifting exercises performed together with phonation, hard glottal attack, and postural adjustment of the head, such as turning the head to the affected side to decrease distance between the vocal folds. The Lee Silverman Voice Treatment (LSVT) program has also recently been employed to increase phonatory effect by taking deeper breaths and carrying out more effortful vocal fold adduction.

Other phonation disorders that may present in dysarthric patients include phonatory instability and phonatory incoordination. Treatment for phonatory instability associated with dysarthria is essentially aimed at achieving steadiness and clarity of phonation, with techniques primarily centerd on breath control exercises. Phonatory incoordination can refer to timing issues of respiration, laryngeal production, and/or articulation as well as prosody disturbances. Delays in voice onset and offset can be affected by a failure to synchronize phonation with exhalation. The presence of phonatory incoordination will also significantly affect prosody of speech due to reduced ability to control speech parameters such as pressure, vocal fold tension, vocal quality, pitch, volume variation, and duration. Therefore, treatment strategies discussed below that outline treatment approaches for prosody and articulation can be applicable to treatment of phonation incoordination.

The accent method has application to treatment of dysarthric patients and associated phonatory disturbances, including hyperadduction, phonatory instability, and phonatory incoordination. Its premise is based on creating an appropriate balance between expiration and the force of the vocal fold muscles, thus improving coordination between the voice produced at the level of the vocal folds and resonance and improving prosody.

As disturbances of pitch, volume, variability, and duration of phonation consistently occur in dysarthric speech, biofeedback tools are an effective method of treatment in these patients. The most useful instruments are those that can consistently display vocal parameters such as the Vocalite (a voice-operated light source that gives feedback on vocal intensity), Visispeech Speech Viewer, and Visipitch. In treating phonation disorders in children, the Speech Viewer, for example, can also provide effective motivation. Children are able to watch a balloon blow up or deflate on the screen by manipulating their own vocal intensity or to help a monkey climb a tree to get coconuts based on pitch levels.

Prosthetic devices available in the treatment and/or maintenance of phonatory/laryngeal disorders in dysarthric patients most commonly include electronic devices designed to compensate for vocal intensity, such as a vocal amplifier. Surgical techniques may be utilized for those patients for whom behavioral, instrumental, and prosthetic techniques do not produce enough improvement. Such intervention may be employed to produce a more appropriate valving mechanism and is followed by other approaches to maximize vocal efficiency. However, the suitability of such procedures needs to be evaluated for each individual, as in some cases such intervention may be inappropriate based on the individual's medical condition or overall disability. Laryngeal nerve section, laser surgery, or botulism toxin injection may be carried out for hyperadduction of the vocal folds to restrict the movement of one or both of the folds. In cases of hypoadduction of the vocal folds, reinnervation of a unilateral paralyzed vocal fold, laryngoplasty, and collagen and Teflon implants may be utilized.

Treatment of Resonatory Disorders   Impaired velopharyngeal function associated with neurological function is characterized by hypernasal resonance and nasal emission of air during speech. In severe cases, improving velopharyngeal function is often the first priority of treatment, as the impairment may contribute to respiratory impairments and articulation imprecision due to air loss through an inefficient velar valve. Determining the amount of palatal closure achieved through therapy tasks requires good self-judgment and in turn relates to effectiveness of treatment and outcomes. Therefore, it is important for the patient to develop an awareness of the velopharyngeal system and an ability to monitor nasality. Visual feedback can be achieved by using a mirror to detect air leakage through the nose. The patient can also obtain information from visual feedback by using a small flashlight and an angled mirror to see and monitor velar elevation during the production of single vowels. A variety of more formal instrumental biofeedback techniques is also employed in the treatment of resonatory disturbances. The use of pressure, icing, brushing, or vibration of the velum may also be of some benefit for patients with flaccid dysarthria. Speech drills using contrastive nasal and non-nasal sounds, as well as drills to correct the timing of palatal elevation in words and phrases, have helped patients progress. The clinician should constantly evaluate the benefit for the patient and be prepared to explore alternative strategies if small or no improvements are made.

In cases where the soft palate is unresponsive to either behavioral or instrumental intervention or is paralyzed, a prosthetic approach to treatment may be adopted and may involve the use of a palatal lift prosthesis. This device attaches to teeth and is designed to improve resonance by partially lifting the soft palate and allowing contact with the lateral pharyngeal walls. This device may be utilized either as a temporary or as a permanent method.

Treatment of Articulation Disorders For most dysarthric and dyspraxic patients, specific articulation training is required in order to establish and/or normalize speech movements. Treatment of articulation in both adults and children should take a functional approach, with compensatory strategies playing an important role in the dysarthric patient. Articulation therapy in dysarthric patients is based on a combination of auditory, visual, and imitation learning as well as speech drills to consolidate and generalize the target sounds.

Based on the underlying physiology for articulatory errors, individual treatment follows a sequential progression from basic sound level through to longer, more demanding, yet more normalized, speech segments. Compensation techniques may include using the blade of the tongue instead of the tongue tip for sounds such as /l/, /n/, /t/, and /d/ if tongue or lip movements remain restricted. When formulating articulation goals for treatment of children, consideration must be given to the developmental acquisition of sounds. However, the general rule should be to choose a sound that the child is able to imitate and that will make the greatest difference to her intelligibility (such as /s/ sounds or in some instances /s/ clusters).

The primary instrumental approach used in treating articulatory disturbances involves electromyography (EMG) biofeedback to alter muscle tone and strength by decreasing or increasing muscle activity. Electropalatography (EPG) and electromagnetic articulography (EMA) involve additional devices that have the potential for use in articulation therapy with dysarthric patients. EPG uses an artificial hard palate embedded with electrodes that is designed to fit into the individual's mouth. This instrument provides details of the location and timing of tongue contact during speech. Such information may be provided to the patient to allow an alteration in tongue position in order to approximate the target sound. In contrast, EMA provides a range of tongue movement data, including velocity, duration, and distance of tongue movement during production of both speech and nonspeech tasks. Impairments in voiced–voiceless contrasts can also be targeted with various instruments that provide feedback regarding intensity, duration, pressure, and airflow that may assist the patient in addition to behavioral techniques. Prosthetic approaches are mainly limited to the use of a bite block, which may assist in stabilizing the jaw and thereby optimizing function of the remaining articulators.

Treatment of Prosodic Disturbances Three key prosodic features—stress patterns, rate, and intonation—play a vital role in treatment of neurogenic speech disorders across all populations. Attention to the area of prosody has many benefits that positively impact other systems (such as articulation) in enhancing intelligibility. Prosodic features contribute to highlighting the type (statement versus question, etc.) or overall tone of an utterance as well as indicating the most important words in a sentence.

The most common behavioral technique for deficits in stress patterning in dysarthric patients involves the use of contrastive stress drills, where increases in pitch, vocal intensity, and duration are utilized to create varying responses to questions. Intonation therapy may require the training of breath group patterning through reading tasks that are marked and practiced in accordance with the most appropriate breath group length. Variation of breath groups may also assist with excessively monotonous intonation. Rate control can be regulated by a number of informal strategies such as tapping or use of a metronome or by more formalized tasks such as controlled reading tasks.

In children, activities designed for syntax therapy may help children to phrase and group words appropriately so as to reduce the amount of words said on one breath. In these activities, sentences are formulated using word boxes, such as *The man / is helping / the lady / across the road.* Older children, however, may benefit from reading strategies similar to those used by the adult population, where predetermined phrasing and breath groups are marked in reading passages. The use of carrier games such as the card game "Go Fish" (*Do you have a rabbit that is eating?*) may also benefit prosodic phrasing or breath group control as well as articulation. Acting out simple plays has also assisted carryover where emphasis on stress, intonation, and rate can be incorporated into the activity.

Instrumental approaches to prosody therapy include the various modes of feedback that present information about parameters associated with stress, rate, and intonation. These include automatically controlled stimulus presentation and altered auditory feedback. The use of prosthetic treatment for prosodic deficits, however, is often reserved for the treatment of speech rate. Such rigid rate-controlling techniques often limit the speaker to a one-syllable/word-at-a-time delivery with devices such as a pacing board. While the naturalness of speech is often forfeited, this approach is beneficial in patients with severe disturbances of rate control.

Treatment of Developmental Neurogenic Speech Disorders

Treatment of Developmental Dysarthria in Children with Cerebral Palsy

Treatment of developmental dysarthria associated with cerebral palsy involves the use of techniques aimed at improving the functioning of the major components of the speech production mechanism to increase overall intelligibility and to develop improved control of components such as the jaw and articulation muscles that impact speech production, language skills, and feeding abilities. An important aspect of strengthening communication skills is to adapt and develop communication methods where necessary. This can involve a combination of speech and the use of an alternative or augmentative communication (AAC) system such as sign language or a communication device.

However, as developmental dysarthria in children with cerebral palsy often consists of a combination of heterogenous features varying from individual to individual, an individualized treatment plan must be employed. While AAC treatment options have been discussed in the treatment section of this chapter and will be covered in greater detail in Chapter 15, a number of additional considerations for therapy will be briefly outlined below. It is, however, important to understand that the capacity of the neuromotor system for improving speech production mechanisms in children with developmental dysarthria is limited.

Treatment of respiratory dysfunction largely focuses on postural control in terms of appropriate positioning that will attempt to counteract abnormal muscle tone interfering with respiration and phonation. Procedures and exercises for assisting children to shift from similar ratios of inhalation and exhalation of at-rest breath control to quicker inhalation and more controlled and prolonged exhalation for speech production are considered essential in managing impairments in respiration.

During positioning, children may be stimulated to produce longer vocalizations such as imitating prolonged vowels and chains of syllables such as *ba-ba-ba* or laughter. Exercises directed at developing cortical control of respiration are also used in order to stimulate deeper breathing, focusing on stimulation and visual cues for deeper inhalation and subsequent prolonged exhalation. Teaching the child to attend to sensations associated with respiration and to practice voluntary inhalation, followed by brief holding of the breath and subsequent controlled exhalation with vocalization, will assist the development of an improved speech breathing pattern in some children with cerebral palsy.

As mentioned above, treatment techniques for laryngeal and respiratory systems are often closely related. Therefore, improvements in respiratory control often also assist phonation in this population. As a result, positioning is incorporated in treatment programs that are directed at improving the ability of the child to initiate and sustain phonation. Facilitating more normalized phonation may be achieved through the use of techniques such as initiating exhalation while in the supine flexed position, which assists in improving tone. Laryngeal tension may also be reduced by singing simple songs as well as imitating whispered and soft vocalization. Smaller breath groups are also useful for assisting children who have prosodic disturbances such as poor control of pitch and loudness. Rising pitch may be counteracted by pausing, inhaling, and relaxing during speech production, as increased stress or emotion commonly results in increased pitch or loudness.

Improving postural tone is often necessary prior to articulation treatment in children with cerebral palsy, as respiration and phonation are significant contributors to overall intelligibility in this population. In cases where only a few speech sounds are able to be achieved through articulatory placement, improvement of syllable shape can provide improvements in intelligibility. When placement is not achieved, use of the appropriate manner of production can enhance effectiveness of communication. As it is often difficult to maintain articulatory accuracy during connected speech in individuals with cerebral palsy, the use of shorter breath groups will enhance intelligibility by slowing rate and allowing grater articulatory control.

While a communication device may be the primary avenue of communication for many individuals with cerebral palsy, it is important to improve intelligibility as much as possible through respiratory, phonatory, and articulatory techniques designed according to the requirements of each individual.

Treatment of Developmental Apraxia of Speech

As developmental apraxia of speech is increasingly recognized to comprise many facets, management of this disorder requires a treatment approach that is multimodal in order to address all levels of the identified underlying deficit. Unfortunately, one of the key identifying features of developmental apraxia of speech is slow progress in treatment programs. Improvement of these children is, therefore, likely to be prolonged over a period of time.

Most therapy programs are individualized to follow a combination of treatment techniques that address the key underlying features of developmental apraxia of speech. Techniques that target the oral motor/speech systems incorporate a variety of techniques including traditional therapy approaches, sensory awareness, reduced rate of speech, motor drills, phonetic placements, and sequencing and systematic drills, as well as the PROMPT system of therapy, which utilizes tactile and kinesthetic stimuli to facilitate phonetic placement and articulatory targets.

Cueing is also an important component of treatment programs for children with apraxia of speech. Techniques include improving spatial targets, total communication, cued articulation, and visual/graphic aids. Melodic intonation therapy is used for prosodic disturbances, whereas phonological rules and phonemic contrasts are incorporated where phonological disturbances are noted. Some examples of multimodal approaches include a combination of visual and tactile cues, exposure to literacy, phonological awareness, and language as well as integral stimulation methods. The Betta Meta program, developed as a combined metalinguistic and motor planning approach, has also been proposed as an effective program for this population.

Summary

Neurogenic speech disorders in adults and children arise from damage to the central and/or peripheral nervous system that disrupts the basic motor processes involved in regulation of the muscles of the speech production mechanism. Such damage may arise from a number of acquired conditions, including trauma, cerebrovascular accidents, tumors, degenerative conditions, and demyelinating disorders, among others, or may result from conditions that affect the functioning of the nervous system present before or shortly after birth (e.g., cerebral palsy). Two major motor speech disorders are recognized: dysarthria and apraxia of speech. In adults, these conditions represent acquired disorders, whereas in children both acquired and developmental forms of dysarthria and apraxia of speech may occur.

Dysarthria results from a disturbance in the muscular control of the speech mechanism and is associated with weakness, paralysis, or incoordination of the affected muscles. All of the basic processes involved in speech production, including respiration, phonation, resonation, articulation, and prosody, may be affected in dysarthria. Depending on the location of the damage to the neuromuscular system, six clinical forms of acquired dysarthria are recognized: flaccid, spastic, ataxic, hypokinetic, hyperkinetic, and mixed dysarthria. Developmental dysarthria is primarily associated with cerebral palsy.

Apraxia of speech is a motor programming disorder characterized primarily by articulatory disturbances with associated compensatory prosodic disturbances. Unlike dysarthria, apraxia of speech is not associated with significant levels of slowness, weakness, incoordination, or paralysis of the muscles of the speech production mechanism.

A range of different techniques is available for the assessment of acquired neurogenic speech disorders, including perceptual, acoustic, and physiologic methods. Likewise, a variety of different treatment approaches has been applied to these conditions, including behavioral, biofeedback/instrumental, surgical and prosthetic, and pragmatic approaches.

case study

CASE 1—ADULT WITH ACQUIRED DYSARTHRIA

Case 1 is a 32-year-old male who sustained a traumatic brain injury during a motor vehicle accident. A Glasgow Coma Score (GCS) of 5 was noted on admission to the hospital, indicating a severe head injury. A magnetic resonance imaging (MRI) investigation revealed bilateral subcortical hemorrhages and multiple contusions.

Perceptual assessment results indicated reduced speech intelligibility, consonant imprecision, reduced breath support for speech, hypernasality, strained-strangled vocal quality, and reduced pitch and loudness control as well as reduced speech rate and impaired stress patterning. Physiological assessment revealed wide-ranging motor speech subsystem dysfunction consisting of reduced respiratory support for speech, hyperfunctional laryngeal activity, velopharyngeal insufficiency, and reduced range and speed of labial and lingual movement.

A combination of both behavioral and instrumental treatment techniques were employed in the management of Case 1. Treatment goals consisted of remediating the physiological dysfunction of the motor speech subsystems and improving speech intelligibility. To target the physiological subsystems, kinematic instrumentation was used to provide visual feedback of chest-wall movement to assist in improving coordination during speech. Techniques such as the chewing/yawn–sigh and gentle voice onset assisted in reducing hyperadduction of the vocal folds, whereas visual feedback from a Nasometer focused on achieving velopharyngeal competence. Isometric and isotonic lip and tongue exercises were employed to increase strength and range of labial and lingual movements.

Modifying stress and intonation patterns, increasing speech rate, and enhancing articulatory precision were also identified as important goals. Techniques included contrastive stress and intonation drills, the PACER technique for speech rate, and articulation drills. Additional treatment strategies were incorporated into Case 1's management to maximize communicative success across varied communication environments. Such strategies included increasing communication-partner awareness of conversational topics and contextual cues, repairing communication breakdowns, and capitalizing on situational and environmental issues (e.g., limiting communicative interactions when fatigued and maximizing opportunities when energy levels are high; avoiding noisy environments). Information was provided to Case 1's family, friends, and coworkers relating to the nature of the communication disability as well as strategies for enhancing communicative effectiveness across a variety of environments.

QUESTIONS

1. In relation to this case, outline the benefits of obtaining both perceptual and physiological information in assessing motor speech function.

2. In addition to the motor speech deficits identified in the description of Case 1, what other features must be considered in planning treatment for the patient?
3. Highlight both the benefits and the disadvantages of providing treatment goals and strategies either concurrently or hierarchically.

case study

CASE 2—CHILD WITH ACQUIRED DYSARTHRIA

Case 2, an 8-year-old female, was admitted to the hospital with severe ataxia. An MRI scan following admission revealed a very large astrocytoma in the posterior fossa. While predominantly located in the midline, the tumor demonstrated some extension to the right and considerable extension into the left cerebellar hemisphere. Marked displacement of the fourth ventricle and considerable dilation of the lateral and third ventricles highlighted the associated increased intracranial pressure.

Six days following admission, the tumor was surgically removed. While no improvement in Case 2's condition was noted for 4 to 5 weeks, a subsequent shunt insertion contributed to an immediate improvement in her condition. Daily speech pathology intervention was initiated soon after the initial surgery with emphasis on decreasing oral hypersensitivity and reducing gag and bite reflex and tongue thrust, which were impeding her ability to feed and swallow.

One month postadmission, Case 2 was receiving daily occupational therapy, physiotherapy, and speech pathology support. Initially, treatment concentrated on feeding and oromotor skills. At 3 months postsurgery, Case 2 was able to produce some babbling sounds, but had difficulty initiating voice. At 4 months postsurgery, Case 2 began to speak in single words, progressing to short sentences within 2 weeks. Volume and pitch were uncontrolled and vocal quality was shaky with pitch breaks. Speech was slow and deliberate and was characterized by omission of final consonants, reduction of clusters, and difficulty with plosives and fricatives. Language comprehension was considered intact at a general level.

From this point, rapid progress was made across all areas. Case 2 demonstrated some perseveration in conversation and had difficulty changing topics and activities.

At 30 months postsurgery, intensive speech pathology intervention focused specifically on Case 2's higher-level expressive language, reasoning, and narrative skills. At this time, her speech was reportedly intelligible with slow rate and stress patterns that were even and equal. When prompted, Case 2 was able to modulate stress for expression and emphasis during storytelling.

Results of a comprehensive perceptual and physiological assessment conducted at 27 months postsurgery revealed that Case 2 had a mild dysarthria characterized by prosodic changes detected by the perceptual assessment. Perceptual assessments revealed mild impairment of alternate lip movements and moderate impairment of alternate tongue movements, volume variability, and reduced rate of speech. Physiological assessment revealed reduced lung volume, capacity, and excursion (indicating a largely abdominal breather) as well as reduced rate of repetition of tongue movements, reduced lip strength, and reduced bilabial lip pressures. Physiological assessment also revealed respiratory and articulatory system difficulties that were not detected perceptually that may certainly have contributed to the major area of concern of reduced rate of speech. Therefore, it was deemed likely that Case 2 was reducing speech rate in order to conserve expiratory output and ensure accuracy and strength of articulatory movements.

Treatment focused on the prosodic aspects of speech, particularly increasing rate and improving intonation patterns as well as respiratory dysfunction (increasing lung volumes and capacities, decreasing abdominal and rib cage termination volumes during speech). Treatment of articulatory dysfunction involved increasing both lip and tongue strength. Treatment of prosodic dysfunction was a priority for Case 2, with treatment techniques including the use of breath group patterning, together with treatment for respiratory-phonatory control, to allow the production of longer breath groups. Additionally, reading and drama-based activities were successful, as Case 2 was able to use modulation techniques for expression.

QUESTIONS

1. Highlight potential developmental issues that need to be considered in the management of this case.
2. Why would assessment of the environment be important to consider in establishing intervention goals?
3. What are the distinguishing features between apraxia of speech and acquired dysarthria in the childhood population?

case study

CASE 3—CHILD WITH DEVELOPMENTAL DYSARTHRIA

A few weeks after birth, Case 3's parents noticed that he was particularly floppy, had difficulty moving and no vocal ability, and was having trouble feeding. At 5 months, Case 3 was diagnosed with cerebral palsy; he was seen by a multidisciplinary team consisting of a physiotherapist, an occupational therapist, a speech pathologist, and a psychologist, and the family was seen by a social worker. All developmental milestones were considered delayed.

Initial treatment goals for communication consisted of engaging Case 3 in vocal play to increased vocal activity, with feeding also a primary goal. Vocal output increased considerably to producing distorted single-word attempts by the time Case 3 was 24 months old. A combined approach of postural support for speech, breathing, and phonation was adopted as well as attention to improving vocalization length and accuracy of articulation. During preschool, Case 3's speech remained highly unintelligible, but a system of teaming one-word signs (Makaton) to vocalizations was used. His speech pathologist also employed a visual cueing symbol system (COMPIC) to enhance communication and increase utterance length. At the age of 7 years, Case 3 was prescribed an electronic communication board. Communicative interaction was largely based on a combination of gesture, an AAC communication device, and limited intelligible speech. Ongoing multidisciplinary management, inclusive of speech pathology treatment, was also continued throughout Case 3's schooling to support his needs.

QUESTIONS

1. What other multidisciplinary team members may also have a role in the communication treatment of children such as Case 3, and how?
2. What considerations are required for socialization in children with developmental dysarthria?
3. How might treatment considerations change based on variations in type of cerebral palsy?

STUDY QUESTIONS

1. Highlight the differences and similarities between adult and child populations in relation to acquired neurogenic speech disorders.

2. Explain why treating the subsystems of speech (respiration, phonation, resonance, articulation) are important within the intervention process for individuals with dysarthria.

3. Why is it important that individuals with a motor speech disorder undergo a comprehensive speech pathology assessment even if a medical diagnosis has already been given? What other factors must be considered in doing so apart from the motor speech components?

4. What are the ongoing resource considerations related to developmental neurogenic disorders and management planning at a multidisciplinary level?

5. What is the expected impact of a developmental neurogenic disorder on language development?

SELECTED READINGS

Barlow, S. M., Finan, D. S., Andreatta, R. D., & Boliek, C. (2009). Kinematic measurement of speech and early orofacial movements. In M. R. McNeil (Ed.), *Clinical management of sensorimotor speech disorders* (2nd ed.). New York, NY: Thieme.

Darley, F. L. (1982). *Aphasia.* Philadelphia, PA: W. B. Saunders.

Darley, F. L., Aronson, A. E., & Brown, J. R. (1969a). Differential diagnostic patterns of dysarthria. *Journal of Speech and Hearing Research, 12,* 246–269.

Darley, F. L., Aronson, A. E., & Brown, J. R. (1969b). Clusters of deviant speech dimensions in the dysarthrias. *Journal of Speech and Hearing Research, 12,* 462–496.

Darley, F. L., Aronson, A. E., & Brown, J. R. (1975). *Motor speech disorders.* Philadelphia, PA: W. B. Saunders.

Knet R. D. (2009). Perceptual sensorimotor speech examination for motor speech disorders. In M. R. McNeil (Ed.), *Clinical management of sensorimotor speech disorders* (2nd ed.). New York, NY: Thieme.

Luschei, E. S., & Finnegan, E. M. (2009). Electromyographic techniques for the assessment of motor speech disorders. In M. R. McNeil (Ed.), *Clinical management of sensorimotor speech disorders* (2nd ed.). New York, NY: Thieme.

Murdoch, B. E. (2009). *Acquired speech and language disorders: A neuroanatomical and functional neurological approach* (2nd ed.). Oxford, England: Wiley-Blackwell.

Murdoch, B. E., Ozanne, A. E., & Cross, J. A. (1990). Acquired childhood speech disorders: Dysarthria and dyspraxia. In B. E. Murdoch (Ed.), *Acquired neurological speech/language disorders in childhood.* London, England: Taylor and Francis.

Zajac, D. J., Warren, D. W., & Hinton, V. A. (2009). Aerodynamic assessment of motor speech disorders. In M. R. McNeil (Ed.), *Clinical management of sensorimotor speech disorders* (2nd ed.). New York, NY: Thieme.

WEBSITES OF INTEREST

www.apraxia-kids.org/indexApraxia-Kids

This website contains articles, frequently asked questions, current research, links, and many resources related to the diagnosis and treatment of acquired and developmental motor speech disorders in children.

www.asha.org/public/speech/disorders/ASHA

This link provides definitions, links, resources, and treatment options. It also addresses a large variety of causes associated with motor speech disorders in both adults and children.

www.uq.edu.au/shrs

This website provides a link to the Centre for Neurogenic Communication Disorders Research, which provides information about the perceptual and physiological techniques described in this chapter as well as current research activity.

Chapter ELEVEN

Developmental Language Impairment During the Preschool Years

Catherine K. Bacon
Arizona State University

M. Jeanne Wilcox
Arizona State University

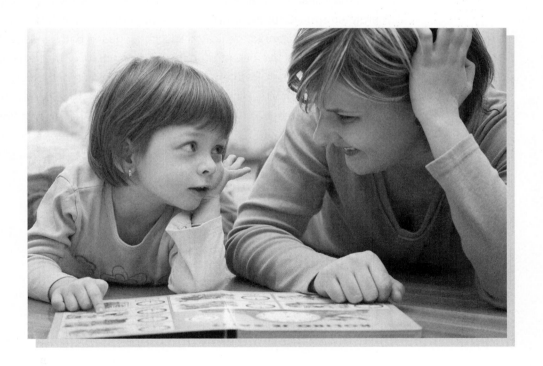

personal PERSPECTIVE

CATHERINE K. BACON

I would like to have a story of a carefully researched, well-planned selection of a lifetime career. Instead, I have the truth: I was an undergraduate at the University of California at Santa Barbara (UCSB), and in order to register for my junior year, I *had* to pick a major. I flipped through the college catalog and found "Speech and Hearing Sciences." It sounded like it would combine my interest in the sciences and love for children, so I registered for a full load of speech and hearing courses. I can honestly say that I have never regretted my hasty decision.

Speech-language pathology is a wonderful profession. It provides opportunities to work in a variety of settings: public schools, hospitals, clinics, private practice, and universities and research centers, to name a few. Speech-language pathologists work with many different people: from young children to the elderly; from individuals with mild articulation problems to those with significant medical and physical challenges. There also tend to be many flexible employment opportunities in the field of speech-language pathology that provide options in life when caring for young children or aging family members.

I have learned so much from this discipline, from my first speech and hearing professors at UCSB, the excellent graduate program at the University of Minnesota, and the many talented, dedicated speech-language pathologists, teachers, and therapists that I have been fortunate to work with over the years. Now I have the opportunity to learn from the future speech-language pathologists and audiologists as I teach and provide clinical training to students in the Speech and Hearing Science Department at Arizona State University. But my biggest lessons still come from the children and families with which I have the honor to work. Every smile and new word never cease to remind me what a lucky decision I made when choosing to major in speech and hearing sciences.

personal PERSPECTIVE

M. JEANNE WILCOX

My path to speech-language pathology was a circuitous one. I began my studies in higher education with a major in philosophy and ancient Greek. Actually, the philosophy was first, and the ancient Greek followed from my desire to read works of Plato and Aristotle in their original language. After developing a working knowledge of this "dead" language, I became interested in language in general, including the philosophy of language and ultimately the emergence of language. This led me to add linguistics to my list of majors. As I was nearing graduation, I happened to overhear someone in one of my linguistics classes talk about speech-language pathology. After learning that the discipline included the study of human language, the development of child language, and the opportunity to conduct language intervention, I felt that speech-language pathology was a perfect fit, and I looked around for a graduate program in speech-language pathology rather than linguistics.

My graduate studies took me to what was then Memphis State University (now the University of Memphis) and the start of a scientific and clinical journey to improve the lives of families and their children with disabilities. In addition to participating in the rich variety of clinical training experiences in the master's program, I developed lasting relationships with a group of clinicians and researchers that continue to inspire me today. My master's thesis experiences set me on a path to pursue a Ph.D. and a career in research. And—as they say—that's how the story goes. My research has always focused on the development and testing of interventions to improve language and developmental outcomes for young children. At present, I am on the faculty at Arizona State University, where I have developed an early childhood laboratory program that includes service delivery, clinical training for persons from multiple disciplines, and ongoing clinical research. I continually get new ideas from interacting with the families and children that receive services through the lab as well as all of the wonderful speech-language pathologists that work with me in the program. The discipline never ceases to amaze me in that there is always something new to learn, a new perspective to investigate, and, of course, families and children who are in need of the best services we can possibly provide.

Introduction: Developmental Language Impairment in Infancy and Early Childhood

From birth, parents begin the process of attributing meaning to their newborn's behavior. For example, many parents quickly identify a type of cry that they believe is an infant's "hunger" signal, and when this cry is produced, they interpret it to mean "I'm hungry" and subsequently feed the baby. Other early signals that parents may identify include "let's play," "my diaper is wet," and "I'm sleepy." While it is clear that infants have not yet learned to talk, or to purposefully convey these specific messages, the point is that their behavior is perceived as communication by their parents.

Between the ages of 8 and 12 months, most infants learn how to use simple gestures to communicate some basic needs and wants. For example, to convey something such as "I want that," an infant might reach toward an item on a high shelf, vocalize, and then look expectantly toward a parent or other adult. In order to convey a message such as "Look at that," an infant might point to a truck and look toward an adult. At approximately 12 months, infants begin to include words with these early messages, and over the next few months, they develop an initial vocabulary of 50 words or so. Typically, children begin to combine words to make early sentences around 18 months of age, and their language continues to develop rapidly during the remaining early childhood years, with a dramatic expansion of vocabulary, sentence length and structure, use of forms to convey specific information (e.g., when, how), and strategies for the socially appropriate use of language. For the vast majority of young children, this process unfolds just as described. However, some infants and young children demonstrate delay in these early processes and are identified as children with a developmental language impairment (DLI).

The American Speech-Language-Hearing Association (1993) defines a language disorder as the impairment or deviant development of comprehension and/or use of a spoken, written, and/or other symbol system. The disorder may involve the form of language (phonology, morphology, syntax), the content of language (semantics), and/or the function of language in communication (pragmatics). Children with language impairment are not developing language skills commensurate with those of their peers. Difficulties may be in comprehension of these aspects of language (receptive language skills) or in production of one or all of these components of language (expressive language skills). The language impairment may be mild, as in a child whose speech contains some grammatical errors, but whose message is easily understood by others, or the language impairment can be quite severe, affecting the child's ability to communicate her wants and needs to others around her. Communication and language disorders are among the most prevalent disabilities in early childhood, occurring in about 10–15 percentage of young children. In this chapter, we will examine the nature of DLI in young children, the factors underlying the language impairment, the general approaches for service delivery to this population, and the identification of and general considerations for intervention during the early years.

Nature of Developmental Language Impairment

Language is a complex system that allows us to exchange meaning efficiently through a shared set of symbols. As we have indicated, there are many components of language, and to use language effectively, a child must master all of these components. The

Diagnostic and Statistical Manual of Mental Disorders, Fourth Edition, Text Revision (DSM-IV-TR) (American Psychiatric Association 2000) identifies diagnostic categories of communication disorders that are usually first diagnosed in childhood:

1. Expressive language disorder
2. Mixed receptive-expressive language disorder
3. Phonological disorder
4. Stuttering
5. Communication disorder not otherwise specified

The first two categories refer to disorders of language (the focus of this chapter) or the ability to understand and use a shared symbols system. The last three categories (phonological disorder, stuttering, and communication disorder not otherwise specified) refer to disorders discussed in other chapters in this book (i.e., articulation and phonological disorders, fluency disorders, and voice disorders, respectively).

The criteria for classification of any of the childhood communication disorders include scores on standardized measures that are substantially below those obtained from standardized measures of nonverbal intellectual capacity. Symptoms for an *expressive language disorder,* according to the DSM-IV-TR, include a limited vocabulary, production of grammatical errors, difficulty with word recall, or production of shorter and less complex sentences than typically produced by children at that age. When thinking about expressive language disorder, it is important to note that recently the accuracy of this diagnostic category has been questioned (e.g., Leonard, 2009). In an analysis of empirical literature that focused on children with language impairment, Leonard notes that children who have been classified as having only an expressive language disorder often have language challenges that are beyond language output and can include subtle problems in language comprehension and word retrieval. Thus, caution should be applied in the use of this diagnostic category.

A classification of *mixed receptive and expressive language disorder* includes symptoms observed for expressive language disorder in addition to difficulties understanding words, sentences, or specific types of words such as spatial terms. The difficulties observed with expressive and mixed language disorders must significantly interfere with academic or occupational achievement or with social communication. In addition to being a primary, or specific, language impairment, DLI does occur secondary to mental retardation, sensory deficit, autism, and environmental deprivation.

Some children with DLI have difficulty acquiring language from birth. During the first months of life, infants communicate with their caregivers through cries, smiles, and vocalizations. As caregivers interpret and respond to these signals, infants learn to use these gestures and vocalizations intentionally to communicate their wants and needs. During this prelinguistic period, most children develop a rich and complex system of communication abilities characterized by increasing competence in conveying messages to their interactive partners. Children's emerging skills (e.g., play, gestures, babbling, coordinated attention) and environmental factors (e.g., adult responsivity) interact to facilitate and support the emergence of a highly functional communication system. For children with well-established communication systems, the acquisition of language has enormous utility; messages are generally exchanged more efficiently with language (Wilcox & Shannon, 1998).

Some children do not demonstrate these early communication skills that appear to form a necessary basis for initial language use, and these children are viewed as at risk for DLI. The rate of intentional communication at this prelinguistic stage of language development may be slower for children with DLI, and this lowered rate has been associated with poorer language outcomes (Calandrella & Wilcox, 2000; McCarthren, Warren, & Yoder, 1996; Wetherby, Yonclas, & Bryan, 1989). The types of prelinguistic intentional communication used by children with DLI may also be different from those used by typically developing children, with children with DLI demonstrating more limited vocalizations and fewer referential and conventional gestures (Capone & McGregor, 2004; McCathren, Warren, & Yoder, 1999; R. Paul, 2007). Finally, the communicative function of these early intentional communications may be different for children with DLI, with some children primarily using communication to regulate the behavior of others and demonstrating fewer communications for joint attention and social interaction (Capone & McGregor, 2004; Mundy, Sigman, & Kasari, 1990). Early intentional communications are important for establishing a meaningful base for subsequent language acquisition and use in interpersonal contexts, and children who demonstrate limited capacity for using early communication for joint attention and social interaction functions may have difficulty learning to use language for these same functions.

Developmental language impairment for other children may not be evident until they begin the process of learning words. As children move into this symbolic stage of language acquisition , they begin to acquire words and can communicate their message more efficiently. First words are typically nouns that are names for objects and people that the child enjoys and interacts with often, although frequent actions (e.g., verbs) may also be among the first words. Phonologically, these early words tend to be simple one- or two-syllable words that contain sounds that are easy to produce (e.g., /m/, /b/, or /d/). Most children understand more words than they are able to produce; their comprehension or receptive language skills precede their production or expressive language abilities. Children with DLI are often slow to produce their first words, with their parents reporting first-word productions around 16 to 18 months of age (or later) rather than the typical report of first-word production around the child's first birthday. Not only do children with DLI exhibit difficulty acquiring initial lexicons, but also some may demonstrate impairment in comprehension of single words and simple phrases (Ellis Weismer, 2007; Thal & Katich, 1996). Often children with DLI are identified in this early-word stage of language development because they are not understanding or producing words as would be expected for children their age.

Children with DLI may continue to demonstrate difficulty acquiring language as they move into the early linguistic stage of language development. Once most children have acquired a vocabulary of about 50 words, they begin to combine words into short phrases to communicate things like "more juice," "my car," and "no night-night"; this typically occurs between 18 and 24 months of age. Children use these early-word combinations to express a variety of semantic meanings (e.g., recurrence, as in "more juice"; possessor–possession, as in "my car"; or negation, as in "no night-night"). These early semantic relations provide the foundation for later syntactic development. Children with DLI, however, may have difficulty developing an initial vocabulary and may be slow to begin using word combinations (Ellis Weismer, 2007; Leonard, 1998; Olswang, Rodriguez, & Timler, 1998). These children may have concurrent difficulties comprehending language, with limited receptive vocabularies and poor comprehension of simple phrases and commands (Deevy & Leonard, 2004; Olswang & Bain, 1996; Thal & Tobias, 1992; Tomblin & Zhang, 2006) Speech production may also be challenging for children with DLI, and they may have a limited number of phonemes (sounds) or syllable shapes that they are able to produce (J. Roberts, Rescorla, Giroux, & Stevens,

1998; Stoel-Gammon, 1989). Children demonstrating slow development of initial vocabularies and a slow transition to using word combinations are demonstrating DLI at the early linguistic stage of language acquisition.

Finally, children with DLI can demonstrate language difficulties during the preschool years, which, for typically developing children, are marked by a dramatic increase in language skills. Children acquire the ability to produce longer and more complex utterances between 2½ and 5 years of age. This period of rapid linguistic expansion is marked by the acquisition of grammatical morphemes, continued vocabulary expansion, and the development of more-complex linguistic structures. By 3, children are adding simple verb endings such as the present progressive (e.g., "walking"), the regular past tense (e.g., "walked"), and the third-person singular (e.g., "walks"). Verb phrase elaboration continues as children add auxiliary verbs, modal auxiliary verbs, and negative forms and learn to embed and conjoin clauses. Most children improve the accuracy of sound production, and the number of persistent sound omissions and substitutions significantly reduces.

By the time a child enters kindergarten, that child has learned 90 percent of the syntax, morphology, and phonology that he will use as an adult (R. E. Owens, 2002). Semantically, the receptive and expressive vocabularies of preschool children increase dramatically, and there is a marked expansion in pragmatic skills (e.g., socially appropriate communication behavior). Preschool-aged children can use language to talk about experiences and to ask and answer questions. Language is used to exchange information and build social relationships. During this time, children develop the ability to accurately relay a story, and they begin building the language foundation needed for learning to read and write. Children with DLI at this stage of language acquisition may have difficulty with all elements of language: pragmatics, semantics, phonology, and especially morphology and syntax (Bedore & Leonard, 1998; Fey, Long, & Finestack, 2003; Leonard, 1998; C. McGregor, Newman, Reilly, & Capone, 2002). For example, preschool children with language impairments have been shown to have difficulties with verb phrase elaboration (Hadley, 1998; Leonard, Camarata, Pawlowska, Brown, & Camarata, 2008; C. A. Miller & Leonard, 1998), past-tense verb forms (Leonard, Deevy, Miller, Rauf, Charest, & Kurtz, 2003; Oetting & Horohov, 1997; M. L. Rice, Wexler, & Hershberger, 1998), and auxiliary verbs (Conti-Ramsden, Botting, & Faragher, 2001; Fey & Loeb, 2002). Problems with retrieval and memory for language processing can interfere with performance across all language domains. A DLI at this stage of language acquisition not only impedes spoken communication, but also can result in problems learning to read (Botting, Simkin, & Conti-Ramsden, 2006; Catts, Fey, Tomblin, & Zhang, 2002; McCardle & Chhabra, 2004; Nathan, Stackhouse, Goulandris, & Snowling, 2004; Scarborough, 2005).

Developmental language impairment during the preschool years has been shown to have a negative impact on a child's social interaction and development. (Brinton, Fujiki, & Higbee, 1998; Brinton, Fujiki, & McKee, 1998; Brinton, Spackman, Fujiki, & Ricks, 2007; Gertner, Rice, & Hadley, 1994; M. L. Rice, Alexander, & Hadley, 1993). Gertner, Rice, and Hadley (1994) demonstrated that children with DLI were less likely to be selected by peers for play than were their normally developing counterparts. In an earlier study, M. L. Rice, Alexander, and Hadley (1993) asked adults to rate audiotaped samples of children with DLI interacting with their same-aged peers. Adults consistently rated the children with DLI lower than they did their peers on variables such as social maturity, leadership abilities, and popularity. Developmental language impairment, regardless of the areas of language affected or the stage of language acquisition in which it occurs, will place a child at risk for challenges not only with verbal communication, but also with social interaction and academic success. We now turn to a consideration of some of the factors underlying DLI.

Factors Underlying Developmental Language Impairment

The acquisition of language is a result of a complex process that depends on innate predispositions as well as responsive, interactive environments. The ease with which most children master complex language behavior may reflect specialized biological mechanisms designed for the purpose of information processing and language acquisition (Tomasello & Slobin, 2005; Wakefield & Wilcox, 1995). However, as Brazelton and Greenspan (2000) suggest, the innate ability to use language requires an emotional foundation. Without reciprocal, enduring, developing, and supportive relationships to add emotional meaning to language, innate language functions don't respond to experiences and stimulation from parents and the environment. Relationships create a context for acquisition of language (Albrecht & Miller, 2001). Language competence is fostered and unfolds when children and adults have frequent, reciprocal conversations. If a child lacks a responsive caregiver or the physical ability to send easily interpreted signals to the caregiver, the development of a foundation in communication is at risk (LaParo, Justice, Skibbe, & Pianta, 2004).

Biological factors (e.g., prematurity, hearing loss, chromosomal or genetic factors) or environmental factors (e.g., deprivation, exposure to toxins during gestation, neglect) can present challenges for a child's development of language. In fact, as Rosetti (1996) states, "anything that interferes with a child's ability to interact with the environment in a normal manner is a potential cause of or contributing factor to the presence of developmental and more specifically communication delay" (p. 2). A baby's care-giving environment may affect development. Factors such as poverty, the mental health of the caregiver, and the caregiver's ability to form attachments can place a child at risk for DLI and subsequent academic challenges. When these biological or environment risk factors are present, we can initiate early intervention to help prevent delays by promoting healthy development (Fowler, Ogston, Roberts-Fiati, & Swenson, 1997; Fox, Long, & Langlois, 1988; Guralnick, 1997).

Nelson (2010) offers a framework for categorizing DLI based on the underlying cause of the impairment:

1. We can examine DLI associated with cognitive-communicative impairment, including developmental disability, intellectual disability, autism spectrum disorders, acquired brain injury, child abuse and neglect, and interactive disorders of attention, emotion, and behavior. These conditions, when present, result in challenges in the acquisition of speech and language skills.

2. DLI can occur as a condition secondary to motor and sensory impairments. Sensory impairments (such as hearing loss, visual impairment), motor disorders (neurological conditions such as cerebral palsy, seizure disorders, head and spinal cord injury), and congenital malformations (such as cleft palate, microcephaly) impede a child's ability to learn language. The pattern of development for children with these conditions is likely to be different than that for other children demonstrating DLI.

3. DLI can occur by itself without any other known problem. Children in this final group have a primary diagnosis of specific language impairment.

In the next section, we review the language acquisition process and deficiencies that are associated the more common cognitive-communicative disorders, motor and sensory disorders, and specific language impairment.

Children with Cognitive-Communicative Disorders

Developmental and Intellectual Disabilities   Several genetic and chromosomal disorders result in global developmental delay that affects the acquisition of speech and language skills. As Nickel and Widerstrom (1997) explain, "genes are the basic unit of inheritance . . . and code for the production and synthesis of proteins and enzymes . . . that result in the infant's physical characteristic and biochemical make-up" (p. 90). Pairs of genes are arranged along chromosomes. Each human cell contains 23 pairs or 46 chromosomes. An alteration or mutation in the chemical make-up of a single gene or gene pair can cause a genetic disorder. Genetic disorders are further classified depending on whether the gene is located on the sex chromosome or not and whether it is dominant (only one parent needs to carry the gene for it to be passed on to the baby) or recessive (both parents must carry the gene for it to be passed on to the baby). Fragile X, a sex-linked genetic disorder, is the most common inherited cause of mental retardation. When abnormalities occur in the number or structure of chromosomes, the result is some type of chromosomal disorder. The most common chromosome anomaly is Down syndrome, or trisomy 21, which results in cognitive disabilities, hypotonicity (low muscle tone), heart problems, and some unique physical traits such as malformation of the eyes, ears, and hands. Because Down syndrome is usually easily identified at birth, babies born with Down syndrome can receive early intervention from the time that they are born in order to promote development in all areas, including speech and language development (Berglund, Eriksson, & Johansson, 2001; Strunk & Fullwood, 2000).

The speech and language behavior of children with global developmental delay related to genetic and chromosomal disorders has been studied closely since the 1960s. In general, the overall sequence of communication and language development in children with global delay is similar to that of children developing typically; however, the rate of development is slower (E. A. Bates, 2004; Caselli, Vicari, Longobardi, Lami, Pizzoli, & Stella, 1998; Pruess, Vadasy, & Fewell, 1987). The relationship between language and cognitive skills is not straightforward. For example, some children with mental retardation demonstrate language skills commensurate with their developmental/cognitive levels, while other children demonstrate delay in the acquisition of speech and language beyond what would be expected for their developmental level. Children with Down syndrome or fragile X syndrome often exhibit poorer language skills than do their typical peers (Abbeduto & Hagerman, 1997; Boudreau & Chapman, 2000; Chapman, Seung, Schwartz, & Kay-Raining Bird, 1998; Eadie, Fey, Douglas, & Parsons, 2002; Kamhi, 1981).

Children with intellectual disability (i.e., mental retardation) usually demonstrate difficulties with all aspects of communication and language acquisition, including pragmatics, semantics, syntax, morphology, and phonology. Children with Down syndrome tend to demonstrate a rate of preverbal intentional communication prior to transitioning to linguistic communication similar to that of children with typical development (Calandrella & Wilcox, 2000; Wetherby et al., 1989); however, they have limited nonverbal requesting abilities as well as selected social-interactive behaviors (Mundy, Kasari, Sigman, & Ruskin, 1995; L. Smith & von Tetzchener, 1986). As Capone and McGregor (2004) point out, "gesture production is a strength for children with Down syndrome relative to their receptive and expressive language skills" (p. 181). Children with fragile X syndrome, however, may show relative strengths in verbal communication and weaknesses in pragmatic skills, use of gestures, reciprocity, and symbolic play skills (J. E. Roberts, Mirrett, Anderson, Burchinal, & Neebe, 2002). Acquisition of linguistic symbols is slower in children with developmental delays and often facilitated by use of augmentative communication such as sign language (Abrahamsen, Cavallo, & McCluer, 1985; Wang, Bernas, & Eberhard, 2001).

In terms of semantics, children with global developmental delay tend to acquire new words more slowly and rely primarily on concrete word meanings. Syntactic development is similar to that observed in typically developing preschoolers; however, children with Down syndrome tend to use shorter, less complex sentences, relying on less mature forms even when they are capable of more advanced syntactic or morphological constructions (Chapman et al., 1998; Eadie et al., 2002; Miles & Chapman, 2002 J. E. Roberts, Mirrett, & Burchinal, 2001). Phonological development is slow in children with Down syndrome, with a tendency to continue patterns of sound simplification (phonological processes) even when they are capable of producing the words correctly (Dodd & Thompson, 2001; Klink, Gerstman, Raphael, Schlanger, & Newsome, 1986; Stoel-Gammon, 2001). For some individuals with Down syndrome, their speech is often unintelligible throughout childhood and adolescence, making it difficult for them to communicate their message verbally. Poor speech intelligibility is also a characteristic of some children with fragile X syndrome, along with problems with rate of speech, stuttering-like repetition of sounds, and perseveration on a word, phrase, or topic of conversation (Abbeduto & Hagerman, 1997; Mirrett, Roberts, & Price, 2003).

Autism Spectrum Disorders (ASD)   Autism and pervasive developmental disorders (PDD) are developmental conditions that are usually identified during the early childhood years and result in language impairment. Autism is a considered a neurological disorder, although the specific genetic or brain dysfunction has not been identified (Akshoomoff, 2000; Towbin, Mauk, & Batskaw, 2002). It affects the functioning of the brain and impacts the development of reciprocal social interaction and verbal or nonverbal communication skills, often resulting in stereotypical behavior, interests, and activities. The prevalence of autism has increased dramatically, and now 1 out of every 150 children may be at risk for ASD (Fombonne, 2007). It affects four times as many boys as girls (Yeargin-Allsopp, Rice, Karapurkar, Doernberg, Boyle, & Murphy, 2003). The chance of autism occurring is not related to racial, ethnic, or social status, nor does it affect children based on family lifestyle, income, or education level. There are three components that must be present for a child to receive a diagnosis of autism or pervasive developmental disorders as described in the (DSM-IV-TR American Psychiatric Association, 2000):

1. The child must demonstrate a qualitative impairment in social interaction (i.e., the child must demonstrate limited inclination to share enjoyment, interests, or achievements with other people).
2. The child must demonstrate a qualitative impairment in communication.
3. The child must demonstrate restricted repetitive and stereotyped patterns of behavior, interests, and activities.

Pervasive developmental disorders include autism, Rett's disorder, childhood disintegrative disorder, Asperger's disorder, and pervasive developmental disorder not otherwise specified (PDD-NOS). The term *autism spectrum disorders*, now used synonymously with PDD, reflects a view that autism includes a range of disorders that all share symptoms affecting social interaction, communication, and patterns of behavior.

The communication and language impairment of children with ASD is often the most devastating aspect of the disorder. Some children with autism never develop any functional communication or language behavior, and others develop functional, but idiosyncratic use of spoken language (Lord & Paul, 1997; Mirenda, 2003; Wetherby, Prizant, & Schuler, 2000). With limited communication skills, children with autism often develop idiosyncratic, unconventional or undesirable behaviors to communicate (aggressive or self-injurious behavior, tantrums).

Wetherby, Reichle, and Pierce (1998) found that children with ASD exhibit unique communication and language impairments relative to other children with DLI as well as to cognitive-matched young children who are developing typically. More specifically, children with autism demonstrate more challenges in the use of (1) communicative functions (e.g., request, comment), (2) gestural communicative means (e.g., point, show), (3) reciprocity (e.g., turn-taking), (4) social-affective signaling (e.g., facial expressions, gaze regulation), and (5) symbolic behavior (e.g., use of signs or spoken words). Mundy and colleagues (Mundy, 1995; Mundy & Markus, 1997; Mundy & Stella, 2000) have found that, typically, children with ASD use contact gestures to communicate (e.g., pulling the adult to an object, manipulating the adult's hand) at significantly higher frequencies than conventional gestures (head nods, waving, pointing). Most children with autism that do learn to communicate with language demonstrate a period of using echolalia, which is the literal repetition of another's speech either immediately following a production (immediate echolalia) or sometime later (delayed echolalia). It has been hypothesized that children with autism may use echolalia as a means to communicate before they are able to generate unique phrases to communicate their wants and needs to others around them (Prizant & Rydell, 1993; Prizant & Wetherby, 1987; Schuler & Prizant, 1985).

Wetherby and collegues (1987, 1998, 2000, 2002) have suggested that the language impairment in children with autism that impacts the social aspects of language (pragmatic skills or use of language) centers around two problems. First, children with autism have a limited capacity for joint attention (e.g., coordinating attention between people and objects); and second, they tend to have a limited capacity for symbol use (understanding that a word or object can represent or symbolize something else). Both of these skills are crucial to language learning. Children with ASD who are able to use gestures to initiate joint attending seem to have the most rapid expressive vocabulary growth (Y. Smith, Mirenda, & Zaidman-Zait, 2007).

Despite significant communication problems for children with ASD, dramatic improvements are possible for these children and their families. An increasing number of children with ASD are being identified during the first 3 years of life, allowing treatment to begin at an earlier age (Woods & Wetherby, 2003). Intervention is successful, particularly behavioral approaches using operant conditioning (sometimes called applied behavioral analysis [ABA] therapies) (Dawson & Osterling, 1997; L. Koegel, 1995; R. Koegel, Camarata, Koegel, Ben-Tall, & Smith, 1998) Evidence-based practice suggests that intervention is most successful when it is embedded in the natural environment, is responsive to a child's lead, and relies upon natural contingencies and reinforcers to promote communication (Hwang & Hughes, 2000; L. Koegel, 1995; Wetherby et al., 2000; Woods & Wetherby, 2003). For children with ASD, the transition from gestural to intentional symbolic communication is the most difficult, and treatment plans should include strategies to facilitate this transition. Oftentimes, signs or picture symbols (i.e., symbols that are less transient than spoken words) can promote the transition from gestural to symbolic communication (Mirenda, 2001, 2003; Schlosser & Blischak, 2001). Children with ASD may also demonstrate hyperlexia (i.e., a precocious ability to read words, but with limited comprehension) and have a greater interest in learning to read and write than to speak (Mirenda & Erickson, 2000). Specific intervention strategies for children with autism need to build on the child's strengths; expand the child's repertoire of communication functions, gestures, and forms; and increase the child's functional social use of communicative behavior.

Traumatic Brain Injury (TBI)   This is defined as an "acquired injury to the brain caused by an external physical force, resulting in total or partial functional disability or psychosocial impairment or both, that adversely affects a child's educational performance" (Individuals with Disabilities Education Improvement Act, 2004, Sec. 300.8[c][12]). TBI can result in impairment in cognition, language, memory, attention, problem-solving, sensory, perceptual, and motor abilities and psychosocial behavior. The impact of traumatic brain injuries on cognitive-communicative processes is related to the location and extent of brain damage and the child's level of functioning prior to the injury, but is not always predictable. Brain damage in TBI can cause symptoms of aphasia as well as motor, cognitive, and sensory deficits (Lees, 2005). Children with acquired brain disorders like TBI often have difficulty with social-emotional judgment as well as with attention, memory, and learning (Nelson, 2010). Children with acquired brain injuries often require the coordinated services of an interdisciplinary team to reteach and facilitate important language and literacy skills, executive functioning, and self-regulatory abilities.

Child Abuse and Neglect   When children are neglected or abused, there is risk for bodily harm that may result in cognitive-communicative language problems. Child abuse or neglect can occur before birth (prenatally) or at any time after birth and includes exposure to domestic violence or maltreatment as well as physical, sexual, and psychological or emotional abuse (Hyter, 2007). We will limit our discussion of DLI in children that are abused or neglected to fetal alcohol spectrum disorder (FASD).

The use of drugs or alcohol during pregnancy can result in damage to the developing fetus and puts the child at risk for DLI and other learning disorders. Fetal alcohol spectrum disorder is a term that describes a spectrum of disorders with a range of symptoms caused by prenatal alcohol exposure. Alcohol use by the mother during pregnancy can result in low birth weight, microcephaly (small head size), changes in the facial features, heart problems, and developmental delay (Howard, Williams, & Lepper, 2010; Widerstrom & Nickel, 1997). The delay may be mild or severe, impacting a child's ability to function and interact with the environment. Infants that have immature or compromised central nervous systems may be easily overstimulated and experience irritability, disrupted sleep/wake cycles, weak sucking, and failure to thrive. Young children with FASD may exhibit delays in walking, talking, and toilet training; often show signs of distractibility/hyperactivity; and often have difficulty following directions and adapting to change (Howard et al., 2010; Streissguth, 1997). Problems with attention, distraction, and memory can interfere with children's acquisition of receptive and expressive language skills as well as their ability to function successfully in social situations. Social communication difficulties are often the most salient problem for children with FASD (Atchison, 2007; J. Henry, Sloane, & Black-Pond, 2007; Timler, Olswang, & Coggins, 2005). For this reason, intervention for the child exposed to alcohol and drugs prenatally needs to facilitate her ability to recognize and communicate her needs, maintain emotional control, and understand cause–effect relationships in daily activities and to create opportunities for her to experience success (Duquette, Stodel, Fullarton, & Hagglund, 2006; Lutke, 1997).

Children with Primary Sensory and Motor Deficits

Sensory impairments, such as hearing loss and/or visual impairment, can be present at birth and create risk for DLI. Children with visual impairments alone don't necessarily demonstrate higher incidence of DLI; however, as one might expect, they have been shown to demonstrate greater delay in early gestural communication development (Preisler, 1995). In addition, there are some birth defects that result in impairments to both the visual and the auditory systems (e.g., Usher syndrome, congenital infections such as rubella and cytomegalovirus).

Hearing loss will impact language development at any age, and early identification of and intervention for hearing impairment are critical. Newborn hearing screenings, mandated and implemented now in all states, have allowed us to identify many babies with hearing loss at birth. It is estimated that 1 in 1,000 babies born will have a profound hearing impairment (Northern & Downs, 2001). These babies are at risk for DLI. The earlier a hearing loss is detected, the better the outcome will be for the child and his family. Hearing aids and cochlear implants are used to enhance or improve whatever hearing the child does have. Over the past 2 decades, studies have shown that children who are deaf and receive cochlear implants have better speech perception and production scores than do children using hearing aids (Fryauf-Bertschy, Tyler, Kelsay, & Gantz, 1997; Peng, Spencer, & Tomblin, 2004), and the younger the child was at implantation, the better the speech and language outcomes (Tomblin, Barker, Spencer, Zhang, & Gantz, 2005). Approaches to early intervention include (1) oral-aural rehabilitation that focuses on verbal speech development, (2) total communication approaches that use both speech and sign language to promote language development, and (3) bilingual (ASL) trainings that focus on teaching the child both American Sign Language and the spoken English language. Hearing disorders and aural rehabilitation are described in Chapters 17 and 18 of this book.

Hearing can also be affected by recurrent and chronic bouts of otitis media with effusion or middle-ear infections during early childhood. The impact of otitis media on language development is complex (see Olswang et al., 1998, for discussion). In general, children with recurrent and persistent ear infection in early childhood are at risk for speech and language delay. It is important that families and pediatricians be aggressive in the management of ear infections to promote the most optimal language outcomes for young children.

Children who are born with multiple disabilities that include *visual and hearing impairment require special consideration*. Usher syndrome, an inherited condition, is the most common cause of a dual visual/hearing impairment, with the hearing impairment present at birth and a progressive loss of vision (Carvill, 2001). Other birth defects that can result in dual-sensory impairment are identified by the CHARGE association, which is an acronym that stands for anomalies presented at birth: *C*oloboma (of the eye), *H*eart anomalies, *A*tresia choanae, *R*etarded growth and development, *G*enital anomalies, and *E*ar anomalies or deafness. Congenital rubella is another common cause of dual visual/hearing impairment; however, the incidence of this type of dual sensory problem has been greatly reduced with the rubella vaccination beginning in the 1970s. This viral infection, when contracted by the mother during the first trimester of pregnancy, can cause multiple defects in the infant, including cataracts, heart problems, inner-ear damage, retardation of growth, and mental retardation. Another virus, cytomegalovirus, can cause eye and heart anomalies plus deafness, mental retardation, and growth deficiency if contracted during pregnancy (Shprintzen, 1997). The age of onset of the hearing impairment and vision loss will impact the developmental outcomes for that child. Language and communication skills are often severely limited or absent in children that are born with dual sensory impairments, especially when these children have accompanying motor and cognitive delays (Carvill, 2001; Rönnberg & Borg, 2001).

As would be expected, assessment and intervention for children with both visual and hearing impairments can be challenging. Standard procedures for assessing hearing, vision, communication, cognition, and motor skills need to be adapted in order to identify functional skills and promote the best outcomes (W. R. Dunlap, 1985; Fewell & Rich, 1987). Intervention includes the use of assistive technology (such as hearing aids or cochlear implants to improve hearing; glasses or eye surgery to improve vision) as well as remediation strategies to train functional skills. With the widespread use of the rubella vaccine, the indidence of dual vision/hearing impairment has dramatically decreased. However, when present, these dual sensory impairments create unique and significant challenges for communication and language acquisition.

Cerebral palsy (or more correctly, static encephalopathy) is a neuromotor impairment resulting from brain injury or anomaly that occurs early in development. It is estimated to occur in two to five children per thousand births. Cerebral palsy (cp) has been classified many ways based on the type of abnormal muscle tone, movement, and coordination that is present and the area of the body affected (see Chapter 10 for a complete description). The injury to the developing brain that causes CP can occur during pregnancy (e.g., as part of a genetic condition), at birth (e.g., due to complications of prematurity or asphyxia), or after birth (e.g., due to meningitis or head trauma). Infants born prematurely (before 36 weeks of gestation) can experience a condition called periventricular leukomalacia, which accounts for approximately 35–40 percentage of the cases of CP. Children with CP are at risk for seizures, feeding problems, speech and language problems, learning disabilities, and mental retardation (Nickel & Widerstrom, 1997).

Developmental language impairment in children with neuromotor conditions, such as cerebral palsy, is often related to limitations in the child's ability to either produce speech or interact with the environment. Movement disorders can interfere with the child's ability to volitionally control reaching, looking, and vocalizing. The baby's signals may be harder for the caregivers to read and interpret, thereby disrupting the flow of caregiver responsivity, which is important to child's development of initial communication skills. When the movement disorder involves the oral musculature, children will have problems developing the ability to generate speech. Chapter 10 describes the type of speech disorders characteristic of children with cerebral palsy and other movement disorders. When oral expressive language skills are severely compromised for children with movement disorders, augmentative communication devices can be used to promote functional communication and language development (see Chapter 15).

Children with Primary language Impairment

Thus far, the discussion of DLI has been associated with an identifiable primary diagnosis (e.g., mental retardation, ASD, hearing impairment, brain damage); however, for many children with DLI the language impairment is the primary diagnosis and occurs in the absence of other identifiable conditions or impairments. The language impairment typically comes to a caregiver's attention as a child approaches 18–24 months and is not talking or is using only a few words to communicate. When children show a significant limitation in language ability that cannot be attributed to problems of hearing, neurological status, nonverbal intelligence, or other known factors, they are diagnosed with specific language impairment, or SLI (Leonard, 1998). It is estimated that 7 percent of 5-year-olds appear to have SLI (Tomblin, Records, Buckwalter, Zhang, Smith, & O'Brien, 1997). SLI occurs more often in boys than in girls, and children with SLI are more likely to have other family members with language and learning problems.

Although SLI has an undetermined cause, subtle irregularities in the brain structure or function have been identified in children with a diagnosis of SLI. Gauger, Lombardino, and Leonard (1997) reported that magnetic resonance images show a higher prevalence of neuroanatomical irregularities in children with SLI. Other studies by Plante and her colleagues have found different patterns of brain region activation and coordination that suggest less efficient patterns of functioning (Ellis Weismer, Plante, Jones, & Tomblin, 2005; Plante, 1991; Plante, Swisher, & Vance, 1989; Plante, Swisher, Vance, & Rapcsak, 1991). These and other studies (see Leonard, 1998, for a review) show fairly high percentages of atypical neuroanatomical and neurophysiological patterns. As Jernigan, Hesselink, Sowell, and Tallal (1991) suggest, the brains of children with SLI may be especially sensitive to the effects of prenatal environmental factors, which, together with genetic, neurological, and environmental factors, interact and may result in language impairment.

Children with SLI have limited vocabularies, use shorter utterances, omit grammatical suffixes and function words, and make more grammatical errors than do children their age. Their phonological abilities can be below age level as well. These children may demonstrate a delay in language production or a delay in both language production and language comprehension, and at times, the delay in expressive language skills is worse than the delay receptive language. Children with SLI may have central auditory processing problems, including difficulty with auditory attention, discrimination, and memory. As a group, children with SLI also demonstrate problems with reading once they begin school (Bird, Bishop, & Freeman, 1995; Catts et al., 2002; Nathan et al., 2004; Rescorla, 2005; M. Rice, Taylor, & Zubrick, 2008).

The specific criteria for diagnosing SLI include language scores below normal limits, with nonverbal intelligence scores within normal limits and no hearing, oral motor, or diagnosed neurological or physical problems. Although children with SLI share these characteristics, they are not a homogeneous group. Some children with SLI may have greater difficulty with morphological elements of language, while other children may have more difficulty with semantic skills, demonstrating limited vocabularies and word-finding problems. As mentioned earlier, children with SLI also vary in the relationship between language production and comprehension, with some children demonstrating a primary delay in language expression and other children demonstrating primary delays in receptive and expressive language. However, as mentioned previously, children with a primary delay in expressive language frequently have other subtle impairment in word retrieval, receptive language, or other aspects of cognitive functioning that supports language (e.g., auditory processing). This also holds true for children who present with receptive and expressive language delay.

Children with SLI have been studied intensely for the past several decades, and successful interventions have been identified that can improve many aspects of these children's language deficiencies (Camarata & Nelson, 2006). Because children with SLI are at risk for reading and academic problems, it is also important to provide or support interventions designed to enhance or promote acquisition of early literacy skills such as phonological awareness, knowledge of the alphabet, recognition of print, and writing (e.g., tracing letters of a name).

Identification of Developmental Language Impairment

As we have noted, some types of DLI are associated with conditions that can be identified at birth; however, many children with DLI do not exhibit conditions that easily distinguish them from their peers. There is a tremendous amount of variability in normal language acquisition: Some children speak their first words before their first birthdays and are using sentences well before they turn 2, while other children are late talkers and seem to be close to 3 before their sentences are understood by people around them. Both groups of children are developing language normally, so how does one identify the child that is outside of this pattern and is at risk for a DLI?

We use much of what we know about typical language development to determine when a child may be deviating from this path or moving along the path too slowly. Table 11.1 provides an overview of receptive and expressive language behavior that can be expected at given ages (see Chapter 2 for more detailed information regarding speech and language development). The information in this table is appropriate when considering children's acquisition of their first language. Children who are learning two or more languages simultaneously may demonstrate patterns in language acquisition that do not conform to these guidelines. (Kohnert, Bates, & Hernandez, 1999; Marchman & Martinez-Sussmann, 2002). Further, children who are learning a second language subsequent to their native, or first, language may not necessarily demonstrate the same patterns of acquisition as they did in their first language (Kohnert & Bates, 2002). However, when children are learning one language and do not show the expected receptive or expressive language skills by certain ages, they should be referred for a complete speech and language assessment.

The lack of language and the limitations in communication development may be the first symptoms noticed by parents and professionals in children with a variety of developmental disorders. A multidisciplinary panel, representing nine professional organizations and endorsed by the American Academy of Neurology and the Child Neurology Society (Filipek et al., 1999), recommended that the following behaviors be used as guidelines for immediate further evaluation for possible autism spectrum disorders:

- no babbling by 12 months
- no gesturing (pointing, waving bye-bye) by 12 months
- no single words by 16 months
- no two-word spontaneous (not just imitated) phrases by 24 months
- *any* loss of *any* language or social skills at *any* age

Although these early language and communication milestones may not be able to distinguish ASD from other DLI, they do provide reasonable criteria for suspecting DLI and referring for a complete speech and language evaluation.

Olswang et al. (1998) identified several factors that can help distinguish children that are late talkers who will catch up on their own from those who are at risk for a DLI. First, the nature of the child's language production and comprehension skills can help predict language change in toddlers. Children with small expressive vocabularies for their age and limited verb lexicons are more likely to demonstrate DLI over time (Olswang, Long, & Fletcher, 1997; Watkins, Rice, & Moltz, 1993). In a recent investigation,

TABLE 11.1   Language Comprehension and Production Skills Expected at Given Ages

When children deviate from this pattern and do not show the expected receptive or expressive language skills by certain ages, a complete speech and language assessment is warranted.

Language Comprehension	*Language Production*
Birth to 3 months	
■ Startles to sound ■ Quiets when spoken to ■ Ceases activity when there is a new sound	■ Has different cries for different needs ■ Coos, gurgles, and makes happy sounds
3 to 6 months	
■ Looks in the direction of your voice ■ Turns to sound ■ Notices toys that have music or sounds	■ Makes sounds like "da," "ga," and "ba" ■ Continues vocalizing when caregiver imitates baby's sounds ■ Begins to repeat sounds like "baba" and "dada"
6 to 12 months	
■ Turns and looks when name is called ■ Responds to "no" ■ Recognizes some words for common objects ■ Responds to simple commands with gestures like "come here"; "give it to me"	■ Vocalizes using longer strings of consonant and vowel sounds together ■ Begins to imitate sounds ■ Uses gestures, points, and looks to communicate ■ By 12 months says a few words like "mama" or "bye-bye"
12 to 18 months	
■ Points to pats pictures in book ■ Follows simple directions such as "go get your shoes" ■ Answers simple questions nonverbally ■ Points to familiar people upon request	■ Uses adultlike intonation patterns ■ Shakes head "yes" and "no" ■ Points to objects desired ■ Uses several words (3–20 words) ■ Tries to imitate simple words
18 to 24 months	
■ Has a receptive vocabulary of 300 words or more ■ Answers "what's that" questions ■ Listens to stories ■ Identifies five to seven body parts	■ Expressive vocabulary includes 50–100 words ■ Imitates two-word sentences ■ Combines words into short phrases ■ Begin to use pronouns ("I," "me," "you," "mine")
24 to 30 months	
■ Understands over 300 words ■ Follows more complex directions ■ Begins to understand prepositions like "on" and "under"	■ Vocabulary increases to 200+ words including nouns, verbs, and pronouns ■ Starts to combine nouns and verbs ■ Asks questions ■ Says name
30 to 36 months	
■ Follows two-step directions ("get the ball and put it on the couch") ■ Understands simple concepts such as "big/little" and "on/off"	■ Uses two- and three-word sentences ■ Uses some grammatical structures such as plurals and the "ing" verb ending ■ 60–70% of the child's is understood by listeners speech ■ Uses age-appropriate consonants (t, d, n, b, p, m, w, h)

(Continued)

TABLE 11.1   (Continued)

Language Comprehension	Language Production
3 to 4 years	
■ Understands simple questions ■ Understands negatives ("not") and descriptive concepts like "same," "heavy," and "empty" ■ Follows two- and three-part commands	■ Produces sentences that have four or more words ■ Uses grammatical structures such as conjunctions, plurals, pronouns, possessives, and past-tense verbs ■ Talks about activities and can tell a simple story ■ Most of the child's speech is understood by listeners
4 to 5 years	
■ Listens to stories and answers questions about them ■ Understands quantitative concepts (whole/half; some/none) ■ Identifies and names colors and some shapes ■ Can follow three unrelated directions	■ Uses adultlike grammar and complete sentences ■ Can define words ■ Tells a coherent story ■ Produces almost all sounds correctly, with the exception of a few like /l/, /s/, and /r/

Source: The information was compiled from a variety of sources, including American Speech-Language-Hearing Association (1983), Bricker and Squires (1999), and Shipley and McAfee (1998).

Ellis Weismer (2007) found that the language comprehension at 30 months of children identified as late talkers was the strongest single predictor of children's language production scores at 66 months. Children with delay in both language production and language comprehension are also at a greater risk for communication disorders (Thal & Katich, 1996). Children with limited speech production skills (e.g., infrequent vocalizations, limited number of consonants, restricted syllable structure) and few spontaneous imitations are less likely to spontaneously catch up in their language skills.

Second, the characteristics of a child's play and social interaction abilities can predict language change in toddlers. Toddlers with DLI demonstrate limited symbolic play behaviors and use fewer communicative gestures than do their late-talking peers. Among toddlers who demonstrate developmental concerns, use of communicative gestures has been shown to be a predictor of language outcomes in that children with low frequencies of early gestural use tend to have poorer language outcomes (Calandrella & Wilcox, 2000). During the early years, children with DLI have been found to initiate communication at low frequencies and often to direct communications to adults rather than peers (H. Craig, 1993; Hadley & Rice, 1991). Finally, factors such as prolonged periods of untreated otitis media, a family history of language and learning problems, and strong parental concern can be indicators that a child is less likely to catch up on his own and more likely to demonstrate DLI that requires intervention.

Various assessment measures are used to identify children with a DLI. Norm-referenced tests are standardized measures that allow the child's behavior to be compared to that of other children the same age. Criterion-referenced tests can also be used to assess a child's level of performance or mastery of a set of developmental tasks or skills. Often both types of measures are necessary to understand a child's abilities. For example, a norm-referenced test in which a child is asked to complete a variety of tasks such as pointing to pictures, manipulating objects, naming items, or repeating sentences might be supplemented with the parents' report of the child's communication strengths and needs. Parent report has been shown to be a valid indication of a child's level of performance when parents are asked to check behaviors currently demonstrated by the child rather than reporting milestones achieved at earlier ages (Dale, 1991; Diamond & Squires, 1993; Meisels & Fenichel, 1996). By including multiple sources of information in the assessment (e.g., norm-referenced or criterion-referenced tests, informal observation, and parent report and observation), a more valid estimate of the child's abilities can be obtained (Bagnato, Neisworth, & Munson, 1997). It is important to talk to the family, other caregivers, and teachers to obtain a complete picture of the child's communication skills and the concerns regarding the child's development. Table 11.2 presents some important questions to ask the family when planning an assessment of a young child. All assessment should include an observation of the child's communication, speech, and language skills with a familiar caregiver in a familiar environment (e.g., home, child-care program, preschool program) to the extent possible. Likewise, assessment of young children's communication skills should include a hearing screening as well as a screen of other developmental skills areas.

For young children, there is often no clear boundary between assessment and intervention. The goal of assessment in early childhood is to provide a comprehensive survey of the child's present levels of skills across or within developmental domains to begin planning intervention. Evidence-based practice encourages assessment that includes *multiple measures, multiple sources, and multiple domains* and accomplishes *multiple purposes* (Bagnato et al., 1997). First, assessment should include *multiple measures;* that is, a battery of developmental scales and instruments should be used to determine the child's and the family's capabilities and needs. Second, assessment should incorporate information from *multiple sources,* including parents, teachers, and other professionals. Third, assessment of young children should be completed in *multiple domains,* including cognitive, adaptive, motor, social-emotional, and language skills, as well as other areas such as parent-child interaction, attention, and motivation, to provide a more complete picture of the range of developmental abilities. Finally, assessment in early childhood

---

TABLE 11.2   Questions to Ask Families When Planning an Assessment of a Young Child

Family-Tailored Assessment

- What questions or concerns do other have? (e.g., sitter, preschool)
- Are there other places where we should observe your child? (Get place, contact person, what to observe)
- How does your child do around other children?
- Where would you like the assessment to take place?
- What time of day?
- Are there others who should be present in addition to parents and staff?
- What are your child's favorite toys or activities that will help him/her be comfortable, be motivated, and become focused?
- Which roles would you find most comfortable during assessment:
    - sitting beside your child; offering comfort and support to your child
    - helping with activities
    - exchanging ideas with the assessor
    - carrying out activities to explore your child's abilities
    - prefer for assessor to handle and carry out all activities

should fulfill *multiple purposes*. For example, the screening tests should identify the areas needing further evaluation, and the results of a comprehensive assessment should provide direction for intervention and program planning. The questions asked in the assessment should provide answers for initial intervention plans. Assessment is an ongoing process wherein the clinician can begin to understand the child's strengths and needs to provide the best possible intervention practices.

Approaches to Providing Services to Young Children with Developmental Language Impairment

Development language impairment impacts social interaction. Because language is used for communication, a child with a language impairment faces real barriers and the possibility of social isolation. Throughout history, children with developmental disabilities, including speech and language impairment, have been treated differently by society. Since 1975, there have been several federal, state, and local laws passed that have provided for educational and therapeutic services for children with developmental disorders, including language delay. Public Law 94-142, the Education of All Handicapped Children Act, passed in 1975, required that all children with disabilities be provided a free appropriate public education. In 1986, Public Law 99-45, the Education of the Handicapped Act, extended these rights to children from birth through 21 years of age. Since 1975, these laws have been reauthorized and amended. The Individuals with Disabilities Education Act (IDEA)—passed in 1990 and amended in 1997 and 2004—sought to improve services for all children with disabilities by requiring early identification, provision of services within the least restrictive environment, and inclusion of parents as partners in the educational process.

There are four service delivery approaches that serve as both a basis and a guideline for provision of services. For many, the most familiar approach is consistent with a medical model of service delivery and is termed remediation. In a remedial approach, the goal of intervention is to improve functioning in the identified deficit area. Aspects of a child's development are evaluated with respect to age-appropriate skills. Areas of delay or disorder are determined, and a plan to remediate or at least mitigate that delay is formulated. Consistent with this approach is the concept of *point-of-diagnosis* access to services, meaning that a child has a diagnosis of a language disorder prior to the commencement of intervention.

Some approaches to intervention focus more on prevention of a deficit. The objective of prevention intervention is to prevent emergence of secondary deficits associated with a primary deficit. Within this approach, children who demonstrate established risk conditions are provided with intervention prior to an actual diagnosis of a language delay or disorder. For example, a child with Down syndrome may receive speech and language intervention at a very early age in hopes of preventing subsequent delay in speech and language development.

Oftentimes the focus of early intervention is to provide compensation for a deficit condition that cannot be remediated or prevented. In this case, assistive devices or services are provided that correct the problem or detour around the problem. For example, a child with a hearing loss may be provided with a hearing aid in an effort to correct the possible speech-language and hearing problems presented by the loss.

Finally, some early interventions for children are designed to facilitate acquisition of typical developmental skills. The focus of intervention is the promotion of developmental skills in children that are believed to be at risk for demonstrating a language delay. Children within this group typically include those with biological or environmental risk factors that may place them at risk for developmental language impairment, (e.g., poverty, low birth weight), but by no means uniformly cause DLI in children with these conditions. In other words, perhaps the children may demonstrate DLI and perhaps not. The promotion, approach, therefore, focuses on creating the optimal context for facilitating development and typically includes caregiver training or caregiver education programs (Baxendale & Hesketh, 2003; Girolametto & Weitzman, 2006; Girolametto, Weitzman, & Greenberg, 2003; Girolametto, Wiigs, Smyth, Weitzman, & Pearce, 2001; Tanock & Girolametto, 1992).

It is important to note that the approaches are not mutually exclusive, and for many children, combinations of approaches may guide service design and implementation. However, irrespective of the approach, there are some key principles of early intervention that are guided by the laws and founded on evidence-based practice. First, the caregiver/family is the center of services provided to young children. Family members are the experts in their children's abilities and are their children's first teachers. Children develop in the context of their family, and the focus of early intervention is to facilitate the family's ability to support their child's development. Figure 11.1 illustrates the role of the speech-language pathologist (SLP) in providing services to young children. When a child is receiving early intervention services, the SLP directs his expertise to the appropriate caregiver to teach that individual how to facilitate the child's language development. When a child is enrolled in preschool classes, the SLP directs his expertise to the child's caregivers and the classroom teacher. The goal of intervention is to promote the child's language development in natural or least restrictive contexts, and for the young child, these contexts include the caregivers or teachers who interact with her on a regular basis and the environment where the child spends most of her time (e.g., home, child-care program, family child-care home, preschool class).

Intervention services can be provided in a variety of settings, including homes, day-care centers, preschools, clinics, and hospitals. Since the 1980s, there has been a move toward providing intervention in the child's natural environment and a move away from traditional "pull-out", therapy, where the child is removed from his classroom so that the

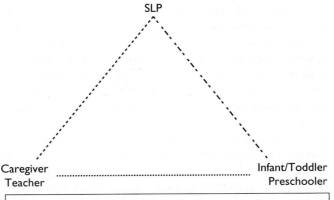

FIGURE 11.1

A model for delivery of language intervention SLP services for infants, toddlers, and preschoolers.

SLP can provide individual speech and language intervention (R. A. McWilliams, 1996; Strain, McGee, & Kohler, 2001; Valdez & Montgomery, 1997; Wilcox, Kouri, & Caswell, 1991; Wilcox & Shannon, 1996; Woods & Wetherby, 2003). In particular, Wilcox et al. (1991) compared the language progress of children who received classroom-based language intervention to that of children who were pulled out of the class for individual intervention. Results indicated that children who participated in the classroom-level program demonstrated superior generalization of learned language skills.

Once a child reaches 3 years of age, speech-language intervention and educational services are typically provided through the public schools. Classroom settings for children with disabilities can be inclusive, in which children with typical development are enrolled in larger numbers than children with DLI. In other cases, children with DLI and other developmental disabilities may be served in self-contained classes that enroll only children with disabilities. Often, with the self-contained model, the children have certain activities in which they participate with children demonstrating typical development. Whenever possible, children with DLI should be placed in an inclusive setting. Inclusive programs provide opportunities for children with DLI to participate in the regular classroom activities with their peers and receive adaptations and support as necessary for them to engage in those activities (M. Rice & Hadley, 1995; Wetherby, 2002; Wilcox & Shannon, 1996). Social interaction is crucial to emerging communication and language skills, and inclusive programs provide for social interaction with typically developing peers. Maximum opportunities for learning appropriate social behaviors should be an integral part of programming for young children with and without disabilities. In many respects, the opportunity to learn socially appropriate behavior and interactive strategies is a primary benefit that children with disabilities derive from inclusive toddler and preschool programs. Through interactions with peers and adults, children are able to learn appropriate social and language skills.

The intervention strategies used to promote communication and language need to reflect the strengths and needs of the individual child and respect the family's concerns and unique sociocultural experiences. It is critical for the interventionist to be aware of potential sources of bias when designing intervention programs for children of varying backgrounds and sociocultural experiences. There are important differences among cultures about how children learn language, the value placed on child talk, social contexts that are appropriate for caregiver–child interaction, and people who are available and appropriate to guide children's learning and participation (Harry, 2002; Lynch & Hanson, 1992; van Kleeck, 1994b; Wilcox & Shannon, 1998). For example, Crago (1990) found that "talkativeness" by young children in the Inuit culture is viewed as a potential sign of a learning problem. Likewise, other studies (van Kleeck, 1994b, and Langdon, 1992) noted that the typical adult–child interaction in Mexican-American culture (and others) is likely to be triadic and include the mother, child, and another adult. Almost all intervention protocols that target early language acquisition include a focus on children's communication interactions in typical settings (e.g., home, playgroup) and rely on adult-interactive techniques known to facilitate children's language acquisition. Van Kleek (1994) provides numerous examples of cultures in which components of typical early language intervention protocols have the potential of conflicting with the prevailing values, beliefs, or typical communication styles of those cultures. It is important for the professionals working in early intervention to develop an awareness of which aspects of an intervention approach or strategy are based on assumptions that may not be held by all families. By providing family-centered services, the potential conflicts are minimized through careful development of goals and intervention strategies in collaboration with family members that respect the unique culture and individual differences of each child.

Summary

Developmental language impairment in infants and young children comes in all shapes and sizes. It can be diagnosed at any point during language acquisition, and it presents in many different ways. There are a variety of biological and environmental factors underlying DLI, including genetic disorders, sensory impairments, neurological disorders, congenital malformations, and other developmental disorders. Over the past 4 decades, researchers have provided substantial information that has allowed us to understand many aspects of the factors underlying and associated with DLI. In turn, this information helps us with early diagnosis in order to promote the best possible developmental outcomes for each individual child.

We considered four management approaches for early language intervention: remediation, compensation, prevention, and promotion. In addition, we discussed the importance of providing services from a family-centered perspective that acknowledges that a child's family is the true expert in terms of her developmental competencies. Further, it is critical to be sensitive to families' sociocultural beliefs and values and to potential mismatches between these values and certain approaches to intervention. Finally, evidence-based practice suggests that the most effective language intervention efforts for young children are those that are embedded within the context of typical activities and routines.

case study

Jake, a 20-month-old boy, was initially evaluated due to parental concerns regarding his expressive language skills. Jake was born at 38 weeks gestation weighing 5 pounds 2 ounces. He experienced difficulty breathing immediately after birth and remained in the hospital for 10 days. Once home, Jake's mother reported that he was a fairly healthy baby, developing and achieving milestones as expected; however, he did experience frequent ear infections. At 16 months of age, pressure-equalizing tubes were placed, and Jake has not had any ear infections since placement of the tubes. Jake's parents became concerned about his language development when he was still not saying any words at his 18-month checkup.

A variety of norm-referenced, parent report, and observation tools were used to assess Jake's communication and language development during the initial evaluation. Jake communicated frequently with his mother using gestures (e.g., pointing, reaching, shaking his head), eye contact, and a few vocalizations. His vocalizations consisted of single-syllable vowel productions with a few consonant–vowel productions that included the /m/, /b/, and /d/ phonemes. He produced a few words (e.g., "ba" for "ball" and "uh" for "up"), and his mother reported that his expressive vocabulary included approximately five different words. Jake demonstrated good language comprehension skills, responding to names of objects, action words, and simple commands during the evaluation.

Speech-language intervention was initiated to increase Jake's expressive vocabulary. The speech-language pathologist (SLP), together with Jake's parents, selected 10 words to begin teaching Jake. These words were names for objects that Jake enjoyed and contained sounds that Jake could produce. The SLP helped Jake's family identify opportunities to use these words during typical daily activities (e.g., bathing, feeding, dressing, and play). Every week, the SLP visited Jake's home and helped his family use strategies to facilitate communication and encourage Jake's use of target words. As Jake learned targeted words, new words were added, and after 4 months of intervention, Jake's expressive vocabulary included close to 40 different words. Jake continues to receive speech-language services to expand his expressive vocabulary and encourage his use of word combinations.

QUESTIONS

1. What are some factors that may be contributing to Jake's DLI?
2. What were some indications that Jake was ready to learn words?
3. Why was it important to solicit the parent's help to select target words, and why did the clinician suggest that Jake's initial target words begin with sounds that he could produce?
4. How did the SLP provide speech and language intervention in natural contexts and social interactions?
5. In what ways did the SLP provide family-centered services?

case study

Jenny was the first child born to Mr. and Mrs. Garcia. She was a beautiful, healthy baby whose development seemed to be right on track. Jenny started talking around 1 year of age, although she seemed to say a word and then never use that word again. She did communicate by leading adults to what she wanted or bringing objects to them when she needed assistance. Jenny was an independent child who seemed to prefer to play on her own, but did not engage in any pretend play. As Jenny approached her second birthday, her parents became concerned that her 12-month-old sister was more communicative, attempted to say more words, and was easier to engage in activities. After many evaluations by a variety of professionals, Jenny received a diagnosis of autism spectrum disorder.

The early intervention team and speech-language pathologist (SLP) began working with Jenny and her family to increase communication and social interaction skills. The SLP showed her family how to use pictures to give Jenny choices and encourage her to communicate. Mrs. Garcia created wonderful opportunities for Jenny to communicate during daily activities, encouraging Jenny to use words or pictures to communicate. By the time Jenny was in preschool, she was able to use words and some rote phrases to communicate. She used her communications to regulate the behavior of others (e.g., request items and protest), but she did not use language to share information or comment on activities. Most of Jenny's communication was directed to adults, and she had difficulty interacting and communicating with her peers. Jenny currently attends a preschool with typical children and children with special needs that is team-taught by a special education teacher and SLP.

QUESTIONS

1. Describe some of Jenny's early behaviors that are characteristic of children with autism spectrum disorders.
2. Why were picture symbols used to facilitate initial communication skills?
3. Identify some of Jenny's strengths in terms of communication and language skills? What are some areas of concern that should be addressed in intervention?
4. What are some typical preschool activities that might provide natural opportunities to facilitate Jenny's pragmatic skills?

SUDY QUESTIONS

1. What is a DLI and what components of language can be affected?
2. Describe the nature of DLI in the prelinguistic stage, the early linguistic stage, and the later linguistic (preschool) stage of language acquisition.
3. What are some of the biological and/or environmental factors underlying DLI?
4. Describe the four approaches to intervention (*remediation, prevention, compensation, and promotion*) discussed in this chapter.

SELECTED READINGS

Blasco, P. M. (2001). *Early intervention services for infants, toddlers and their families.* Boston, MA: Allyn & Bacon.

Fryauf-Bertschy, H., Tyler, R. S., Kelsay, D., & Gantz, B. J. (1992). *Performance over time of congenitaly deaf and postlingually deafened children using a multichannel cochlear implant.* Journal of Speech and Hearing Research, *35*, 913–920.

Hulit, L. M., & Howard, M. R. (2006). *Born to talk: An introduction to speech and language development* (4th ed.). Bostonm, MA: Allyn & Bacon.

McCauley, R. J., & Fey, M. E. (2006). *Treatment of language disorders in children.* Baltimore, MD: Paul H. Brookes.

Nelson, N. W. (2010). *Language and literacy disorders: Infancy through adolescence.* Boston, MA: Allyn & Bacon.

Owens, R. E., Jr. (2008). *Language development: An introduction* (7th ed.). Boston, MA: Allyn & Bacon.

Owens, R. E., Jr. (2010). *Language disorders: A functional approach to assessment and intervention* (5th ed.). Boston, MA: Allyn & Bacon.

Paul, R. (2007). *Language disorders from infancy through adolescence* (3rd ed.). St. Louis, MO: Mosby/Elsevier.

Peng, S-C., Spencer, L.J., and Tomblin, J. B. (2004). *Speech intelligibility of pediatric cochlear implant recipients with seven years of device experince.* Journal of Speech, Language, and Hearing Research. 47: 1227–1236.

Tomblin J. Bruce, Barker Brittan, A., Spencer Linda, J., Zhang Xuyang, Gantz Bruce, J. (2005). *The effect of age at cochlear implant initial stimulation on expressive language growth in infants and toddlers.* Journal of Speech, Language, and Hearing Research. 2005; 48(4): 853–67.

WEBSITES OF INTEREST

www.cdc.gov/ncbddd

The National Center for Birth Defects and Developmental Disabilities promotes the health of babies, children, and adults to enhance the potential for full, productive living. This site includes information on causes of and treatment for birth defects and developmental disabilities including autism spectrum disorders, cerebral palsy, mental retardation, and vision and hearing impairment.

www.asha.org

The American Speech-Language-Hearing Association website provides information on speech, language, and hearing development and disorders for the public and for professionals in audiology, speech-language pathology, and speech and hearing science.

It includes activities to encourage speech and language development as well as referral information for families concerned about their child's language development.

www.nichcy.org

The National Dissemination Center for Children with Disabilities, funded by the U.S. Department of Education, Office of Special Education Programs, provides information to the nation on disabilities in children and youth; programs and services for infants, children, and youth with disabilities; IDEA, the nation's special education law; No Child Left Behind, the nation's general education law; and research-based information on effective practices for children with disabilities.

Chapter TWELVE

Language Disabilities in School-Age Children and Youth

Barbara Culatta
Brigham Young University

Elisabeth Wiig
Boston University

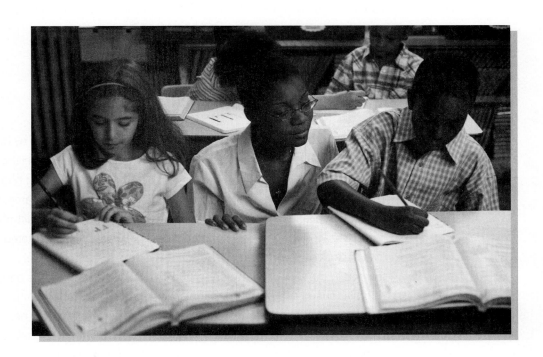

personal PERSONAL PERSPECTIVE

BARBARA CULATTA

I selected speech pathology as a college major because I wanted to be in a helping profession and because my parents insisted that I major in something "marketable." I chose speech pathology because I liked the prospect of working individually with children as opposed to teaching in a whole-class setting. I was also intrigued with learning about causes, effects, and interventions for disordered communication. I have loved my career choice, and I now enjoy working in classroom settings helping teachers to impact what happens to children in their academic and social classroom experiences. While I am still fascinated with disorders and strategies, my curiosity has been replaced with understanding and with a deep passion for the field. I continue to be fascinated with how psychological, cognitive, and sociocultural factors impact communication. And although I had always wanted to help people, I hadn't anticipated the amount of gratification I would experience from observing children with impairments functioning well when given the right supports. It has truly been a blessing to contribute to improving the lives of children. I am continually grateful for the profession I selected so many years ago.

personal PERSONAL PERSPECTIVE

ELISABETH WIIG

It is difficult for me to remember a time when I was not intrigued by human communication, with its intricacies, variations, and sometimes debilitating interferences. I grew up in a bilingual, bicultural family. Listening to and learning two languages in parallel was to me like a fun, puzzling, and always entertaining game. I used my listening and language skills to the max for 2 years to cover the fact that I could not make any sense of written or printed letters or words. When I entered the third grade, I was diagnosed with dyslexia and spent the next 3 years in special education. What I learned in the special education setting probably directed my life's path. I learned that good language and communication abilities provide a firm foundation for learning and using what has been learned. I learned that students with special needs progress at different rates and reach different heights. I learned that the specialists who taught us had an inner glow and a sense of personhood that was unique and that gave us courage and hope. Last, but not least, I learned some of the skills of the trade of a detective that I could later apply in evaluating students, identifying their needs, and providing interventions. Speech-language pathology has provided me with professional opportunities that have been broad in range, offered practical and intellectual challenges, and given me both personal and professional rewards.

Introduction

Speech-language pathologists must know how students function in school contexts in order to understand and address their language needs. Since language is the primary medium for functioning both academically and socially, it is not surprising that students with language impairments have difficulty keeping up with curricular expectations and/or establishing close friendships. Good language skills are essential for comprehending texts, following directions, solving problems, learning to read and write, and negotiating interactions with others. This chapter will focus on the language abilities that students must obtain if they are to meet the demands they encounter in school. It will describe the language challenges students face in school, explain the nature of the language problems they may encounter, and describe what speech-language pathologists (SLPs) do to assess language problems and help students succeed.

To put a personal face on communication contexts, examples of one student's difficulties will be interspersed throughout the chapter. Connor, a 7½-year-old first grader, struggled in school because of language problems. Despite having repeated kindergarten, he experienced great difficulty acquiring early reading skills. He also exhibited significant expressive language problems and had trouble establishing close friendships. Due to the discrepancy between Connor's language skills and the language demands he faced, the SLP played an important role in his educational program.

Nature of School Language

To understand the impacts of language impairments, it is important to know the language demands associated with acquiring information and mastering skills. This section describes the complex language that students encounter in school and identifies the breakdowns in language that students may experience.

Demands Students Encounter

The language students encounter in school is much more complex than the language they experience at home. In school, students need to represent abstract ideas, connect units of information, simultaneously process multiple pieces of linguistic information, and flexibly alternate among the communication modalities of listening, speaking, reading, and writing.

Represent Abstract and Remote Events   Just as a map symbolizes faraway places, school language represents events removed from personal experience (Britton, 1990; Cazden, 1988; Silliman & Wilkinson, 1991). The ability to represent abstract ideas and remote events permits students to learn about historical events, understand how to perform math operations, and comprehend how feelings and beliefs relate to characters' actions in stories. Things that are remote and abstract can be communicated because language rules (words and syntactical relationships) can represent recurring aspects of events as well as specific situations. A student who knows the words *first* and *paragraph* and hears them in the sentence "There's a hint in the first paragraph about what happened to the man's dog" will know where to look in the story for needed information. Likewise, students who know syntactical rules will be able to recognize relationships signaled in sentences they've never heard before. A student can hear "If the doctor had taken his job seriously, he wouldn't have made that kind of mistake" and know there is a cause/effect relationship between the problem created and something the doctor had done previously. With well-established knowledge of grammatical and vocabulary rules, students can acquire new information and understand how ideas relate.

Combine Smaller Components into Larger Ones   To function in school, students must be able to combine the structural components of language, such as sounds and words, to form larger units. They must also be able to connect the sentences they hear and understand to particular functions or reasons for communicating. The structural and functional components of language combine to form complex communication units.

The smallest structural component of language, a phoneme or speech sound, combines with other phonemes to form words (e.g., /d/ plus *–og* forms *dog*; /th/ plus *–ink* forms *think*) and word parts (e.g., morphemes such as *ing* and *un*). Words and syntactical patterns combine to form sentences, and sentences come together to form larger discourse units or texts. The terms *text* and *discourse* refer to groups of related utterances that convey connected or organized information about a topic—such as paragraphs, essays, stories, explanations, class presentations and discussions, and conversations (Blank, Marquis, & Klimovitch, 1994; N. W. Nelson, 1998; Roseberry-McKibbin, 2007).

The functional components of language also combine to form higher, more complex communication events. The highest functional level, the discourse event, refers to the overall purpose of the exchange or communicative act, which is influenced by the topic and context (Peets, 2009). Different types of discourse events include conversing socially (e.g., sharing experiences and feelings), relating information (e.g., giving reports about happenings), instructing (e.g., explaining how to perform a procedure or conveying information about an event in history), and telling stories (e.g., entertaining and sharing information through fictional texts).

Within a discourse event, students must integrate the structural and functional components of language and/or the smaller units with the larger ones. The structural components of language (i.e., the rules for combining sounds into words, words into sentences, and sentences into texts) signal meanings and intentions that arise from the purpose and topic of the discourse event. The higher-level purpose and topic bear upon the words and sentences selected and the ways sentences are tied together. The overall topic and purpose of the discourse event influence meanings signaled, functions conveyed, and sentences formed to communicate particular ideas and achieve specific functions. The integration of structural with functional parts of language to achieve intents complicates its use. Tables 12.1 and 12.2 illustrate how the structural and functional components of language combine within particular discourse events.

Process Different Components Simultaneously   Constructing larger discourse units, such as conversations and texts, requires students to operate on different components of language at the same time. This simultaneous or parallel processing of multiple language parts and levels, which generally needs to occur very rapidly, makes school language challenging (Carroll, 2008; R. Chapman, 1992).

As students receive linguistic messages, they attach meanings and functions to words and syntactical rules, and they relate those meanings to what they already know about the topic. As additional parts of the message are received, students continue to

TABLE 12.1   Functional and Structural Components of Language

Functional Components

Discourse events

- Inform or instruct (Convey information, teach, explain, read expository texts; listen to lectures)
- Negotiate (Engage in impersonal exchanges; participate in class discussions)
- Tell fictional stories (Read, write, or listen to narratives about imagined events)
- Tell personal narratives (Relate experiences or recount shared events)
- Engage in social conversations (Talk with family members or friends about common, familiar events in supported contexts)

Mechanisms for Managing the Topic and Turn Exchange

Discourse-level functions or turn types

- Extend (Add something relevant and new to a partner's utterance)
- Maintain (Acknowledge or answer a question without adding new information)
- Initiate (Talk about something new, change the topic)

Decisions about what to say in context

- Select utterances that fit social roles, goals, situations; identify when to talk, how much to say, what is relevant to say

Explicit statements about the exchange, repairs

- Comment on whose turn it is to speak or the relevance of a turn; announce changes in a topic; alter a message when breakdowns occur (Restate, rephrase, or repeat an idea; increase the volume, add stress, or slow production)

Utterance-Level Functions (reasons for producing particular utterances)

Higher-level, more complex functions

- Predict, plan, problem solve, negotiate, and state beliefs

Lower-level, more simple functions

- Request information, actions, or objects; answer; make comments or statements

Structural Components (largest to smallest units)

- Texts (Connected utterances organized around a topic, such as chapter books, stories, informational texts or passages, conversations, discussions, paragraphs, explanations, class presentations)
- Several related sentences (Two or three adjacent utterances referring to the same topic or context)
- Sentences (Combinations of words, phrases, and clauses that signal relationships among the ideas in those units)
- Clauses and phrases (Word combinations that signal relationships among words)
- Words (Ideas expressed in sound combinations that stand for ideas, meanings)
- Morphemes (Parts of words that combine to make larger words)
- Sounds (Phonemes of language that are not meaningful unless combined to form words that have shared meaning among members of a community)

Integration of Functional and Structural Components

- The discourse event (overall purpose and topic of communication) influences selection of lower-level functional and structural components.

(Continued)

TABLE 12.1 (*Continued*)

■ The discourse event creates demands to connect smaller structural units (sounds, words, sentences) into larger units (texts, discourse).

■ Higher-level discourse events influence or dictate selection of words and sentences needed to signal meanings that relate to the topic and purpose of the communication.

■ Producing language at the discourse level is more difficult than producing isolated components of language in simple contexts.

■ The ability to function at lower structural levels (know words, combine words into sentences) is important for functioning at higher levels of discourse.

■ In school, lower-level components of language (sounds, words, phrases, sentences) rarely operate in isolation (without connecting to form discourse or text units and without fitting into authentic communicative situations).

■ More-difficult instructional discourse events require more-demanding language skills than do simpler social conversations that occur in familiar, supported contexts.

Source: Based on Dore (1979, 1986), Grice (1975), Nelson (1998), Tough (1977), Wallach & Butler (1994).

attach meaning to the new parts, while relating that new information to what was already processed. Students continue to process incoming sentences in light of what they already know, while concurrently attempting to understand the text as a group of connected utterances (Ashcraft, 1994; R. Chapman, 1992).

Comprehending stories, through either listening or reading, is a language task that requires simultaneous processing of different types of information. A student listening to a story must understand incoming words and sentences, connect ideas in sentences to each other, and construct a larger connected "whole" representation of the story. This is accomplished by relating information in the words and sentences to the story's theme and plot—that is, the character's problem, goal, plans, and attempts to solve the problem as well as the story's eventual resolution (N. L. Stein & Glenn, 1979; J. P. Williams et al., 2002). Reading rather than listening to stories involves accessing word meaning through printed letters, while attaching meaning to words and sentences. In reading, students attach sounds to letters and sound combinations to letter patterns. Recognizing the letter pattern *gate* as a real word requires blending or integrating three separate sounds (/g/, â [long *a*], and /t/) and understanding that the final *e* is silent. Making letter–sound associations and blending sounds into words permit access to word meaning. After attaching meaning to words, students must also be able to combine words and sentences into larger connected texts (C. Scott, 1994). This ability to combine words into sentences and sentences into topically related ideas is essential for story comprehension in either the oral or the written mode.

Participating in class discussions also requires parallel integration of components and levels of language. Students must process the utterances they hear during a discussion, relate the participants' contributions to what they know about the topic, keep track of the topic as the discussion progresses, decide what information would be relevant to add, and select language needed to make a contribution. In addition to following what other participants say about the topic, students must monitor and manage the turn-taking process. Because of the linguistic challenges involved in participating in a class discussion, some children with language difficulties may make irrelevant comments or be unable to participate.

TABLE 12.2   Language Demands in Simple and Complex Discourse Events

Component or Task (High to Low)	Discourse Event	
	Social Conversational Exchange (Simple, Familiar Context)	Instructional, Informational Exchange or Text (Complex School Context)
Identify and organize the discourse	Identify and signal temporal and causal relationships; use context and shared experience to identify the topic	Identify and signal the text's organization, purpose, and theme; judge whether information fits the theme and organization of the text
Manage turns, topic	Rely on context, gestures, familiarity with the topic to connect turns; add to or acknowledge partner's prior utterance; repair breakdowns by repeating or rephrasing information; monitor listener's level of interest	Signal changes in the topic; reflect on relevance and appropriateness of specific content to the topic; provide listener with important background information; introduce subtopics; reflect on listener's perspective
Relate utterances to each other	Connect utterances to immediate context or familiar, shared experience; use simple pronouns and conjunctions to connect ideas in adjacent sentences	Connect ideas together using pronouns, synonyms, conjunctions, conditional words (*if, while, because, therefore, but, however, before*); monitor sentences for topical "thread"; fill-in assumed information; connect new information to previously stated information held in memory
Signal functions	Signal basic functions (labeling, commenting, answering questions, requesting actions or information, greeting, calling, protesting)	Achieve higher-level functions (hypothesizing; predicting; solving problems; planning; stating rules, beliefs, and thoughts)
Produce related ideas in sentences	Produce simple and compound sentences; modify verbs and nouns	Relate ideas within a sentence using complex syntax; produce relative and subordinate clauses; Judge correctness of sentences
Combine word parts (morphemes)	Add basic plural, possessive, and tense endings to words (*-ing, -ed, -s*)	Create new words with additional prefixes and suffices (*un-, in-, anti-, dis-, ism-, er-*)
Identify and retrieve words	Know and use familiar, common, concrete words	Understand abstract words; use metaphorical expressions; talk about words in metalinguistic ways (give definitions; judge appropriateness)
Produce speech sounds	Produce intelligible words	Produce intelligible words; produce multi-syllabic words

Source: Based on C. Scott (1994), Silliman & Wilkinson (1994), Wallach & Butler (1994), Van Meter & Nelson (1998), Westby (1994), Williams et al., 2002.

Move Across Modalities and Adapt to Changes   In addition to simultaneously processing different components of language, students must flexibly move across the communication modalities of reading, writing, listening, and speaking. In school, students often need to relate information they receive in one modality to what they produce in another (N. W. Nelson, 2007). For example, after reading stories, students are often required to write a response paper or dramatize a character's actions. After listening to or reading an informational text, students may need to generate questions about the passage or to discuss or write about how they feel about the topic. Even if the students aren't required to make a verbal response, they still need to generate internal thoughts and questions about what they read or hear.

In addition to connecting the modes of verbal communication, students must adapt to changes that arise in discourse events. Within a conversation, for example, shifts may occur in communicative purpose, discourse topics, and participant roles (Bernstein & Tiegerman-Farber, 2009; R. Chapman, 1992). One discourse event often evolves into another or reveals embedded subgoals. A teacher-directed class discussion can be followed by a peer-led work session. Or during a factual presentation on electricity, students may encounter a personal story about someone having actually seen lightning strike a tree. Students need to process the changes in discourse events and make adjustments in their own language to meet those changes (Damico, 1991a).

In addition to the requirements of comprehending and producing connected discourse units, dynamic changes in language require fluent and efficient integration of different communication modalities, components, and levels of the language system. The many complicated language processes that occur in school make the language tasks students encounter very demanding. School language is particularly demanding for students with language impairments.

Breakdowns in Language Use

Understanding the complexity of language makes it possible to predict where students with language disabilities are likely to break down when they must use language to communicate, gain knowledge, and acquire academic skills. Communication difficulties occur more often at the higher and larger discourse levels than at the lower word and sentence levels and with abstract topics and/or limited contextual supports.

Students with language impairments who are processing complex school language have much in common with second language learners who lack concrete, simple, supported communication contexts. Many foreign language learners are able to understand and generate enough sentences in their second language to order food in a restaurant, ask the time, or comment on the weather, but are unable to follow conversations, read a newspaper, understand explanations, or establish deep relationships. They may recognize individual words without being able to comprehend sentences. At other times, they may understand individual sentences without being able to connect them to a whole conversation, story, or discussion. When they encounter complex language in school, students with language impairments often process discourse units or passages as isolated, unrelated parts. If the language demands become too complex, the individual will stop attempting to process the input altogether and may resort to pretending to understand, daydreaming, or withdrawing from the situation.

Definition and Identification of Language Impairments

Understanding the difficulty of school language is necessary for comprehending the challenges students with language impairments face and the nature of language impairments. This section will provide information about what language impairments are, how they are identified, and how they relate to academic and social difficulties.

Specific Language Impairments

Children with Specific Language Impairments experience particular difficulty using language to communicate. The terms *Specific Language Impairment* (SLI) and *Language-Learning Disability* (LLD) refer to language difficulties that are not caused by emotional disorder, cognitive delay, sensory impairment, or language difference (Bernstein & Tiegerman-Farber, 2009; National Joint Committee on Learning Disabilities, 1994; Pence & Justice, 2008). Various types of language impairments can involve different modes of communication (listening, speaking, reading, or writing) or different components of the language system (structural, functional, or semantic) (Bashir, Conte, & Heerde, 1998; National Joint Committee on Learning Disabilities, 1994; N. W. Nelson, 1998).

Identification of Children with Language Impairments

An important job of the SLP is to identify students with SLI and determine which students should receive services. For identification, the SLP can draw upon three frameworks: (1) look for a discrepancy between language performance and nonlanguage performance, (2) view how students function in important settings, and (3) determine how children respond to intervention (R. Paul, 2007).

Discrepancy in Performance Traditionally, language impairments have been identified in terms of a gap between students' levels of nonlanguage and language function. Nonlanguage cognitive levels are assessed by performance-based intelligence tests that include such tasks as finding similarities in visual displays and replicating block designs. Language levels are demonstrated by tests that assess word and grammar knowledge, word retrieval, and sentence production. With this form of diagnosis, students receive language services only if they demonstrate a measurable gap between language and nonlanguage scores (Fey, 1986; Krassowski & Plante, 1997). A weakness of this discrepancy model is that the lower levels of language use (e.g., word knowledge and sentence production) are easier to measure accurately than are conversational or text comprehension abilities.

Ability to Function in the Environment Heavy reliance on test scores to determine who receives services excludes useful information and is prone to error (Ehren, 2000; N. W. Nelson, 2000). In contrast, an environmental perspective bases identification on students' performance relative to expectations in academic and social contexts (Fey, 1986). Tools used in this identification model include interviews with teachers and parents, observations of the students' performance, analyses of schoolwork, and discussions with the students about how they experience school tasks. The environmental model reveals how students communicate in real contexts, including the functioning of some language components that cannot be measured with standardized tests (Merritt & Culatta, 1998; N. W. Nelson, 1998).

Connor, the 7½-year-old first grader with SLI referred to earlier in this chapter, performed more poorly using language in context than he did on language tests. While Connor had borderline low scores on tests of his knowledge of vocabulary and sentence structure, he experienced greater difficulty comprehending texts, expressing himself in class discussions, and relating past events. The discrepancy between his test scores and his performance in the classroom illustrates the value of observing how students function in a language environment rather than relying on tested knowledge. Observing how Connor functioned in classroom contexts more accurately revealed the extent of his language problems.

Response to Intervention   The third model for identifying children with language disorders, referred to as *response to intervention (RTI)*, involves providing interventions to struggling learners with the goal of matching level and type of intervention to student need. RTI involves monitoring a student's progress at various stages of intervention and using the data in making decisions regarding the level and type of further intervention required to help the student succeed (Justice, 2006; RTI Action Network, 2009).

Problems Encountered in School

Students with language impairments may communicate well when talking about familiar events shared with classmates, such as making cookies or going to the store. In contrast, they struggle with the complex language demands outlined in Tables 12.1 and 12.2 and have difficulty acquiring information, learning to read and write, and maintaining social relationships (Bashir et al., 1998; Catts & Kamhi, 2005).

Difficulty Acquiring Information   Since language is the medium by which knowledge is acquired, it is not surprising that children with SLI have difficulty keeping up with the curriculum (Bashir et al., 1998). Children with language impairments often perform poorly in content areas, such as history and social studies, because much of the information is conveyed in written texts, class discussions, and oral presentations (Donahue & Pidek, 1993; Tiegerman-Farber & Radziewicz, 2008). In addition, expressive problems may limit students' ability to convey the content information they know. Teachers can underestimate the knowledge of students who have difficulty relating information in an organized manner or retrieving information needed to answer questions or explain relationships among ideas. If children's comprehension abilities are significantly below the level of complexity of their texts or class presentations, then acquisition of knowledge is compromised. In addition, school will not be motivating or interesting for students who do not easily understand what is presented.

Reading and Writing Problems   Reading and writing depend on strong language skills. Students have difficulty reading if they have trouble knowing the meanings of words, relating ideas in sentences, or connecting ideas across sentences to construct an understanding of a text as a whole (Catts, 1997; C. Scott, 1994).

Literacy problems also result from difficulties with lower-level letter and sound components (recognizing letters, associating sounds with letters, and blending and segmenting sounds into words). Children with poor phoneme awareness skills (i.e., difficulty analyzing words into sounds) and poor decoding or phonics skills tend to be poor readers (Catts, 1997; S. Hall & Moats, 1999; National Institutes of Health, 2000; R. Owens, 2010).

In first grade, Connor experienced reading problems related to poor letter–sound knowledge and deficient phoneme awareness skills even though he had repeated kindergarten. While he could identify a small core of letters and sounds and blend simple sounds into words (/g/ and –*um* into *gum*), he could not identify initial sounds in words, make new words by changing the initial consonant (e.g., *at, bat, mat, sat,* or *cat*), or identify the common sound pattern in *top* and *drop*. Connor needed intensive instruction to learn how to "crack the code" before he could gain meaning from printed text.

Limited Social Relationships   Children with language problems often have social difficulties (Bashir, Wiig, & Abrams, 1987; Brinton & Fujiki, 2004; Conti-Ramsden & Botting, 2004). Children find it difficult to interact with someone who can't express needs and feelings, make relevant responses to others' comments, or talk about a variety of topics. Because of difficulty using language, students with SLI may express themselves in nonverbal (physical) ways, produce inappropriate or irrelevant behaviors, or become passive and withdrawn (Brinton & Fujiki, 1993; Fujiki, Brinton, Morgan, & Hart, 1999). Peers are less likely to include students who don't make relevant contributions to social situations (Fujiki, Brinton, Hart, & Fitzgerald, 1999). In addition to difficulties with comprehension and self-expression, students with language impairments may have difficulty recognizing social cues or fail to perceive intent in others' messages (Fujiki, Spackman, Brinton, & Illig, 2008; Timler, 2008b). Thus, students with SLI can have difficulty fitting in with peers.

Types of Language Impairments

Despite variability in the manifestations of language impairments, an SLP needs to recognize students who are experiencing a particular language difficulty. He must consider language impairments in terms of the modes of communication involved, the aspects of language that present difficulty, and the presence of environmental and cognitive factors that interfere with performance.

Modes or Channels of Communication

In observing students in school contexts, the SLP watches for signs of difficulty comprehending or producing messages (Creaghead & Tattershall, 1991). Specific problems can be in either the receptive or the expressive mode of language or in both.

Receptive Problems   Students with specific receptive or comprehension problems have difficulty attaching meaning to messages they receive. These students are likely to have difficulty carrying out directions, following explanations, and gaining information presented via language. They may have difficulty reasoning in language, identifying information that is needed to solve problems, detecting inconsistent or missing information in passages, and connecting ideas in stories. Receptive problems can also be reflected in how students talk about information they receive: They will have difficulty retelling stories, providing explanations, and participating in conversations and class discussions. If they cannot process language, they will have difficulty paraphrasing information and making relevant contributions. Students who have difficulty understanding may dominate a conversation or change the topic of a conversation because it is easier to talk about familiar events than it is to process what others say about unfamiliar topics.

An SLP will also watch for nonverbal indications of receptive difficulties. To compensate for language difficulties, students may be passive and agreeable in order to avoid using language to assert and defend their positions. They may watch their peers in order to know how to respond instead of relying on the information presented in the teacher's directions or explanations. In addition to observing how they respond to language, the SLP who suspects receptive language problems will observe the students' reliance on visual and contextual cues (Coggins, 1998; R. Paul, 2000a; Silliman & Wilkinson, 1991).

Expressive Problems   Students with expressive problems have difficulty producing well-formed sentences and other connected utterances. They have difficulty selecting or retrieving words and grammatical forms to convey ideas and may revert to using gestures in expressing ideas that are complex, abstract, or relational. In conversations, students with specific expressive impairments may not give sufficient background information or specify how their ideas relate to the topic. If they have difficulty formulating responses to a partner's comments, they may passively agree with or simply acknowledge what the partner says instead of extending or elaborating the topic as an active conversational participant (Fey, 1986; German & Newman, 2004).

Since students with specific expressive problems understand language better than they produce it, their written or oral responses are likely to be relevant and appropriate even though they might be simple and without detail or organization. These students will be less likely than students without SLI to produce complex sentences or to tie sentences together (Donahue, 1994; C. Scott, 2004) due to difficulty in signaling subtle relationships, coordinating phrases, or adding emphasis. For example, they may use only common contracted forms of negative expressions, such as *didn't* or *don't*, instead of occasionally using the uncontracted *did not* or *do not* to emphasize a point. They may have difficulty using embedded clauses to efficiently connect ideas (e.g., the man *who almost won the race* was very disappointed). And they may have difficulty specifying conditional and causal relationships with conjunctions such as *instead of, but, if, so,* and *because.*

Students with expressive problems will experience particular difficulty talking about events that occurred in the past or are removed from personal experience. Connor, who exhibited great difficulty with expressive language, had difficulty telling his mother about a game he had played with the SLP in which he received points for finding objects in a "feely" box. He told his mother that he had played a game, but he did not tell her what the game was. Without context or shared knowledge, Connor's mom resorted to guessing and asking questions, but she was not able to determine what had happened.

Mom: Tell me about the game you played.

Connor: Get little block. Then her [the SLP] try to hide it from me. (Long pause)

Mom: Did anything else happen? (Long pause)

Connor: (No response)

Mom: How did you figure out who won?

Connor: By scores ... by piece uh paper.

Mom: Who won?

Connor: Her. Her got one. I got none.

Mom: How did you keep score?

Connor: Pencil.

Mom: With a pencil?

Connor: Uh huh.

Mom: You were the one who did the counting?

Connor: (No response)

Mom: How high did you count?

Connor: Three.

Mixed Receptive and Expressive Problems   Students with mixed language impairments have difficulty with both receptive and expressive language. Although Connor's expressive language skills were very poor, he also exhibited difficulty comprehending connected utterances, such as stories and class discussions.

The SLP watches for behavioral indications of difficulty understanding language and also determines if expressive performance is noticeably poorer than receptive, giving careful attention to how students respond to what they hear and how they retrieve or use the aspects of language they know when they are talking about events. Reliable observations of receptive and expressive language performance provide a helpful starting point for identifying language impairments.

Aspects of Language Performance

Language problems can be described in terms of students' knowledge and skills in the different components of language. The SLP is interested in knowing how students perform on isolated vocabulary or sentence construction tasks as well as how students integrate components at higher levels—for example, comprehending or generating stories or informational texts. Students with SLI are likely to have more difficulty with higher-order complex language than with a simpler isolated component, such as vocabulary. The SLP must know how students function at the word, sentence, and text levels.

Vocabulary Knowledge   Students with language impairments tend to have more-limited vocabulary knowledge and to experience more difficulty acquiring words than do their peers (Wiig & Secord, 1992). While school-age students with SLI are likely to know the meanings of simple concrete words (such as *heavy, hard, wipe, cut, shake, missing,* and *tip*), they are less likely to know words for temporal, spatial, and quantity relationships (*each, more than, before*), internal states (*wonder, expect, ponder, speculate*), or generic categories (*reptiles, utensils, bodies of water*). They also are less likely to know many synonyms (*deposit* and *make payment*) or to understand subtle differences between words with similar meanings (*discouraged* and *disappointed* or *frustrated* and *irritated*) (Wiig & Secord, 1992).

In addition to difficulty in developing vocabulary and learning abstract words, students with SLI often gain only partial understanding of words. A student with partial or shallow knowledge of the word *dangerous* may think the word refers only to specific harmful events such as starting a fire or crossing a busy street, not understanding how things can be psychologically or emotionally harmful, how almost anything can be dangerous if misused, or how something like hanging out with the wrong crowd could lead to harmful incidents. In contrast, peers who have deep and well-formed knowledge of words can apply them and talk about them in many different situations (Carroll, 2008).

Connor displayed a limited knowledge of words for abstract ideas and spatial, temporal, and quantity relationships. Although he knew hundreds of common nouns and verbs, he had difficulty understanding words for internal states (*greedy, discouraged*) and relational terms (*equal, beyond, middle*). He often failed to comprehend some of the important words he encountered in lessons, class activities, and stories.

Retrieval of Words   While most people experience occasional difficulty recalling word names, students with SLI frequently have extreme difficulty remembering names for objects, actions, or attributes. While students with retrieval problems understand the meanings of many words, they can have great difficulty selecting words to use when they want to convey an idea or describe a situation (Denckla & Rudel, 1976; German & Simon, 1991).

Students with word retrieval problems may incorporate gestures to aid their communication or use excessive pauses or fillers (e.g., *um* or *ok*). They may abandon ideas, be slow in naming things, or use indefinite words such as *some, stuff, or thing* instead of specific words. The ideas these students express may be more sophisticated than the language they use to convey them. They find it difficult to use a variety of different words to express ideas (C. Scott & Windsor, 2000).

Connor exhibited difficulty retrieving words. He understood more words than he produced, displayed long pauses and false starts, and had difficulty describing or referring to events explicitly. In the sample below, Connor was telling his mother how to arrange a set of objects to match an arrangement hidden by a screen. Although Connor understood words and expressions for such relationships as *upside down, inside, on its side, line up,* and *in a row,* he did not use these terms to describe the arrangements to his mom to help her replicate it.

Arrangement of Objects	*Connor's Instructions*
	Put one block on top. Put the other one . . . down in. Put zero in the other one. One cup—in the first. Put a block in the second. Put down. And put block in. Third one, put nothing. Zero.

Sentence Comprehension and Processing   Sentence comprehension requires one to attach meanings to words and grammatical forms and then integrate those meanings. Students with language problems may have difficulty processing the relational meanings signaled in grammatical structure or noticing the subtle alterations of meaning signaled in grammatical forms such as pronouns, conjunctions, prepositions, and tense endings (Conte, 1993; Fey, Long, & Finestack, 2003). A student with SLI might hear the sentence "The boy who knocked into the teacher dropped the plate" and think that the teacher dropped the plate.

To comprehend sentences in school, students must pay close attention to grammatical structures. Although Connor was able to comprehend most simple sentences, at times he failed to understand complex sentences. Sometimes he misinterpreted meaning because he did not attend to small grammatical elements. For example, when asked to "find something a boy wouldn't want to eat," Connor picked a cookie until the sentence was rephrased, using and emphasizing the uncontracted *would **not*** for *wouldn't*.

Use of Grammatical Rules   Students with language impairments have problems in acquiring and using complex grammatical rules—for example, marking tenses, coordinating ideas between sentences, and producing embedded and conditional phrases such as "The girl who brought the box doesn't go to this school" or "If the part is loose, you can get more glue" (Bedore & Leonard, 1998; Cleave & Rice, 1997). They produce a limited variety of sentence types, relying on a small set of familiar structures. Syntactical difficulties may cause them to express ideas in awkward or immature ways, perhaps using only skeletal sentences without modifying words or phrases. They may fail to signal subtle differences in meaning or be unable to express related ideas in an organized, efficient manner—requiring the listener to guess intended or implied relational meanings.

Connor exhibited difficulty producing grammatical forms and structures: coordinating ideas with conjunctions such as *then*, *but*, and *because*; producing negative sentences; differentiating subject and object pronouns (e.g., using *her* for *she*); inverting the verb in questions; and using helping verbs like *is*, *are*, and *am*. He signaled future tense with the simple *wanna* and *gunna* instead of using the forms *will* or *going to*. The language sample below is typical; Connor was commenting on toys he found on a table.

> There a dog. Dog hidin. There ain't no more. Money ain't toys. Money can buy things. How many you want? I don't wanna play with babies. Her can't eat this. Pig make a face at me. Him bite a dinosaur up. I don't want no skunk. Take the skunk away. These two the same. Got one more. Her ain't got room. That supposed to be out. That go to that.

Story or Passage Comprehension　Comprehending connected utterances in stories or informational texts is a complicated process. Reading or listening to stories, for example, requires attaching meaning to words and sentences; connecting sentence ideas with conjunctions, pronouns, and synonyms; relating story information to a theme; and holding information in memory while these connections are being made (Field, 2004; Marton & Schwartz, 2003; Meltzer, 2007). Understanding a story also requires identifying information that pertains to the story's plot structure, such as the problem that initiates the story, the character's plan and attempt to solve the problem, and the resolution or consequence of that attempt (Merritt & Liles, 1987; N. L. Stein & Glenn, 1979; J. P. Williams et al., 2002). Readers must distinguish important ideas and plot components from irrelevant information. In addition, readers or listeners must relate information to previously acquired experiences and knowledge (Britton, 1990). This prior knowledge allows them to fill in information that isn't stated, to infer unstated ideas and feelings, and to remember important information presented early in a story as it becomes relevant to events that occur later on (Merritt, Culatta, & Trostle, 1998).

Understanding a story is like constructing a building. Builders start with an idea of the type of structure (the story's theme), create a blueprint (the organization or plot structure), and then construct supportive beams (elements in the plot)—made functional by braces and joints (cohesive connections like conjunctions and pronouns that tie story ideas together). With the structure in place, bricks, wallboard, and flooring (story information) can be added to complete the form and give substance; finally, decorative fixtures such as wallpaper and moldings (details or descriptions) are crafted for imagery and interest. Story comprehension involves considering the theme and plot structure and then fitting ideas and eventually "the fun stuff" into that organization.

Given the complexity of text-level language, it is not surprising that Connor had problems comprehending stories. He had difficulty making predictions and inferring unstated information, such as guessing how characters felt from descriptions of their actions or experiences. Although he could answer simple questions about concrete facts, such as the main character's name, he could not easily find causal relationships, relate internal thoughts and feelings to story events, or project plans or attempts the character might make to solve the problem.

Narrative Production　Narrative production, such as telling personal or fictional stories, requires students to retrieve words and syntactical forms and to signal important story elements (McCabe, 1995). Like story comprehension, narrative production requires establishing the plot elements, indicating important temporal and causal relationships, and connecting ideas between sentences with conjunctions and pronouns (Liles, 1987; Merritt & Liles, 1987).

Connor had difficulty producing stories. As the following story retellings show, he did not include temporal, causal, or disjunctive relationships (*because*, *so*, *then*, and *but*). He remembered a few salient ideas from the beginnings and endings of the stories, but eliminated information from the middle. In the second passage, he altered an important idea.

Story Tasks	*Connor's Retelling*
A brown puppy was sitting in his yard. He saw a cat. He ran after the cat because he wanted to play. But the cat did not want to play. The puppy wanted to go home, but he was lost. He found a little girl, and the girl took him home.	A brown puppy … was sitting … running down the … no …. Him found a girl. Him went to the girl. The girl took him home.
A Momma cat had five little kittens. She took them to the park because they wanted to play. At the park, a dog came to play with the kittens. But the Momma cat did not want the dog to stay. So she hissed at the dog and the dog ran away.	The cat had … three or four kittens. And the dog came by and kittens run away.

Connor also had problems in relating personal narratives. Although he usually understood what he wanted to convey, he often lacked the language to relate his experiences. For example, in trying to tell his mother that he had held slides up to a window so he could see the pictures and trace them, he said, "We had little cards and had draw stuff. I had a draw two window and a man and … man hammering. I copy these things."

Social Conversations   Conversational turn-taking is a high-level language skill that presents problems to children with SLI (Brinton & Fujiki, 1989, 2005; Brinton, Robinson, & Fujiki, 2004). They may have difficulty understanding others' contributions, managing the turn-taking exchange, identifying or noticing shifts in the topic, making relevant additions to the topic, or retrieving the language needed to express ideas and achieve conversational functions. They may also be awkward in social situations. To interact appropriately, students must recognize how what they say and do fits the social context, including the roles, goals, and perspectives of their peers. They must monitor social interactions, including others' reactions to their contributions, in order to know what to talk about, how much to say, and what not to say (Cheng, 2007; Grice, 1975; Timler, 2008a). Students with SLI may lack a sense of the informal rules of social interactions and conversation, and they may have difficulty taking on the perspective of others (Hughes & Leekam, 2004; Watson, Nixon, Wilson, & Capage, 1999).

Connor rarely engaged in conversations or social interactions with his classmates. When he did converse, he did so passively, filling his turn by answering questions or agreeing with his partner, but not expanding the topic. His answers to questions were generally appropriate, but he rarely added new information or initiated new topics. He participated only in a few back-and-forth exchanges. The following exchange illustrates Connor's passive style, mostly responding to specific questions.

Adult: Are you going to go trick-or-treating?
Connor: Uh huh.
Adult: Where do you go trick-or-treating?
Connor: You don't know what houses.

Adult: What about the house that's right next door to your house?

Connor: We don't have no next store neighbors.

Adult: You don't? How are you going to go trick-or-treating if you don't have any neighbors?

Connor: Drive to people houses.

Adult: Just anywhere?

Connor: People we already know.

Adult: Do you have trick-or-treaters coming to your house?

Connor: Uh huh.

Adult: What are you going to give them?

Connor: Candy.

Metalinguistic Skills   Many school tasks require students to have conscious awareness of language (Nippold, 2007; van Kleeck, 1994a; van Kleeck & VanderWoude, 2003). *Metalinguistic skills* relate to the ability to reflect on and talk about how language works; for example, phoneme awareness enables students to learn to identify sounds and syllables in words. Other complex metalinguistic tasks children encounter in school include giving definitions; stating multiple meanings for words such as *band*, *draw*, and *bat*; understanding synonyms; correcting grammatical errors; revising paragraphs; identifying missing information; reflecting on conversations; identifying topic sentences and main ideas in passages; illustrating how passages are organized; and differentiating important from irrelevant information in texts.

Phoneme awareness tasks, like analyzing words into their parts, were challenging for Connor. He had difficulty counting syllables and sounds in words, identifying initial and final sounds, and determining what sounds would be left if the initial consonant was taken away (getting *end* by taking the /b/ off the word *bend*). He made errors on worksheets that required him to mark all the words that started with the same sound and could not make new words by adding or changing sounds (make *bat* by adding a /b/ to *at*).

Metaphorical Language Abilities   Metaphorical language use involves understanding figurative expressions (similes, metaphors) and jokes. The expression "nothing succeeds like success" is amusing to students who can perceive the word similarity. Students frequently need to interpret metaphors used in curricular contexts (a hot topic) and in humor or sarcasm expressed in social contexts ("oink, oink" for a greedy classmate) (Reid, 2000). Students with language impairments have trouble processing messages at a nonliteral level (Milosky, 1994; Nippold, 2007) and interpreting sentences in stories that have symbolic meanings, as in an allegory or a fable.

Students who do not have the ability to use language at a simple literal level should not be expected to use it metaphorically. Even some students with basic language knowledge have great difficulty with figurative language.

Cognitive Knowledge and Skills

In addition to language skills and abilities, cognitive factors influence a student's communicative performance.

Conceptual Knowledge   Because language is used to represent events and conditions in the world, a student must understand the environment in order to select appropriate words and sentences. A teacher or SLP should know what students understand about the events in their world and about information presented in curricular texts and discussions (Hyter, 2008). They need to consider how well students' knowledge is organized by and connected to words (N. W. Nelson, 1998).

Many students with SLI understand the world around them in ways they are unable to represent in words, sentences, or larger connected units such as conversations or written paragraphs. This nonverbal knowledge is indicated by their ability to participate in events, act appropriately on objects, and express ideas in gestures or very simple language. Sometimes students with SLI use words they have heard without accurately understanding what those words mean—for example, saying "this is between" when pointing to a block at the top of a stacked pile.

Connor's knowledge of conditions and events went beyond his ability to describe or talk about them. The language samples already given illustrate how much Connor's understanding exceeded his ability to express what he knew. Exerting effort and considering context, listeners can identify some ideas that are well formed, but poorly expressed. However, since information about abstract and remote events is acquired through language, Connor's poor language skills interfered with his ability to learn about things he hadn't directly experienced.

Cognitive Processes and Strategies   The cognitive processes of attention, memory, and perception greatly influence language performance (Gillam, 1998). Most students go through these processes subconsciously in listening to or reading stories, participating in class discussions, and completing school assignments. They are unaware of attending to incoming signals, recognizing and attaching meanings to words and syntactic patterns, and holding meanings in memory as they process incoming sentences.

There are also more-conscious and -deliberate metacognitive skills that influence performance. In school, students must actively control or allocate their cognitive resources in order to perform certain tasks and monitor their own performance (B. Singer & Bashir, 1999). They must purposefully focus attention, rehearse or hold information in memory, reflect on what they know about a topic, and determine what steps they need to take in order to complete an assignment. The abilities to keep track of, organize, and purposefully remember information, referred to as *executive control functions*, affect how students perform. Students with deficits in metacognition or executive control have difficulty "putting things together" (Im-Bolter, Johnson, & Pascual-Leone, 2006). Inaccurate comprehension, fatigue, and distractibility are likely when students have difficulty controlling and organizing the flow of information and tasks with multiple components (Lahey & Bloom, 1994; Stevens, Sanders, & Neville, 2006).

Attention and memory problems interfered with Connor's language learning and processing. If not alerted, he would miss important or incongruent information. It was hard for him to hold information in memory in order to repeat it back or operate on it at a later time.

Environmental and Cultural Influences

Environmental and cultural factors also influence students' functioning. Students bring experiences, beliefs, skills, and feelings to school, which can be either in tune or out of sync with what they encounter there.

Cultural and Linguistic Background   Students' individual experiences, cultural expectations, and attitudes can be as significant as their communication knowledge and skills. Those from nonmainstream cultural and linguistic backgrounds may not have facility in the same dialect, language, or content base as classmates from the mainstream culture (Damico & Hamayan, 1992; Genesee, Paradis, & Crago, 2003; Hyter, 2008). In addition, students from low-income families may have had little access to educationally stimulating outings, books, or discussions due to limited resources and high family stress. Students whose cultural, linguistic, or low socioeconomic background may have prevented them from experiencing events discussed in typical mainstream classrooms are at risk for academic problems (National Center for Education Statistics, 2008).

Connor, who lived on a farm, went to school with children living in a small city nearby. Connor's peers were more knowledgeable and animated when talking about computer games, shopping, and skateboarding, while Connor was more knowledgeable and engaged when talking about the county fair, farm chores and farm equipment, and animal care. An observant teacher or SLP could relate a concept such as *cooperation* to both playing computer games and working together to feed animals.

Teachers must avoid misinterpreting culture-based language differences as specific learning disabilities or language impairments. However, they must be aware that students from different backgrounds who also have specific disabilities are particularly vulnerable to academic difficulties if their prior knowledge and interactional expectations are not considered. When language disorders are mixed with nonmainstream backgrounds or low socioeconomic status, the risk for educational difficulties increases (Learning to Read and Write, 1998; N. W. Nelson, 1998).

Attitudes and Self-Esteem   Along with differences in experiences, students have different attitudes about learning. Students with language impairments become discouraged when they are not successful in school. Previous difficulties reading, writing, listening, or speaking reduce their interest in learning or communicating—they feel inadequate and dislike school. Students with good reading skills read often and improve; students with poor skills lag further and further behind (Stanovich, 1986).

Many children with language problems don't think of themselves as capable learners and don't enjoy reading, writing, or giving class presentations. This poor self-esteem can be turned around if teachers and SLPs provide students with successful learning experiences by making sure tasks are not too difficult, relating instruction to children's interests, and providing sufficient supports and encouragement.

Context   Along with abilities and attitudes, performance is influenced by contextual demands and supports (Kovarsky & Maxwell, 1997). Performance improves when students are presented with interesting activities and materials; content they can relate to; and engaging, responsive, interactive facilitators.

Connor's experiences in various contexts show how successful communication depends on environmental modifications and supports. Connor could function relatively well when he received contextual support and when his communicative partners were responsive to his needs by slowing their speech, saying things in different ways, using gestures, illustrating the content with objects and demonstrations, and reducing the complexity of their language. In contrast, when a teacher would relate remote events and abstract ideas without providing objects or actions to illustrate the content, Connor had great difficulty comprehending language. For children with SLI to function well in school, sufficient supports must be provided to meet task-by-task demands.

Individual Performance Profiles

Students with SLI vary in language performance. Once SLPs and teachers understand a student's individual performance profile (modes of strength, levels of functioning, aspects of language that present difficulty, knowledge, experiences, and attitudes), they can adjust demands and supports to fit that profile.

Assessment and Planning

Assessment guides intervention. After an SLP has assessed a student's language knowledge and use, intervention strategies can be individualized. This section will present assessment frameworks and procedures that support intervention and improve students' functioning.

Curriculum-Based and Dynamic Assessment Models

Curriculum-based and dynamic assessment models work well in schools, designating what students can do within the curriculum and identifying factors that influence performance. Both models help SLPs make important intervention decisions.

In curriculum-based assessment, SLPs determine students' abilities to handle the content and processing demands encountered in curricular tasks. Students' responses to the language of texts, class presentations, and assignments provide important information about performance capability (Cirrin, 1994; E. Jones, Southern, & Brigham, 1998; N. W. Nelson, 1998).

Dynamic assessment, based on the work of Vygotsky, assesses students in the process of learning (Merritt & Culatta, 1998). The SLP determines how a student functions without support and then compares that baseline performance, known as the student's Zone of Actual Development (ZAD), with how the student functions with instructional supports (e.g., suggestions, models, prompts, guiding questions). The student's improved level of performance with supports, known as her Zone of Proximal Development (ZPD), reveals what she is capable of doing and under what circumstances. Specifics about the amounts and kinds of supports that facilitate performance guide intervention programs.

Used together, curriculum-based and dynamic assessment models determine intervention goals. Skills students can perform with support may be considered as possible goals. In contrast, content or skills students cannot understand in a supportive context, being beyond the student's ZPD, would be unrealistic expectations. By using both forms of assessment, SLPs identify instructional procedures that will enhance students' school performance.

Strategies and Procedures

Various assessment procedures within the curriculum-based and dynamic assessment models provide important information. In addition to formal assessment tools, SLPs interview teachers and parents, observe students in relevant contexts, analyze products, and talk with students about school experiences.

Tests and Formal Tools   Tests can determine what students know about some aspects of the language system, as they isolate vocabulary knowledge, sentence structure capability, phoneme awareness, and metalinguistic skills. However, tests isolate components of language and don't reflect how students perform in real contexts. Higher-level components of language and simultaneous processing of components cannot be easily tested. Additionally, a test developed for middle-class English speakers will not be valid for students from other cultural or linguistic backgrounds.

Onlooker Observations   Observations of student performance during classroom tasks can provide valuable information (Silliman & Wilkinson, 1991). When communication breakdowns occur, SLPs analyze the demands that are operating at the time and then follow up by exploring what students understand about those specific task components (Donahue, 1994).

Although some students can hide difficulties by passively agreeing to what others say or imitating what classmates do, a trained observer is sensitive to subtle indicators and will use students' reliance on contextual support and their ability to follow the behavior of others in detecting problems.

Probes and Informal Tasks   During assessment, SLPs analyze the language of teacher presentations, texts, and tasks in order to determine what students understand of those demands (Merritt & Culatta, 1998). After analyzing tasks, SLPs create probes: tasks or activities that isolate knowledge or use of a rule or skill. If a teacher tells the "Ice Cream" story from the book *Frog and Toad All Year* (Lobel, 1976), the SLP would want to know what important ideas and relationships the student understands. In this story, Toad tries to surprise Frog on a hot day by bringing him ice cream, but the ice cream melts, and Toad gets lost on his way back to Frog. The SLP could create probing questions: "Why does Toad start to walk fast when the ice cream begins to drip?" or "Why doesn't Toad eat the ice cream when it starts to melt?" These questions assess the student's understanding of Toad's goal to bring the ice cream to his friend and of the cause/effect relationship between the melting ice cream and the need to return to Frog quickly. Probes can be created to assess understanding of the parts of any curricular task.

Analysis of Students' Products and Language Samples   The SLP also looks at students' school products and samples of their language performance (Ukrainetz, 2006a). Samples of retelling or paraphrasing texts can reveal grammatical constructions, content understanding, and expressive ability. Written stories and homework assignments reveal students' knowledge about language and their ability to organize language components into larger units. Students' invented spellings reflect their phoneme awareness skills because students will spell what they hear. Useful information can be obtained by analyzing anything the student says, does, or creates (Damico, 1991b, 1992).

Interviews and Participant Observation   SLPs will want to interview parents and teachers about students' performance. They will also want to conduct interviews with the students themselves.

In participant observations, SLPs interact with students while they are performing curricular tasks (Lidz, 2005; Lidz & Pena, 1996), probing for understanding of specific parts of a task. They might ask students to interpret or explain the meaning of words, statements, explanations, or information encountered in directions or texts. By asking how story ideas are related, they can determine if students have connected or fragmented understanding.

Another aspect of participant observation is to notice how functioning is influenced by supports such as modeling correct responses, giving suggestions, and providing prompts and cues. When SLPs can determine how various levels and types of support help students reach higher and deeper levels of understanding, future supports can be more judiciously chosen.

Participant observation, like the other curriculum-based and dynamic assessment procedures, enables SLPs to analyze the fit between students' abilities and the curricular requirements and to identify ways to improve that fit.

Language and Literacy Intervention

Language and literacy intervention, including participation of the SLP, should result in improved student functioning and enhanced instructional services. This section will discuss the goals of intervention, the roles of SLPs in various service delivery models, and various approaches and procedures for intervention.

Goals of Intervention

Intervention should enhance students' participation and learning in important contexts, improve communicative functioning, facilitate the development of academic skills, and help students to maintain close social relationships and eventually to attain gainful occupation (N. W. Nelson, 1998). To achieve these goals, intervention is designed to teach knowledge and skills and to make adjustments in important contexts.

Role of SLPs in Language and Literacy Instruction

The SLP can make significant contributions to education by applying what he knows about how language influences curricular knowledge and literacy skills. The SLP's intervention strategies apply to the development of reading and writing skills as well as listening and speaking skills (Spracher, 2000; Wallach & Ehren, 1997; Westby, 1998). Because literacy depends on integrating the modalities and components of language, the SLP's understanding of high-level processing of connected discourse (texts, discussions, class presentations, and conversational exchanges) is extremely valuable. Students need to understand the purpose of reading and to activate personal meanings from the printed materials they encounter. The SLP's ability to focus on small "code" components of language, such as patterns in words and sounds, while maintaining meaning and purpose, is an invaluable contribution (Catts, Fey, Tomblin, & Zhang, 2002; Neuman, Copple, & Bredekamp, 2000). It is important to ensure that both code skills (phoneme awareness and decoding) and meaning skills (vocabulary and comprehension) are supported when students participate in guided reading encounters with more-competent readers. Instructors need to know how to manipulate language in order to facilitate reading performance (Catts, 1997).

Service Delivery Models

To improve students' language and literacy functioning in school, SLPs must be thoroughly involved in the curriculum and classroom instruction. This section, along with Table 12.3, explores SLPs' options for providing services in school settings.

TABLE 12.3   Comparison of Pull-out and Curriculum-Based Service Delivery Models

	Separate Pull-Out Services	*Collaborative and Classroom-Based Services*
Intervention Contexts	Isolates students from authentic contexts Presents intervention in a separate room	Includes students in authentic social situations Presents intervention in functional contexts (classroom, playground, lunchroom)
Role of the SLP	Serves as primary service provider Presents the intervention	Plans an intervention program (decides where, when, and who will facilitate language)
Relationship of the SLP to Parents and Teachers	Serves as the expert Engages teachers and parents as helpers	Collaborates with and values the expertise of parents and teachers Draws upon parents and teachers as change agents
Goals and Objectives	Selects goals on the basis of test measures and language analyses Determines content and tasks arbitrarily, without regard to curriculum	Bases goals on curricular content and tasks Individualizes expectations Determines need for adaptations or supports
Language Focus	Addresses components of language removed from real discourse events	Focuses on language components as they relate to functioning in whole discourse events Integrates language parts
Assessment Mechanisms	Relies on standardized measures Identifies students' weaknesses, what they can't do Compares students' performance to test norms	Assesses performance within curricular tasks Identifies abilities and influence of supports Determines functioning relative to curricular demands
Evaluation Methods	Re-administers tests periodically Charts attainments of specific targets	Monitors outcomes continually Assesses functioning in context Analyzes products
Student Roles	Places students in structured one-on-one interactions Leads to limited, passive roles	Draws upon an array of communicative events Permits active social roles and varied types of participation
Communicative Options, Demands	Limits or structures response options and participation in types of communication events	Requires flexible use of communication skills Leads to participation in a variety of "whole" communicative events

Pull-Out Services   Traditionally, SLPs provided one-on-one or small-group intervention outside of the classroom. Removing students, however, eliminated functional reasons for using language (DiMeo, Merritt, & Culatta, 1998), making intervention goals seem less relevant. The pull-out model also reduces opportunities to support students' interactions with peers, so that relevant social situations do not provide contexts for intervention.

While instruction should be tied to the classroom as much as possible, at times assistance with curricular content can be provided in a separate setting—for example, when preteaching a skill in order to prepare a student to use it in the classroom. Some students with SLI may need direct instruction in a particular language rule before encountering it in a complex context. Some may need opportunities to notice and practice using social rules, such as when and how to change topics, in supportive "scripted" role play before applying those rules in real settings. Even if some instruction is provided in a separate session, the main goal should be to improve classroom performance and help children transfer skills to authentic contexts.

Consultative Services   In consultative, indirect services, SLPs advise and direct teachers in applying intervention strategies. To help students benefit from classroom instruction, suggestions to teachers should pertain to relevant curricular content and expectations (DiMeo et al., 1998). The more removed the SLP input is from the curriculum and the classroom, the less likely it is to fit the teachers' or the students' needs.

Collaborative Classroom-Based Intervention   In collaborative classroom-based service delivery, the SLP participates as a member of the classroom team, uses the curriculum as the content for intervention, and provides intervention in the classroom. The intervention is thus relevant to students' needs.

By integrating the expertise of teachers and SLPs, collaboration results in effective instructional programs (DiMeo et al., 1998; N. W. Nelson, 2007). Teachers and SLPs acquire skills and competencies from each other, language-teaching capabilities increase, and all students benefit. Strategies that support students with SLI are not limited to students with SLI. English language learners, for example, have many similar needs.

The goal of collaboration is to strengthen students' participation in the curriculum. Students with SLI will not always have the same goals as their peers, but curricular expectations can be altered without removing students from the classroom. Adapting the curriculum and context to keep students learning and participating is an important goal of collaborative classroom-based intervention.

Intervention Approaches

From their repertoire of effective intervention approaches, SLPs select the approach that best fits the needs of individual students. As team members, they draw upon teacher-directed, child-centered, hybrid, or combined approaches to language and literacy instruction.

Teacher-Directed Instruction   *Direct instruction* involves structuring experiences and tasks to highlight specific skills (Fey, 1986; Goeke, 2009) by focusing children's attention on particular rules or patterns and by presenting systematic opportunities for students to practice skills. Language goals addressed through direct instruction can include knowledge of relational concepts (*middle, least, equal*), production of speech sounds, and use of grammatical rules and some comprehension strategies. Direct instruction has also been shown to improve phoneme awareness, spelling, and reading skills (Blachman, 1994; National Institutes of Health, 2000). Systematic direct phonics instruction highlights letter–sound associations and exposes students to patterns in words (such as the *op* word ending, the silent *e* in *ake* and *ate*, and *un* and *dis* suffixes) in a proper developmental order.

Programmed or controlled texts, such as basal readers, are direct instruction programs for teaching decoding (associations between patterns in printed and spoken words). In such programs, students have frequent opportunities to recognize and practice print–sound associations they encounter in books and stories (M. J. Adams, 1990; S. Hall & Moats, 1999). This systematic exposure to patterns in stories is provided at varying levels of complexity.

Naturalistic, Child-Centered Approach   Students can learn a lot about language and literacy from exposure to patterns in stimulating environments (Beck, McKeown, & Kucan, 2002). When given reasons for sending and receiving messages (e.g., making shopping lists, advertisements, and invitations; creating stories; or writing notes to family and friends), students are motivated to read and write, and they practice using rules in the process. And when participating in shared reading with engaging and competent partners, students can be guided in their skill development (Dinkins, Norris, & Hoffman, 2006). Because authentic language and literacy activities are inherently meaningful, they provide students with opportunities for developing skills.

Child-centered intervention is effective with students who are able to abstract rules and regularities from authentic language examples. Some students readily notice patterns highlighted as they participate with facilitators in interactions centered around interesting books and other printed material. Students with SLI, however, may not be able to learn all necessary language rules and skills by incidentally participating in naturalistic tasks.

Focused Stimulation, Hybrid Instruction   Focused stimulation (hybrid instruction) draws on both naturalistic and direct instruction principles (Fey, 1986). Students encounter motivating reasons to notice or practice using examples of systematically selected target rules within meaningful contexts. They engage in role play, explore stimulating materials, and discover compelling reasons to communicate within real or contrived interactive contexts. Exchanges with facilitators guide them in practicing rules in functional ways. For example, an SLP could provide practice using *because* by setting up a role play in which a customer must give reasons to a store clerk for not liking certain products.

A project entitled *Systematic and Engaging Early Literacy Instruction* (Culatta & Hall, 2006; K. Hall, Bingham, & Culatta, in press; Project SEEL) illustrates effective use of the hybrid approach to teach emerging literacy skills of rhyming, sound blending, and letter–sound associations. The project systematically exposes children to examples of literacy targets in such meaningful activities as eating a snack, making art projects, enacting stories, participating in dramatic storytelling, and exploring interesting hands-on materials. In teaching rhyming and reading words that end in -*ack*, for example, the children read about a careless man named Jack who scatters snacks on train tracks (toy or paper) that lead to a cardboard box serving as a shack, encountering many other –*ack* words on the way. After watching adults enact the story in rhyme, the children take turns playing Jack and then read and write about their experiences.

Instead of presenting specific linguistic elements in isolation without social context, programs such as Project SEEL highlight patterns *in* context (Kovarsky & Maxwell, 1997). The children who participated in the "Jack Stacks Snacks on the Tracks" enactment eagerly interacted with the facilitators, enjoyed playing with the materials, produced their own –*ack* rhymes, and were eager to read and write about their experience. Exaggerated examples of targets in situations where students take on roles, have social goals, and encounter reasons to communicate make rule learning meaningful. All instruction should be made as functional and naturalistic as possible, even when instructors control aspects of the context and provide systematic opportunities for students to practice (Woods, 2008).

Combined Instruction   A current trend in speech-language pathology is to use both naturalistic and structured approaches in teaching language and literacy skills. SLPs and educators are encouraged to address both code (spelling, phoneme awareness, word recognition) and meaning (vocabulary and story comprehension) components when developing language and reading programs. Figure 12.1 provides an example of components included in combined and balanced instruction.

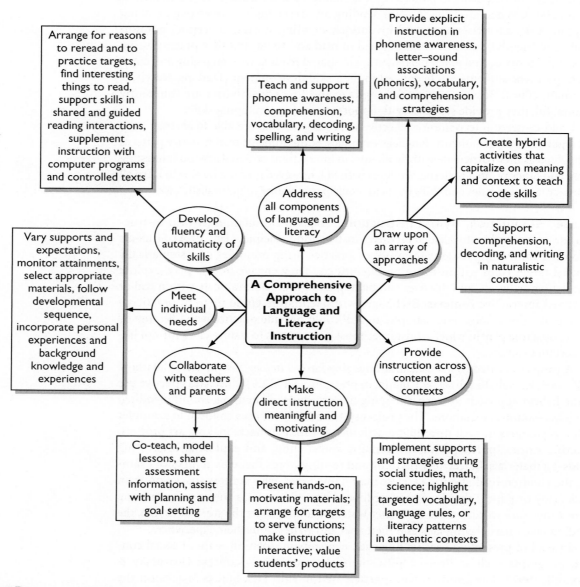

FIGURE 12.1   A comperhensive appraoch to language and literacy instruction.

This combination approach emerged from research demonstrating that the most effective way to teach reading is to use a comprehensive method including explicit phonics instruction, phoneme awareness training, interactive shared reading, and comprehension training strategies (National Reading Panel, 2000). Strong meaning and code skills have been found to be important for reading success (Snow, Burns, & Griffin, 1998; Ukrainetz, 2006b). The ability to comprehend and retell stories, participate in decontextualized conversations, and identify meanings of words are important *meaning skills*, while letter knowledge, phonics and phoneme awareness are important *code skills*. Since students with language impairments can have difficulty with both code and meaning components of reading, combined instruction is important in meeting their needs.

Intervention Strategies or Procedures

Some intervention strategies or procedures can be used with any instructional approach to facilitate language and literacy skills. Basic facilitative procedures include modifying linguistic complexity, providing supports and prompts, providing contextual cues, activating prior knowledge and experience, and modeling use of strategies.

Modify Language Complexity and Expectations   Children with language problems can improve performance if goals are developmentally appropriate and matched to students' individual needs and if accommodations are provided. Once adjustments are made in the complexity of language input, students will develop language and literacy skills more readily.

An SLP must assure an appropriate match between each student's language abilities and the adapted language demands (Gruenewald & Pollack, 1990; Simon, 1998; Wallach & Butler, 1994) if students are to benefit from classroom activities. Children with SLI are likely to be challenged by complex sentences, abstract vocabulary, and connected discourse units. *Recasting* (saying the same thing in multiple ways) provides additional opportunities to process the language and permits the input to be adjusted to different levels of complexity. As students who do not have prerequisite concepts for high-level performance are at a great disadvantage, students with SLI need a curriculum that permits them to build complex skills onto a firm foundation of lower-level skills.

Connor was able to process language in explanations and stories when the complexity of the language he received was adjusted. For example, he could understand first-grade-level stories when the storyteller highlighted important ideas, paired complex words with simpler synonyms, filled in important background information, and repeated and rephrased key information. When information was presented in multiple ways, information was repeated, and connections between ideas were clear and redundant, Connor could understand most of the stories presented to his class.

Provide Supports and Prompts   SLPs and teachers must learn to provide effective supports. For example, the SLP may help students understand and remember stories by assisting with recall of the events and by highlighting important information as students listen to, read, discuss, or enact them. Pictures, verbal clues, repeated encounters, leading questions, and graphic representations of story elements are among the supports that help a student remember and retrieve important elements. Highlighting known information and calling attention to characters' feelings and thoughts can help students infer or predict goals or plans and understand cause/effect relationships. Supports can also help a student understand informational texts. For example, in reading a text about pets students can fill in a chart that identifies how cats and dogs are alike and different and thereby learn that some informational texts are organized with a comparison/contrast structure.

Strategies for processing tasks and language can help students in compensating for cognitive deficits, including SLI (Fisher, Schumaker, & Deshler, 2002; Wiig & Secord, 1990). Some strategies that students deliberately use to make performing school tasks and comprehending texts easier include attending to headings, outlining major organizational parts of a text, identifying information that doesn't make sense, paraphrasing texts, asking questions, and purposefully thinking about how content relates to what is already known.

Provide Contextual Cues   Educational team members can reduce the limitations or impact of students' language difficulties by providing contextual cues (N. W. Nelson, 1998). First-hand experiences, gestures, demonstrations, pictures, and graphic representations (such as maps and timelines) give meaning to language and aid the processing and recognition of language that is not well stored or well established (Merritt & Culatta, 1998).

Students with SLI will acquire and process language better when clear nonverbal information—from objects, actions, gestures, pictures, and demonstrations—can accompany explanations and verbal presentations. First-hand experiences activate interest, motivate and engage students, and readily relate to what students already know about events. Contextual information compensates for difficulties students have in processing content that is abstract, remote, or unfamiliar. One important strategy for helping students process abstract or remote content is to talk about how immediate and familiar experiences relate to events that are removed in time and space (Blank et al., 1994; Cummins, 1984; Merritt & Culatta, 1998).The immediate experience becomes a bridge to understanding remote and abstract information.

Activate Knowledge and Experiences   In order to process or understand texts, students must relate information they hear or read to what they already know. In order to generate language, students must also base what they write or say on their existing knowledge. Information that does not relate to prior experiences will be learned as isolated facts that are quickly forgotten. An important intervention strategy, therefore, is to relate new information to what students know about a topic. Intervention that does not acknowledge, value, and include information from students' own lives will not be meaningful or motivating and will not be processed or understood.

The need to address students' prior knowledge is particularly important when dealing with children who come from diverse cultural and linguistic backgrounds. Students' interests and backgrounds should be acknowledged in the experiences, topics, and materials presented. In addition, any contributions that students make about their interests or experiences should be incorporated as much as possible. For example, students from Mexico in a classroom taught in English eagerly participated in identifying initial sounds in words when targets included *taco*, *tortilla*, *tostado*, and *torta* as well as *tomatoes*, *toast*, and *tarts*. In addition, the students enjoyed reading and talking about similar stories written from different cultural perspectives, such as *The Gingerbread Man* (Kimmel, 1994) and *The Runaway Tortilla* (Kimmel, 2000). Even when students don't share experiential backgrounds, comments about how particular content relates to what they know activates their interest and helps them construct personal meanings. Discussing events relative to the backgrounds of the characters in books can help students understand differences and find commonalities in feelings and experiences (Barton, 1996). Students can understand how different backgrounds can influence people's reactions, attitudes, actions, and decisions.

Model Strategy Use   A conscious understanding of how to handle the language demands of curricular tasks can improve school performance. Students can be taught to actively apply strategies that will enhance the processing, learning, and remembering of information (Wiig & Secord, 1992). Facilitative strategies that can be taught include outlining important ideas, illustrating information graphically, webbing or mapping relationships among ideas, rehearsing important information, talking through tasks, identifying topic sentences, attending to headings, generating questions about a text or task, and referring to a listing of the steps involved in carrying out a task.

In teaching a targeted strategy, team members first model use of the strategy in clear ways. Facilitators guide students' implementation of the strategy in simple tasks with simple content before expecting them to use the strategy without support. Students are given many opportunities to practice using a strategy before being expected to apply that strategy to complex tasks, with new information, or without support. After demonstrating strategy use in multiple contexts, teachers and SLPs gradually decrease supports and increase student responsibility for applying strategies in new situations. The goal is for students to become independent in their use of strategies so they have empowering tools that can guide their learning.

Teaching strategy use is one way SLPs can support students' language and academic functioning. Decisions about when and how to implement strategy training, along with the other facilitative intervention procedures and approaches, result from the desire to create an individualized program that addresses a student's profile of performance. An intervention program should be tailored to meet the individual needs of each student.

Summary

Most classroom and social contexts require students to operate on complex connected discourse units, such as conversations and stories, and to integrate components of language to meet high-level communication demands. In order to help students with language problems function in these contexts, SLPs must understand the complexity of school language as well as the factors that influence language and academic performance.

Students will have difficulty in school when curricular tasks are not in tune with their skills, interests, knowledge, attitudes, and experiences. In contrast, students can perform beautifully when given a supportive teacher, hands-on activities, multiple ways to access information, and expectations that are developmentally appropriate. A primary role of the SLP is to determine how contextual and linguistic input either supports or interferes with what students know, believe, feel, and can do.

SLPs should remember that the ultimate purpose of intervention is to help students develop language skills they need to participate in relevant, important contexts (N. W. Nelson, 1998). This chapter has demonstrated how the value of an intervention program depends on the degree to which it fits students' needs and contributes to their functioning. SLPs draw upon different approaches and intervention strategies to facilitate student performance. While SLPs may teach or support some isolated skills, they also help students deal with the higher-level, more complex language demands that students encounter in authentic school contexts. The needs of children with language difficulties can be addressed successfully by balancing intervention methods, along with adjusting demands, inputs, objectives, and supports.

STUDY QUESTIONS

1. What are the differences between language encountered in school and language encountered in interpersonal, familiar contexts?

2. What makes school language difficult? What types of problems are children with language impairments likely to have in school?

3. When communication breakdowns are likely to occur in school? What kinds of language-related school tasks would be difficult for students with language impairments?

4. How are language impairments defined? How are children with language impairments identified?

5. How are language problems described or characterized? How are different types of language problems differentiated? What are some indicators of an expressive problem? What are some indicators of a receptive language problem?

6. Give some examples of cognitive strategies that could help children with language impairments process the language demands encountered in school.

7. What is meant by curriculum-based assessment? What is meant by dynamic assessment?

8. What are the differences between teacher-directed and naturalistic or child-centered intervention?

9. What is meant by combined or balanced literacy instruction?

SELECTED READINGS

Bishop, D. V. M. (2006). What causes specific language impairment in children? *Current Directions in Psychological Science*, 15, 217–221.

Johnston, J. (2007). *Thinking about child language.* Greensville, SC: Thinking Publications.

Nelson, N. W. (1998). *Childhood language disorders in context: Infancy through adolescence* (2nd ed.). Boston, MA: Allyn & Bacon.

Paul, R. (2007). *Language disorders: From infancy to adolescence* (3rd ed.). St. Louis, MO: Mosby.

WEBSITES OF INTERNET

education.byu.edu/projectseel
Project SEEL (Systematic and Engaging Early Literacy Instruction).

www.cec.sped.org//AM/Template.cfm?Section=Home
The Council for Exceptional Children's website includes a page on communication disorders.

www.asha.org/public/speech/development/default.htm
The American Speech-Language-Hearing Association provides information on typical speech and language development.

Readingrockets.org
This website includes ideas for language arts interventions/activities for school-aged children.

ReadWriteThink.org
This website offers ideas for language arts interventions/activities for school-aged children.

Chapter THIRTEEN

From Emergent Literacy to Literacy

Development and Disorders

Froma P. Roth
University of Maryland

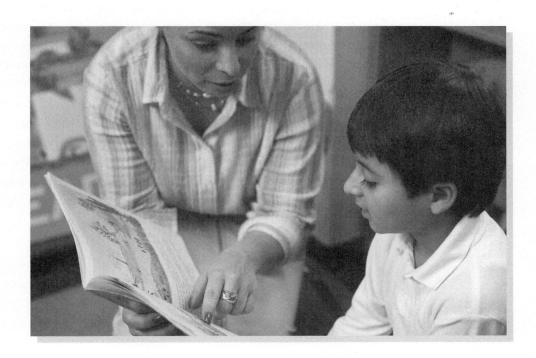

personal PERSPECTIVE

FROMA P. ROTH

I discovered the field of communication sciences and disorders indirectly when my plans to become a medical doctor were hampered by my less than stellar undergraduate performance in the physical sciences and mathematics prerequisite coursework. My academic advisor suggested that I pursue an area of strength rather than one of struggle and guided me to enroll in an introductory course in the hearing and speech sciences. I was immediately captivated by the material, particularly the information pertaining to childhood language disorders. At that time, clinical practicum was part of the undergraduate major in the field, and my first client experience was with Matt, a 4-year-old boy with autism. My clinical supervisor (who I would later learn was a master clinician) had me observe the session through a two-way mirror. She energetically engaged Matt in what appeared to be a casual free-play session with an array of toys. I thought to myself, "Gee, that looks easy enough." She then invited me into the room, suggested that I interact with Matt, and quietly faded into the background. Almost immediately, the session deteriorated into mayhem as Matt began screaming, banging his head, and throwing the toys about the room. My clinical supervisor reappeared and quickly regained control of the session, and Matt returned to being a happy, agreeable child. At that instant, I realized that there was a plan underlying this "free-play session," and my career path was clear.

From that moment on, I have maintained my enthusiasm for the field of speech-language pathology through teaching, conducting research, mentoring students, collaborating with colleagues, and staying involved in the clinical process. A fundamental fascination with human language development, the interdisciplinary nature of the profession, continual advances in scientific knowledge, and the uniqueness of each young person perpetuate a bounty of new challenges and learning opportunities.

M ost children arrive at school prepared to learn to read and write, having acquired the basic building blocks for literacy acquisition during their preschool years in a developmental period known as *emergent literacy*. Emergent literacy can be defined as the period between birth and 5 years, in which children become increasingly aware of the forms and functions of print and develop attitudes about literacy (Roth & Baden, 2001; Roth & Troia, 2009). Children acquire this basic knowledge about print through everyday, natural experiences in their home, day-care, and/or preschool environments. For example, they learn to understand and express themselves verbally in everyday conversations, recognize environmental print such as familiar street signs and restaurant logos, identify some letters of the alphabet, write some letters or words, and demonstrate sound sensitivity by recognizing that certain words rhyme or begin with the same sound. The experiences gained throughout this period prepare them for formal instruction in reading and writing that begins in the early elementary school grades and paves their transition into conventional literacy (the adult form of reading and writing behaviors of the members of a particular society).

The Essential Elements of Literacy

As stated previously, conventional literacy involves reading and writing. Reading consists of two interrelated and sequential processes: *decoding* and *reading comprehension*. To **decode**, a child must be able to analyze words into phonemic (sound) elements and translate the phonemes into their corresponding letters (graphemes). This conversion from phonemes to graphemes is known as the *alphabetic principle*. To read fluently, a firm grasp of the alphabetic principle is essential so that a child can decode accurately and automatically. Without decoding fluency, children have to sound out each word individually, and reading occurs in a halting and stumbling fashion. *Reading comprehension* involves deriving meaning from printed words and text and depends, to a great extent, on fluent decoding skills. Writing also involves two interconnected processes: *spelling* (encoding) and *written composition*. To spell, a child must segment words into syllables and sounds and generate their corresponding graphemic representations (letters and letter sequences). *Written composition* requires the ability to produce longer segments of written language (sentences, paragraphs) and different genres of text (e.g., stories, compare-contrast essays, poems, letters, persuasive essays). To compose, children need the ability to plan, write, revise, and edit written material as well as knowledge of the conventions of the writing system such as punctuation and paragraph organization.

Relationship Between Oral Language and Literacy

Oral language supports literacy, and there is a strong connection among oral language, later literacy, and overall academic achievement. Several avenues of evidence have demonstrated these links. Children with delayed language development in the preschool years show a significantly higher incidence of reading problems than do children without language problems (e.g., M. A. Coleman, Roth & West, 2009; Gallagher, Frith, & Snowling, 2000; Rescorla, 2009; Snowling, Bishop, & Stothard, 2000). This means that children who enter school with weaker verbal abilities are much more likely to experience difficulties learning to read and write than are their typically developing peers (Scarborough, 2001; Scarborough & Dobrich, 1990). In fact, problems in oral language skill in preschool and kindergarten predict reading ability in the early elementary grades (e.g., Roth, Speece, & Cooper, 2002; Torgesen & Davis, 1996). Moreover, early literacy difficulties are persistent. It is estimated that between 65 and 88 percent of children identified as having reading problems in the early grades continue to read poorly throughout the school-age years and into adulthood (Gallagher et al., 2000; Scarborough, 1998). Furthermore, the oral language–literacy relationship is reciprocal, meaning that attainments in one domain continually influence attainments in the other (Scanlon, Vellutino, Small, Fanuele, & Sweeney, 2005). For example, the oral language ability to recognize speech sounds as separate units (e.g., that the word *dog* is composed of three phonemes: /d/, /o/, /g/) is a prerequisite for reading, but reading instruction and practice promotes continued awareness of sounds.

Extrinsic Factors Contributing to Emergent Literacy

A broad range of factors contribute to the development of emergent literacy. Those that are present in the household or community are referred to as extrinsic, or family-based, factors and include socioeconomic status (SES), the linguistic/cultural background in which a child is raised, the home literacy environment, and the family history of language or learning disabilities.

Socioeconomic Status (SES)

Children who are reared in poverty or are from low-income families are at considerable risk for delays in emergent literacy development (Barnett, 2001; Whitehurst, 1996). Many of these children are raised in homes that do not provide sufficient experiences to promote print-related skills, and consequently, they enter school without the knowledge necessary to successfully engage in academic learning. Economic disadvantage is also one of the strongest predictors of reading achievement differences in children beginning first grade on measures of reading achievement as well as several measures of emergent literacy (Juel, 1988). These early performance differences compound over time and create an ever-widening gap between those who have good literacy skills and those who do not. Hart and Risley (1995) describe the link between economic disadvantage and school failure, in part, in terms of the quantity of language addressed to children from different SES backgrounds in the first 2 years of life. These researchers showed that the number of words spoken to children per hour was related to the children's language and cognitive abilities at 3 years of age and their expressive language development at 9 years.

Linguistic/Cultural Background

The multifaceted process of emergent literacy development becomes even more challenging for children whose native language or culture differs from the language of literacy instruction (Linan-Thompson & Ortiz, 2009). In the United States, children for whom English is a second language face potentially significant obstacles. These English language learners (ELLs) perform more poorly on tests of language and literacy achievement and demonstrate overall lower literacy levels than do native-English-speaking children from equivalent SES backgrounds (Abedi, 2002; Hammer, Lawrence, & Miccio, 2007). In fact, recent results from the National Assessment of Educational Progress (NAEP) (U.S. Department of Education, 2007) show that fourth-grade students from culturally and linguistically different backgrounds are much more likely than their peers to lack even the most basic reading skills. According to these statistics, for instance, ELLs whose first language is Spanish or who are African American are twice as likely as their non-Hispanic Caucasian peers to read below age level (C. Snow, Burns, & Griffin, 1998).

Cultural differences and parents' degree of acculturation in the literacy learning society also affect emergent literacy development. Literacy expectations for children entering school vary across cultures. Thus, children's first/native language is embedded in the culture, traditions, values, beliefs, and attitudes of their home.

Home Literacy Environment

Well-developed emergent literacy skills are the result of a stimulating and responsive environment in which children are exposed to print, observe the uses of print, and are encouraged to engage with print-related materials (Oxford & Spieker, 2006). Children with limited access to and infrequent experiences with literacy activities and materials (e.g., shared book reading) display lower levels of early literacy than do children with more frequent exposure and experience (Frijters, Barron, & Brunello, 2000; Neuman & Dickinson, 2001; Oxford & Spieker, 2006; C. Snow et al., 1998; Whitehurst & Lonigan, 1998). However, the number of literacy materials available is not as important as the amount of direct interactions a child has with these materials (Senechal, LeFevre, Hudson, & Lawson, 1996). Thus, the term *print-rich environment* is used to refer to both the artifacts and the experiences that promote the development of emergent literacy skills.

Shared/joint book reading is an aspect of the home literacy environment that contributes to children's oral language development and provides a fertile source for the acquisition of other emergent literacy skills. It most commonly involves a reading experience between a child and parent (or other caring adult) in which the two share the content, language, and images of children's books (Justice, Kaderavek, Fan, Sofka, & Hunt, 2009; Ninio & Bruner, 1978). The child associates the reader with a pleasurable experience, while the adult provides a reading role model and a reservoir of vocabulary. Frequent, regular storybook reading that begins at an early age is a factor that distinguishes children who go on to perform well on reading and writing tasks from those who struggle (e.g., Whitehurst, Epstein, Angell, Payne, Crone, & Fischel, 1994).

Adult modeling of literacy activities is another home literacy environment factor that is positively linked to children's later literacy achievements (Whitehurst & Lonigan, 1998). Children's interests often reflect those of their parents, and the same seems to be true for literacy. Children whose parents view literate activities as a source of entertainment and read and write for pleasure tend to have more positive attitudes toward reading and better reading skills than do children of parents who do not (Britto & Brooks-Gunn, 2001).

Of course, it is difficult to completely separate home literacy factors from other variables such as household income because frequently children with more-limited home literacy environments are those from low-SES families. Further, the relationship among all of the factors that contribute to and make up emergent literacy is complex. One window into the relationship is the finding by D. H. Cooper, Roth, Speece, and Schatschneider (2002) that family literacy measured in kindergarten predicted oral language development of children in kindergarten through second grade, while kindergarten oral language performance predicted their phonological awareness skill between kindergarten and second grade. So it may be that the home literacy environment and children's oral language proficiency affect reading ability indirectly through their influence on phonological awareness development.

Family History of Language Impairment

Children from families with histories of language and learning impairments are significantly more likely to display difficulties in these areas. This fact has fueled the search for a gene or combination of genes that is linked to or causes developmental learning disorders. Several studies have revealed high familial (family) concentrations (Lyytinen, Erskine, Tolvanen, Torppa, Poikkeus, & Lyytinen, 2006). For example, Neils and Aram (1986) reported that 20 percent of children with language impairment had affected family members, in comparison to 3 percent in the control group. Other studies have reported estimates between 30 and 40 percent (e.g., Tallal et al., 2001). Also, about 50 percent of children with preschool language impairments go on to develop reading problems (Catts, Fey, Zhang, & Tomblin, 1999, 2001). Findings also reveal, however, that a substantial proportion of the risk remains unexplained by genetics alone.

Further, familial problems are not always due to genetic factors, which means that not all children with language and literacy impairments have a positive family history of these problems. Another line of thinking is that a genetic predisposition may exist in all cases within a family, but that not every family member exhibits the genetic trait. This within-family variation suggests that language and learning problems result not from a single genetic root, but from multiple chromosomal sites. Moreover, language problems do not arise from genetic influences alone, but from an interaction between genetic and environmental factors, in which the environment can influence the expression or nonexpression of the genetic risk. For example, children who have a weak expression of an affected gene combined with a print-rich environment may be less likely to express the language impairment than are those with sparse linguistic environments. It is most likely that multiple factors (genetic and environmental) interact to predispose a child toward or away from emergent literacy deficits (Gilger & Wise, 2004).

Summary

The information that has been accumulated thus far indicates that extrinsic, or family-based, factors create a significant divide in emergent literacy knowledge when children enter kindergarten. Further, the gap is greater for children who enter school with a combination of risk factors (economic disadvantage, primary language other than English, sparse home literacy environment, family history of impairment, lower level of maternal education, single-parent home). Finally, the literacy achievement gaps remain stable over time, at least through the end of high school, making it increasingly more difficult to successfully tackle the problem.

Aspects of Emergent Literacy

Emergent literacy comprises several components, or areas of knowledge. These knowledge components interact with the contributing factors discussed earlier and converge to form emergent literacy (Lonigan, Burgess, & Anthony, 2000). This section will describe some of the key indicators of emergent literacy development.

Oral Language Development

Throughout the preschool years, children acquire the ability to understand and express themselves in their native language(s), which is composed of several subsystems: phonology, morphology, semantics, syntax, and pragmatics. Table 13.1 provides definitions of each subsystem.

In addition to the acquisition of basic linguistic knowledge, children begin to develop higher-level linguistic abilities, often referred to as *metalinguistic awareness:* explicit knowledge of and ability to manipulate subsystems of language independently of the meaning conveyed by the message. Metalinguistic awareness allows children to consciously reflect on and think about language as an object unto itself, as when a 3-year-old boy announced about his brother's name, "'Nafan' is hard to say. It has a 'th' in it"; or when a 2-year-old girl stated, "Hey, boots and toots—that matches!" (van Kleeck & Bryant, 1983; van Kleeck & Schuele, 1987). "Meta" language skills are developed within each language subsystem (i.e., metaphonology, metamorphology, metasemantics, metaysntax, metapragmatics) and are the areas of oral language that are most closely linked to literacy acquisition. One key aspect of metaphonological ability, phonological awareness/sensitivity, has received much attention by researchers, educators, and clinicians because of its direct link with the acquisition of early literacy skills.

TABLE 13.1 Subsystems of Language

Subsytem	Definition
Phonology	The sound system of a language; the individual phonemes that comprise the sound system of a particular language (e.g., /p/, /g/, /t/, /a/, /i/) and the rules for permissible sound combinations into longer sequences such as words (e.g., vowel-lengthening rule, in which vowel sounds are longer in duration before voiced final consonants than when preceding voiceless final consonants, as in *mob* vs. *mop*).
Morphology	The structure of words and the construction of word forms from the basic elements of meaning (i.e., morphemes); these include word endings that indicate plurality (e.g., *boys*), tense markers (e.g., *walked*), possessives (e.g., *daddy's*), and so on.
Semantics	The meaning of individual vocabulary words and the rules that govern the combinations of word meanings to form meaningful phrases and sentences. For example, the sentence *Colorless green ideas sleep furiously,* while syntactically correct, violates semantic combination rules.
Syntax	Rules governing the order and combination of words to generate well-formed sentences.
Pragmatics	Rules governing the use of language in everyday social contexts such as conversation.

Phonological awareness is a phonological processing ability that involves manipulating the sound structure of spoken language, and young children engage in a variety of oral language activities that require phonological awareness. These include rhyming (e.g., _bake_—_take_); alliteration (e.g., _mean monkeys make a mess_); blending sounds (e.g., _c-a-t_ → _cat_); isolating sounds (e.g., _dog_ → _d-og_); segmenting words into their individual sounds (e.g., _fish_ → _f-i-sh_); deleting sounds (e.g., _spill_ → _pill_), and substituting sounds (e.g., _top_ → _mop_). As children play with the sound properties of language, they acquire the building blocks necessary for learning to read and write. Of the variety of phonological awareness skills, it is those that involve phonemic awareness—knowledge that spoken words are made up of individual sounds and the ability to manipulate these sounds—that are most critical to early literacy acquisition. Recall that beginning reading requires children to be able to map individual speech sounds onto their corresponding letters in order to decode the written word, while basic spelling necessitates that a child encode discrete sounds into single letters or letter combinations. Thus, phonemic awareness enables children to develop the alphabetic principle (the concept that letters in written words correspond to sounds in written words) (e.g., Liberman & Shankweiler, 1985). Knowledge of the alphabetic principle promotes basic reading and spelling skill, which in turn furthers the development of phonemic awareness. Thus, the relationship between phonological awareness and literacy is mutually dependent and reciprocal (Torgesen, Wagner, & Rashotte, 1994).

Studies consistently show that children who perform well on phonological awareness tasks become successful readers, while those who perform poorly often struggle with reading and spelling, regardless of other factors such as a child's intelligence (IQ) or SES (Adams, 1990; Blachman, 1989; Stanovich, 1986; Vellutino & Scanlon, 1987; Wagner & Torgesen, 1987). In fact, phonological awareness in kindergarten is the single best predictor of reading and spelling achievement at the end of first and second grade (Cooper et al., 2002; Perfetti, Beck, Bell, & Hughes, 1987; Roth, Speece, et al., 2002; Torgesen et al., 1994).

Significant growth in phonological sensitivity occurs during the preschool period, even as young as 3 years of age. The earliest phonological awareness skills demonstrated by children are rhyming and alliteration and are among the first indications that children are sensitive to the fact that speech is made up of separate units. Rhyming and alliteration serve as important building blocks for more-explicit forms of phonological awareness, which emerge in the following order: blending → segmenting → manipulation. Blending and segmenting syllables is easier than segmenting or blending individual sounds, so a task that requires a child to clap hands for each syllable of a word like _telephone_ is easier than a phonemic awareness task that asks a child to indicate the individual number of phonemes in a word such as _bat_. Even more difficult are manipulation tasks such as "Say 'fat'; now say it without the /f/" or "Say 'table'; now take away the /t/ and put a /f/ at the beginning."

In addition to phonological awareness, other aspects of oral language development are important to literacy acquisition. Among the most critical is lexical semantics, or vocabulary. A child's vocabulary knowledge has immediate and long-term effects on the development of both oral language and written language and is thus an important emergent literacy foundation for literacy learning and later achievement. Most well documented is its influence on reading acquisition in terms of both the ability to read words (decode) and the ability to understand what is read (reading comprehension). For example, Scarborough (1998) showed that receptive and expressive vocabulary size at 3 years was predictive of subsequent decoding ability at the end of second grade. Others have shown that vocabulary at 3 years predicts both reading and spelling achievement in kindergarten through third grade (Walker, Greenwood, Hart, & Carta, 1994). Vocabulary knowledge also has been linked to children's phonological sensitivity (McGregor, 2004). Finally, based on a thorough examination of the research literature, the National Reading Panel (2000) concluded that oral vocabulary is essential to word-and text-level reading development.

From about 18 months of age, typically developing children learn about eight to nine new words per day (Baumann & Kameenui, 1991; Beck & McKeown, 1991). So by the time they enter school, children have developed a vocabulary (**lexicon**) of thousands of words. These words are learned through natural, daily interactions and conversations with others in their environment. The rapid pace and ease with which young children acquire vocabulary have been referred as a process in which the child's brain is a "vocabulary sponge" that "soaks up" several new words each day (G. A. Miller & Gildea, 1987; N. W. Nelson, 1998). Young children with language delays do not have the same experience. They have difficulty learning new words and retaining the meaning of newly learned words and, thus, exhibit vocabulary deficits early on. For example, Rescorla and Lee (2000) reported that the expressive vocabulary size of toddlers with language impairments was fewer than 50 words, in comparison to 130 to 160 words for their typically developing peers. In addition to arising early, vocabulary differences widen over time (Stanovich, 1986). Children with vocabulary deficits frequently have difficulty learning to read and, therefore, lose out on opportunities to learn new vocabulary words from written texts. This is important because once children learn basic reading skills, most new words are learned as children engage in the act of reading itself.

Sense of Story

In literate cultures, children develop a "sense of story" during their preschool years through their everyday experiences with various forms of narration (storybooks, personal stories, oral anecdotes). Narrative discourse involves extended units of spoken or written language such as storytelling, the relating of a personal experience, written composition, and the retelling of a previously heard story. Narration is considered a "literate" discourse form because it requires a more abstract grasp of language than does everyday conversational discourse. Apparently, children proceed from the conversational or communicative use of language to narration, the more formal, literate language use. As such, narratives are thought to function as an important transition between oral and literate language styles (Westby, 1991). The basis for this thinking is that oral narration and written text share many of the same properties and abilities. Unlike conversation, narratives are monologues rather than dialogues. Oral narratives and written texts also share a concise and complex syntactic style, focus on topics that are frequently unfamiliar or abstract, and contain rich and rare vocabulary. Further, like written text, narratives are a decontextualized language form because they require distancing from immediate experiences—reflecting on past experiences or making up event sequences (C. E. Snow, 1991).

Sense of story reflects a child's growing knowledge of the internal structure of narratives. It is believed that joint book reading promotes the development of story knowledge because it is through repeated exposure to stories that children begin to internalize a framework for understanding and generating narrative sequences (Justice et al., 2009; Roth, 2009). From a developmental perspective, children's earliest stories are personal narratives or "scripts" that involve recounting very familiar experiences such as going to a birthday party or taking a trip to the zoo. By about 5 years of age, children acquire the basic structure of stories—the story schema—knowledge that a story has a beginning, middle, and end with a theme or plot that logically ties events together. This knowledge gives rise to fictional narratives, and children begin to understand and produce stories about made-up experiences that are not part of the immediate context. By the time children enter school, their stories contain physical descriptions of the characters and have simple, but well-developed plot structures, with story events logically connected to one another and linked to a central theme. Based on the work of Applebee (1978) and N. L. Stein and Glenn (1979), five stages characterize children's early story development. Table 13.2 shows these stages, along with examples that illustrate the kinds of stories children tell at each stage.

Presumably, children bring a basic knowledge of story structure to literacy learning tasks, and apply this knowledge in their efforts to understand, compose, and remember text. It has been repeatedly demonstrated that children (and adolescents) with reading and writing deficits have difficulty understanding stories, producing stories of their own, and retelling stories told or written by others (Newcomer & Barenbaum, 1991; Roth & Spekman, 1986; Roth, Spekman, & Fye, 1992). Thus, narrative discourse is an emergent literacy skill that demonstrates the interrelatedness among the domains of speaking, reading, and writing (Roth, 2000, 2009).

TABLE 13.2   Stages of Story Development

Heap	Simple listing of ideas in no particular order. Example: *The cat is climbing on the tree. It's raining and the children are there and the cats. The sky is all blue and the clouds. The end.*
Description	Contains information about the personality and physical characteristics of the main character. Example: *Once there was a big black cat who lived in a house. He was mean and scary. He had giant black eyes and big claws and scratched people in the face. And he chased dogs. The end.*
Action Sequence	Story events are connected through temporal relationships, but not causally. Example: *Once there was a big black cat. Every day, he came out and chased dogs. Then he played with his friends. Then he found some lunch. Then he purred and licked his fur. Then he went home and went to sleep. The end.*
Primitive/Abbreviated Narrative	Events are linked temporally and causally, but there is no goal-based action. Example: *Once there was a dog named Fella who lived by the train tracks. Fella was playing by the tracks, hopping over the rails, when along came a train, and Poosh, that was the end of Fella. The end.*
True Narrative	Events are chained logically to one another and to a central character or theme. Example: *Once there was a big black cat who lived in the city. One day he decided that he was very hungry and that he needed to get something for dinner. So he went into the alley and spotted a little bird, caught him, and had him for dinner. The end.*

Print Knowledge

Various strands of development are involved in learning to process print, all of which are paths to children's growing discovery that print communicates. These include knowledge of concepts/conventions of print, recognition of environmental print, and alphabetic letter and sound–symbol knowledge.

Children demonstrate *concepts of print* when they recognize print conventions and accepted standards or practices for interacting with print. This includes understanding that spaces between words represent word boundaries; understanding that English print runs left to right and top to bottom; understanding that books are read from front to back; and realizing that there are different forms and functions of print such as to tell a story, write an email, and make a shopping list.

Recognition of environmental print is evident when children identify familiar symbols and demonstrate knowledge that print carries meaning (e.g., street signs such as *STOP, EXIT*; logos on cereal boxes; familiar words in their natural contexts such as *Happy Birthday* on a greeting card). *Alphabetic knowledge* is demonstrated when children recognize and can name individual letters. The ability to accurately and rapidly identify letter names in kindergarten is strongly associated with later reading success. In alphabetic reading systems like English, a basic requirement for beginning reading (decoding) and writing (spelling) is the ability to differentiate the letters of the alphabet. A beginning reader who cannot recognize and distinguish among alphabet letters will have trouble learning the sounds that correspond to the letters they represent. By early to mid-kindergarten, a majority of typically developing children from middle-class homes can name most or all alphabet letters (Justice, Invernizzi, & Meier, 2002). Children as young as 3 years can identify almost half of the letters.

However, knowledge of letter names alone does not guarantee reading acquisition. Children also learn *sound–symbol correspondences*—the alphabetic principle. Knowledge of the systematic relationships between alphabet letter names and sounds enables children to discover, for example, that the letter *f* is the sound in both the /f/ and the /ph/ graphemes. Developmentally, children show continued growth in this skill in the early elementary school years and master the alphabetic principle by about 8 years of age. Preschool children's grasp of letter knowledge also seems to play an influential role in the development of phonological awareness, which in turn is closely linked to growth in the alphabetic principle, an essential element for learning basic reading and spelling skills.

Emergent Writing Development

When we observe very young children absorbed in scribbling and drawing undecipherable lines on a piece of paper and then pretending to read it, they are showing an awareness that writing communicates even though these toddlers do not yet know the conventions of writing. In fact, children's earliest writing is most commonly in the form of wavy lines, picturelike scribbles, and pictures, which eventually become transformed into letters, wordlike sequences, conventional word spellings, and short sentences, which become more "readable." Most children enter kindergarten knowing how to write a few words. By the end of first grade, children can write a few sentences in a manner that can be read by another person without much difficulty.

To write effectively, children must learn to spell fluently. The development of spelling begins long before children start spelling instruction in school. Their early writing efforts demonstrate a fascinating and creative process called invented spelling. A term coined by Read (1971), *invented spelling* describes children's attempts to write words using a more

TABLE 13.3   Stages of Emergent Writing Development

Stage	Description/Example
Drawing	Child holds a crayon or marker and writes by drawing using scribbles, wavy and circular lines.
Prephonemic	Child understands that writing has a purpose; uses random strings of pictures, squiggles, letters, and numbers with no meaningful correspondence between letters and sounds (e.g., BmKTO = candy; XAb6UL = train); letters and numbers may be mixed in together as well as upper- and lowercase letters.
Semiphonemic	Writes 1 to 3 letters to stand for a word, sentence, or idea (e.g., T = train; MR = monster; PTE = pretty); child knows that letters stand for sounds due to emergence of the alphabetic principle, but only has partial mapping of the phonetic representation of words; may be able to print own name.
Phonetic/Letter Name	Child spells words the way they sound; all of the phonemes are represented in a word, but spellings are unconventional (e.g., LETL = little; EGL = eagle; NIT = night).
Transitional	Spellings conform to the conventions for English writing; vowels are included in each syllable (e.g., FAFRIT = favorite; ALUGADOR = alligator), but letters may not be in the correct order (e.g., NIHGT = night).
Conventional	Basic rules of spelling are mastered; child can spell a large number of words automatically (e.g., EAGLE = eagle; MONSTER = monster).

Source: Information from Bear and Templeton (1998) and Gentry (2000).

or less phonological strategy as opposed to a random strategy. It indicates that children have started to develop an awareness of the internal structure of words—and specifically that words are made up of phonemic segments represented by letters of the alphabet. Invented spelling helps children figure out the alphabetic principle, is a robust indicator of children's phonological awareness skill (Torgesen & Davis, 1996), and is strongly related to early word-reading ability (Ehri, 1987, 1989; J. A. Scott & Ehri, 1990). Ehri and her colleagues demonstrated this reading–writing connection by showing that young children who could spell words phonetically (invented spelling) learned to decode similar-sounding words much better than did the peers who could not.

The developmental pattern of children's early writing and spelling is outlined in Table 13.3. In reviewing this table, one notes that children begin by scribbling and drawing using wavy lines and pictures, progress to writing more conventional letterlike forms that represent the phonetic properties of speech, and finally master the principles of conventional spelling.

Children at Risk for Literacy Problems

By 5 years of age, most typically developing children have a broad range of emergent literacy abilities that reflect a growing recognition of the forms and functions of print and the relationship between oral and written language. These include

(1) understanding and using oral language in everyday speaking and listening situations; (2) having "word awareness," or knowledge that words are separate units of language; (3) exhibiting early phonological awareness; (4) using context to recognize environmental print; (5) distinguishing between printed letters and words; (6) identifying some or all of the letters of the alphabet; and (7) having knowledge of book and other print conventions.

By comparison, many children with disabilities do not acquire these basic emergent literacy skills. These children tend to acquire emergent literacy skills at a slower rate than do their same-age peers. Delays are prevalent in children whose primary disability is language impairment, children who demonstrate other disabilities that affect communication development (e.g., mental retardation, autism spectrum disorders, hearing impairment and deafness, attention deficit disorder, or other behavioral difficulties), and children with motor or other disabilities who use nonspeech or augmentative/alternative communication systems. Still others are at risk due to poverty, limited English proficiency, limited access to print, and/or history of language or reading disability. The deficits exhibited by these children cross all of the key areas of emergent literacy.

The challenges for researchers and practitioners are to reduce the probability that such deficits will occur, identify potential problems early, and provide effective emergent literacy instruction to reduce/avoid the cycle of failure.

Prevention, Assessment, and Intervention Processes

Speech-language pathologists (SLPs) have been called upon to take an active role in promoting the emergent literacy development of all children—and particularly those at risk for literacy-related learning difficulties (American Speech-Language-Hearing Association, 2001b). This role includes preventing literacy problems, identifying and assessing children at risk for reading and writing problems, and providing intervention to remediate literacy-related difficulties.

Prevention

The main goal of prevention is to promote opportunities for meaningful and successful interactions with the world of print. Prevention is a process requiring collaboration among SLPs, teachers, families, and administrators to ensure that young children have high-quality and ample opportunities to participate in emergent literacy activities, both at home and in the preschool/day-care environment. Prevention also involves providing access to such experiences to older children or those with developmental delays who have missed these opportunities. Importantly, the process of prevention reflects the increased attention being paid to the early identification of children who are vulnerable to literacy learning difficulties. Once identified, children can then be provided with needed additional supports and services or be referred for further assessment so that early interventions can be implemented. Adoption of a preventative model entails taking a proactive stance to identify problems before children enter first grade and are enmeshed in formal literacy instruction, unequipped to maintain the pace of instruction.

Assessment and Intervention

Evaluation and treatment of emergent literacy are guided by a number of common principles, which are outlined below.

  1. Emergent literacy assessment and intervention should address the domains of both oral language and written language because of their reciprocal and continual influence on one another. For example, phonological awareness intervention is most effective when accompanied by instruction in the alphabetic principle (National Reading Panel, 2000) because phonological awareness itself is not sufficient for learning to read.
  2. Assessment and intervention activities must be developmentally appropriate, based on a child's age and level of functioning. For example, rhyming and alliteration are developmentally appropriate tasks of phonological awareness for 4-year-old children, while phoneme segmentation is typically considered beyond the firm grasp of children at this age. Further, different tasks require differing levels of processing; in general, receptive tasks are easier than expressive tasks, so that identifying pictures that rhyme is easier than generating a word that rhymes with a target word produced by the clinician.
  3. Clinical procedures must be sensitive to the child's cultural and linguistic background because these variables directly influence all aspects of the assessment and intervention processes. Clinical tools and procedures inherently are culture bound because they reflect the linguistic and social beliefs, values, and interaction styles of a society. Further, different cultures have different expectations about when children should learn to read and write. As a result, ELLs from linguistically diverse backgrounds may demonstrate depressed performance on emergent literacy measures that are not representative of their actual ability (Gutierrez-Clennen & Pena, 2002).
  4. Emergent literacy assessment and intervention practices must be based on scientific evidence. This necessitates incorporating and translating the best and most recent research information into clinical decision making and procedures. Assessment measures must be well constructed with strong psychometric properties, including reliability (consistency of results over repeated administrations) and validity (extent to which a test measures what it claims to measure). For intervention, this means that the best instructional practices are evidence based—strategies and procedures that have been shown to be effective in well-designed research studies. Clinicians then select and implement these tools using their own judgment and knowledge acquired through professional experience. It is the continual advancement of our knowledge that helps SLPs deliver the most effective clinical services and bridges the research-to-practice gap between what science shows to be beneficial and what is currently implemented in early childhood instructional settings.

Assessment   Evaluation should encompass a broad array of emergent literacy skills that are strongly and reliably linked to later literacy achievement so that they are sensitive to differentiating between those who are at risk and those who are not (Fawcett & Nicolson, 2000). An ideal test battery includes measures administered directly to the child; observation of the child's emergent literacy skills in different contexts (e.g., structured classroom activity vs. free time); and family interviews, checklists, or questionnaires to ascertain information about the availability of and opportunities for participation in print-related activities outside the school environment.

Intervention   The importance of early intervention cannot be overstated. Emergent literacy instruction needs to occur early in the preschool period for children to harvest meaningful gains in oral and written language that will prepare them for reading and writing instruction and allow them to access the education curriculum. This instruction can draw on the growing number of studies demonstrating the effectiveness of emergent literacy training for at-risk children (e.g., Justice & Ezell, 2002; Justice et al., 2009; Roth, Troia, Worthington, & Dow, 2002, 2006).

For SLPs, the overall goal of emergent literacy instruction is to build on and foster the reciprocal relationships between oral language and literacy development discussed throughout this chapter. Emergent literacy instruction is most effective when SLPs work in collaboration with teachers, families, and others to provide children with the highest-quality literacy experiences. Promoting emergent literacy development is not confined to young children. Older children, particularly those with speech and language impairments, may be functioning developmentally in the emergent literacy stage and require intervention aimed at establishing and solidifying these essential precursors.

SLPs assume a variety of instructional roles in emergent literacy. The most obvious is to provide direction and intervention for children with identified language and communication impairments. But clinicians serve numerous other important functions: collaboration with classroom teachers to incorporate developmentally sensitive emergent literacy activities into general education preschool and kindergarten curricula, professional staff development through continuing education workshops for teachers and others working with children at the emergent literacy stage, family and community education, advocacy on behalf of children and their families to ensure the provision of appropriate services, and policy development to educate school and district administrators and shape policy decisions regarding the importance of emergent literacy skills for all students.

Several factors require consideration in the development and implementation of emergent literacy instruction, including the language development status and cognitive functioning of the child, because both of these variables have been shown to be excellent predictors of long-term language and literacy skills. For example, preschool children with receptive and expressive language disorders often perform significantly more poorly on measures of language, reading, and writing 12 years later than do children with only expressive language deficits. In addition, their preschool scores on measures of nonverbal intelligence strongly predict later literacy achievement (Bishop & Adams, 1990). So it is imperative to know the specific language subsystems that are affected and the overall cognitive status of children when designing and planning instructional programs. Instruction/intervention also needs to address the needs of children with different types of disabilities. Children with autism may benefit from an emphasis on written expression through a writing center approach (Koppenhaver & Erickson, 2003), AAC users require early access to assistive-technologies for early writing and drawing opportunities (Light & Kent-Walsh, 2003), children with motor disorders such as cerebral palsy may need special adaptations of standard writing materials, and children with attention disorders may benefit from increased repetition and use of visual cues to maintain their attentional focus (Lonigan et al., 1999).

Emergent literacy instruction/intervention is informed by several "best practices" principles:

1. Provide direct and explicit instruction for all children. Children with language impairments do not learn and generalize through their everyday, natural experiences with print. They require explicit, direct, and repeated guidance. Explicit instruction is also advantageous with typically developing children because they may not use their entire skill repertoire unless specifically prompted to do so.

2. Embed instruction in natural—authentic—contexts. Young children learn best through active exploration, meaningful experiences, and interactive participation with materials that sustain their interest. Classroom-based or small-group instruction is most well suited to the developmental capabilities of young children and older children functioning at an emergent literacy level. Authentic learning contexts also foster an enjoyable learning atmosphere, unlike drill-like instructional formats.

3. Foster family engagement in the instructional program. The type and quality of early everyday interactions between adults and young children influence the acquisition of emergent and early literacy skills (Dickinson & Tabors, 2001; Dodici, Draper, & Peterson, 2003).

4. Use scaffolding to guide a child's understanding beyond his or her current level of knowledge. In scaffolding, an adult (or more mature learner) provides systematic support to enable a child to progress one step further than what the child can accomplish on his own. For example, in storybook reading, parents of 9-month-old infants tend to draw the baby's attention to the book and the pictures, but do not request a label; at 17 months, a label is requested; by 27 months, a toddler's responses are followed by an adult comment on the same topic.

Guided by these principles, several aspects of emergent literacy can be targeted to increase a child's awareness of print. Below is a brief sampling of these areas along with evidenced-based practices that have been successfully used to foster the development of emergent literacy skills.

Shared Book Reading and Sense of Story

- Expose children to developmentally appropriate high-quality literature.
- Use dialogic reading: interactive book reading between an adult and a child in which the child is an active participant. The adult (or more mature reader) engages the child in the book-reading experience through questions posed throughout the reading.
- Read a variety of different kinds of books: stories that contain frequent pairs of rhyming words, alliterative sequences, or other interesting sound patterns; books with repetitive themes or predictable patterns; books with appealing illustrations; alphabet-letter books.
- Direct the child's attention to the printed word rather than focusing solely on the pictures.

Vocabulary

- Introduce new vocabulary during dialogic book reading; use definitions (e.g., *He built a cocoon—a warm comfy blanket*), synonyms (*thief—robber*), and comparisons (e.g., *chimney—He came out of the chimney like Santa Claus*) to teach and strengthen newly learned words.
- Use visual supports such as semantic webs or maps to sort words by categories (e.g., color, action, location); connect new words with existing vocabulary.

Phonological Awareness

- Use nursery rhymes, fingerplays, and songs with rhythmical or alliterative patterns.
- Identify/generate words that rhyme or begin with a target word.

- Play games such as "I Spy," focusing on different sounds of words as clues (e.g., "I spy something that begins/ends with /p/").

Concepts/Conventions of Print

- Engage children in book-handling experiences such as turning the pages during storybook reading.
- Point out/model reading conventions such as the left-right orientation of print, front-back directionality of book reading, spaces between words, and different types of punctuation (e.g., question mark, exclamation point).

Emergent Writing

- Provide an assortment of attractive writing materials (e.g., pens, markers, crayons, chalk, children's writing software), writing surfaces (e.g., paper, tagboard, dry-erase board), and daily opportunities to engage in writing.
- Encourage scribbling, drawing, and use of invented spelling.
- Have children dictate stories, letters, emails; write pretend notes (e.g., to the tooth fairy), after which the adult reads back the child's message.
- Display alphabet letters on foam board or put up magnetic letters for children to see.

Alphabetic Letter Knowledge

- Name letters in highly familiar and frequent words.
- Sort pictures by the same letter; make lists of words that begin with the same letter.

Adult Modeling of Literacy Activities

- Provide frequent opportunities for children to watch adults engaged in reading and writing in everyday situations (e.g., reading a book or newspaper, writing down a phone number, following a recipe from a children's cookbook).
- Point out and read print in environmental contexts (e.g., traffic signs, restaurant logos, familiar words such as *Cheerios* on a cereal box).

Summary

This chapter described emergent literacy acquisition in typically developing children and those at risk for literacy learning difficulties. A central theme of the chapter was the critical relationship between oral language development and literacy acquisition that begins early in the preschool years and continues throughout childhood and into adolescence. Factors that influence the acquisition of emergent literacy were discussed, as were the key components that form the construct of emergent literacy. Although we know many of its chief components, a definitive developmental model of emergent literacy is not yet apparent. Delineation of such a model awaits further understanding in at least three areas: the developmental origins of different emergent literacy skills, how these skills interact with one another at different points in development, and the long-term effects of these skills on language and literacy achievement.

In this chapter, it was emphasized that most literacy problems have their roots in the preschool years before children begin formal instruction in reading and writing. Children who start out behind their classmates in learning to read and write usually remain behind, even when provided with high-quality special education and language intervention services. This fact underscores several important points: (1) All professionals working with young children must be knowledgeable about the developmental connections among language, literacy, and associated risk factors; (2) preschool curricula must incorporate developmentally appropriate and systematic, high-quality instructional opportunities for children to learn and practice key emergent literacy skills in all early childhood education settings; and (3) the early identification of children who may be susceptible to literacy problems is critical to ensure appropriate referral for assessment and timely provision of needed educational/intervention services. To this end, the concluding sections of this chapter focused on the prevention, assessment, and intervention to foster emergent literacy and on the variety of collaborative roles that SLPs may assume in these clinical processes.

case study SUSAN

Susan is a 4½-year-old child whose native language is English. She comes from an economically disadvantaged family and attends a Head Start preschool program in her community. Susan has difficulty learning and understanding vocabulary words. She does not seem to follow classroom lessons or activities that focus on rhyming and alliteration, and she cannot name any letters of the alphabet. When asked to retell a simple story, she cannot recall the events in a logical sequence. When "writing" her name, Susan scribbles in wavy lines across the page.

Following a comprehensive assessment, the classroom teacher and the SLP worked together to develop and implement an effective plan for Susan. Their collaborative partnership resulted in the selection of three initial areas of focus: (1) phonological awareness/rhyming, (2) sense of story, and (3) vocabulary. To facilitate rhyming, the teacher and SLP co-taught a lesson in the classroom, which involved storybooks (e.g., *Mouse Mess*) and fingerplays (e.g., "Teddy Bear, Teddy Bear") that contained many rhyming words. The SLP explained the concept of rhyming to the class, providing examples of word pairs that do and do not rhyme. The teacher then read the story, using exaggerated articulation of the rhyming words. After finishing the book, the teacher read it again, this time asking the children to provide the rhyme word at the end of the sentences. After a third reading, the teacher went around the class, asking for volunteers to rhyme the names of each student. In a follow-up activity led by the SLP, the class made a "rhyming tree," in which the rhyming words of the book constituted branches of the tree. Children took turns saying the rhyme pairs and attaching them to the tree. Once completed, the SLP led the class in playful rapid repetition of the rhyming words to reinforce the concept of rhyming.

Sense of story and vocabulary were targeted through dialogic reading in a classroom lesson led by the SLP. The book selected for the activity was taken from the school curriculum. The SLP engaged in dialogic reading, posing questions throughout the book reading (i.e., before, during, and after). The questions focused on the objects, events, and actions on individual pages (e.g., *What is this? What is the lion doing?*) and questions about the relationship between the storyline and the children's own experiences (e.g., *Do you remember at the zoo when we saw the lion roaring?*). The SLP then asked the children to recap the main events of the book by asking them to identify the beginning, middle, and ending parts of the story. Throughout the reading, the SLP identified new vocabulary words (e.g., *roaring*) and provided simple definitions of each term. She also provided short descriptions and synonyms to strengthen the vocabulary words (e.g., *He built a cocoon—a warm comfy blanket*).

Susan also received direct intervention services from the SLP to reinforce and build upon the areas of emergent literacy targeted in the classroom.

STUDY QUESTIONS

1. What is emergent literacy? How is it related to conventional literacy?

2. Identify and briefly describe (a) factors that contribute to emergent literacy development and (b) the key components of emergent literacy.

3. Explain the importance of the relationship between oral language and literacy for typically developing children and for children at risk for literacy deficits.

4. Identify and briefly explain the principles of (a) emergent literacy assessment and (b) emergent literacy intervention.

SELECTED READINGS

Bennett-Armisteaa, V. S., Duke, N. K. & Moses, A. M. (2005). *Literacy and the youngest learner.* New York, NY: Teaching Resource.

Burns, M. S., Griffin, P., & Snow, C. E. (1999). *Starting out right: A guide to promoting children's reading success.* Washington, DC: National Academy Press.

Dickinson, D. K., & Tabors, P. O. (2001). *Beginning literacy with language.* Baltimore, MD: Paul H. Brookes.

Rhymer, P. M. (2009). *Emergent literacy and language development.* New York, NY: Guilford Press.

WEBSITES OF INTEREST

www.nifl.gov
   The National Institute for Literacy administers The Partnership for Reading and other programs to promote child and adult literacy.

www.nationalreadingpanel.org
   To obtain a copy of *Teaching Children to Read*, the 2000 report of the National Reading Panel.

www.asha.org
   The American Speech-Language-Hearing Association's site has introductory information on reading and writing development and disorders.

Chapter FOURTEEN

Aphasia and Related Acquired Language Disorders

Audrey L. Holland
University of Arizona, Emerita

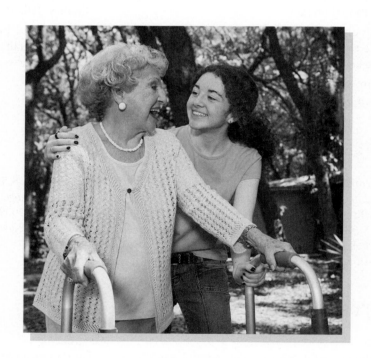

personal PERSPECTIVE

AUDREY L. HOLLAND

I once thought I wanted to be a music teacher in the public schools, but decided against it before college because I was sure that I didn't have the patience for it. This should make it harder to understand why I ended up choosing Aphasiology as my area of research and clinical involvement. It certainly has left me wondering on more than one occasion because being an aphasia clinician requires a commitment to being patient. Since my days as an undergraduate psychology student, I have always been interested in the brain generally, but most specifically, in *mind*—that is, those aspects of neural activity that encompass thinking, talking, problem solving, and creating.

When a close high school friend suffered severe brain damage in a car accident, I watched the resulting devastation of his aspirations, his social relationships, his entire family's quality of life. My need to know more about how the brain works and, now, what happens when it is damaged began to shape my career. I also had the pleasure of watching my friend and his family survive, flourish, and grow, if not in the planned directions, at least in satisfying and valid ones. My need to be part of such a thing also became apparent. And here I am, many years later, still asking questions about the brain and perhaps best of all, still being instructed and energized by the patients and families with whom I work.

Students often view aphasia as a mysterious disorder. Consequently, their initial encounters with aphasic individuals are sometimes filled with dreaded anticipation of the unknown. We hope that this chapter eliminates much of the mystery of the disorder and provides you with comfort as you encounter your first aphasic individual. The chapter begins with an illustrative case history and continues with descriptions of brain–language connections, aphasia syndromes, diagnostic procedures, and intervention alternatives.

case study **MS. J**

Ms. J, age 46, was hospitalized following a sudden onset of right-side weakness and loss of speech. Following a complete neurological examination and series of tests, she was diagnosed as having had a thromboembolic stroke involving the left middle cerebral artery.

Prior to this, Ms. J had led an active life working in the public relations department of the Pittsburgh Steelers, raising two teenage sons, and managing the household with the help of her husband. She was an avid potter, and her other interests included professional sports, scuba diving, and reading.

One week following her stroke, Ms. J was transferred to a rehabilitation center, where she was engaged in a full-scale rehabilitation program that included physical, occupational, and speech-language therapy. Following 3 weeks of intensive therapy, Ms. J was able to walk with the aid of a short leg brace and had regained some use of her right arm and hand. A formal speech and language evaluation indicated a mild-to-moderate Broca's aphasia. Ms. J's spoken output was limited in quantity; she spoke in short phrases that had many grammatical errors. She also had marked word-finding difficulties, which were quite frustrating to her. Ms. J's auditory comprehension was considerably better than her spoken language; however, she had some problems understanding complex instructions and messages. Reading was affected minimally, but writing content was similar to spoken language. Because of a mild residual muscle weakness in her right arm and hand, Ms. J's writing was not as clear as it was prior to her stroke.

Ms. J began to receive 1 hour of daily individual speech-language therapy. Therapy was designed to increase her functional communication and decrease her anxiety about her faltering speech and language skills. At the onset of treatment, Ms. J was mildly depressed. But the gains she had made in physical therapy began to lift her spirits, and she worked with determination in speech-language therapy. Her family visited her every other day. Her husband began to attend the rehabilitation center's family group sessions that prepare families for patients' return to the home. Both the social worker and the clinical psychologist were alerted to Ms. J's depression and initiated brief counseling sessions. The social worker centered his activities on realistic appraisal of potential for return to work, while the psychologist focused her sessions on restoring Ms. J's self-concept in relation to her problems.

Ms. J was dismissed from the center following 6 weeks of intensive rehabilitation. At that time, she was walking with the assistance of a cane and was able to use her arm and hand to perform most of the activities of daily living, including cooking. She had made many gains in speech-language therapy. Most notable was the improvement in auditory comprehension, which was now near normal. Problems with word finding and writing persisted, however, and it was recommended that speech-language therapy be continued on an outpatient basis. Arrangements were made with the local university clinic for treatment.

Ms. J received 2 hours per week of individual and group therapy for the ensuing year. Consistent, but slow progress was maintained for approximately 10 months, with no apparent progress after that time. At the end of 1 year, Ms. J agreed to be discharged from treatment. At the time of discharge, Ms. J demonstrated minimal speech and language problems in most communicative situations. Occasionally, when under pressure, her word-finding problems resurfaced, but she was able to use strategies to overcome these problems.

During her time in the clinic, a number of family decisions influenced her treatment. Although Ms. J was determined to return to work initially, she and her family later decided against this. She did not, however, retire from life. In addition to returning to her major managerial role at home, she joined her local aphasia group, where she participates in many activities.

Within the year, Ms. J's family resumed its normal functioning. Her teenage children, almost ready for college, felt that they had had a significant learning experience. They were impressed by their mother's courage and strength in pursuing her recovery. Ms. J's husband, who felt the major financial and emotional burden of the stroke, was optimistic about the future. "We've learned a lot. We've learned to handle adversity. We've learned what we're made of. I'm terribly sorry it happened. But we've survived—and survived well."

This chapter is about a communication disorder called **aphasia**, which is usually acquired in adulthood. Aphasia is not simply a speech disturbance. In addition to affecting spoken language, it produces disturbances in comprehending the speech of others, reading, and writing. *Aphasia* is a general term used to describe a number of related, but separate problems, as we shall see later. It refers to a breakdown in the ability to formulate, retrieve, or decode the arbitrary symbols of language. Aphasia's onset is usually abrupt, occurring without warning to people who have no previous speech or language problems. Although injury to the head, brain tumors, and other neurologic diseases may produce language disturbances, aphasia is most frequently caused by stroke. Most of us know a relative or neighbor who has experienced one or more of its disastrous consequences.

The purpose of this chapter is to acquaint you with the mechanisms that produce aphasia, the various forms of the disorder, and treatment for the problem. Aphasia is a fascinating topic, not only to speech-language pathologists, but also to neurologists, linguists, and neuropsychologists. This is because aphasia affords a unique opportunity to study some of our most perplexing questions about ourselves. These include the nature of brain–behavior relationships, the interaction between thought and language, and the neurologic underpinnings of cognitive activities. As a result, there is much, often contradictory, literature concerning aphasia that has been accumulating for more than a century. We will merely scratch the surface here, but in the process, we hope to share with you our excitement about studying aphasia and working with aphasic adults.

Aphasia and the Brain

Basic Neuroanatomic Considerations

Although damage to many different parts of the brain can cause some sort of communication problem, the cortex, or covering of the cerebrum, is of most interest to aphasiologists. This wrinkled and crumpled gray surface appears to be the body's major network for implementing and carrying out our most complex cognitive activities. Speaking, reading, writing, and comprehending are all cognitive activities; therefore, damage to the cortex (cortical damage) is most likely to produce aphasia. Damage to some of the structures that lie underneath and are connected with the cortex (subcortical damage) also can result in aphasia. Damage just anywhere in the cortex is not sufficient to produce aphasia. Controversy still exists over what particular sites of damage produce which form of language problem. We have limited understanding about how the damage exacts its toll, yet some principles of neurologic function allow us to speculate about cortical damage and aphasia.

We begin with a review of the cerebral hemispheres. Like some other organs (e.g., the kidneys), the cortex-covered cerebrum appears to be a pair of organs. The cerebrum consists of two halves that are roughly similar in size and shape. Most normal brain functioning requires both halves to be operating properly; however, the functions of the halves of the brain are not totally the same. Each half does some unique things. We will discuss three broad types of cortical activities—motor, sensory, and cognitive—in terms of their hemispheric control.

Movement or Motor Behavior

Our only means of affecting our environment is through movement. Even our thoughts are inaccessible to the world around us unless we can move our speech muscles to put our thoughts into words or move our bodies to communicate them wordlessly. Movement seems the most obvious of our abilities; yet movement—how the brain controls the body's muscles—remains at the scientific frontier. The enormous complexity of neuromotor control is not yet satisfactorily explained. For highly skilled motor behavior, nature plays an interesting trick. The left half (left cerebral hemisphere) controls movement of the right side of the body, and the right half (right cerebral hemisphere) controls the left side of the body. If cortical brain damage results in some motor impairment (and it frequently does), we can observe a paralysis of the side of the body opposite the brain damage. **Hemiplegia** is the paralysis of one side of the body. Slight or incomplete paralysis is called **hemiparesis**. We can use hemiplegia and hemiparesis to predict the side of brain damage. If a left hemiplegia is noted, we can infer right-hemisphere damage; if a right hemiplegia is noted, we can infer left-hemisphere damage. In the case of Ms. J., we could predict from her right-side weakness that she had sustained damage to the left hemisphere. She also experienced a mild degree of sensory loss in her right arm and leg, which further indicates left-side brain damage. Sensory changes may also occur after stroke.

Sensation or Sensory Behavior

Although all the senses are important in perceiving the world around us, we will limit our discussion to the sensory systems that are most important to language: vision and audition. Let us first consider vision. In animals or birds with monocular vision, such as pigeons, vision in the left eye is the province of the right hemisphere, and vice versa. But human beings, along with a few other animals, have binocular rather than monocular vision. In humans, the visual pathways are partially crossed. This crossing occurs just behind the eyeballs. Beyond this crossing point, damage either to the optic pathways or to the area of the cortex that receives visual impulses causes a loss of vision of one-half of what is being viewed. This loss is called **hemianopsia**. An interruption of the left optic tract or occipital lobe, therefore, causes loss of the right half of the visual space. The loss of the same visual half-field of both eyes is identified by the term **homonymous**—hence, *right homonymous hemianopsia*.

As with vision, there is something strange about the manner in which auditory information is relayed to the cortex. The circuitry involved can be difficult to demonstrate due both to the nature of sound waves and to the fact that auditory information is quite generously distributed to both hemispheres. Roughly 70 percent of the auditory fibers from each ear cross to the opposite hemisphere. Few, if any, effects on hearing sensitivity are caused by purely cortical damage. Deafness in one ear occurs as a result of damage to the ear itself or the sensory pathways below the level of the cortex. In audition, the cortex serves to interpret auditory signals and messages; that is, it makes sense out of the signals received by the ears.

In the case of visual and auditory information, nature appears to have been careful to protect these two major avenues for comprehending the world around us. First, by giving us two eyes and ears, nature has arranged it so that if one member of either pair is damaged, we are not totally cut off from its sensory contributions. Second, nature has protected us by arranging for each member of the pair to have access to both cortical hemispheres. This further ensures some access to vital visual and auditory information, even in cases of unilateral brain damage.

Cognition

We have seen how sensory input from the eyes and ears is received differentially by the left and right hemispheres. We also have been alerted to the manner in which motor output is controlled differentially by the hemispheres. What about the cognitive functions of these two halves of the brain? Is there a difference in the hemispheres' respective roles in integrating, processing, and computing information?

It has long been recognized that aphasia usually occurs with damage to the left hemisphere and that people with right brain damage usually escape it. Thus, language appears to be a function of the left hemisphere. Because language is typically localized to the left hemisphere, and because language was so prominent in Western society's beliefs about how humans think, the left hemisphere was considered to be the *dominant* hemisphere for many years. There was the added implication that the right hemisphere was sort of a spare part, to be called into thinking operations only when the left was damaged. Further, it was believed that in left-handed people, the situation was reversed, with the left being the cognitive spare part.

Recent advances in cognitive neuroscience altered this simple view. Far from being subservient, the right hemisphere is now considered to make its own distinctive contribution to our thinking skills. Briefly, the right hemisphere is thought to play a major role in nonverbal aspects of cognition, such as visuospatial problem solving and artistic and creative mental activities. Thus, for most of us, neither hemisphere is dominant. Each is different and appears to support different types of cognitive activity.

A great deal of the research that is changing our view of brain functioning uses techniques such as functional magnetic resonance imaging (fMRI) and positron emission tomography (PET). Neuroscientists can now observe the normal and abnormal brain when it actually performs complex activities. Many of our traditional beliefs (including some that we have just mentioned), which limit particular activities to specific parts of the brain, are being challenged. A much more complex picture is beginning to emerge. For example, the right hemisphere appears to be involved in language to a greater extent than was previously thought. Even parts of the brain that were thought to play very limited roles in cognitive processing, such as the cerebellum, are often shown to be active in fMRI or PET scans, depending on the specific nature of the task. There is much more to be learned from imaging studies about how the brain does the computations that constitute language and other cognitive activities. Therefore, it is important for beginning students to be aware that we live in an unusually brisk time for research concerning the brain processes that underlie language and that this new information could change dramatically the way we understand some of the very basic concepts of our field.

Along with imaging work, studying what happens to behavior following destruction of part of the brain still is a fruitful source of information about cognitive function and the brain. But there are problems. Over 100 years ago, Hughlings Jackson, a renowned neurologist, warned that localizing a symptom is not the same thing as localizing a function. What he meant was that by interrupting an area of the normally working cortex with its complex interconnected circuitry, one also disrupts the integrity of the whole brain. The cortex probably does not physically map cognitive events; that is, there is probably not a tiny spot of cortex that controls nouns, or verbs, or other units of language. Yet it would require that sort of discrete mapping for us to conclude that, because area q, for example, was damaged and the patient could no longer produce nouns, nouns must reside in area q. Our best leads are that the brain works in the much more complex ways being demonstrated with our new imaging techniques. What we see in the cognitive behavior of a brain-damaged person is a result of how the brain adapts to the damage, and of how the remaining tissue is affected by the insult, in addition to being a manifestation of the damage itself. With brain-imaging methods, we can complement this view of behavior with a view of the adaptive brain networks themselves. We have stressed language here, but language is only one of a store of cognitive events, such as making music or doing math, reading maps, and remembering events. Jackson's warning applies to all.

The Left Cerebral Hemisphere and Aphasia

Figure 14.1 shows a lateral (side) view of the left hemisphere. The lobes of the brain are named after the bones of the skull that overlay them and are not anatomically distinct. The regions of the cortex posterior to (behind) the fissure of Rolando and above the Sylvian fissure are primarily responsible for analyzing sensations coming in from the outside world. The occipital lobe is specialized for vision, the parietal for somatic sensory analysis, and the temporal lobe for audition. The area directly anterior to (in front of) the fissure of Rolando initiates movement. The functions of the areas even more forward in the frontal lobe are more subtle and harder to describe. Both right and left frontal lobes play an executive role in initiating, planning, and integrating the whole spectrum of behavior, and they receive their inputs from the three other lobes as well as some structures lying deep within the brain. The frontal lobes appear to have responsibility for directing individuals as they negotiate their environments.

Notice in Figure 14.1 that the area surrounding the Sylvian fissure is shaded. This is the general area of the left hemisphere thought to be primarily responsible for speech and language functions. Notice the portions that are even darker. The dark spot in the temporoparietal lobe is termed **Wernicke's area**. The one in the frontal lobe is called **Broca's area**. (The latter is the area of Ms. J's damage.) Each area was named for a nineteenth-century researcher who began to delimit that area's special roles in language: the German neurologist Karl Wernicke and the French physician Paul Broca, respectively. We begin our discussion of how speech and language are affected by damage to the general shaded area by discussing the posterior speech areas first and then the anterior areas.

Posterior Speech Areas   Remember that the posterior cortex is concerned with reception and analysis of stimuli from the outside world. Note that Wernicke's area lies in the temporal lobe (with its relationship to auditory stimuli), and the posterior speech region extends upward into the parietal area (where somatic sensation is integrated). Brain damage in this particular location is associated with the input of

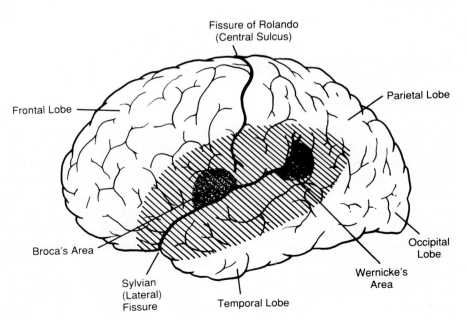

FIGURE 14.1
The left cerebral hemisphere.

language—that is, with understanding speech. Damage to Wernicke's area produces difficulties with comprehending speech and in many cases difficulties with reading as well. Still further back in the posterior language area is the place of a convergence for visual, auditory, and other sensory stimuli. Difficulties in reading, writing, naming, and so forth are associated with damage here. It is important to note that posterior brain damage does not affect the area of the brain responsible for initiating and producing speech. Thus, patients with posterior lesions speak at rather normal rates with patterns that are appropriate for their native language. Aphasiologists call the disorders associated with posterior lesions *fluent aphasias*. A variety of aphasias, depending on the location and extent of the damage that produced them, comprises fluent (posterior) aphasia syndromes. We will discuss them later. But the points emphasized here are that individuals with posterior aphasias speak fluently. Many also have difficulty with the input side of language, such as auditory and reading comprehension. Difficulties in retrieving words are also common.

Anterior Language Area   Remember that the frontal lobe is responsible for movement and its initiation. The anterior language area is thus responsible for speaking. Damage here is much less likely to interfere with comprehension; instead, it disrupts fluent, well-articulated speech. The speech of a person with Broca's aphasia is slow and labored and lacks the flow and intonation of normal speech. Aphasiologists refer to the speech patterns of anterior aphasias as *nonfluent*. Please note that for aphasia, the words *nonfluent* and *nonfluency* have different meanings than they do for stuttering. In addition to slow and labored speech, damage to the anterior language area often results in the articulatory problems and motor programming deficits that are described in Chapter 10. These two problems accompany nonfluent aphasia because the anterior language area lies adjacent to the areas of the cortex responsible for motor control of speech. The anterior language area is also near the cortical areas responsible for other motor movement. As with Ms. J, individuals with nonfluent aphasia often have an accompanying right hemiplegia. Finally, word-retrieval difficulties are common. However, the pattern and types of word-retrieval errors might differ in anterior and posterior aphasia.

Syndromes of Aphasia

Principles of Typing

We have implied already that many language variations occur in aphasic patients. These variations are often discrete and can be referred to as *syndromes*. The type of aphasic syndrome that a patient manifests is largely related to the location of the damage that produced it. It is also related to the extent of damage, age, and general health and to poorly understood neurophysiological, metabolic, and neuropharmacological dynamics that relate both to normal and to disturbed brain functioning. Here are some ground rules to keep in mind as you read about the syndromes (or types) of aphasia. First, aphasic symptoms are not bizarre or mysterious—they seem to be extreme variants of everyday occurrences. For example, all of us have misspelled a word we know well; all of us have experienced difficulty in remembering a name or a word or have heard or read something, even in our own language, that we couldn't understand. It is quite useful to keep these experiences in mind when you explore the world of aphasia.

Second, regardless of the cardinal symptoms, people with aphasia have some basic underlying problems with two aspects of language—auditory comprehension and word retrieval. You should know that some authorities emphasize the features that are common to most aphasic patients, while others approach the analysis by identifying distinguishing characteristics. Each approach may serve a useful function in the attempt to find rules and patterns of organization that help further our imperfect understanding of the mechanisms. These differing approaches may suggest new ways to test, as well as treat, aphasic patients.

Hildred Schuell and Frederic Darley, both distinguished speech-language patholo-gists, were major proponents of the view that aphasic patients' similarities are more important than their differences. They viewed aphasia as a unitary disturbance of lan-guage. Schuell and Darley's work, which emphasized the role of auditory comprehen-sion in aphasia, is of enormous rehabilitative significance and will be discussed in detail later. While acknowledging the impact and importance of this point of view, we must also acknowledge our preference for a multidimensional view of aphasia; that is, we prefer to differentiate symptom complexes as specifically as possible. Even among workers who prefer to describe aphasia multidimensionally, different terminology and differing points of view exist. Rather than discouraging you by these inconsistencies so early in your study of aphasia, we wish only to alert you to the problem. We use the ter-minology of Geschwind, Goodglass, and their coworkers because of its currency in the United States. Because aphasia is a language disorder rather than a speech disorder, it is appropriate to describe details about other language modalities in addition to spoken language. Therefore, relevant details of speaking, comprehending, reading, writing, and repeating are included in the following discussion of aphasia syndromes.

Finally, as we have seen, lesions involving the posterior portions of the left hemi-sphere (temporal-parietal-occipital lobes) produce fluent aphasias, and lesions involv-ing the anterior or frontal lobe produce nonfluent aphasia. This is not a law, however; some people escape aphasia altogether, even if their damage is in these regions, while others show minor language difficulty in the presence of large areas of damage. The left hemisphere is usually afflicted when aphasia occurs, even in left-handers, although right-hemisphere lesions can produce aphasia in left-handers, and even more rarely in right-handers. Finally, aphasias also occur as a result of subcortical rather than cortical brain damage. Lesions to the left thalamus or the basal ganglia, for example, have been shown to produce aphasic behaviors.

With these ground rules in mind, the following major patterns can be described.

Fluent Aphasias

Wernicke's Aphasia   Individuals with Wernicke's aphasia speak fluently and often excessively, a condition sometimes referred to as *press of speech*. The speech of such a patient often lacks content; in the most severe cases, spoken output is composed of incomprehensible and incoherent utterances that are fluent, well articulated, and phonologically correct and are known as **jargon**. The unsophisticated listener often initially mistakes the fluent output of the individual with Wernicke's aphasia for nor-mal speech. Even for those whose speech is jargon, the prosody of the native language is maintained, and to a large extent, the speaker's jargon observes the sound-combining rules of the native language. She shows reduced ability to comprehend not only the speech of others, but often her own speech as well. In most of the more common types of aphasia, reading and writing abilities are similar to the auditory comprehension and speech patterns on which they are built. The person with Wernicke's aphasia is a good example: Reading, especially reading aloud, is often poor, but occasionally, a person with Wernicke's aphasia may have better preserved reading comprehension than his oral reading might suggest. This feature is a useful cornerstone on which treatment can be built. The mechanics of handwriting are minimally affected (hemiplegia is usually absent in this type of aphasia); however, the content of writing is disturbed.

Repetition, as we will see, is often a sensitive diagnostic sign regarding the nature of the aphasic syndrome. In the case of the individual with Wernicke's aphasia, her repetition skills are impaired as a result of the comprehension impairment. In fact, one can derive a clue about what a patient with Wernicke's aphasia might be hearing by listening to what she says in her repetition attempts.

Here is an example of Wernicke speech from Gardner (1975) in response to the question, *What brings you to the hospital?*

> Boy, I'm sweating, I'm awful nervous, you know once in a while I get caught up. I can't mention the tarripoi, a month age, quite a little, I've done a lot well, I impost a lot, while on the other hand, you know what I mean. I have to run around, look it over, trbbin and all that sort of stuff. (p. 68)

Anomic Aphasia   Another fluent aphasia is called *anomic aphasia*. Individuals with anomic aphasia have otherwise almost normal language, but it is marred by word-retrieval difficulties. Auditory and reading comprehension is usually near normal, but the inability to produce substantive words is also evident in writing. When the word that the anomic person is searching for is furnished, she usually recognizes it immediately and can take advantage of it momentarily. Thus, her repetition is usually better than her spontaneously produced speech. Word-retrieval problems that typify anomic aphasia are common to all aphasias, but only in these patients are they the salient symptom. Word-retrieval problems allow us to speculate about the role of memory in the generation of aphasic problems. Although aphasia can hardly be explained as a language-specific memory loss, verbal memory plays a role in aphasia, and some likely memory difficulties often coexist.

Here is an example of a person with anomic aphasia. He is describing a busy scene from a picture in the Boston Diagnostic Aphasia Examination (Goodglass & Kaplan, 1983) in which a little boy and girl are stealing cookies. The boy is standing on a stool about to topple, and their mother is serenely washing dishes, oblivious both to the cookie theft and to the fact that her sink is overflowing.

> This is a boy an' that's a boy an' that's a . . . thing! (Laughs). An' this is goin' off pretty soon (points to toppling stool). This is a . . . a place that this is mostly in (Examiner: "Could you name the room . . . a bathroom?") No . . . kitchen . . . kitchen. An' this is a girl . . . an' that something that they're running an' they've got the water going down here . . . (p. 86)

Conduction Aphasia   *Conduction aphasia* is another fluent aphasia syndrome in which comprehension of language is high, but speech is frequently marred by inappropriate words. The majority of these inappropriate words are the result of the speaker's inclusion of incorrect sounds in words; for example, calling someone named Suzie, "Satie," or incorrectly ordering the sounds in words—calling Suzie, "Seezu." Errors such as these are called *literal* or *phonemic paraphasias*. Other errors include the use of inappropriate words (*table* for *chair*) and are called *verbal* or *semantic paraphasias*. In the rare patient with severe conduction aphasia, these sorts of errors can occur frequently enough to result in spoken output that is incomprehensible to the listener. Since the individual with conduction aphasia has good comprehension and is aware of these errors, she makes frequent and often unsuccessful self-correction attempts. The hallmark of this syndrome is a disproportionate inability to repeat or make use of verbal cues supplied by others. Reading and writing are usually good in conduction aphasia. Here is an example of a person with conduction aphasia describing the cookie-theft picture.

> Well, this um . . . somebody's . . . ah mathher is takin the . . . washin' the dayshes an' the water . . . the water is falling . . . is flowing all over the place, an' the kids sneakin' out in back behind her, takin' the cookies in the . . . out of the top in the . . . what do you call that? (Examiner: "Shelf?") Yes . . . and there's a . . . then the girl . . . not the girl . . . the boy who's getting the cookies is on this ah . . . strool an' startin' to fall off. That's about all I see. (Goodglass & Kaplan, 1983, p. 90)

Nonfluent Aphasias

Broca's Aphasia   *Broca's aphasia* is the more common of the two nonfluent aphasias. It is characterized by paucity of speech, difficulties in word retrieval, and a labored and slow rate of speech. Individuals with this disorder often omit small grammatical elements such as *the*, *is*, and *on* and word endings such as *-ing*, *-s*, and *-ed*. This condition is called **agrammatism**.

Comprehension of spoken and written language is surprisingly better than an individual's spoken output would suggest. Repetition is marred by the fluency problems, and writing mirrors the speech output. The mechanics of writing are also impaired because most patients with Broca's aphasia also have right-arm and -leg paralysis. They must often learn to use the left hand for writing. Here is an example of the speech of a person with Broca's aphasia:

Q.   What happened to make you lose your speech?

A.   Head, fall. Jesus Christ, me no good, str, str ... oh Jesus ... stroke.

Q.   I see. Could you tell me what you've been doing in the hospital?

A.   Yes, sure, me go er up P. T. nine o'cot, speech two times . . . read . . . wr . . . ripe, er, rike, er, write . . . practice . . . getting better. (Goodglass & Kaplan, 1983, p. 61)

Mixed and Global Aphasia

The majority of aphasia cases result from lesions that encompass both the anterior and the posterior speech areas. The result is likely to be a mixed or global aphasia. The distinction between mixed and global aphasia is a practical one, typically made on the basis of the severity of the presenting problems. *Mixed aphasia* usually refers to aphasia that involves both comprehension and production, but is not more than moderately severe. *Global aphasia* refers to severe comprehension and production deficits. Global aphasia produces the scarcity of speech typical of nonfluent aphasia and the difficulties with comprehension typical of the Wernicke patient. Often global-aphasic individuals have only a few utterances available to them, and these are used both appropriately and inappropriately. They are called *stereotypys*. **Stereotypys** may be real or nonsense words and phrases that are produced involuntarily and carry little, if any, meaning. We know a global-aphasic patient whose entire verbal repertoire was "weema-jeema." Both reading and writing are seriously compromised, and repetition is poor. Global aphasia is generally considered to be the most severely debilitating of the common aphasic syndromes.

Mechanisms of Aphasia

Let us turn now to the manner in which a person might become aphasic. We have been using the term *lesion* frequently in this chapter. As used here, a lesion is an injury that leaves an area of cortical tissue incapable of functioning in its normal way. Brain tissue may be destroyed directly, as in the case of a wound resulting from a bullet. It may be rendered incapable of functioning because other tissues push on it and distort it in some way, as when a tumor grows into or displaces the brain. And tissue may die as the result of an infectious process or as the result of being denied the nourishment necessary to its healthy function, usually by interruption of the blood supply.

We mentioned earlier that a stroke is by far the most common cause of aphasia. *Stroke* is the term used by physicians to describe the abnormal neurologic function that occurs when a brain artery is blocked and blood can no longer nourish a given part of the brain. Figure 14.2 shows the arteries that feed the left cerebral hemisphere. Note especially the area supplied by the middle cerebral artery. Because its territory encompasses the speech areas we have been discussing, it is easy to see that problems with this artery are frequently responsible for aphasia-producing strokes.

Strokes are of three basic types: (1) thrombotic, (2) embolic, and (3) intracerebral hemorrhage. In thrombotic strokes, a buildup of plaque blocks a vessel, which then thromboses (clots). An embolic stroke results when a clot, or thrombosis, forms elsewhere—perhaps the heart or blood vessels of the chest or neck—and breaks off to become an embolus (clot) that may then be carried to a brain artery. Such an embolus often arises from a location in the carotid artery in the neck—a site predisposed to blockage and embolus formation. Since the basic processes are the same, the term *thromboembolic stroke* is sometimes used to describe these two types. Hemorrhages are

FIGURE 14.2
Blood supply to the left cerebral hemisphere.

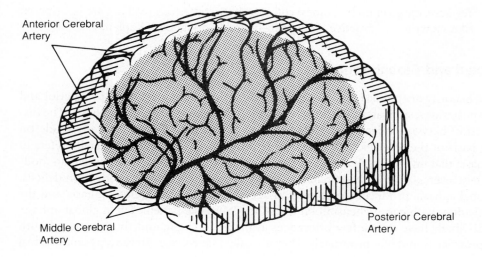

Anterior Cerebral Artery

Middle Cerebral Artery

Posterior Cerebral Artery

different. Arterial walls, weakened by the effects of high blood pressure or losing elasticity due to aging, occasionally burst under pressure. The blood rips into the brain tissue, dissecting it and causing intense inflammation and swelling.

Another cause for hemorrhage that is less common, but that may occur in young adults as well as in older individuals, is the rupture of aneurysms. These are blisterlike balloonings of arteries occurring at vessel branch points. They develop through early adult life. When aneurysms rupture, they often bleed into the fluid-filled space surrounding the surfaces of the brain. Although bleeding into this space may damage the brain or even cause death, it is only when the bleeding is directly into the brain tissue itself that characteristic stroke syndromes like aphasia are likely. Even less common is bleeding into the brain from abnormal arterial and venous tangles of vessels occasionally present from birth—called an *arteriovenous malformation.*

Why does localized rather than more general damage to the brain occur in the stroke process? Shouldn't the whole cortex, beyond the point of disruption, be affected by arterial occlusion? You can answer this question by referring again to Figure 14.2. Note the rich intertwining of the vascular tree and the possibilities it affords for developing secondary pathways. The complexity of the vascular network also helps to explain the differences in both extent and severity of damage and the variability of symptoms we find in individuals with aphasia. Part of this variability is due to how effective alternative routes are in supplying an individual's cortex with blood.

At the beginning of this section, we mentioned other causes for aphasia, including trauma to the head and tumors. While damage to the speech areas by injury can certainly occur and tumors can grow in such a way as to put pressure directly on the speech areas, it is quite likely in these cases that other cortical areas are also damaged. With progressive neurologic disorders and infectious disease, more-generalized cortical involvement is the most typical result. Thus, while aphasic symptoms are found in these conditions, many other changes in cortical function are almost always present as well. Describing the person with traumatic brain injury (TBI) or the postencephalitic person as aphasic is often likely to be inaccurate; disturbances in language complicated by generalized brain damage often produce a more complicated problem than does aphasia occurring as the result of a focal brain lesion.

Bilingual and Multilingual Aphasia

When it occurs in individuals who speak more than one language, aphasia presents intriguing problems, most of which remain unsolved. For example, how language is represented in the bilingual brain is not thoroughly understood, thereby complicating the aphasia picture. Some researchers have argued that the language first learned is best recovered; others say that the language most used, regardless of when learned, recovers best. In the pluralistic society in which we live, these issues loom large for speech-language pathologists. For example, even the relatively rare clinician who is bilingual in the same languages as a particular patient may have few leads about which language should be the focus of treatment or whether something is to be gained by treating both. Further, the question of how to work with patients for whom English is weak presents real barriers to effective intervention. There is a great need for bilingual clinicians, as well as for clinicians who have been well trained in multicultural issues across the profession, but probably nowhere more urgently than for those who intervene in aphasia.

The Person with Aphasia

We know a great deal more about aphasia than we do about people with aphasia. In recent years, however, many clinicians and researchers, as well as aphasic individuals and their families, have begun to change this picture. Growing awareness of the effects of chronic aphasia on the quality of life, the growth of consumer advocacy groups such as the National Aphasia Association, and recognition by the World Health Organization (WHO) of the personal and societal consequences of many disorders (including aphasia) all have begun to shift the focus away from the impairment itself and onto how to live with aphasia.

At the beginning of courses in aphasia, we often ask students to describe how they would react if injury or illness resulted in their becoming aphasic. Frequently, students attempt to advance the problem in time to some future date when they are older. This suggests that students (like their teachers) have some fear of the problem. When asked to retry the task, the expected descriptions begin to emerge. Students commonly use words like *afraid*, *frustrated*, *angry*, *anxious*, *depressed*, *crazy*, *stupid*, and *useless*. The list goes on, mostly in the same vein, never getting more optimistic than the wistful word *challenged*. We believe students' initial reticence and final descriptions of their responses to aphasia are similar to what aphasic patients themselves first feel. Once they have discovered their own survival, the devastating effects of aphasia begin to emerge.

Our own most precious skills, often unappreciated and taken for granted, include our ability to communicate our needs and wants to others and our power to present ourselves to and affect others by our words. When these skills are suddenly withdrawn or limited, a person becomes less powerful. One's self-concept is threatened and/or seriously compromised. It is important to understand these reactions to a language problem. Even though these reactions may lessen with the passage of time and with learning to make adjustments, they are a formidable aspect of aphasia and must be dealt with in therapeutic interactions, particularly in the early stages of recovery.

In addition to the patient's reaction to language loss, there are other factors to contend with in the aftermath of stroke. We have already mentioned the likelihood of sensory and motor problems, particularly hemianopsia and hemiplegia. In the case of hemiplegia, a person's loss of mobility may pose a seemingly insurmountable obstacle to returning to normal life. Even the person who escapes aphasia after stroke perhaps has to learn to get around in a wheelchair, use a cane and a leg brace, or use her left hand for eating, dressing, and writing and faces some amount of depression and fear.

Brain damage often subtly changes some aspects of a person's cognition regardess of aphasia. Included among these changes are tendencies to think more concretely—that is, more literally—than previously, to be more sensitive to emotional events than before, to lose some initiative, or even to be less inhibited. Other effects of brain damage may possibly be some **agnosia** (loss of the ability to perceive, integrate, and attach meaning to incoming stimuli) or **apraxia** (loss of the ability to progam, plan, sequence, or initiate movement). Many people speculate, but there is little hard evidence concerning the overall effects of aphasia on a person's personality. My own experience is that aphasia does not produce many personality changes; rather, it tends to exaggerate a person's cognitive and social style.

Aphasia is a problem that actually affects a whole family. It takes its toll not only on the aphasic person, but also on those around him, primarily because it seriously disrupts a family's sense of balance and requires a restructuring of familiar family roles. Financial changes and role reassignments may be the most obvious, but other roles may be affected as well. Clinicians must know something about the aphasic individual's culture and family structure before aphasia. This will provide greater insight into the *family* nature of the problem. Webster and Larkins (1979) report four family problems to be paramount: (1) the nonaphasic spouse has no time alone, (2) finances, (3) getting used to the new roles that aphasia creates for both spouses, and (4) finding ways to deal with the issue of dependence/independence for the aphasic spouse. Rehabilitation involves helping the family members to work through their feelings. It is also necessary to mobilize other members of the community to help the family in the restructuring of roles and responsibilities that may be required in the wake of aphasia. Finally, for both the aphasic person and the family, it is important to remember that aphasia does not occur only to previously well-adjusted people and families. It occurs to people who have the same chances as the rest of us for having unresolved personal, financial, social, and family problems. And aphasia cures none of them. It merely adds another dimension to them.

We have been stressing, up to this point, the darker side of aphasia—there is a brighter side. We find work with aphasic patients and their families to be most rewarding. If aphasic individuals work through their earliest reactions successfully, they often have an impressive tenacity for solving their own problems. Such persons permit their clinicians to see the basic strength and ability to rise to a challenge that dignifies us all. In many encounters with such patients, it is possible to have an almost constant awareness of the indomitability of the human spirit. Perhaps the best summary of this can be found in the words of the husband of a remarkable aphasic woman:

> When she first got her problem, we [the family] were real scared and we all helped out too much. Then we got angry at her because she needed the help. We finally worked all that out, due to her. I really didn't know who I was married to 'til she became aphasic. I thought she was a nice, passive housewife. Instead, she is this tough, gutsy, talented, independent person. It's not at all bad.

This quote is from the husband of the real person on whom Ms. J's story was based.

The Natural Recovery Process in Aphasia

Immediately following stroke, aphasia is at its worst. This is related to the severity of the event and to the extent of brain damage incurred. Within a few days, however, the natural recovery process gets under way. Swelling begins to reduce, and some injured cells begin to function more normally again. A clearer picture of the residual damage begins to emerge. Nonetheless, in the early few weeks after damage, it is difficult to predict the course and the degree of a patient's recovery.

Natural recovery is influenced by a number of factors, including age, general physical condition, the extent and location of brain damage, and to some extent the quality of care he receives. Despite these uncertainties, we may be sure that some improvement will occur as the repair process continues for some months. This naturally occurring improvement is called **spontaneous recovery**. It is most rapid soon after the onset of brain damage; as time progresses, the rate of change slows down. Spontaneous recovery occurs not only for speech and language, but for other cognitive, motor, and sensory abilities as well.

During the period of spontaneous recovery, the whole presenting syndrome may evolve into another, usually milder, form of aphasia. The most likely expectation of evolution is with global aphasia, which may evolve into any of the other types of aphasia that we discussed. For example, at 1 week poststroke, Ms. J had a mild-to-moderate Broca's aphasia that evolved into anomic aphasia by 1 year poststroke. Although there is some controversy over just how long the period of spontaneous recovery continues, most changes occur during the initial 2 months. The degree to which they continue is likely to depend on a variety of individual factors.

There is also controversy over when formal speech and language intervention should begin. The traditional view is that therapy should be initiated as early as possible to take advantage of spontaneous recovery. However, changes in chronic aphasia are increasingly being reported. In addition, so that changes are not attributable to spontaneous recovery, new treatment techniques are validated using aphasic patients whose period of spontaneous recovery is long past. This makes a strong case for late, as well as early, intervention.

The Assisted Recovery Process in Aphasia

Successful rehabilitation in aphasia is essentially interdisciplinary, requiring cooperation among medical and paramedical specialists. The optimal team includes a neurologist, a psychiatrist, a physiatrist, physical and occupational therapists, a neuropsychologist, a social worker, and a speech-language pathologist.

Evaluation

Before undertaking treatment, the speech-language pathologist conducts a detailed evaluation. The first goal of evaluation is to determine if clinical intervention is feasible. The case history is one of the most important features of the evaluation, but more direct assessment of language is also critical. This direct assessment includes detailed analysis of the aphasic patient's language performance, aimed at defining and describing the type of aphasia the patient has and measuring the extent of auditory comprehension and/or motor programming deficits. It also includes identification of other disorders that can co-occur along with aphasia. Motor speech disorders such as apraxia of speech and dysarthria are identified as well. The speech-language pathologist must also check for signs of dysphagia, or swallowing disorder. When dysphagia is present, speech-language pathologists are typically responsible for its treatment as well (see Chapter 16.)

The formality of the initial evaluation will be directly related to how long after brain damage the evaluation is made. Early evaluation tends to be less structured and often relies on observation of the individual at bedside. Table 14.1 provides an example of a brief bedside assessment and a guide for determining the type of aphasia and location of lesion. After the aphasic patient's condition has stabilized, observation is supplemented with formal tests of language ability and comprehension of speech, reading, and writing. Among the more common tests used by speech-language pathologists are the Porch Index of Communicative Abilities (PICA; Porch, 1967), the Boston

TABLE 14.1   A Guide for Evaluating and Labeling Aphasia

Get a sample of each of the following:

1. Ability to comprehend spoken language
   a. Does the patient appear to follow the conversation?
   b. Ask the patient to follow one-, two-, and three-stage commands. For example,
      "Point to the ceiling and then to the door."
      "Put an X on this paper, fold it in half, and give it to me."
   c. Ask the patient a few yes/no questions. For example,
      "Are the lights on in the room?"
      "Do helicopters eat their young?"
2. A conversational speech sample
   a. Check for fluency. Does it sound like normally spoken English, even if it is not comprehensible? If so, the aphasia is fluent. Does it sound slow, labored, amelodic? If so, it is nonfluent.
3. Naming ability
   a. Confrontation naming: "What is this?"
   b. Associative naming: "Table and _____."
   c. Responsive naming: "Where do you buy stamps?"
   d. Using names: "Who is president?" "What is your favorite TV show?"
4. Repetition
   a. "Aluminum."
   b. "Muff, earmuff, muffler, muffin tin."
   c. "The dog chewed a bone."
   d. "Three plus six equals nine."
   e. "The Chinese fan had a rare emerald."

Labeling and Localizing

1. Up to 40% of all aphasias are mixed or global. On a probability basis alone, you can guess that the aphasia is one of these. Although any lesion may produce a mixed aphasia, larger lesions affecting anterior and posterior regions are associated with intractible global aphasias.
2. If speech is fluent, the patient likely has a posterior lesion. If comprehension is good, the type may be anomic. If comprehension is poor, it is Wernicke's.
3. If speech is nonfluent, the patient likely has an anterior lesion. If comprehension is good, the patient likely has Broca's aphasia.
4. If repetition is disproportionately worse than performance on the other three tasks, then the aphasia is conduction. Location of lesion is posterior—possibly in the arcuate fasciculus.
5. If repetition is disproportionately better than performance on the other three tasks, then the aphasia is transcortical sensory or transcortical motor. The lesion is located outside of the perisylvian area.

Diagnostic Aphasia Examination (BDAE; Goodglass, Kaplan, & Barresi, 2001), the Western Aphasia Battery (WAB; Kertesz, 1982), and the Aphasia Diagnostic Profile (ADP; Helm-Estabrooks, 1992).

These tests all sample aphasia at what the WHO refers to as the "impairment" level. That is, they provide a snapshot of basic language skills, not how those skills might be used in actual communication. As such, they are useful in disentangling what might be causing a particular patient to have difficulty in communicating and provide an inventory against which subsequent treatment might be measured.

Different measures are used to assess what effects these basic impairments are likely to have on everyday communication. (These types of tests measure how the impairments constrain functioning.) One such measure is Communicative Activities of Daily Living (CADL-2; Holland, Frattali, & Fromm, 1999) Rating scales are also used to judge communication skills rather than language performance. An example is the Functional Assessment of Communicative Skills (ASHA FACS; Frattali, Thompson, Holland, Wohl, & Ferketic, 1995). Finally, scales that look to quality of life and burden, for both aphasic individuals and spouses, are beginning to emerge. Two examples are the Burden of Stroke Scale (BOSS; Doyle, 2002) and the Quality of Communicative Life scale (QCL; D. Paul, Frattali, Holland, Thompson, Caperton, & Slater, 2004). Measures such as these represent the WHO's concern not only with the effect of an impairment on daily activities, but also on how activity constraints affect one's ability to function in society.

Finally, special tests are sometimes used with aphasic individuals as well. The Psycholinguistic Assessment of Language Processing in Aphasia (PALPA; Kay, Lesser, & Coltheart, 1992) is a good example. The PALPA provides detailed information about the processing of minimal language units.

Treatment

Treatment for people with aphasia, as currently practiced in the United States, is a relatively new field. It had its beginning during World War II, with the impetus being the large number of head-injured military survivors. In 1951, Wepman wrote a careful description of these intensive rehabilitation efforts, and his work is still influential. Such early efforts developed the model of treatment for American aphasiology that is still in effect today.

All the evaluation information is brought into play in determining the exact nature of and goals for clinical intervention. Although planning rehabilitation is dictated mostly by the extent of the impairment, other aspects of the patient's lifestyle, motivation, medical needs, and so on are also important. Techniques and goals for treatment will differ for a person with global aphasia and for a person whose residual language deficits are minimal. In the ideal case, these goals are made clear, set, and mutually agreed on by the aphasic person, his family, and the speech-language pathologist.

Approaches to aphasia rehabilitation can be characterized as *restorative*, *compensatory psychosocial*. All these general approaches provide many specific clinical techniques that can be used to improve language and communication in aphasia. They also commonly rely on the fact that the damaged brain remains capable of learning and adapting. As a result, practice is an important part of aphasia treatment. We are not able to specify with certainty how learning and adaptation actually occur in the brain as a function of treatment. Nevertheless, cognitive neuroscience, as well as the growing sophistication of neuroimaging techniques, is beginning to further our understanding in this regard. Also to date, no pharmacological treatments for aphasia have proven efficacious, although a number of drugs continue to be investigated. The following sections will provide examples and rationales for all these treatment approaches.

Restorative Approaches   When clinicians use restorative techniques, they are counting on the ability of the brain to recover some of its previous skills, possibly by some form of cortical reorganization within the damaged hemisphere, or by increased involvement of the undamaged hemisphere. Restorative techniques are broad in scope and range from approaches that emphasize underlying processes such as memory or auditory comprehension to practical practice of specific abilities rendered difficult by aphasia. For example, Helm-Estabrooks, Fitzpatrick, and Barresi (1982) developed a technique for use with globally aphasic individuals called visual action therapy (VAT). VAT is a carefully sequenced series of activities designed to help the patient reestablish representational behavior. Patients are trained to use gestures to represent objects. VAT is a silent technique—neither patient nor clinician talks as its steps are performed. Patients profit not only by learning some iconic gestures, but by improving auditory comprehension as well. This latter improvement, since the treatment is silent, underscores the notion that training in a basic process (in this case, reestablishing a system of representation) generalizes to other behaviors.

One technique that specifically appears to recruit the undamaged hemisphere is melodic intonation therapy (MIT; Sparks, Helm, & Albert, 1974). This approach capitalizes on aphasic individuals' usually unimpaired ability to sing or intone (both thought to be activities that occur in the nonlanguage-dominant hemisphere). MIT is most effective with individuals who have Broca's aphasia. The person is taught to intone words and phrases, and gradually intonation is faded out toward more normal speech prosody. Some approaches are directed specifically to impaired sentence processing. Among the most promising recent approaches is that of Thompson, Shapiro, Kiran, and Sobecks (2003) in which complex structures are used for training, with generalization to simpler forms resulting. This approach, called the complexity account of treatment efficacy (CATE), has also used training with rare nouns to generalize to more common ones (Kiran & Thompson, 2003).

Many approaches to helping aphasic persons retrieve words have been developed, and drills designed to train people in regaining former language skills have been described. One example is training people to use a well-practiced telephone script for getting help in emergencies (Holland & Hopper, 1998). Another example is constraint induced language therapy (CILT), an approach originally developed for the treatment of arm paralysis that has been modified for treatment of aphasic naming problems with promising results (Maher et al., 2006; Pulvermüller et al., 2001).

Finally, treatment involving computer use (both restorative and compensatory) is equally promising, with techniques ranging from simple drill and practice of difficult scirpts (Cherney, Halper, Holland, & Cole, 2008) grammatical structures derived from the work of Thompson et al. (2003) described earlier.

Compensatory Approaches   Aphasia treatment seldom produces full recovery from aphasia, and much of the work of clinicians is geared to lessening problems or finding ways to circumvent them. This is the territory for compensatory solutions to aphasia. The goals for compensatory approaches are to develop and train alternative approaches to circumvent the language skills that have been affected by aphasia. In using them, clinicians are counting on the brain's ability to learn alternative ways to negotiate in a communicating world and to learn to use other, often nonverbal, forms of communication. Compensatory approaches include teaching aphasic individuals to use a relatively intact language skill (say, writing or drawing) to substitute for talking. A specific technique is called promoting aphasic communication effectiveness (PACE; G. A. Davis & Wilcox, 1981, 1985). Using a controlled analogue to the give and take of everyday requesting, the aphasic person is required to transmit information to another person using a variety of communication strategies, including gestures and writing. The effectiveness of these communications is measured simply by whether or not a naïve listener understands what the message is, regardless of its form of communication. Some clinicians teach the use of communication boards or simple augmentative devices where they are appropriate. Some approaches concentrate on conversational partners, teaching them how to communicate in such a way as to increase the effectiveness of the aphasic person's attempt. One particularly effective approach is supported conversation for aphasia (SCA; Kagan, 1998). Conversational coaching is similar, but it simultaneously provides training for both the aphasic individual and a partner (Hopper, Holland, & Rewega, 2002).

Psychosocial Approaches   All of the above examples involve one-to-one treatment for aphasic individuals by speech-language pathologists. Such treatment should always be accompanied by some form of psychosocial involvement of families and individuals with aphasia. It is important to point out that group treatment for aphasia has been shown to be effective, not only as an accompaniment to individual treatment, but also as a primary mechanism for positive change (Elman & Bernstein-Ellis, 1999). Group work in aphasia is grounded in the notion that groups provide strong psychosocial support. Indeed, consideration of the psychosocial needs of aphasic persons and their families is perhaps the most rapidly growing change in the aphasia treatment landscape; aphasia centers and programs, both small and large, are being developed. In addition to conversation groups and special interest activities, programs in most such centers are designed to train others to be effective communicative partners, and programs to help families adjust are often included. In most instances, these programs are staffed by speech-language pathologists, which makes knowing about them important.

Efficacy of Treatment

It is not enough for us to believe that aphasia treatment is beneficial. For ethical reasons, we must demonstrate that treatment works. Third-party reimbursers require us to demonstrate it as well. There is a large database concerning the effects of treatment. The evidence suggests that intervention for people with aphasia is useful. The data come from many sources: large, well-designed, and carefully controlled studies as well as smaller studies grouped together. These smaller studies can be examined using two approaches: meta-analysis and systematic reviews. Robey (1998) examined studies of small groups of participants using meta-analysis and concluded that treatment in general is valuable. Beeson and Robey (2006, 2008) reached similar conclusions for single-subject studies. Systematic reviews are less well known, but are beginning to be used in aphasia treatment research. CILT has recently undergone such a review that found positive effects for individuals with anterior lesions. A systematic review is currently under way to evaluate partner training. All of this work does not mean that all treatment is effective, and there are more questions that demand attention, such as timing and intensity of treatment and which treatments work best with which persons. The field of aphasiology continues to have a responsibility to demonstrate the value of treatment for aphasia.

Related Disorders

Traumatic Brain (TBI) Injury in Adults

Symptom Pattern   Although cerebral trauma may occur at any age, adolescents and young adults are at greatest risk. The mechanism of injury is a blunt blow to the head that most often is associated with a motor vehicle accident. Unlike stroke, TBI is nonfocal. Many areas of the brain may be compromised as a result of primary damage (bruises, lacerations) or secondary damage (swelling, increased pressure). What results is a diverse conglomeration of motor, sensory, and behavioral deficits. Although aphasic syndromes are rare, cognitive-linguistic impairments are common. Attentional problems and difficulties with concentration often result in reduced auditory comprehension. Memory and learning disturbances may be associated with word-finding problems, while poor organizational skills may result in disorganized verbal expression. Decreased inhibition and errors of judgment may also have an effect on the pragmatics of language. For example, individuals may swear or laugh inappropriately, talk excessively, interrupt others while they are talking, or be unable to maintain a topic of conversation.

Diagnosis and Treatment   Recovery following TBI differs from stroke recovery. Individuals with closed-head injury evolve through distinctive stages of recovery and require ongoing diagnosis of their cognitive-communicative deficits. There are few assessment batteries specifically designed to evaluate the individual with TBI. Rather, the speech-language pathologist uses portions of language and neuropsychological test batteries to assess attention, perception, concentration, verbal and nonverbal memory, language, problem-solving, and a variety of other intellectual skills. Performance typically depends on the stage of recovery.

Hagen (1981) described an eight-stage recovery scale, the Rancho Los Amigos (RLA) Hospital's Levels of Cognitive Recovery, that is widely used today. During the early stages (RLA 2–3), the individual begins to respond to the environment. Treatment consists of sensorimotor stimulation with the goal of increasing recognition of objects, people, and events. During the middle stages (RLA 4–6), sensorimotor stimulation may have to be muted to reduce the individual's agitation. Highly structured therapy sessions should focus on reducing confusion, increasing orientation and goal-directed behavior, and improving memory. In therapy, specific language tasks might include listening to increasingly long and complex language samples; following directions; describing objects, events, people, and places; defining words; classifying ideas according to a theme; and improving the organization of conversational speech. During the late stages (RLA 7–8+), the goal is for patients to reach their maximum level of independence. Treatment is designed to help the individual compensate for residual deficits, which may include word-finding difficulties; problems with comprehension of complex materials; shallow reasoning and problem solving; memory disturbances; impulsive and socially awkward behavior; and impairments in goal setting, inhibiting, self-monitoring, and self-evaluation (Ylvisaker & Feeny, 1998). Treatment may also focus on improving the efficiency of language processing in real-life and stressful situations.

Given the diffuse damage associated with TBI, the swallowing function may also be compromised. Dysphagia evaluation and treatment may be part of the diagnostic and therapeutic process.

Right-Hemisphere Disorders (RHD)

Symptom Pattern   Unlike the symptoms of aphasia, the symptoms of RHD may be difficult to detect during an initial, casual encounter with an individual with RHD. One might have the impression that the person has an optimistic response to stroke, only to discover in subsequent encounters that the patient has an unrealistic appraisal of her deficits. For example, she may minimize or deny the existence of left hemiplegia and refuse to participate in physical or occupational therapy. She may be disoriented and confused about what has happened. The individual with RHD may not appear to be concerned about her confusion.

Attentional and visuospatial disturbances have also been associated with right-hemisphere damage. One of the most fascinating is **unilateral neglect**. Patients with this condition fail to respond to stimuli that are contralateral to the side of brain damage. Although neglect may follow left-brain damage, left-side neglect (resulting from right-brain damage) is more frequent and more severe. In mild cases, persons with RHD may omit or provide little left-side detail on drawings. In more severe cases, they may ignore people and objects on their left side and may be unwilling to look in that direction, even with assistance. In addition to unilateral neglect, RHD individuals may demonstrate other visuospatial difficulties. Among the more common are difficulties reading maps, remembering familiar routes, and recognizing familiar faces.

Right-hemisphere–damaged individuals may also have communication problems. They may make aphasiclike errors on auditory comprehension, naming, repetition, and reading and writing tasks. As Tompkins (1994) points out, these deficits are not a major source of their communication impairment. Rather, individuals with RHD have difficulty in appropriately expressing and comprehending the emotional contexts of communication. Their speech lacks the normal prosody used to express sadness, surprise, confusion, elation, and disappointment. Comprehension of these prosodic features, in addition to other representations of emotion (e.g., facial expression), is also impaired. Right-hemisphere–damaged persons tend to respond to the more literal or superficial aspects of stimuli and have trouble making inferences. Thus, their communication may be filled with irrelevant, repetitious detail and lack organization and an overall theme. The following is an example of speech from a person with RHD. The patient is describing a picture from the WAB that shows a family having a picnic at the lake.

> See him flying a kite. Sitting there. Sailboat. See a guy flying a kite. Sitting by a nice big elm tree. Out in the country. A guy in overalls, he's sitting in a barge in a boat or in a schooner out ready for arrival taking in a boatride headed for down toward the river somebody flying a kite. Man, woman, and child. Two of 'em riding a river down in a boat. Boy might have a place set out to eat.

Diagnosis and Treatment   The Rehabilitation Institute of Chicago Evaluation (RICE; Burns, Halper, & Mogil, 1985) includes tasks for assessing visual scanning and tracking, writing, pragmatic communication, and metaphorical language in right-hemisphere dysfunction in addition to ratings of attention, orientation, and awareness of illness. Naming, auditory comprehension, reading, and writing deficits can be captured by standardized aphasia batteries. The spontaneous speech and picture-description subtests of these batteries are also particularly useful in revealing the communication problems that characterize this population. During a picture-description task, we are interested in the abilities of individuals with RHD to use contextual cues to provide a well-organized, efficient, relevant, and coherent description. Similarly, we may also observe patients communicating with family, nursing personnel, and other rehabilitation specialists to assess the pragmatics of their communication.

In treating individuals with RHD, we may work initially on improving attention and orientation. Tasks that emphasize visuospatial perception may also be included to aid reading and writing abilities. Tasks that focus on the comprehension and production of emotional tone can be included as well. For example, we might ask a person to point to the face that goes with an angry voice, or sad voice, and then to produce sentences that convey similar emotions. Sequencing tasks are often effective for organization of verbal material. Persons with RHD may be asked to select critical items of a picture or story and then to specify the relationships among these items. Limits might be imposed on speaking time to help the individual avoid digression and perseveration. The clinician may also use cues to assist with eye contact, topic maintenance, and turn-taking during conversational exchanges.

Dementia and Primary Progressive Aphasia

Language disorders also occur in dementing conditions such as Alzheimer's disease (AD) and multi-infarct dementia. These dementias are among a larger group of age-related declines that result in many irreversible changes in all aspects of cognition, including language. The majority of dementias are irreversible. It is beyond the scope of this chapter to provide much detail about these conditions, but the nature of the language disorders in progressive dementias and the possible role for speech-language pathologists in their management need to be mentioned. AD is the best described dementia, so it is highlighted here. Like TBI, AD seldom has a focal point of brain damage. Rather, the disease process is diffuse and often affects many areas of the brain.

One of the frequent early signs of AD, in addition to difficulties with memory, is change in language. Some experts believe that the language of individuals in early phases of AD is essentially similar to that of persons with aphasia; others disagree. Particular difficulties in word retrieval occur, and many persons with AD demonstrate disturbed abilities to use language appropriately. As AD progresses, more and more aspects of language are affected, and in late-stage AD, many individuals are essentially mute and unresponsive to the speech of others. In these latter stages, dysphagia is often present.

With the grim prognosis of worsening language and cognition over time, whether there is a direct role for the speech-language pathologist might be questioned. However, it is apparent that speech-language pathologists can help to bolster remaining language in these individuals. For example, working to improve the communication of those who interact with AD individuals and playing a role in manipulating the environment to meet communication needs are both useful approaches. Counseling families about communication and how to promote it is also helpful.

A related disorder, in which the role of the speech-language pathologist is much clearer, is primary progressive aphasia (PPA). PPA is currently not well understood, but unlike the declines in general cognitive function and memory found in AD, individuals with PPA show initial declines only in language. Individuals with PPA have not had strokes or other diseases that could cause their language problems. Some persons with PPA eventually develop dementia, but approximately half of them do not. Counseling is an important part of managing an individual with PPA and his family. Another important aspect of management in PPA involves helping the person learn to use augmentative and alternative modes of communication early enough in the course of the disorder that they are experienced and comfortable with them before their use becomes absolutely necessary.

Summary

This chapter introduced you to the problem of aphasia in both its academic and practical aspects. We have also differentiated the disorder from related neurogenic communication disorders that result from traumatic brain injury or right-hemisphere stroke. Aphasia is a common disorder that brings many challenges to patients and their families. With the rehabilitative and supportive efforts of the speech-language pathologist, many individuals rally to regain aspects of the language they have lost, while maintaining their personal, familial, social, cultural, vocational, and recreational interests and activity levels. We hope that you, too, will be challenged to work with aphasic patients and their families and find reward in helping them achieve these goals.

case study MR. QZ

Mr. QZ suffered a stroke and when seen by the speech pathologist evidenced the following impairments and preserved abilities on each of the following evaluation tasks, as indicated on Table 14.1:

1. Ability to comprehend spoken language
   a. Mr. QZ was capable of following simple conversational speech.
   b. He could follow one- and two-stage commands, but was inconsistent on his ability to follow longer commands.
   c. His performance on yes/no questions was moderately good, but overall he appeared to have more difficulty when asked complex as opposed to simple questions.
2. A conversational speech sample
   Mr. QZ spoke fluently, but there were frequent disruptions to the flow of his speech due to his failures at retrieving words he was searching for.
3. Naming ability
   Mr. QZ had difficulty with all forms of naming (confrontation, associative, responsive) tested and difficulty using names in response to questions.
4. Repetition
   Mr. QZ's repetition ability was excellent.

QUESTIONS

1. Are you sure about what type of aphasia Mr. QZ has? What is the basis for your answer?
2. If you said yes, what type is it? If you said no, what features give you problems with assigning a type to his aphasic disorder?
3. Whether you said yes or no, what additional observations might help you to decide what is wrong with his speech?
4. Where do you think his brain damage might be located?

STUDY QUESTIONS

1. How does one become aphasic?
2. What is spontaneous recovery? What factors influence its extent?
3. List the major syndromes of aphasia and their defining characteristics.
4. Differentiate between impairment and the effects of impairment on activities of daily living and the ability to participate in society.

SELECTED READINGS

Basso, A. (2003). *Aphasia and its therapies.* New York, NY: Oxford University Press.

Brookshire, R. (2003). *An introduction to neurogenic communication disorders* (6th ed.). St. Louis, MO: Mosby.

Davis, G. A. (2000). *Aphasiology: Disorders and clinical practice.* Boston, MA: Allyn & Bacon.

Helm-Estabrooks, N., & Albert, M. L. (2004). *Manual of aphasia and aphasia therapy.* Austin, TX: Pro-Ed.

Lyon, J. (1997). *Coping with aphasia.* San Diego, CA: Singular Publishing Group.

Pound, C., Parr, S., Lindsay, J., & Woolf, C. (2000). *Beyond aphasia: Therapies for living with communication disability.* Bicester, England: Winslow.

Tompkins, C. (1994). *Right hemisphere communication disorders.* San Diego, CA: Singular Publishing Group.

Worrall, L., & Frattali, C. (2000). *Neurogenic communication disorders: A functional approach.* New York, NY: Thieme.

Ylvisaker, M., & Feeney, T. (1998). *Collaborative brain injury intervention: Positive everyday routines.* San Diego, CA: Singular Publishing Group.

WEBSITES OF INTEREST

Following are important websites for learning more about neurogenic language disorders as well as support, research, education, advocacy, and prevention of those disorders.

Aphasia and Primary Progressive Aphasia

www.aphasia.org
www.aphasiahope.org

Traumatic Brain Injury

www.biusa.org

Dementia

www.alz.org

DVDs OF INTEREST

Picturing Aphasia. A fine videotape in which aphasic people describe their problems, accompanied by pictures of their experiences, which makes this an "aphasia friendly" DVD for people with aphasia. DVD available from moresmc@aphasia.tv.

Inside Aphasia: An exploration of the problems of aphasia, and living with them, with aphasic speakers telling their stories. DVD available through the Callier Center at the University of Texas at Dallas: www.utdallas.edu/calliercenter.

Project Simple: A large videotaped collection of the variety of speech errors aphasic speakers make as well as some examples of aspects of aphasia that can make the problems of aphasic speakers clearer. Speech samples are provided that can augment your classroom understanding. Available to instructors by contacting Michael J. Flahive, Ph.D., Department of Communication Sciences and Disorders, Saint Xavier University, 3700 W. 103rd Street, Chicago, IL 60655.

Chapter FIFTEEN

Augmentative and Alternative Communication

Kathleen A. Kangas
Idaho State University

Lyle L. Lloyd
Purdue University

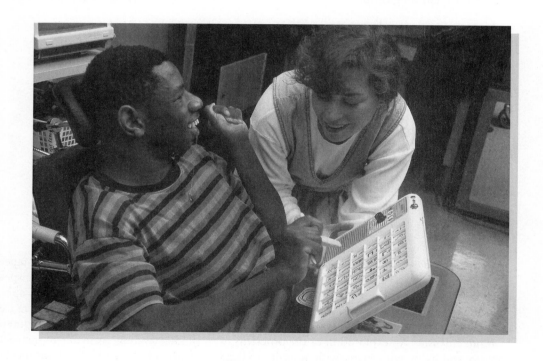

personal PERSPECTIVE

KATHLEEN A. KANGAS

My first professional experience with individuals with multiple and severe disabilities was a terrible experience for me, and it was probably only slightly more positive for my clients. I spent one-half day per week at a residential facility teaching early speech and language skills to adults with severe mental retardation. Even for those few residents who made progress on my goals, I came to feel that there was no real benefit to them in their daily lives. They continued to live in a sterile, institutional environment with little meaningful activity. I left that setting determined never again to work with individuals who had severe disabilities.

It was by accident that I later found myself working in a school-based program for children with multiple and severe disabilities. The school curriculum focused on functional and community-based activities. Teachers never asked me to expand a student's sentence structure or repertoire of phonemes. They asked me to help a student order in a restaurant, or request change in a video arcade, or comprehend instructions in a janitorial job. These requests led me to the varied materials and strategies known as augmentative and alternative communication (AAC). In this setting, I found that working with people with severe disabilities was challenging, exciting, rewarding, and fun!

Since then, my skills and experiences have expanded to include a wider range of clients, both children and adults. The individuals I see share one characteristic: Each experiences severe difficulty in communicating thoughts and ideas to other people. Communication keeps us connected and in touch with other human beings. It is the excitement of focusing on that fundamental need to communicate that continues to drive my work in AAC.

I once provided help to a man who was in the advanced stages of amyotrophic lateral sclerosis. His family later told me that on the day of his death he used the alphabet eye-gaze board I had recommended to leave his parting words of love and inspiration to his children. Moments such as these leave me speechless.

personal PERSPECTIVE

LYLE L. LLOYD

In 1956, I entered the field as a public school speech-language pathologist ("speech correctionist" in those days) and later became a school audiologist. My undergraduate professor, Wayne L. Thurman, had inspired me to do my best to meet each client's needs, to work collaboratively, to critically read the books and journals, and to be active in professional associations. His mentoring and teaching provided a foundation for meeting the professional challenges that awaited me.

In 1963, I encountered, for the first time, an individual with no functional speech. A young man with mental retardation taught me that I had much to learn about observing behavior and assessing individuals who do not speak. In 1964, I went to Parsons State Hospital and Training Center (Kansas) as Director of Audiology. In this position, I was able to critically evaluate our current practices. It was believed at that time that individuals with severe mental retardation were innately unreliable and untestable. With Joe Spradlin, Psychologist and Research Director, we were able to combine sound audiological practices and behavioral principles to obtain valid test results with individuals previously considered untestable. This was the beginning of Tangible Reinforcement and Visual Reinforcement Operant Conditioning Audiometry.

Also about that time, I first engaged in what was to become known as AAC. We were faced with a girl who could not use typical speech and language. She had attended the state school for people who are deaf, but she was transferred because she was classified as mentally retarded and was presenting behavioral problems. It was believed at that time that individuals with mental retardation could benefit little, if any, from our services. In opposition to the common mythology, we initiated a program of signing. As this young woman learned to communicate through a visual mode, she became less aggressive and revealed abilities that were previously hidden. It is not that her diagnosis was in error; she did have both severe hearing impairment and mental retardation. But she was still able to establish elaborate and reliable manual communication skills.

I had been in the field almost a decade before encountering the challenges of individuals with severe disabilities. The field has changed since then. Most speech-language pathologists now expect to encounter such clients, and our profession supports many approaches to meeting their communication needs. But the principles I gained from my first undergraduate professor are as important today as they were then. Our field continues to evolve as clinicians and researchers critically question prevailing myths and assumptions. We should continue to view new and demanding situations not as threats, but as challenges.

Potential Users of AAC

Augmentative and alternative communication (AAC) strategies are used by a wide range of individuals who may share only one common denominator: Some disability or impairment inhibits their ability to communicate through conventional means. It is important to recognize that both spoken and written communication needs may be involved. Many types of impairments, including cognitive, motor, and sensory impairments, may cause an individual to have little or no functional speech. Users of AAC may have congenital disabilities such as autism, mental retardation, or developmental apraxia of speech. Other AAC users acquire their disabilities later in life, after an experience with typical communication. Examples of acquired disabilities include brain injury due to traumatic injury or cerebral vascular accident and progressive diseases such as amyotrophic lateral sclerosis (ALS) or Parkinson's disease. These categories of potential AAC users will be discussed later in this chapter.

Prevalence

The prevalence of people with severe communication impairments is difficult to determine because a variety of disabilities may lead to a communication impairment and because there is no single reliable definition of a severe communication impairment. After reviewing existing data, Beukelman and Ansel (1995) concluded that approximately 1 percent of the general population in the United States, or a range of 0.8 to 1.2 percent, currently experiences impairments that require AAC interventions. It appears that the prevalence is lower among younger people and increases among groups of older individuals. Using population estimates and the figure of 1 percent of the population, Soto, Huer, and Taylor (1997) projected that there will be over 3 million individuals in the United States who will have disabilities requiring AAC intervention by the year 2020.

Categories of AAC

AAC is a set of strategies and methods to assist people who are unable to meet their communication needs through speech or conventional handwriting. Many of these strategies will be introduced in this chapter. The defining characteristic that places all of them under the category of AAC is that they are strategies that either are not used by most individuals or are not relied on by most individuals to meet communication needs of daily life.

The term *augmentative and alternative communication (AAC)* encompasses two aspects of practice. An augmentative communication strategy is one that is used in combination with residual speech skills and that enhances, aids, or supplements speech. For example, an individual who has speech that is difficult to understand might use a communication board to set the topic or an alphabet board to indicate the first letter of each key word. By adding these means, the person improves the intelligibility of speech. An alternative communication strategy is one that completely replaces the more typical communication mode. For example, a person might use a device that has computerized speech output to communicate the full intended message. This use is an alternative to speech.

In general, AAC techniques may be divided into two broad categories, **aided** and **unaided** (Lloyd & Fuller, 1986). Unaided techniques are those that require no additional pieces of equipment. These are techniques that use only the individual's own body as the mode of communication. One of the most common examples of this is manual signing. Gesturing, pantomiming, pointing, and using eye gaze are also unaided communication techniques. Aided strategies of communication involve some external device or equipment. These may range from a simple picture board or wallet to a complex electronic device with synthesized speech.

AAC Model

AAC may be viewed in terms of a broad communication model including (1) a sender who has the intention of communicating (e.g., a message to send or communicate); (2) a receiver who is engaged in an interaction with the sender; (3) a set or system of symbols to represent messages (e.g., feelings, requests, information); (4) a channel through which one sends the message (e.g., acoustic, optic, vibratory); (5) the broader context or environment in which the communication act is taking place; and (6) complex feedback systems within and between individuals (Lloyd, Quist, & Windsor, 1990). The success of communication depends on many factors, including the degree to which the sender and receiver share common verbal and nonverbal symbols, their cultural backgrounds, and their experience levels with combining the symbols. Although AAC basically fits into the traditional broad communication model, it entails some specialized considerations.

AAC can be modeled as a process composed of three aspects:

1. Means to represent a symbol
2. Means to select a symbol
3. Means to transmit (Lloyd et al., 1990)

Each of these three aspects may be aided or unaided (Lloyd & Fuller, 1986; Lloyd et al., 1990). Although the three aspects are discussed sequentially, they usually do not occur in this order. They are typically interactive and frequently occur concurrently.

Means to Represent

In typical communication by nondisabled individuals, meanings are represented by symbols, usually spoken or printed words. In AAC, meanings must also be represented by symbols, but often these symbols are especially designed for this type of communication. Symbols may be described as *sets* or *systems*. Furthermore, symbol systems and sets may be unaided (e.g., gestures or sign language) or aided (e.g., objects, Braille tactile alphabet or graphic symbols). Lloyd and Fuller (1986) listed 31 distinct AAC symbol sets and systems. Of these, 22 were aided and 9 were unaided.

Symbol Sets and Systems   Symbol sets are collections of symbols, in which each symbol has one or more specified meanings. Although the set may be expanded, there are no specified rules for expansion. Examples of graphic symbol sets include highly pictographic sets such as Picsyms (Carlson, 1984) and Picture Communication Symbols (PCS) (R. Johnson, 1981, 1985), which are shown in Figure 15.1. These graphics are examples of aided symbol sets. Gestures such as Amer-Ind (Skelly, 1979), a set of gestures based on American Indian hand talk, may also constitute a set. Gestures are unaided symbol sets.

Many graphic symbol sets have been produced specifically for communication boards and other picture-based communication aids. These include the Oakland Picture Dictionary (Kirstein & Bernstein, 1981), PCS (R. Johnson, 1981, 1985), Communicaid (Gethen, 1981), and Compics (Bloomberg, 1985). Some symbol sets such as Picsyms

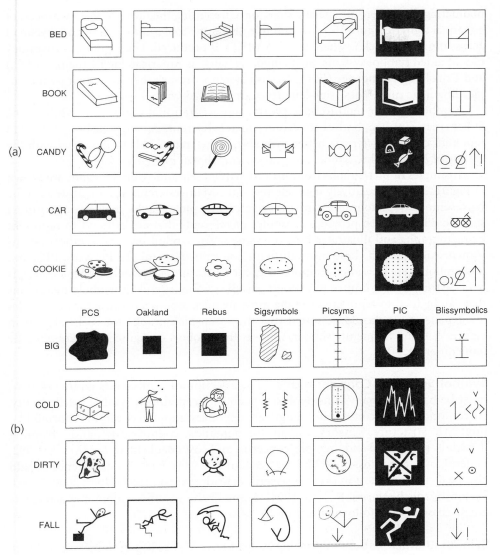

(a) — rows labeled BED, BOOK, CANDY, CAR, COOKIE

Column headers: PCS · Oakland · Rebus · Sigsymbols · Picsyms · PIC · Blissymbolics

(b) — rows labeled BIG, COLD, DIRTY, FALL

FIGURE 15.1
Examples of graphic symbols. Selected symbols are from the sets and systems of Picture Communication Symbols, Oakland Pictures, Rebus Symbols, Sigsymbols, Picsyms, Pictogram Ideogram Communication, and Blissymbolics. Figure 15.1a shows pictographs for relatively common concrete referents. Figure 15.1b shows symbols for somewhat abstract referents.
Source: Modified from Vanderheiden and Lloyd (1986).

(Carlson, 1984) and Pictogram Ideogram Communication (PIC) symbols (R. Johnson, 1981, 1985) contain ideograms as well as pictographic symbols. **Ideograms** are constructed to represent an idea, but they are not necessarily a picture of how the referent looks in the real world. For example, *big* is represented by a shapeless blob in PCS (see Figure 15.1) and by a ruled line in Picsyms, but these are not pictures of any actual object.

   Symbol systems, in contrast to sets, have a rule-governed structure, which gives them an internal consistency. When the system is expanded, the rules of the system determine how new symbols are created. Examples of rule-based graphic systems are Blissymbolics (Bliss, 1965; S. McNaughton, 1985; Wood, Storr, & Reich, 1992) and Sigsymbols (Cregan, 1980; Cregan & Lloyd, 1990). In Blissymbolics, there are approximately 100 basic elements, each with a specific meaning, such as a heart for *feeling* and a wavy line for *water*. To create a symbol for a specific concept, one combines the elements for the related ideas: For example, the heart combined with a down arrow represents *feeling down*, or *sad*, and the wavy line combined with a down arrow means *water that comes down*, or *rain*. In Sigsymbols, some of the symbols are a system based on manual signing. There are specific rules for representing the most important aspects of a manual sign. In Figure 15.1, for example, the Sigsymbol for *dirty* shows a movement across the chin, which is where the sign DIRTY is produced. These graphics are examples of aided symbol systems. Sign languages, such as American Sign Language (ASL) and British Sign Language (BSL), are also systems because they have their own complex linguistic rules. These sign languages are unaided symbol systems.

Symbol systems tend to have greater representational range than symbol sets. Systems can represent both abstract and concrete referents equally well, but sets tend to represent concrete referents better than abstract referents. This is illustrated with the variety of AAC graphic symbol sets and systems shown in Figure 15.1.

Examples of pictographs from various symbol sets and symbol systems are shown in Figure 15.1a for relatively concrete referents. Many referents are too abstract to be represented by pictographs; for other referents, pictographs may be too context specific. Figure 15.1b provides examples of referents that are difficult to represent by pictographs and illustrates how the same seven symbol sets and symbol systems shown would depict these more difficult concepts. Sigsymbols, Picsyms, PIC, and Blissymbolics are presented as approaches for representing the more difficult concepts because they are not limited to pictographs. Blissymbolics and Sigsymbols are systems that can be used to represent even the most abstract concepts because they have rules for expansion. It should be noted that the seven pictographs for each referent in Figure 15.1a are frequently similar, whereas the symbols in Figure 15.1b are typically quite different.

Symbol Selection Considerations The selection of symbol sets and/or systems must be based on many considerations such as acceptability, symbol intelligibility, correspondence to community language, openness, rapid accessibility, portability, linguistic structure, sensory and motor demands, cognitive demands, training demands, perceptual and memory concerns, and cost (Beukelman & Mirenda, 1992; Fuller, Lloyd, & Schlosser, 1992; Lloyd & Karlan, 1984). Cultural experience should also be a consideration in symbol selection (Bridges et al., 1994; Huer, 2000; Lloyd, Taylor, Buzolich, Harris, & Soto, 1994). Some of the specific symbol characteristics are discussed in the following section.

Symbol Characteristics A growing body of research has begun to investigate characteristics of the symbols used in AAC. Several studies have focused on the characteristic of iconicity, with less research on other characteristics. (See Lloyd and Fuller, 1990, for a summary.)

Iconicity refers to the degree to which a symbol resembles its referent or some aspect of the referent. For example, most people would agree that the books in most of the picture sets in Figure 15.1a look very much like a book and are, therefore, highly iconic. On the other hand, the Blissymbol for *book* looks a little like a book, so it has some degree of iconicity, but the Blissymbol for candy doesn't look like candy at all and so is low in iconicity. In paired associate learning tasks (i.e., the subject must learn to associate a symbol with a referent), iconicity has been found to be related to learning success in nondisabled children and adults and in individuals with mental retardation.

Another graphic symbol characteristic, **complexity**, was quantified by Fuller and Lloyd (1987) as the number of lines or strokes used to make up the Blissymbol. In his study of prereading preschool children, Fuller and Lloyd, 1987 found that iconicity was an important factor in learning, but that complexity appeared to play a role only when the symbol was not highly iconic. This may be because a complex symbol provides additional information and redundant morphemes, which become useful clues when iconicity cannot be relied on. Clinical observations suggest that complex manual signs may be relatively difficult to learn, but this has not been corroborated by more controlled experimental research. Although more research is needed, it is important for clinicians to realize that in some cases complex symbols are easier to learn and retain and in other cases they are more difficult.

Perceptual distinctness of symbols refers to the degree to which several symbols seem obviously different and distinct. If perceptual distinctness were low, then different symbols might easily be confused. For example, among the Blissymbols shown in Figure 15.1, the symbols for *candy* and *cookie* may appear to be the same unless one looks carefully at the details of the symbols. *Abstractness* of the concept is another characteristic that has been thought to affect symbol learning. The noun referents in Figure 15.1a are all highly concrete, whereas the adjectives and verbs in Figure 15.1b are slightly more abstract. Even more abstract would be emotional or mental concepts such as *excited, frustrated, love,* or *imagine.* Although these characteristics may be important in symbol learning, no experimental studies with AAC symbols have investigated these effects. (See Lloyd, Fuller, Loncke, and Bos, 1997, for discussion of issues relevant to the selection of aided and unaided symbols.)

Symbols should also be consistent with the cultural experience of the AAC user and the important communication partners (Bridges et al., 1994; Huer, 2000; Lloyd et al., 1994; Nakamura, Newell, Alm, & Waller, 1998). The meanings we attach to symbols are influenced by our culture. For example, the majority of children in the United States have positive associations with a frog, due in part to a character on a popular children's television show. Frogs may seem to be gentle, friendly, and kind. Similarly, for most Americans an owl is a symbol of wisdom and intelligence. However, for some Native Americans, frogs and owls are symbols of evil, and these animals are portrayed as villains in cultural myths. It would be inappropriate and insensitive to place these symbols on a communication board or device without considering the cultural implications. Gestures also have meanings and associations derived from cultural experience. A gesture that signals "OK" in some cultures may be viewed as obscene or taboo in another culture.

Means to Select

Regardless of the symbols used, the individual must have some means to select the symbols to convey a message. Selection may be aided or unaided (Lloyd et al., 1990). Selection techniques are often divided into direct selection and scanning (Quist & Lloyd, 1997; Vanderheiden & Lloyd, 1986).

Direct Selection   **Direct selection** means the individual has the ability to pick out and indicate the desired symbol from a selection of available symbols. The most common method of unaided direct selection is simply pointing to a symbol. The selection in this example is unaided; that is, individuals use only their own bodies to select the symbols, even though the symbols themselves are aided (Vanderheiden & Lloyd, 1986). Thus, the means to represent the message is aided, while the means to select the symbol is unaided.

There are other unaided selection techniques. An individual may use another body part such as the foot to select a symbol. Using eye gaze to select is also unaided. The individual might use an eye-gaze board and look at a symbol on a clear acrylic board held between the two communication partners. A user might also gaze directly at a desired object (Goossens & Crain, 1987).

Direct selection can also be aided. Some individuals use a hand splint or short dowel rod to activate keys. Pointing sticks can be used by hand, mounted on the head, or held in the mouth. These are all approaches that allow direct selection of the symbols by touching them with a device that is external to the user's body.

Electronically aided direct selection techniques use a light pointer, light sensor, or tracking device. A light pointer is much like a small flashlight: The user focuses the light on the desired selection. Although the light sensor looks much like the light pointer, the sensor is a device that receives signals rather than emitting light. When a light sensor is focused on a particular key, it reads a signal flashed by that key. The information regarding which key has been selected is then transmitted back to the device. Light pointers and light sensors are most frequently used in a head-mounted position. A more recent development for computer systems and electronic devices is the tracking device. The person wears a small reflective dot, usually on the forehead or attached to eyeglasses. A tracking device, which looks like a small camera mounted on the computer monitor or device screen, can track the head movements by sensing the reflective dot. In this way, head movements are translated to movements of the cursor on the screen.

Scanning   **Scanning** selection methods are those in which the possible choices are offered in sequence and the individual must indicate when the desired choice is offered (Quist & Lloyd, 1997; Vanderheiden & Lloyd, 1986). Commonly, **electronic scanning** devices provide a switch-operated scanning method. An example of a scanning system is shown in Figure 15.2, in which the child can select any message available on the device simply by moving his head to the right to touch the round switch plate.

Visual scanning occurs when the individual watches for the item to be indicated. **Auditory scanning** is a similar process, except that the choices are presented auditorily, and the user waits to hear the desired item (Fried-Oken & Tarry, 1985).

Partner-assisted scanning is similar to device-driven scanning, but instead of a device offering choices, the communication partner offers the choices and waits for a signal when the desired choice is offered. In visual partner–assisted scanning, the communication partner points to the possible items. In auditory partner–assisted scanning, the partner voices the options on the array.

Scanning options are generally used by people who do not have sufficient motor skill to manage a direct-selection technique. Scanning is generally a slower means of communication, and considerable attention and concentration may be needed to monitor the scanning and wait for the desired selection to be presented.

Usually, **linear scanning** is introduced first because it is conceptually the most simple. In linear scanning, each item is presented one at a time. Other scanning arrays might later be introduced to increase the speed and efficiency of selection by allowing the individual to scan large groups first and then narrow the selection to a single item. **Row–column scanning** is probably the most commonly used array. Items are arranged in horizontal rows, and after the user selects the desired row, the items of that row are individually scanned. (See Quist and Lloyd, 1997, or Beukelman and Mirenda, 1998, for discussion of scanning.)

Switch Access   A variety of switches can be used with most electronic communication aids (Berliss, Borden, & Vanderheiden, 1989). Common switches include those activated by pressure from the hand, head, or foot. Less frequently used activations include the eyebrow wrinkle switch (activated by the action of raising the eyebrows); electromyographic switch (activated by sensing any tensing or tightening of a muscle);

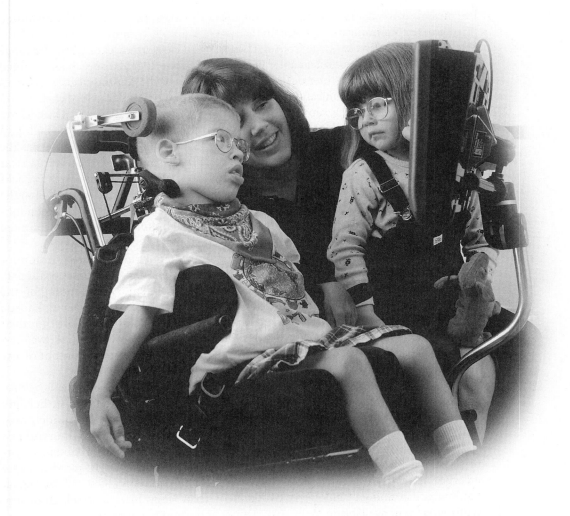

FIGURE 15.2   Young boy using a scanning device. By moving his head to the right and touching the round switch plate, this boy activates a Vanguard communication device. The possible choices on the Vanguard screen are highlighted, and the boy touches the switch when his desired choice is highlighted. The front of the Vanguard device is shown in Figure 15.3.
Source: Courtesy of Prentke Romich Company.

eye-gaze switch (activated by sensing the muscle activity of turning the eyes); and the sip-and-puff pneumatic switch (activated by intra-oral pressure changes). In selecting the method of switch activation, one would usually choose the type that is easiest and fastest for the user to operate without accidental activations.

Means to Transmit

Transmission relates to how the AAC user sends the selected message to a listener, and this leads to a consideration of output methods. In the case of unaided communication, such as manual signs or speech, the transmission is direct, and the listener interprets the message directly. In aided communication, the message is typically transmitted through the communication device. In the case of a simple, communication board, the listener must read the message from the board. With electronic devices, a wider range of transmission methods is available. These include computerized speech and printed messages by hard-copy printer or liquid crystal display. If the communication symbols are aided, then the communication transmission will always be aided (Lloyd et al., 1990).

Computerized speech can be categorized into three types: digitized, synthesized, and combined. **Digitized speech** is simply a computer recording and replaying of speech as it is spoken into a microphone. Given high-quality equipment, this has the potential to produce extremely good-quality speech, sounding to the human ear exactly like the original speech signal that was recorded. There are two main drawbacks to this type of speech. First, there is little flexibility; that is, the user is restricted to the exact words or phrases that were previously recorded. Second, it takes a tremendous amount of computer memory to store the speech signal; thus, the user will be limited in the number and length of messages that can be stored.

In **synthesized speech**, the computer program contains rules or an algorithm for the parameters of a speech signal. Instead of recording a specific word or speech signal, only the rules are stored, which reduces the demand for memory. Depending on the algorithm, the synthesizer can produce speech based on either the proper alphabetic spelling or a phonetic spelling of the desired speech. The computer algorithm then generates the speech from the set of rules. This type of speech synthesis allows for a highly flexible system incorporating text-to-speech capability or speech output of any typed message.

The earlier versions of speech synthesizers were produced purely as synthesis by rule. In these systems, however, the quality of the speech was artificial, and the intelligibility was generally affected. The Echo speech synthesizers were probably the most widely used examples of synthesis by rule. Improved quality was achieved when the synthesis approach was combined with the benefits of the digital approach. In the combined synthesizers, digital recordings of diphones, or transitions between pairs of phonemes, are incorporated into the algorithm, or rule, system of the synthesizer. DECtalk by Digital Equipment Co. and ETI-Eloquence by Eloquent Technology, Inc., are two high-quality synthesizers now available in many AAC devices and computer applications.

These high-quality synthesizers provide preprogrammed variations or distinct voices for the user to choose from. In addition, it is possible to program additional variations in pitch, quality, and prosody to create emotional emphasis, unique voices, and even singing. Computer-generated speech is discussed more thoroughly by Cohen and Palin (1986) and Schlosser (2003d).

Examples of Representation, Selection, and Transmission

Figure 15.3 shows a sample of **dedicated communication devices** produced by some leading manufacturers. A dedicated communication device is one designed primarily for communication instead of adapting a standard computer for the added function of communication. The devices shown here are only a small sample of the wide variety of devices currently available. Glennen (1997) listed 78 different dedicated communication devices.

The Talk Trac from AbleNet (Figure 15.3a) is an example of a device designed for limited use. It uses digital recording and allows the user to have five messages available for use. It might be appropriate, for example, to have a few important messages ready

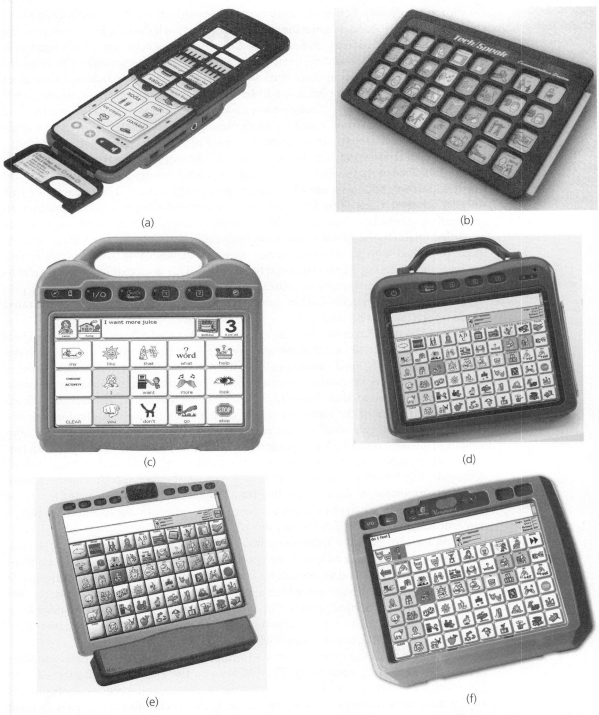

(a)

(b)

(c)

(d)

(e)

(f)

FIGURE 15.3   Examples of dedicated communication devices. These photos illustrate only a small fraction of the many varied devices available. *Sources:* (a) Lingo, courtesy of AbleNet, Inc.; (b) TechSpeak, courtesy of DynaVox Mayer-Johnson (www.dynavoxtech.com); (c) SBL 15, courtesy of Prentke Romich; (d) VTL, courtesy of Prentke Romich; (e) ECOpoint, courtesy of Prentke Romich; and (f), Vanguard Plusr, courtesy of Prentke Romich.

to communicate with a clerk in a store or with a bus driver. The Talk Trac is designed to be worn as a wrist band, illustrating the portability of such devices. Similar devices are designed to be carried in a purse or tote bag, clipped to a belt, or carried as a notebook. There are also digital recording devices that allow for a single message to be recorded on a switch. These are sometimes used as calls for attention or for taking a turn in an activity where a repetitive phrase might be used, such as playing games, reading children's stories, or singing. Although independence on such devices is limited because they require that someone record the exact messages, an advantage is their great flexibility in that the messages can be changed quickly to adjust for the situation.

The Tech Speak from Advanced Multimedia Devices Inc. (Figure 15.3b) is similar to the Talk Trac in that it also relies on digital speech recording, and it is designed for limited and introductory use of a speech-generating device. The capacity of this device, however, does allow for a more systematic and comprehensive approach to expanding vocabulary. This device has 32 locations, and a different message can be recorded for each one. Short phrases can be combined to increase the variety of messages produced. The power of the device is further expanded by use of a level system where different sets of 32 messages can be recorded. This does require someone else to take responsibility for setting the correct level and changing the overlay with 32 pictures or symbols to match the set of messages selected. The Tech Speak can be operated by direct selection or by scanning.

The MT4 from Dynavox Systems (Figure 15.3c) is also a level system. An important difference in the MT4 is that the levels or pages are presented on a computer-type screen and can be changed automatically by the AAC user. This is known as a dynamic display, and it allows for powerful storage of many different sets of messages. The symbols can be picture based as shown in Figure 15.3c, or they could be letters or printed words, and the size of the locations can be changed based on the individual's needs. The MT4 is a relatively small device, with a front size of approximately 6″ by 8″, and weighs just over 3 pounds. A companion device, the DV4, has the same operating features but is larger, with a front size of approximately 9″ by 12″, and weighs almost 6 pounds. These devices are usually operated with synthesized speech. However, there is also an option to use digital recording for a few special messages such as the start of a song or a favorite catch phrase that may depend on inflection for its full effect (e.g., a sarcastic exaggeration of "I'm sooooo sorry.")

Link Plus by Assistive Technology Inc. (Figure 15.3d) uses a standard keyboard, and the user must be able to spell. Word prediction is available to increase the speed of typing, and the letters and words can be selected by direct selection or by scanning. It also has abbreviation expansion, which allows the user to store favorite messages. This device includes synthesized speech. The Link Plus may be a comfortable choice for a person who loses speech later in life because it relies on a familiar keyboard rather than requiring new learning of other symbols.

Pathfinder from the Prentke Romich Company (Figure 15.3e) represents another approach to accessing vocabulary. The 128 keys on the Pathfinder are marked with Minspeak icons. These icons each have multiple meanings, and words or short phrases are accessed as a sequence of two or three icons. It also has the ability to type with word prediction. It also offers direct selection by touching the device, using a headpointer, and using the scanning options. As does the MT4 from Dynavox described above, the Pathfinder operates with synthesized speech, but also allows for digital recording for a select set of messages.

Vanguard II, also from the Prentke Romich Company (Figure 15.3f), is a good illustration of the increasing power of devices to offer multiple options within the same device. Vanguard II has a dynamic display screen similar to the MT4 and DV4, but like the Pathfinder, it also maintains the use of Minspeak icons for storage of words and phrases in short sequences of meaning-based icons. The Vanguard II offers both synthesized and digitized speech, and it can be accessed by touching the screen, scanning, or using a tracker system.

The six items in Figure 15.3 are examples of dedicated communication devices, meaning each was designed primarily as a communication device. Each of these devices is also a **speech-generating device**, and they demonstrate many of the features now commercially available on dedicated communication devices.

Another approach is to begin with a standard computer (laptop or other) and to use software and hardware to provide access and communication functions for use by individuals with disabilities. Examples of this approach are shown in Figure 15.4. Software can provide a range of graphic symbols and turn any computer into a communication device.

As shown in Figure 15.4a, any laptop computer can function as a communication device when a speech synthesizer such as the Micro CommPac from Words+ is added to it. In this example, the EZ Keys software allows for typing with word predication and abbreviation expansion, and the speech synthesizer allows the message to be spoken aloud. Word prediction means that as the user begins typing a word, the software predicts and offers likely choices for completing that word, similar to the way that a spell checker offers choices. If the correct choice is offered, the user may select it instead of completing the letter-by-letter typing. Abbreviation expansion means that selected letter combinations are pre-stored and will be replaced with the expanded text every time they are used. For example, I might store my initials as an abbreviation for my own name; thereafter, I would never type my full name, only my initials, but my full name would appear every time.

The TuffTalker Convertible, shown in Figure 15.4b, is based on a Panasonic ToughBook computer. As shown, Talking Screen software is installed, and a page of pictures is ready for use in a fast-food restaurant. On this device, one can access the standard keyboard, or the screen can be turned and folded so that it becomes a tablet computer with a touch-screen function. An advantage of computers is that the user has standard computer functions, such as a word processor, Internet access, and game programs, available along with a speech-generating device.

Figure 15.4c illustrates the remarkable versatility of size of the computer. In this case, Say-it! SAM software has been added to a handheld computer, the Hewlett Packard iPAQ 5000, allowing it to function as a speech-generating device. This is a highly portable system; however, the user would need excellent visual acuity and fine motor skills to select the small targets.

Some individuals require special help to access a computer not for speech, but for standard computer functions or to replace handwriting. Intellikeys from IntelliTools Inc., shown in Figure 15.4d, is one example of an alternate keyboard. This enlarged panel can be configured to emulate the entire keyboard or only selected keys.

A difficult challenge for people with motor disabilities is to control a mouse. Several options are available to replace a standard mouse. These include the Expert Mouse from Words+ Corporation (Figure 15.4e) and the roller and joystick from Traxsys (Figure 15.4f).

Assistive communication device technology is changing rapidly, and the items discussed are only examples of the many items now available. The reader is encouraged to keep up with this changing technology by exploring the exhibits at major conventions and by contacting manufacturers individually or through the Communication Aid

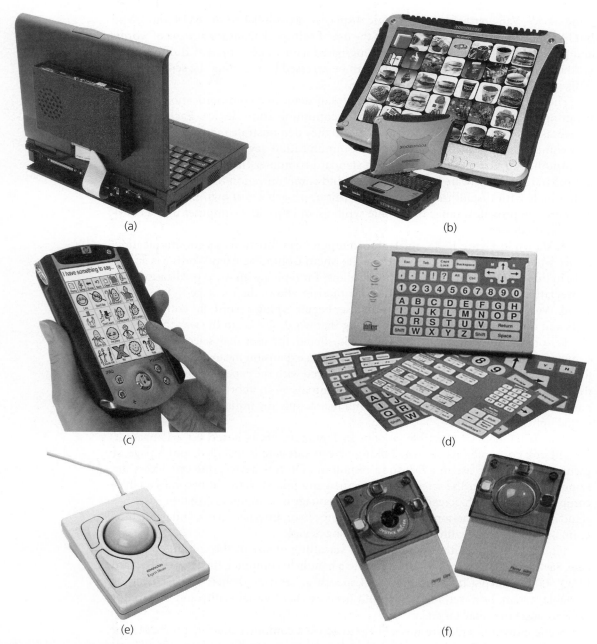

FIGURE 15.4   Examples of computer adaptations. The first three items are illustrations of the use of computer systems to function in place of dedicated communication devices. The remaining three items illustrate options to allow persons with disabilities to access computers for the same functions that other people use the computer. (a) Micro CommPac by Words+, courtesy of Words+ Corporation; (b) TuffTalker Convertible by Words+ Corporation, courtesy of Words+ Corporation; (c) Say-it! SAM software by Words+ Corporation, courtesy of Words+ Corporation; (d) Intellikeys from IntelliTools Inc., courtesy of Words+ Corporation; (e) Expert Mouse, courtesy of Words+ Corporation; and (f) Joystick Roller II (left) and Roller (right), courtesy of Dynavox Mayer-Johnson (www.dynavoxtech.com).

Manufacturers Association, 205 W. Randolph Street, Suite 1830, Chicago, IL 60606
www.aacproducts.org.

Multimodal Communication

Some researchers have observed that most people (both disabled and nondisabled) use
multimodal communication (Vanderheiden & Lloyd, 1986). People may speak to
convey thoughts, but additional meaning is conveyed by facial expressions, gestures,
tone of voice, and even posture. A typical person might use speech, but also use some
gestures, writing, typing, and a recording such as a telephone answering machine.
People easily switch from one modality to another and combine modalities.

Users of AAC systems should also be viewed as multimodal communicators
(Blischak & Lloyd, 1996). Their communication systems should include both unaided
and aided strategies. They should include both the communication modes they have
developed naturally without formal intervention and those strategies that can be facilitated or taught by clinicians/educators. A variety of techniques may be needed to
address a varied audience. For example, a person who uses manual signing with familiar listeners would need some other approach to communicate with store clerks or
bank tellers who might have no knowledge of signing. In addition, when one uses an
electronic device, it is important to have a backup system for times when the device
may be broken or the battery needs charging.

One outcome of viewing an AAC user as a multimodal communicator is that
whatever communication mode the individual chooses will be respected and accepted.
It is often reported that clinicians and teachers, in their enthusiasm to teach what they
view as more effective communication modes, sometimes refuse to accept simpler,
more effective modes. For example, a teacher might put the words *yes* and *no* on an
individual's communication device. When the student attempts to answer a question
by nodding or shaking the head, the teacher might respond with "Use your device to
tell me." This is an unnecessary refusal because the teacher probably understood the
gesture. Incidents such as this are reported by users to be very frustrating (Huer &
Lloyd, 1988a, 1988b) and may have the inadvertent, negative effect of causing the
student to become discouraged about even trying to communicate.

Reasons for AAC Success

AAC facilitates communication development. There are at least six general aspects
that could account for the facilitative effects of AAC (Fristoe & Lloyd, 1979; Lloyd &
Karlan, 1984).

First, there appears to be a simplification of input when AAC symbols are presented. Clinicians and teachers may eliminate extraneous comments when modeling
AAC use, and the rate of presentation can be slowed.

Second, there are advantages related to producing a response. When using AAC,
the negative pressure to improve speech production is eliminated. The motor requirements for AAC are less complex and can be selected to match the motor skills of the
individual. There is an opportunity to provide physical assistance to help a person
access AAC symbols or to produce signs and gestures. In contrast, we can do only limited physical manipulation to assist in producing speech sounds. The visual nature of
AAC symbols also facilitates the use of shaping as a teaching strategy.

Third, there seem to be advantages related to the cognitive abilities required. In most AAC systems, the vocabulary is somewhat limited and is highly functional. It is possible that the visual nature of the symbols also aids in maintaining attention to the symbols.

Fourth, there are advantages related to language and auditory processing abilities. Because the input of AAC messages may be simplified, the language may be easier to process. For an individual with limited auditory short-term memory or with auditory processing problems, the visual symbols bypass the auditory channel and may, therefore, be more successful.

Fifth, there are other aspects of the symbols that are beneficial for processing and association. The figure–ground differential is enhanced, the consistency of stimuli optimized, and the temporal duration of the symbol is greater. Compared to the rapid flow of speech, these are advantages in learning to associate symbols with their referents.

Finally, there are advantages related to the symbolic representation. Most AAC symbols can be used simultaneously with speech, and, therefore, they serve as a supplement to the speech input. Because the symbols are visual, a symbol may be iconic (i.e., it looks like its referent).

From the above discussion of factors, it can be seen that there are many reasons to believe that the use of AAC symbols will enhance the development of language and communication skills. This has been shown to be the case. In a review of the literature, D. Miller, Light, and Schlosser (2000) concluded that improvements in speech skills were observed in the majority of cases of AAC intervention reported in the literature.

Communicative Competence

Janice Light (1989) discussed the important concept of communicative competence related to AAC use. She put her discussion within the framework of the purposes of communication expressed by people, both disabled and nondisabled. According to Light, all individuals use communication to (1) express basic needs, (2) exchange information, (3) establish social closeness, and (4) engage in social routines. Each of these functions should be considered for the AAC user. Different strategies may be more effective for one or another of these four functions. According to Light, four distinct competencies contribute to overall communicative competence. These are linguistic competence, operational competence, social competence, and strategic competence. (See Light, Beukelman, and Reichle, 2003, for a detailed discussion of competence.)

Linguistic competence refers to knowledge of the language, or linguistic code. According to Chomsky (1965), *linguistic competence* refers to the internal abilities of the individual. It includes everything the person knows about the language and how the units can be combined. Light (1989) points out that for the AAC user, linguistic competence may include knowledge of both the native language used in the environment (e.g., English or Spanish) and special AAC symbols (e.g., Blissymbolics or Minspeak icons).

Operational competence is a unique concern of AAC, especially for aided communication. *Operational competence* refers to the user's ability to manage the specific devices or techniques that are used in the communication process. This might include the ability to turn a device on or off, adjust the device's volume, operate a scanning system, and so on.

Social competence refers to the broad communication skills addressed by sociolinguistics (Hymes, 1971). This includes discourse strategies, interaction functions, and pragmatic adjustments to context. Examples include maintaining a topic, using transitions to change topic, adjusting the type of language used to the ability of the listener, gaining someone's attention, and giving appropriate feedback to the communication partner. Social competence may be a serious issue that is easily overlooked for an AAC user. It is not unusual for AAC approaches to be introduced to an individual who has had extremely limited communication abilities for many years. Social competence abilities that are developed quite naturally for typically developing children may be problematic for AAC users simply because AAC users have not experienced successful communication to facilitate these abilities.

Social competence should be considered in the cultural context (Hetzroni & Harris, 1996; Soto et al., 1997; Wall & Barnett, 1998). Expectations of how one communicates, when, and with whom will vary for different cultural groups. Additionally, families from different cultures will have differences regarding the role of children, attitudes about disability, and the acceptance of AAC approaches.

Strategic competence (defined by Canale, 1983) refers to adapted strategies that are called into play when there is some breakdown in the communication process. Examples include asking for additional information, recognizing when the listener has not understood, and repeating or changing a message to clarify the error. As pointed out by Light (1989), this is especially important for AAC users. There are probably a greater number of difficulties and barriers to achieving efficient communication when AAC strategies are being used.

Types of Impairments

In order to select strategies and techniques that will enhance competence, abilities in a range of domains must be considered. Understanding the strengths and weaknesses of the individual will allow for feature matching—that is, matching features of an AAC approach to the needs of the individual.

Clearly, motor abilities must be considered. For unaided approaches such as gestures and signs, sufficient fine and gross motor skills must be present. If aided communication is considered, the motor abilities will determine which modes of access are possible. Direct selection devices require both range of motion and accuracy of selection to be effective. While scanning systems can be used with very limited motor skill, accurate timing of switch activation is a significant concern.

Cognitive abilities must be considered. As discussed earlier, AAC communication involves the use of symbols to convey meaning. The more arbitrary the symbols, the greater the cognitive demand to learn and use the symbols. Successful AAC users must understand not only the language of their communication partners, but also the particular symbols of their AAC approaches (Light, 1989). It can be extremely difficult to assess the cognitive ability of some individuals because, by definition, they have great difficulty communicating. Those who have never experienced success with communication may seem quite limited in their efforts to comply with tasks usually used for the assessment of cognitive and language abilities (i.e., they may show little awareness of the demands of a test setting and have little motivation to complete a standardized test).

Sensory abilities are, of course, important in all types of communication intervention. In the case of persons who experience severe and multiple disabilities, however, it may be very easy to overlook sensory impairments; yet this is a very important area because some AAC strategies will not be appropriate if sensory disabilities are present. For example, a child with cerebral palsy may rarely respond to speech. The family and teachers may attribute the lack of response to the lack of speech or a lack of cognitive skill. If there is an undetected hearing loss, the introduction of a voice output communication device might meet with little success, and the intervention team might conclude that the child does not have the cognitive ability to learn the symbols and the device presented. The real problem might be that the child cannot process the speech. (In fact, there is some evidence that the presence of sensorineural hearing loss may have a greater impact on the understanding of computer-synthesized speech than on natural speech [Kangas & Allen, 1990].)

Problems in visual acuity and visual perception should also be considered. An inability to deal with visual symbols might be easily confused with a vision problem. Visual tracking and the ability to maintain focus are very important in managing a visual display of many symbols and may be especially important for scanning systems. As individuals learn to manage communication symbols used in AAC interventions, it is not unusual that the displays they use become progressively more complex as a greater number of smaller symbols are made available. This may challenge the visual skills of acuity and figure–ground discrimination.

Congenital Disabilities

A variety of congenital disabilities may lead to a need for AAC intervention. Disabilities that fall into this category include autism, cerebral palsy, developmental apraxia of speech, mental retardation, and specific language disorder (Mirenda & Mathy-Laikko, 1989). These disabilities truly require a lifetime perspective; individuals may have the disability throughout their entire lives, although their need for AAC may or may not be a lifetime need.

For a very young child, the family is most likely facing some very basic issues such as the survival and physical health of the child. If the disability is clearly diagnosed when the child is an infant, it is likely that the family would not have begun to think about communication. One role of early intervention should be to enhance any natural abilities the child has to communicate. Helping the parent or other caregiver to understand how interaction with an infant leads to later communication development may allow the caregivers to enhance the child's active role in social interaction (Reinhartsen, Edmondson, & Crais, 1997).

In many cases, such as autism or specific language disability, the child's lack of expressive language at the expected age may be the parents' first indication suggesting the presence of a disability. In these cases, the child may be 2 or 3 years of age when the parents seek professional help. Here, the parents may be very motivated to address communication issues, but they are likely to be focused on questions of why the child is delayed and may be looking for ways to bring the child's skills up to age level. If the prognosis for speech development is quite poor, it may be difficult for parents to accept AAC approaches because of fear of delaying speech development.

With the infant and toddler population, it is important to focus on the communication, regardless of the level at which the child performs. In the past, some authors suggested specific prerequisites to introducing any AAC approach, such as a certain level of cognitive ability (Shane & Bashir, 1980), social skills, and receptive language abilities (R. E. Owens & House, 1984), or a gap between receptive and expressive language (Chapman & Miller, 1980). The evidence to support the prerequisite approach was mainly based on observations of correlates of expressive language, with no evidence of cause-and-effect relationships, and much of the data was based on typically developing children, not children with disabilities. The prerequisite approach, therefore, was challenged and rejected (Kangas & Lloyd, 1988; Reichle & Karlan, 1985). Currently, early use of AAC approaches is directed to increasing the child's participation in daily routines, expanding the repertoire of communication behaviors, and/or developing intentional and symbolic abilities (Cress & Marvin, 2003; Kangas & Lloyd, 1988).

For the school-age child, access to interaction with peers and school curriculum becomes of greater concern (McCormick & Wegner, 2003). With current trends in education increasing the opportunities for mainstreaming and full inclusion in school programs with nondisabled children, it becomes very important for the child to have a means of communication that is effective with both disabled and nondisabled peers. Figure 15.5 shows an example of an interactive application. This boy uses an AAC device to interact with a friend. For the young child, this must be a form of communication that does not require reading because the child will be communicating with children who do not yet read. Access to the curriculum is also of great importance for school-age children. This is true whether the children are receiving the standard curriculum for all children in their age group or an adapted or special education curriculum.

An important consideration for children is the development of literacy (Koppenhaver, Evans, & Yoder, 1991; Mirenda & Erickson, 2000; M. M. Smith, 1992; M. M. Smith & Blischak, 1997; Sturm & Clendon, 2004). Recent research has

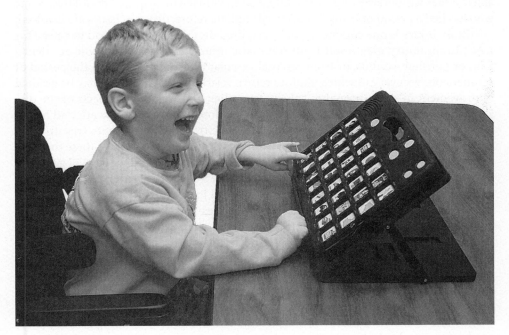

FIGURE 15.5   Boy using a speech-generating device to interact with a friend. The ability to communicate with peers is critical to the successful integration of a student with disabilities into a regular education classroom. This boy uses a Go Talk device from Attainment Company. The device has digital speech output for each of nine messages on each level, with up to four levels available.
Source: Courtesy of Attainment Company.

demonstrated the importance of early experiences in the development of literacy skills for nondisabled children. This literature has been applied to programs for children with disabilities as well. It has been recognized that children with the intellectual capability to learn to read need a nurturing environment and appropriate training from a young age if their ultimate potential is to be achieved. Computers and other electronic devices have given access to the printed word for many children and have opened the door to reading and writing programs.

For the adolescent and adult, the transition to adult roles will be critical. Intervention should be geared to providing access to the most independent living situation possible and to participation in a wide range of community activities. For those who have the ability, university or other higher education should be considered. AAC intervention can be effective in assisting adults to find and to keep meaningful employment (Light, Stoltz, & McNaughton, 1996; A. C. Odom & Upthegrove, 1997; Storey, Ezell, & Lengyel, 1995). Through the use of AAC and other assistive technology coupled with telecommunication networks and distance learning programs, individuals with disabilities now have access to a world of achievement potential.

Acquired Disabilities

Acquired disabilities may require attention to issues somewhat different from those raised by congenital disabilities (Beukelman & Yorkston, 1989; Beukelman, Yorkston, & Reichle, 2000; Garrett, Beukelman, & Low-Morrow, 1989). Anyone may become disabled, either temporarily or permanently. An individual with acquired disabilities is one who has had a period of being nondisabled, and, therefore, different issues are involved.

Brain injury is one common type of acquired disability that may lead to a need for AAC. Brain injury may result from traumatic injury, such as automobile accidents, falls, or gunshot wounds, or from cerebral vascular accidents. Following the period of spontaneous recovery in which abilities return relatively rapidly, there may be gradual improvement in skills throughout the person's life; however, some aspects of the disability may remain relatively stable. Communication abilities might be affected by the motor abilities (resulting in dysarthria), by specific language deficits (resulting in aphasia), by general cognitive impairments, or by some combination of these three.

Spinal cord injury presents mainly a motor disability. The individual will generally have impaired motor control below the level of the injury. If the injury is high enough to affect arm and hand movement, the person will have difficulty using written communication in addition to losing the use of the legs and the ability to walk independently. If the muscles of respiration are involved, then reliance on a respirator will become an issue, and speech may also be affected.

Living with the results of brain injury or spinal cord injury will mean adjusting to permanent changes in life situations. Family roles will have been established based on an individual's previous, nondisabled status, and the entire family will likely have to make adjustments to the person's new status of being disabled (Beukelman & Yorkston, 1989). Communication may be one of the keys to addressing some of these needs. If the disabled person can regain ways to communicate with the family, this may help to re-establish emotional bonds and support roles and may help to prevent frustration. A man who is used to being self-sufficient may become enraged when he needs help and has difficulty requesting it for simple tasks such as getting a cup of coffee. Some of the frustration might be relieved by introducing efficient communication strategies.

Social roles are also very important. Adults generally have a well-established social network, which may include relatives, neighbors, longtime family friends, business acquaintances, and members of clubs, churches, or committees. One goal of AAC intervention might be to return to social interactions with the same network of people. It will be important to provide strategies that are acceptable in a variety of situations by a network of listeners. An adolescent who was active in a particular sport may need the vocabulary to discuss that sport. An older adult might wish to share information about children and grandchildren.

Generally, people living with brain injury or spinal cord injury will want to return to their previous roles as much as possible. For many adults, this may mean returning to their previous work or choosing a new vocation (McNaughton, Light, & Gulla, 2003). For children and adolescents, this may mean returning to the same classroom they attended before the injury. Any AAC strategy selected for a person who hopes to return to work or school should take into account the type of communication needed in that setting. For example, in some businesses, it may be possible for individuals to return to the same or a similar job if they can access the usual computer programs such as word processors and accounting spreadsheets. For others, use of communication devices or computers may be initiated to replace communication skills that were previously accomplished through typical communication modes. For example, a student might return to an active role in the classroom by using a communication device with speech output to give oral reports or to participate in group discussions.

Certain conditions may give rise to temporary, but severe disabilities. For example, the type of brain injury event discussed previously may sometimes create very severe conditions initially, but the person affected may progress to complete or nearly complete recovery in a matter of weeks or months. Temporary dependence on a respirator precludes any production of natural speech (Beukelman & Garrett, 1988). A neurologic disease known as Guillain-Barré syndrome often causes very severe disabilities, but in most cases, these will be temporary (Beukelman & Garrett, 1988). For temporary conditions, the individuals' immediate needs are most important. They may need immediate ways to express physical needs and to communicate symptoms to medical staff. In addition, they may feel great fear about what is happening, and the ability to ask questions related to their immediate care and future recovery may be very important. In these cases, simple strategies that do not require any time to learn will be most effective. A simple wipe-off board or child's "magic slate" toy might be effective for those who retain the ability to write. An eye-gaze board fitted with the alphabet might be the simplest immediate strategy for individuals with severely restricted movement (Fried-Oken, Howard, & Stewart, 1991).

Some acquired disabilities are the result of progressive diseases, such as amyotrophic lateral sclerosis (ALS), multiple sclerosis (MS), and Parkinson's disease (Beukelman & Garrett, 1988). In these cases, considering current and future needs is a different picture because a person with a progressive disease faces a future of diminishing skills. AAC needs might not be apparent immediately, but in many cases, AAC interventions will improve the quality of life for these patients in the later stages of the diseases. The intervention in these cases should be directed to anticipating the status of physical and mental abilities in the future and to meeting the needs about which the person is most concerned. Maintaining a wide circle of contacts for as long as possible might be an appropriate goal of AAC intervention. For example, a communication device that allows a person to talk on the phone might help to maintain frequent contact with friends when leaving the home becomes difficult. One should consider that communicating highly personal and emotional messages to a spouse, however, might be far more important than the ability to greet casual friends.

One challenge for the speech-language pathologist working with this population is that the patient may be unwilling or unready to accept the prognosis for future disabilities. In the case of ALS, for example, the person will be faced with accepting the reality of death in the near future. The emotional impact of accepting this reality might prevent the person from recognizing that there will be a stage near the end of life when natural speech is not possible. Some patients will be unwilling to accept AAC strategies until their need is immediately critical. Beukelman and Garrett (1988) recommend introducing possible strategies to the patient early, but then allowing the patient to determine when to begin using these approaches.

Assessment

As in all areas of speech-language pathology, careful assessment will be critical when developing an appropriate intervention plan. Assessment of the existing communication abilities, abilities in related domains such as cognition and motor development, and sensory acuity will be important, as will the understanding of the cause of the impairments. The typical AAC assessment focuses on the strengths and needs of the AAC user relative to the current and probable communication partners and environments or contexts (Wasson, Arvidson, & Lloyd, 1997).

Attention to auditory, visual, and motor abilities is especially important in AAC because of the nature of means to represent (symbols), select, and transmit messages in AAC approaches. Many individuals with AAC needs have sensory and/or motor impairments resulting from their disabilities. A feature-matching approach is an effort to match the needs and abilities of a client to the specific features needed in the individual's AAC system, including both aided and unaided means to represent, select, and transmit (see Wasson, et al., 1997, for a discussion of assessment).

The choice of a means to represent messages (for both expressive and receptive communication) is influenced by sensory abilities. When using graphic symbols, the individual must have sufficient visual abilities to perceive the symbols presented on any communication aid. Vision is also important in the use of unaided communication. For the use of gestures and signs, the need for motor ability for expression is obvious, but it is also important to consider whether visual skills are sufficient to perceive and understand the gestures and signs of a communication partner.

Cognition also must be considered in relation to symbol selection. As discussed previously, symbol sets and systems vary in several characteristics such as iconicity, complexity, and abstractness. These features must be matched to the learning abilities of the individual.

The means to select a message, especially in aided communication, depends particularly on motor abilities. For direct selection, the user must have sufficient range of motion to reach the extremes of the display or keyboard to be used and enough motor coordination to select the desired symbol. These abilities will in part determine the size of the symbols that can be used as well as the number of symbols that can be available. In scanning selection, a major task of assessment will be to identify one or more movements (e.g., eye blink, eye gaze, finger movement, head movement) that are sufficiently well controlled so that the user can activate a switch reliably without extreme fatigue.

Transmission of messages not only affects the listener, but also provides feedback to the AAC user during expressive communication. For example, if a person uses a device with synthetic speech output, careful consideration must be given to the user's auditory acuity and perception. If the user cannot use the auditory feedback, it will be more difficult to provide feedback that allows the user to know accurately what has been communicated.

Accommodation in Testing

The preceding comments relate to ways in which sensory and motor abilities affect the selection of AAC strategies. But it is also critical to consider the type of response required in the assessment of cognitive and both receptive and expressive language abilities. Obviously, for most AAC clients, spoken responses will not be possible. Furthermore, cognitive and language tests frequently involve motor control and timing aspects. This means that one may not obtain an appropriate index of the ability of many AAC users by using standard assessment procedures. Test modification may be necessary to reduce demands for motor control or speech (Thurlow, Elliott, & Ysseldyke, 1998). Applying different procedures for testing may also change the linguistic and cognitive demands of the test or may create greater fatigue. The interpretation of results must take into account how this may affect the results.

In many respects, AAC may be viewed as accommodations and modifications to improve accessibility and full participation. In assessment, there are frequently accommodations or modifications of standardized and norm-referenced test procedures so that some information can be obtained. However, there is a general psychometric rule that when one deviates from the standardization used for developing the normative information, the norms should not be used unless there is additional standardization or other empirical forms of validation (e.g., concurrent or construct validity). This does not mean that one may not employ standardized tests with accommodations to gain some information about an individual. Such information may be of value for monitoring. The problem arises when one makes accommodations in standardized tests without appropriate validation of those accommodations and then uses the norms provided under the original standardized procedures (Code of Fair Testing Practices in Education, 1988).

Recent education legislation underscores the importance of identifying and validating accommodations during the administration of testing. The Individuals with Disabilities Education Act (IDEA, P.L. 108-446) mandates that every child be included in statewide assessments. Under IDEA, students with disabilities may participate by taking the same assessments as other students and under the same conditions, or they may be allowed accommodations to the testing process but with the same standards, or they may be allowed to demonstrate progress through alternate assessments. However, the No Child Left Behind Act of 2001 (P.L. 107-110) has restricted the number of students who may be allowed to substitute alternate assessment procedures for the statewide standardized measures. The full implementation of this law adds urgency to the demonstration of validity in modifying test procedures or substituting alternate assessments.

In assessment for AAC, it is particularly critical to include the environment and the communication partners as part of the assessment focus. AAC techniques are quite different from typical speech, and the techniques selected must be well matched to the real communication needs of individuals and their environments. In many cases, it is the communication partners in the environment who will determine if the communication program fails or succeeds. For example, AAC techniques are slow compared to typical speech, and unless communication partners are prepared to allow more time for AAC users to respond, it is likely that AAC users will not have the opportunity to express original ideas, even if they have the skills needed for expression. The culture of the environment must also be considered (Bridges, 2004; Soto et al., 1997). For example, many cultures teach children to be quiet unless spoken to when in the presence of adults. In such a culture, a strategy designed to give assertive powers to a child will probably not be supported by the environment.

Intervention

Team Intervention

Severe communication disabilities can affect all aspects of an individual's life. Furthermore, these communication disabilities usually occur concomitant with a wide variety of other disabilities. As a result, intervention programs should reflect input from a team that represents expertise from several disciplines in conjunction with the personal interests and desires of the individual (Beukelman & Mirenda, 1998; Mirenda & Iacono, 1990).

Disabilities that may occur along with severe communication disabilities include cognitive disabilities, motor disabilities, linguistic disabilities, and sensory impairments. The individual may need services from the fields of regular and special education, audiology, ophthalmology, physical therapy, occupational therapy, rehabilitation engineering, computer science, social work, psychology, and career counseling as well as speech-language pathology. Each of these disciplines offers knowledge and expertise that may be important to understanding the complete picture of the individual's needs and developing appropriate intervention strategies. However, there is a danger that the total program for the individual may become fragmented and disjointed rather than being coherent and holistic (Beukelman & Mirenda, 1998; Mirenda & Iacono, 1990). In the past, individuals were often removed from their natural environment to receive special services from each of the appropriate specialists. Thus, a school-age child might have spent large amounts of time receiving individual therapy and, therefore, may have missed many classroom events. A more current approach is to view the classroom (or other natural setting) as the individual's basic environment and to incorporate services into that natural setting. The individual is removed from the natural setting only when it seems necessary to provide appropriate services.

One focus of team intervention is to have access to a variety of perspectives to fully understand an individual's impairments and disabilities and to recognize their implications. Each team member would have unique information and skills, and the total program for the individual should incorporate these various perspectives.

Another focus of team intervention is to coordinate services. It is not unusual for a person with severe disabilities to receive services from many specialists, and, unless carefully coordinated, the various professionals might inadvertently undermine each other's efforts. A particularly common example related to AAC intervention is the need to coordinate motor access to a communication device with needs for linguistic and communicative aspects. A speech-language pathologist might position a communication device where it appears that the individual can access the device quickly and easily. The physical therapist, however, might have a concern that this position encourages a detrimental movement pattern, such as triggering an abnormal reflex pattern.

Similarly, the physical therapist might decide that this device should be used to motivate practice for difficult motor patterns, such as expanding range of motion, and might place the device in a position that requires increased effort to activate. Effective team functioning requires these professionals to coordinate their efforts and avoid hindering progress in each other's areas.

Intervention Priorities

Effective intervention must be directed to meeting both long-range and short-range objectives (Beukelman & Mirenda, 1998). A long-range perspective would include concerns for where the individual wishes to live, his expected employment, and his family and social network. Also of long-range concern is the prognosis, whether for improving skills and abilities or declining skills in the case of progressive diseases.

Short-term priorities might address more immediate concerns, such as the ability to be part of a classroom or to discuss immediate medical and care needs. Immediate concerns are directed to the participation needs that are obvious now and usually must make use of current skills.

In many respects, AAC intervention will follow the same principles and practices as other forms of communication intervention (Zangari & Kangas, 1997). Goals will be based on careful evaluation of current abilities and on the prognosis for improvement. Teaching strategies will be based on the same learning principle as other forms of intervention are.

The disabled individual and family members should be viewed as critical members of the team, and their input must be a part of the decision-making process. At all times, it must be remembered that the focus of intervention is a person who has human and civil rights. It is the individual who will live with the results of intervention for a lifetime. Success of intervention should be viewed from the perspective of the individual, not from the perspective of the professional. For example, communication strategies that help a child to take part in playful and emotional interactions with family members might be viewed as successful if this is the family's concern. On the other hand, if these needs are generally well met by the family without professional intervention (i.e., the family has worked out its own patterns of interaction that meet emotional needs), the family might select a different aspect of communication as the focus of intervention. Perhaps the family is concerned that the child does not interact with other children in the neighborhood. The focus of AAC intervention should be to address the needs and concerns of the individual and the family.

It should also be recognized that priorities differ in different settings. It is not unusual to hear professionals complain that they do not receive cooperation from the family. These professionals may fail to recognize that they are asking family members to impose on the home environment the strategies that work in an outside setting. For example, a parent might be able to anticipate that the child would like a snack when first arriving home and might choose to establish the selection of a snack by offering two or three choices and interpreting the child's facial expression. It would be unreasonable to insist that the parent delay this important opportunity for communication to provide access to an electronic device to accomplish the same goal. For this same child, it might be appropriate to target expressing specific requests via a communication device in a school or community setting where others are not readily able to anticipate needs. By considering the viewpoints of the family, plans can be made to enhance the individual's success in all settings, thereby avoiding the frustrations inherent in setting up unreasonable expectations (Beukelman & Mirenda, 1998; Reichle, York, & Sigafoos, 1991).

Communication Partners and Environmental Interventions

An important aspect of intervention with AAC users involves the communication partners and the environment (Beukelman & Mirenda, 1998; Buzolich & Lunger, 1995; Zangari & Kangas, 1997). The environment in which the individual participates can be adjusted to enhance the ability to engage with others in that environment (Goossens & Crain, 1987). This includes arranging the physical environment so that the person is physically close to potential partners and able to establish eye contact. It may also include structuring activities so that the AAC user has the opportunity to communicate in meaningful ways.

The role of communication partners is critical to AAC users (Culp & Carlisle, 1988). This focus on the communication partners is important across the age range, for preschool children (Goossens & Crain, 1987), school-age children (Dowden & Marriner, 1995; Sigafoos, 1999), and adults (Garrett & Beukelman, 1992; Sigafoos, 1999). Partners should be assisted in recognizing and interpreting the AAC user's efforts to communicate. They can be encouraged to structure the conversation in a way that encourages the AAC user to take part. It should be recognized that all forms of AAC are slower than the use of typical speech. In some cases, a significant pause is created as the AAC user selects an appropriate message. A communication partner who pauses and gives sufficient time for communication will have a positive impact on the individual's communication patterns.

AAC and Challenging Behavior

Some individuals with little or no functional speech exhibit challenging behaviors that may include aggressive behavior (Talkington, Hall, & Altman, 1971), self-injurious behavior (Schlosser & Goetze, 1992), and stereotypical behavior (Moersch, 1977). To address these serious concerns, several researchers (e.g., Carr & Durand, 1985; Durand, 1990; Horner & Budd, 1985) developed the strategies of functional communication training as an assessment and intervention approach. Functional communication training involves the replacement of excess behavior by teaching an alternative communicative behavior that has the same function or pragmatic relationship as the challenging behavior (Baumgart, Johnson, & Helmstetter, 1990; Donnellan, Mirenda, Mesaros, & Fassbender, 1984; Doss & Reichle, 1989; Vaughn & Horner, 1995). Once it has been determined that the problem behavior serves a communicative function such as gaining attention, requesting, protesting, or negating (e.g., escaping from task demands), intervention should focus on the teaching of a communicative behavior that serves the same function as the problem behavior (e.g., teaching the request for a break). For these individuals, selection of an AAC system that provides immediate change is critical. When a response is needed to replace problem behavior, long-term development may be of secondary concern. In selecting an AAC system, it is preferable to use gestures or other communication symbols that are already in the individual's repertoire. When a functional communicative alternative to the problem behaviors is established, longer-range communication objectives can resume primacy.

(For more thorough discussion, see Mirenda, 1997; Reichle and Wacker, 1993; or Schlosser, 1997.)

Funding and Individual Rights

Funding

Funding of communication devices is a frequently voiced concern of speech-language pathologists and others involved in AAC interventions. Funding should include not only the initial purchase of equipment, but also the ongoing costs of maintaining and repairing the equipment, staff time needed to set up vocabulary or display options, and training to educate the individual in using the device. (See Ourand and Gray, 1997, or Zangari and Wasson, 1997, for discussion of funding issues.)

A variety of sources may be approached, depending on the needs of the individual and the expected outcomes for using AAC techniques. Medical agencies (Medicaid, Medicare, private medical insurance) might fund AAC interventions that are directly related to medical needs or that are clearly related to a prosthesis for the lost function of speaking or writing skills. Educational agencies fund equipment that is needed for the student to benefit from an educational program. Vocational rehabilitation agencies are concerned with providing the opportunity for an individual to develop job skills or to return to a previous work setting. If funding cannot be obtained through any of these agencies, many philanthropic and charitable organizations have sometimes purchased AAC devices. Low-interest loans may be available to the family that chooses to purchase a device with personal funds. In applying for funding, it is always important to present well-documented needs of the individual as well as the expected outcomes of the AAC program being recommended. The person who applies for funding must clearly understand the goals of the funding source that is being asked to pay for the AAC intervention, and the guidelines of the intended funding agency should be followed strictly. According to one booklet that deals with seeking funding for AAC equipment, "Funding success is 100 percent dependent upon the perseverance of the client-advocate. Funding is always available!" (Prentke Romich Co., 1989).

Rights of Individuals

Communication is a right. Access to appropriate methods of communication is a right of every individual. The national Joint Committee for Meeting the Communication Needs of Persons with Severe Disabilities (1992) has issued guidelines for meeting communication needs. These guidelines, endorsed by the American Speech-Language-Hearing Association (ASHA) and several other professional organizations, state that "all persons, regardless of the extent or severity of their disabilities, have a basic right to affect, through communication, the conditions of their own existence" (p. 2).

Access to appropriate AAC techniques and services is not just a matter of best practices; it is also a matter of respecting the basic human rights of individuals with severe communication disabilities. The civil rights of persons with disabilities are now protected by federal law in the United States (Americans with Disabilities Act of 1990, P.L. 101–336). Children have a guaranteed right to a free and appropriate public education as protected by the Individuals with Disabilities Education Act (P.L. 108–446). For children with severe communication impairments, AAC devices and support services may be required so that these children can benefit from their guaranteed education.

Speech-language pathologists have a legal and ethical responsibility to provide appropriate services for clients in need of AAC interventions. Those speech-language pathologists who lack the necessary skills and training to manage AAC interventions must pursue additional training and/or make appropriate referrals to other professionals. Support for professionals engaged in AAC practice may be found through the International Society for Augmentative and Alternative Communication (ISAAC) and its national chapter, the United States Society for Augmentative and Alternative Communication (USSAAC). As noted in Chapter 1, ASHA is the major national professional association for speech-language pathologists. Within ASHA, Special Interest Division #12 is dedicated to AAC. Other professional associations that include divisions on communication disorders include the American Association on Mental Retardation, the Council for Exceptional Children, and the Rehabilitation Engineering and Assistive Technology Society of North America.

Outcomes Measurement and Evidence-Based Practice

As in other areas of practice, professionals engaged in AAC are increasingly concerned with outcomes measurement and evidence-based practice (EBP). These are two frameworks concerned with ways in which academic research interacts with interventions for typical clients. One significant challenge to these efforts within AAC practice is the relative recency of AAC as a recognized field of study.

As recently as the 1970s, AAC was considered to be in its early stages, with a few professionals engaged in new and innovative efforts (McNaughton, 1990). By the 1980s, AAC was more widely accepted and was becoming recognized as an expected form of intervention. The technology offered in commercially produced AAC devices has changed dramatically in recent years. The rapidly changing knowledge base in the profession, the acceptance by the general public, and the changing technology combine to create an especially challenging situation as we examine the results of AAC interventions.

Outcome measurement in AAC refers to efforts to document changes before and after AAC interventions (Schlosser, 2003c). According to Schlosser, it is important that outcomes measurement be reported for intervention under ideal conditions (e.g., when treatment is provided intensively by highly trained clinicians), but it is also critical that outcomes be reported for average and marginal conditions, which may be typical of how most intervention is presented (e.g., when sessions are intermittent or when treatment is provided by a clinician or teacher who is not a specialist in AAC).

While outcomes measurement is only in its beginning stages in AAC, there are some beginning efforts to document results in some important areas. Measures of participation document the level of integration and participation in real-world settings and events. For example, we might apply AAC intervention for a school-age child so that the child can be active in answering questions in class. A somewhat similar area of focus is to document group membership. Membership refers to a sense of belonging to a group. There is a difference, for example, in how classmates view a child who "comes into" their classroom versus a child who "is part" of their classroom. Membership is sometimes measured as being chosen by other group members or as being the result of a judgment of status in a group. A third focus of study is the measurement of quality of life. According to Schlosser (2003c), there are more than 100 instruments that claim to measure quality of life. These measures include both objective measures (e.g., measures of health status or income) and also subjective measures (e.g., reports of satisfaction with number of friends).

Good clinicians have always attended to outcomes. It is especially true in AAC practice that the severe nature of the disabilities involved causes us to reflect on our true purpose and the value of services we provide. In most cases, we know that clients who use AAC strategies will never be like their nondisabled peers, so we are forced to ask ourselves what outcomes we do expect from our efforts. The development that is relatively new to our practice is the call for systematic demonstration of these outcomes. According to Schlosser (2003c), only a few studies have begun to investigate each of these important aspects of outcomes measurement.

EBP for AAC practice is defined as "the integration of best and current research evidence with clinical/educational expertise and relevant stakeholder perspective to facilitate decisions for assessment and intervention that are deemed effective and efficient for a given direct stakeholder" (Schlosser & Raghavendra, 2003, p. 263). EBP is a systemtic approach to examine the evidence available and to use that evidence to make good clinical decisions for an individual client.

In AAC practice, the level of evidence does not meet the standard expected in some areas of practice, and it is unlikely that it ever will. The "gold standard," or highest level, of evidence in medical practice is a review of randomized group studies comparing a treatment group to a control group. In AAC, however, it is not feasible to design a randomized group study. AAC clients are considered to be a low-incidence population, and they tend to be a very heterogeneous group. Even if a sufficiently large and homogenous population could be identified, ethical issues would make it difficult to withhold treatment from a control group.

The absence of randomized control group comparisons does not mean, however, that the clinician must abandon the EBP model. Best available evidence must be defined in relation to the field. Although we do not have randomized group trials, we do have some group designs that are considered "quasi-experimental." For example, we might have a group treatment and compare pretreatment and posttreatment measures. We also find many single-subject designs used in AAC research. One example of this is an ABAB design, where a baseline is measured with no treatment in the A-phase; the behavior continues to be measured during the B-phase or treatment segment; and then the pattern is repeated. We should be able to see the effects of the treatment changing the behavior measured only during the B-phases. These approaches do have some ability to demonstrate that treatments have specific effects, even though some questions of validity may be raised. Schlosser and Raghavendra (2003) proposed a hierarchy of evidence with meta-analysis of multiple quasi-experimental designs and single-subject designs as the top level of evidence. A second level would be a single study of one of these types. Lower levels of evidence would include literature reviews, case study reports, and expert opinions. It is important to remember that the EBP framework refers to using the best evidence available, not to waiting for the ideal level of evidence to answer clinical questions.

Schlosser (2003b) has presented the most extensive review yet directed to applying EBP in AAC. He included several literature reviews designed to assist the clinician in making treatment decisions for presymbolic communicators (Olsson & Granlund, 2003), beginning communicators (Sigafoos, Drasgow, & Schlosser, 2003), and adults with aphasia (Koul & Corwin, 2003). Also, many aspects of practice were studied, including the effects of AAC on natural speech (Schlosser, 2003a) and the impact on literacy

(Blischak, Gorman, & Lombardino, 2003). While it interesting to note that the literature does provide some important information in each of these areas, it is also noted that evidence is most often judged to be "suggestive." That is, in rating the quality of information available, the authors consistently found that there were strong suggestions that AAC interventions had positive outcomes, but that the level of evidence was not strongly conclusive. This clearly shows the need for additional research in AAC outcomes.

case study AMANDA

Amanda is 7 years old and shows profound developmental delay in all areas. She communicates much the way a 6-month-old baby would, in that she fusses if she is unhappy and smiles or laughs when she is happy. Motor development and self-help skills are similarly delayed to infant levels.

Amanda participates in a typical first-grade classroom, although she cannot match the skills of the other children in the class. She learns to do things that are in predictable routines. For example, when she first comes to school each day, she is helped to take off her coat and hang it on the hook beside her name; then the class gathers for "opening circle" time during which Amanda will help to put the number cards on the calendar board. She is frequently offered choices, such as choosing a book to represent library time or a sweater to represent that she will go outside. Simple gestures are encouraged, so she has a ready way to indicate "I want that" by pointing and holding out her hand or "I don't want that" by holding up her hand with the palm out. Teachers also model the use of basic vocabulary in manual signs. She uses a Go Talk communication device for some of her activities; for example, during art activities she can touch one of the picture symbols to activate recorded messages to say, "Help me"; "I'll do it myself"; "I need more"; "I'm done"; and "I want the pink one." Her classmates quickly learned that pink is her favorite color.

QUESTIONS

1. Identify at least four different AAC strategies that Amanda uses. Describe these strategies in terms of aided or unaided means to represent, to select, and to transmit messages.
2. Why might these AAC strategies be successful for Amanda even when her speech and overall development have not reached age-appropriate levels?

case study BRIAN

Brian is 14 years old and looking forward to high school next year. Throughout his early years, school staff have worked to help him to be active in his classes, even though he has severe cerebral palsy, uses a wheelchair, and needs physical assistance throughout the day. He can vocalize to get someone's attention and to show when he is angry or excited, but he does not make any words that can be understood by others. He is at or near grade level for most academic subjects, although assignments and tests have to be modified for Brian. In his early school years, he required the constant development of simple strategies for him to communicate his thoughts, such as using many picture boards to keep up with topics in first-grade classes. He now does his school work through a Pathfinder communication device. This device allows him to access thousands of words and phrases by selecting sequences of picture icons, or he can use the keyboard function to type new words. The device has high-quality synthesized speech that allows him to take part in group conversations and to answer questions in class. It also connects to a computer so that he can print out class assignments such as book reports. During some activities, such as lunch, items are placed within his reach, and he can use simple pointing to indicate what he wants next. His friends are used to responding to his facial expression that indicates he wants something or has a joke to tell.

QUESTIONS

1. Identify five different strategies that Brian has used to communicate. Describe each strategy in terms of means to represent, to select, and to transmit messages.
2. Imagine the activities and settings in which Brian will want to participate in high school and as a young adult. How will Brian's AAC strategies help him to be an active and competent participant?

case study MR. CHARLES

Mr. Charles is a retired school teacher diagnosed with amyotrophic lateral sclerosis (ALS), a degenerative neuromuscular disease. Currently, his speech remains useful in most situations, although his voice has dropped in both pitch and loudness, and his articulation is increasingly slurred. Late in the day or when he is especially tired, even his family members cannot understand him, and it feels like too much effort to continue talking. His most recent complaint is that people cannot understand him on the telephone, and this interferes with keeping contact with his children and grandchildren. He is also experiencing difficulty with handwriting, as the ALS affects all parts of his body.

Currently, Mr. Charles has opted for using a laptop computer with specialized software. By using EZ Keys software, the demands of typing are somewhat reduced already. In the future, if necessary, he can access the computer by one-finger typing. He also has the Micro CommPac, which allows the computer to function as a speech-generating device. This is useful when he is tired or on the telephone. His speech-language pathologist is introducing him to scanning options in connection with this computer. He may one day require scanning to continue accessing all of the computer functions with a simple switch control instead of keyboard access. He is also experimenting with eye-gaze systems because control of eye muscles is sometimes the last volitional motor control as ALS progresses to the final, fatal stage. By working with various AAC options now, Mr. Charles has confidence that he will continue to have a means to communicate and a way to make important decisions about his own life throughout the course of his disease.

QUESTIONS

1. Identify at least four different AAC strategies that Mr. Charles has used or experimented with. Describe each strategy in terms of means to represent, to select, and to transmit messages.
2. What priorities do you think Mr. Charles will set as the intervention team discusses options with him? How will his AAC strategies help him to address his priority concerns throughout the course of his disease?

Summary

This chapter has presented a brief overview of the many strategies and techniques referred to as AAC. AAC strategies may be aided or unaided, and they differ from typical communication in the use of a means to represent a message, a means to select a symbol, and a means to transmit a message. Users of AAC strategies are a diverse population, including those with congenital disabilities or acquired disabilities; these impairments may affect motor, cognitive, and/or sensory abilities. While expanding technologies provide many exciting options for helping individuals to participate in a full range of life experiences, communication continues to be an interpersonal interaction between two or more people. The success of AAC depends upon carefully matching the strategies to the needs of the individual, effectively presenting and teaching the client to use the AAC strategies, and developing an environment that provides opportunities and support to the AAC user. Continued research is needed to develop more-effective and more-efficient strategies and to assist professionals in matching intervention strategies to the needs of clients they serve.

STUDY QUESTIONS

1. Use the framework of the AAC communication model (means to represent [symbols], to select, and to transmit messages) to compare and contrast AAC with typical communication.

2. Identify the four distinct communicative competencies related to AAC use presented by Light (1989) and elaborate on their roles in contributing to effective communication.

3. Compare and contrast the AAC needs of an individual with a congenital disability, such as cerebral palsy, with the needs of an individual with an acquired disability, such as aphasia.

4. How is AAC related to the rights of individuals with disabilities?

SELECTED READINGS

Beukelman, D. R., & Mirenda, P. (1998). *Augmentative and alternative communication: Management of severe communication disorders in children and adults* (2nd ed.). Baltimore, MD: Paul H. Brookes.

Beukelman, D. R., Yorkston, K. M., & Reichle, J. (Eds.). (2000). *Augmentative and alternative communication for adults with acquired neurologic disorders.* Baltimore, MD: Paul H. Brookes.

Kangas, K. A., & Lloyd, L. L. (1988). Early cognitive prerequisites to augmentative and alternative communication use: What are we waiting for? *Augmentative and Alternative Communication, 4,* 211–221.

Koppenhaver, D., Evans, D., & Yoder, D. (1991). Childhood reading and writing experiences of literature adults with severe speech and motor impairments. *Augmentative and Alternative Communication, 7,* 20–33.

Lloyd, L. L., Fuller, D. R., & Arvidson, H. H. (Eds.). (1997). *Augmentative and alternative communication: A handbook of principles and practices.* Boston, MA: Allyn & Bacon.

McCormick, L., & Wegner, J. (2003). Supporting augmentative and alternative communication. In L. McCormick, D. F. Loeb, & R. L. Schiefelbusch (Eds.), *Supporting children with communication difficulties in inclusive settings: School-based language intervention* (2nd ed., pp. 435–459). Boston, MA: Allyn & Bacon.

Mirenda, P., & Erickson, K. A. (2000). Augmentative communication and literacy. In A. M. Wetherby & B. M. Prizant (Eds.), *Autism spectrum disorders: A transactional developmental perspective* (pp. 333–367). Baltimore, MD: Paul H. Brookes.

National Joint Committee for the Communication Needs of Persons With Severe Disabilities (1992). *Guidelines for meeting the communication needs of persons with severe disabilities* [Guidelines].

Reichle, J., Beukelman, D. R., & Light, J. C. (2002). *Exemplary practices for beginning communicators: Implications for AAC.* Baltimore, MD: Paul H. Brookes.

Williams, M. B., & Krezman, C. J. (Eds.). (2000). *Beneath the surface: Creative expressions of augmented communicators.* Toronto, Ontario: International Society for Augumentative and Alternative Communication.

WEBSITES OF INTEREST

www.aac.unl.edu

This homepage for the Munroe Barkley Memorial Center at the University of Nebraska–Lincoln has a wide variety of resources in AAC, including demographic information, presentations, resources, and links to other related sites.

www.aacproducts.org

The Communication Aid Manufacturers Association provides links to many companies that produce AAC devices as well as information about workshops on AAC technology.

www.isaac-online.org

This homepage for the International Society for Augmentative and Alternative Communication (ISAAC), an organization of more than 3,000 members in 50 countries, includes links to 15 national chapters, including one in the United States. ISAAC includes many different professions as well as AAC users and their families; it sponsors biennial international conventions; and it publishes a quarterly journal devoted to AAC.

Chapter **SIXTEEN**

Swallowing

Process and Disorders

Barbara C. Sonies
University of Maryland and George Washington University

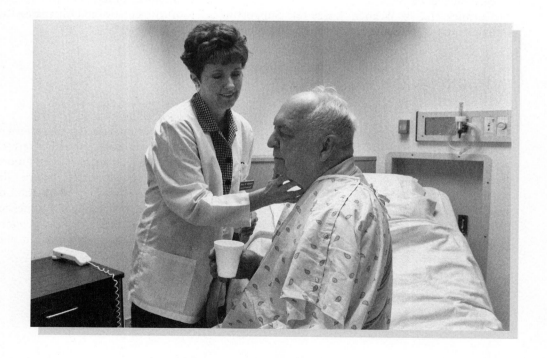

personal PERSPECTIVE

BARBARA C. SONIES

As a teenager I wanted to be an actress or a TV personality, but I realized that I just was not suited to be a starving artist. When I was a senior in high school and had to write a paper for my psychology class, I chose cerebral palsy. I began to visit school programs in the community for children with cerebral palsy. In addition, I visited the local university clinic that trained speech therapists and was introduced to the therapist. Her work was quite fascinating to me, so I made more on-site visits. This field, although not the theater, required good communication skills and seemed to be challenging. After some reflection and more talks with therapists and university students, I was sold on the field as being a match for my aptitude and interests. When I entered college at the University of Minnesota, I knew I was going to enroll in the speech pathology program. It was one of the premier programs in our field, and I was so lucky to have a group of renowned scientists/teachers (Arnold Aronson, Bryng Bryngelson, Gerald Seigel, Frederick Darley, Hildred Schuell, Clark Starr, Jon Eisenson, Willard Zemlin) who were role models for the career that has been mine for 40 years.

After working in the schools and hospitals with both children and adults, I went back and earned my Ph.D., knowing that dysphagia was going to be my main focus. My two-decades-long presence in dysphagia grew from working with a patient who could not swallow and from my work with children with cerebral palsy with oral motor and swallowing disorders. I found that we did not fully understand swallowing physiology and that I could use a variety of instrumental techniques to image the oropharynx during the swallow. I learned about a new technology, ultrasound imaging, and developed it as a way to view the oropharynx. I have enjoyed being able to create new methods and models of swallowing behavior. Dysphagia is exciting for me because we can help patients in relatively few sessions. Personal satisfaction, service to others, and intellectual stimulation are what keeps me in this field.

Engaging in social situations remains one of the most pleasant interactions of family, religious, and community life. Most of these pleasurable activities revolve around the interactions that occur during eating. When the ability to eat is impaired, the quality of life is seriously impacted. Dysphagia (difficulty swallowing) is common to a variety of conditions and is seen across the life span from infancy to old age. Swallowing difficulty presents in a wide spectrum of clinical settings from acute inpatient hospitals to outpatient rehabilitation departments, long-term care facilities, skilled nursing residences, and schools. The incidence of dysphagia in nursing homes ranges from 50 to 70 percent and is more common among the elderly who require hospitalization and those with neurological conditions (Langmore, Skarupski, Park, & Fries, 2002; Marik & Kaplan, 2003). The incidence of dysphagia has been estimated at 15 million per year, and it is estimated that one-third of the 650,000 to 700,000 new stroke patients will have swallowing difficulty (Teasell, Foley, Fisher, & Finestone, 2002). The care for persons who are unable to eat normal diets and thus require supplemental tube feedings is expensive, making swallowing rehabilitation a medical priority.

The speech-language pathologist has in-depth training to both diagnose and treat individuals with swallowing disorders. Treatment of dysphagia is complicated and requires a team of professionals in addition to a speech-language pathologist, who is often the coordinator. Teams may include a radiologist, gastroenterologist, nurse, nutritionist, dentist, neurologist, respiratory therapist, occupational therapist, pharmacist, nurse, or physical therapist. To understand and treat persons who have dysphagia, knowledge of normal and abnormal swallowing is essential, as are cultural issues, effects of aging, instrumental assessments, clinical evaluations, and treatment options.

Cultural Competence and Swallowing

To adequately assess those with a complaint of swallowing difficulty, we must understand cultural backgrounds. Culture can be defined as "thoughts, communications, actions, customs, beliefs, values, and institutions of racial, ethnic, religious or social groups" (ASHA Leader, 2004). During an evaluation of swallowing, we need to be aware of how our interactions and our suggestions for therapy may be interpreted by persons from differing culture. An interpreter may be needed to answer questions. Specific to dysphagia are ethnic or religious dietary preferences, use of spices, textures of foods, food preparation practices, when and where meals are served, and who is present during eating. Some societies have rigid rules as to the mixing of genders during meals, and in some cultures, it would be difficult for a nonoral diet to be followed for the head of a family, who is used to being an authority figure. In relating to persons from varied cultures, it is important that medical terminology be explained.

Normal Swallowing

An understanding of the normal anatomy and physiology of the upper aerodigestive system is required before evaluation and treatment for dysphagia can begin. The speech-language pathologist needs to know what anatomic structures are affected and how the muscles, joints, nerves, and other organ systems interact in a swallow. In addition, we must have a working knowledge of the cranial nerves that innervate these structures and must know the cortical control processes that govern the swallow. Knowledge of medications, neurologic disorders, aging, infant development, cognitive function, memory, cultural diversity, and sociocultural implications of the various diseases that impact on our ability to swallow is also required.

Anatomy of the Normal Swallow

The gross anatomical structures of the upper aerodigestive tract involved in swallowing, including the oral cavity, pharynx, larynx, and esophagus, can be seen in Figure 16.1. The specific structures of oral cavity that are used during a swallow include the lips, teeth, tongue, hard palate, soft palate or velum, hyoid bone, mandible, maxilla, floor of the mouth, and faucial pillars. The tongue can be divided into two components: (1) the oral tongue and (2) the pharyngeal tongue. The oral tongue consists of the tongue tip, blade, front, center, and back, and the pharyngeal base of the tongue forms the top of the vallecular space in the pharynx. The pharynx consists of three constrictor muscles—superior, medial, and inferior—which make up the posterior and lateral pharyngeal walls (Netter, 1953).

The pharynx, an open air-filled column, is divided into the *nasopharynx, hypopharynx (oropharynx), and laryngopharynx.* The structures in the laryngopharynx include the undersurface of the epiglottis, which forms the superior border of the laryngeal additus or vestibule, the pyriform sinuses, and the upper border of the cricopharyngeus muscle also referred to as the upper esophageal sphincter (Netter, 1953). The spinal cord and cervical vertebrae form the posterior support for the pharynx, while the laryngeal cartilages give support to the anterior of the laryngopharynx. The majority of the many muscles activated in the oral and pharyngeal swallow attach

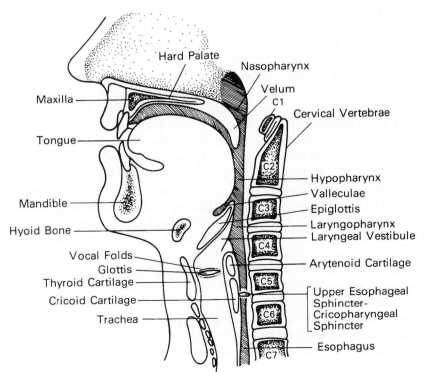

FIGURE 16.1

Schematic of the oropharynx.

to the hyoid bone. Although the glottis and the trachea form the top of the airway, as shown in Figure 16.1, these structures are not involved in the swallow; rather, they need to be protected from material entering into the airway by closure of the vocal folds and lowering of the epiglottis. The esophagus is a closed structure composed of striated muscle in the upper third and smooth muscles in the lower two-thirds. Peristaltic activity is initiated throughout the esophagus to move the swallowed material to the stomach for further digestion.

Physiology of the Swallow

Phases of the Swallow   The normal swallow consists of four phases or stages: the *oral preparatory phase*, the *oral phase*, the *pharyngeal phase*, and the *esophageal phase*. These sequential phases are overlapping. For example, when tongue activity occurs in the mouth, activity may also be detected in the pharynx and esophagus. Swallowing behavior is predictable and follows a replicable pattern that is both reflexive and volitional. In the volitional phases (oral preparatory and oral phases), the swallow can be terminated at will if the taste or smell is unpleasant or if food is spoiled. Once the reflexive swallow (pharyngeal and esophageal phases) occurs, it is difficult to impede the flow of a bolus. Although the swallow pattern is highly repeatable, there are variations in how we swallow depending on the texture, volume, and viscosity of a bolus. Because swallowing patterns change due to bolus variations, swallowing is not considered a truly reflexive behavior; rather, it is termed a patterned or programmed response. However, it is important to remember that rather than each phase being temporally discrete, swallowing is an interdependent, overlapping, and dynamic process where activity may exist simultaneously from the mouth through the pharynx.

Oral Preparatory Phase.   In the oral preparatory phase, food is manipulated and chewed. This phase is variable in duration and is stimulated by the sensory inputs of the cranial nerves (V, VII, IX) that control taste, smell, and temperature. In this voluntary phase, the swallow can be terminated at will if the material does not taste good or if it is spoiled, too hot, or otherwise undesirable. In the *oral preparatory phase* of the swallow, the lips remove food from a spoon, fork, straw, or cup to form a tight seal that will prohibit any leakage of food out of the mouth. To initiate a swallow, the tongue tip and blade elevate behind the incisors, placing the bolus in position to begin to swallow. Whereas no preparation is needed for liquids, for solid materials the food is moved from side to side over the tongue to the molars, chewed, and mixed with saliva into a "swallow ready" consistency. The secretions of the three sets of salivary glands—parotid, sublingual, and submandibular—mineralize the teeth, aid in control of oral infection, and promote digestion. The prepared material rests on the medial surface of the tongue in a central groove with the lateral borders of the tongue touching the molars and the tip of the tongue elevated to the central incisors. The lips remain closed to eliminate oral dripping. Timing of the oral preparatory phase of the swallow is highly individualized. Once the bolus begins to move over the surface of the tongue, the oral phase of the swallow begins. There is considerable overlap between the oral preparatory and the oral phases of the swallow.

Oral Phase.   During the oral phase, the tongue propels the food bolus backward through the oral cavity until the pharyngeal swallow is triggered. As the tongue transports the bolus backward over the surface of the tongue, the back of the tongue contacts the velum to protect the nasal passages from entry of food. Tongue retraction also helps force the bolus into the upper pharynx. At the same time, the hyoid bone begins its forward/upward trajectory, causing the floor muscles of the mouth (geniohyoid, mylohyoid) to contract and the epiglottis to lower over the entry into the airway (laryngeal vestibule).

When the bolus reaches the faucial pillars, tactile sensation stimulates the swallow response, and the bolus is propelled into the pharynx. The bolus rests for a short time in the valleculae at the base of the tongue while the epiglottis continues to descend, covering the airway. The cranial nerves involved in the oral phase are V (trigeminal), VII (facial), and IX (glossopharyngeal). (See Table 16.1 for details.)

Pharyngeal Phase. This phase begins when the bolus head passes over the base of the tongue into the hypopharynx and begins its vertical descent. The velum elevates and contacts the posterior wall of the pharynx to seal off the nasopharynx and prevent nasal regurgitation. Gravity, combined with changes in interbolus pressure and the forces of the muscles of the pharyngeal walls, creates a stripping wave that transfers the material through the pharynx. Contractions of the pharyngeal constrictor muscles create this stripping wave. The movement of the tongue and hyoid that began in the oral phase helps to elevate the larynx and depress the epiglottis, protecting the laryngeal vestibule from entry of food. Just before the bolus enters the hypopharynx, the floor muscles of the mouth (geniohyoid and mylohyoid) contract, bringing the hyoid bone forward and upward as the tongue moves the bolus posteriorly into the pharynx. Food is directed laterally to both sides of the epiglottis, resting momentarily in the pyriform sinuses in the cricopharyngeal area. There is short period of apnea when respiration stops and the airway is protected by vocal fold adduction. Studies have shown that the elevation of the hyoid in the oropharyngeal phase causes the floor of the mouth muscles to contract, the epiglottis to lower, the larynx to elevate, the vocal folds to oppose, and the upper esophageal sphincter to relax and open (Shaker et al., 1993; Shaw et al., 1995; Sonies, Parent, Morrish, & Baum, 1988). As the hyoid bone elevates, the arytenoid cartilages tilt toward the base of the epiglottis and aid in protecting the airway. Although the pharyngeal swallow is thought to be involuntary, there are several volitional maneuvers such as a cough or clearing of the throat that can stop material from entering the airway. The oropharyngeal swallow (a combination of the oral and pharyngeal phases) occurs within 1 to 1.5 seconds. At the end of the oropharyngeal swallow, the epiglottis returns to its original upright position, the hyoid returns to rest, and the velum returns to a lowered resting position with an entirely open airway.

Esophageal Phase. Esophageal peristalsis (rhythmic involuntary contractions) carry the bolus to the stomach. There is no evidence of volitional or cortical control during the esophageal phase of the swallow, which is under the control of the vagus nerve (X). As the cricopharyngeus (CP) muscle of the pharyngo-esophageal (PE) segment, also called the upper esophageal sphincter (UES), relaxes and opens due to traction, or pull, of the hyoid motion, the bolus head enters the esophagus. Gravitational force and the weight of the bolus help to relax and open the UES. When the UES opens, the laryngeal vestibule is closed off, and the airway is protected. It takes approximately 8 to 10 seconds for the bolus to move through the esophagus into the stomach.

TABLE 16.1   Role of the Cranial Nerves in Swallowing Function

Cranial Nerve	Phase	Sensory	Motor
V Trigeminal Nerve	Oral Preparatory	■ Sensation to the anterior 2/3 of tongue ■ Sensation of hot and cold ■ Sensation of oral pain	■ Somatic motor for muscles of mastication: temporalis, masseter, pterygoids
	Oral	■ Sensation to all oral mucosa, teeth, and gums ■ Salivary flow to major and minor glands	■ Innervates floor muscles, which aid in elevation of the larynx
	Pharyngeal	■ None	■ Indirectly same as the 4 above
VII Facial Nerve	Oral Preparatory	■ Taste to the anterior 2/3 of the tongue ■ Sensation to the soft palate	■ Somatic motor for facial muscles: digastric, mylohyoid, geniohyoid ■ Lips—closure/seal, shape, motion ■ Cheeks—seal with lips and tongue
	Oral	■ Salivary glands	■ Preparation of bolus and lip seal for the removal of the bolus ■ Visceral—lingual gland
	Pharyngeal	■ None	■ Assists in elevation of the hyoid bone ■ Raises larynx to protect the airway
IX Glossopharyngeal Nerve	Oral Preparatory	■ None	■ None
	Oral	■ Taste to the posterior 1/3 of the tongue ■ Sensation to faucial pillars and soft palate ■ Innervates parotid gland	■ Provides sensation during velopharyngeal closure to prevent nasal regurgitation
	Pharyngeal	■ Sensation to the pharynx and larynx	■ Innervates stylopharyngeus muscle
X Vagus Nerve	Oral Preparatory	■ None	■ None
	Oral	■ None	■ None
	Pharyngeal	■ General sensory from pharynx, larynx, and trachea	■ Somatic motor to base of the tongue, pharynx (middle/inferior constrictors, upper/lower)
		■ Visceral sensory from mucosa of the valleculae, pharynx, larynx, and lungs	■ Larynx (external and internal), diaphragm/lungs, peristalsis

(Continued)

TABLE 16.1   (Continued)

Cranial Nerve	Phase	Sensory	Motor
	Esophageal	▪ Visceral sensory from mucosa of the stomach and abdomen	▪ Somatic motor—peristalsis and constriction of esophagus
XII Hypoglossal Nerve	Oral Preparatory	▪ None	▪ Somatic motor for tongue muscles (except palatoglossus): To seal oral cavity; preparing bolus size; removing food particles from buccal sulci, palate, and molars; mixing bolus with saliva
	Oral	▪ None	▪ Somatic motor for tongue muscles: alveolar-palatal contact, bolus from mid-palate to posterior tongue, tongue/palate contact to close airway as reflex begins, transport bolus to pharynx
	Pharyngeal	▪ None	▪ Somatic motor—raise and lower hyoid and larynx to protect the airway

Neurology of the Swallow

Cortical and Subcortical Innervation

Daniels (2004) stated that "evidence from anatomical and functional imaging indicate[s] involvement of a widely distributed neural network for swallowing." Swallowing was once regarded as a function controlled by the swallowing center in the medulla and pons, part of the brain stem; however, recent studies using functional imaging of brain activity have revealed numerous areas of cortical regulation of the swallow (Daniels & Foundas, 1997, 1999; Daniels, Foundas, Iglesia, & Sullivan, 1996; Dziewas et al., 2003; R. E. Martin & Sessle, 1993; Suzuki, et al., 2003). A schematic of these structures is found in Figure 16.2. According to Bass (1997), the volitional components of the oral and pharyngeal swallow are modulated by "the supramedullary structures, such as pons, mesencephalon, and limbic and cerebral cortex" (p. 23). Studies examining brain activation during the normal swallow using functional magnetic resonance imaging (fMRI) and positron emission tomography (PET) have found strong evidence for cortical activation of the following cortical structures: sensorimotor cortex, insula, cerebellum, putamen, globus pallidus, thalamus, anterior cingulate gyrus, and supplemental motor area, with evidence for localized involvement of the

FIGURE 16.2
Schematic of the
cortical and subcortical
components of the
swallow (after Bass,
1997).

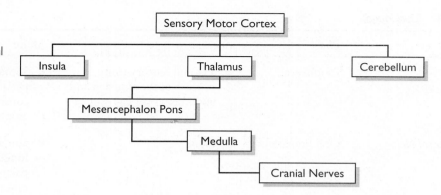

basal ganglia, pons, and medulla (Daniels & Foundas 1997; Daniels et al., 1996; Dziewas et al., 2003; Hamdy et al., 1999; R.E. Martin & Sessle, 1993; Suzuki et al., 2003). A schematic of these structures is found in Figure 16.2.

There is also evidence of differences in the type of dysphagia found in patients with either right or left-hemisphere lesions. It has been found that damage to the left hemisphere in stroke will cause oral or oral preparatory phase problems and that damage to the right hemisphere will cause pharyngeal problems and an increase in aspiration (Alberts, Horner, Gray, & Brazer, 1992; Robbins & Levine, 1988; Robbins, Levine, Maser, Rosenbek, & Kempster, 1993). As more neural imaging studies are done with more sophisticated technology, more information on cortical swallowing will emerge.

Cranial Nerve Innervation

Because sensation precedes movement, damage to sensory, motor, or both components of the cranial nerves may adversely affect swallowing. The cranial nerves involved in swallowing provide both sensory and motor innervations for the muscles of the oral cavity, pharynx, larynx, and esophagus. They are called *cranial nerves* because they originate from the cranium and differ from spinal nerves, which originate from the spinal column. Cranial nerves can be specialized, so that individual nerves can be either sensory or motor. There are five cranial nerves that are responsible for the swallow: trigeminal V, facial VII, glossopharyngeal IX, vagus X, and hypoglossal XII (Perlman, 1991). They all emerge from the swallowing center in the brain stem's medulla and pons (Netter, 1953). Although the cortex has a role to play in the volitional components of the swallow, it is primarily a brain stem and cranial nerve behavior. We will discuss the function of each cranial nerve and its participation in swallowing separately (see Table 16.1).

Trigeminal, Cranial Nerve V   This nerve supplies the main sensory (afferent) input during the oral and oral preparatory phases of the swallow by providing oral sensation to the anterior two-thirds of the tongue, soft palate, cheeks, floor of the mouth, teeth and gums, temporomandibular joint, lips, nasopharnx, soft palate, hard palate, and tonsils and visceral sensation to the salivary glands. Facial and dental pain, touch, and temperature are also stimulated by the trigeminal nerve. The trigeminal nerve has a role in the motor (efferent) function of the oral phase of the swallow, as it innervates the temporalis, masseter, and pterygoid muscles during mastication. It also innervates the floor muscles of the mouth—the mylohyoid, geniohyoid, and digastric—to assist in elevation of the hyoid bone.

Facial, Cranial Nerve VII   The facial nerve conveys taste sensation to the anterior two-thirds of the tongue and sensation to the soft palate and salivary glands. The facial nerve supplies the majority of the motor input to all of the muscles of the face, including the lips, cheeks, floor of the mouth, and submandibular salivary glands. It provides the innervation for lip seal, lip rounding, removal of a bolus from utensils, sucking from a straw, and preparation of the bolus before the actual swallow occurs.

Glossopharyngeal, Cranial Nerve IX   This cranial nerve activates the posterior portion of the tongue and oral cavity by providing taste to the posterior portion of the tongue and sensation to the faucial pillars and soft palate. It also innervates the parotid glands, which are the major salivary glands, and provides sensation to the upper pharynx. It innervates the stylopharyngeus muscle of the upper pharyngeal constrictor muscle to aid in bolus transfer through the upper pharynx.

Vagus, Cranial Nerve X   This cranial nerve is often termed the *major,* or primary, cranial nerve for swallowing, as it has both sensory and motor fibers and provides innervation to the entire upper and lower digestive system, including the pharynx, larynx, esophagus, and stomach, as well as to the gastrointestinal system from the stomach to the colon. It also has fibers that convey general sensation and taste to the pharynx, laryngopharynx, epiglottis, vocal folds, and even the posterior part of the tongue. The motor fibers innervate the base of the tongue, the middle and inferior constrictor muscles that contract the pharynx, the lungs, the diaphragm, and the esophagus, causing peristaltic activity.

Hypoglossal, Cranial Nerve XII   The hypoglossal nerve provides the major motor input to all of the lingual muscles during the oral preparatory, oral, and pharyngeal phases of the swallow. It is important in that it innervates the tongue to seal the oral cavity, prepare the bolus, and remove food particles from the buccal sulcus, palate, and teeth in the oral preparatory phase of the swallow. This cranial nerve implements the motion of the tongue for alveolar palatal contacts before the swallow, during bolus transfer from mid-palate to tongue dorsum and base of the tongue, and during bolus transfer into the pharynx. This nerve is essential for stimulation of the elevation and depression of the hyoid bone during the swallow and during airway protection.

Swallowing and Normal Aging

Age alone does not predispose a person to swallowing disorders. There are, however, numerous changes that can impact the ability to swallow. Because more people are living longer, most older persons will have several chronic conditions and multiple health problems that can cause swallowing impairments (Compher, Kim, & Bader, 1998; Fucile & Wright, 1998). We will first review normal age-related changes and how age affects the oral pharyngeal structures.

Common Effects of Aging and Swallowing

There is a general effect of age on swallowing, especially in persons over age 70, including longer duration of total swallow, delayed elevation of the hyoid, longer duration of opening of the upper esophageal sphincter, decline in overall pressure reserves, and

TABLE 16.2   Age-Associated Effects on Swallowing

Morphologic Changes	*Effects of Change on Swallow*
Poor dentition	Altered size of bolus
Decreased perception of viscosity	Preference for softer foods
Reduced smell	Changed food preferences
Increased taste threshold	Addition of spices
Muscular atrophy	Cricopharyngeal bar and pain
Decreased muscle tone	Diverticula and reflux
Reduced tone in pharynx	Delayed pharyngeal clearance-pooling
Reduced contractions in esophagus	Delayed cricopharyngeal opening
	Slowed esophageal transport
Degenerative osteophytes and spurs	Painful swallowing
Ligamentous laxity	Delayed laryngeal adduction and penetration
Hiatal hernia	Gastrointestinal reflux and pain

Source: Information from Sonies (1992a).

decreased tongue pressure and strength due to general muscle wasting or sarcopenia (Evans, 1995; Nicosia et al., 2000; Robbins, Hamilton, Lof, & Kempster, 1992; Robbins, Levine, Wood, Roecker, & Luschei, 1995; Sonies, 1991b; Sonies et al., 1988). The effects of some of these changes on swallowing in the elderly are shown in compensations during eating or subtle subclinical changes in swallowing (see Table 16.2).

Respiration   During swallowing, it is essential that the timing of breathing be coordinated with swallowing events to prevent aspiration of material into the lungs. Structures involved in respiratory function include the larynx, thorax, diaphragm, internal and external intercostals, and abdominal muscles (Boone & McFarlane, 2000). Aging may result in postural changes adversely affecting respiratory function (Rammage, Morrison, & Nichol, 2001). This is attributed to thinning of the vertebral column and degeneration of the vertebral vertebrae resulting in the ossification and inward sinking of the thorax and reducing vital capacity (Sonies, Stone, & Shawker, 1984).

Breathing and swallowing are highly integrated and coordinated. During a normal swallow, there is a brief moment of less than 1 second when breathing ceases (apneic interval) and the airway is protected from entry of food (B.J. Martin, Logemann, Shaker, & Dodds 1994). Normal swallowing occurs during expiration or when air is exiting from the respiratory system. In order for this to occur, there must be normal activity of the larynx to close off the airway at the level of the ventricular folds and to cause forward displacement of the arytenoid cartilages and lowering of the epiglottis (Martin et al., 1994). In contrast, studies have shown that, when the airway should be closed and an expiratory pulse should occur, most elderly persons instead have an inspiratory pattern of air intake *during* or just following a swallow that causes material to enter the laryngeal vestibule, thereby producing a cough to clear material. (Martin-Harris, Brodsky, Price, Michel, & Walters, 2003; H. Nilsson, Ekberg, Olsson, & Hindfelt, 1996). In addition, it has been found that normal elderly persons have a pattern where there is bolus retention in the pharynx and the swallow is delayed, but the bolus eventually clears (Dejaeger, Pelemans, Ponette, & Joosten, 1977; Perlman, Schultz, & VanDaele, 1993).

Larynx   The larynx comprises one bone and several cartilages (Boone & McFarlane, 2000). While changes to the larynx commonly affect voice, ossification of the laryngeal cartilages may adversely affect swallowing.

As documented by case reports, the cricoarytenoid joint and laryngeal cartilages are susceptible to the same age-related changes that other joints in the body experience (Sonies, 1991b). These changes may affect vocal function and swallowing (Sonies, 1991b). According to Rammage et al. (2001), most changes affecting the cricoarytenoid joint result from intubation trauma and acute injury. The joint can become inflamed, arthritic, or fibrotic, which can stiffen the joint, limiting mobility (Rammage et al., 2001). Laryngeal elevation is essential for swallowing safety, so if the cricoarytenoid joint is immobilized, airway protection can be jeopardized.

Oral Mucosa   The mucosa becomes thinner, loses its elasticity, and becomes less firmly attached to the underlying bone and connective tissue with age (Bruestedt, 1983). Environmental effects from years of smoking, chewing, wearing poorly fitted or poorly maintained dentures, and taking medications cause change in the oral mucosa (Sonies, 1991b). Healthy older nonsmokers with excellent oral hygiene do not appear to experience changes to the oral mucosa (Sonies, 1991b).

Saliva   Saliva is an essential bodily secretion that serves to maintain oral moisture, prevent tooth decay, lubricate the oropharynx and esophagus for digestion, mineralize the teeth, assist in digestion, and neutralize stomach acid (Logemann, 1998a; Stuchell & Mandel, 1988). As one ages, there is diminished salivary flow (xerostomia), which causes dryness and changes in oral sensation (Baum, 1989; Sonies, 1991b). Tooth decay and caries may become more prevalent with advanced age (Baum, 1989; Sonies, 1991b). Xerostomia is the major cause of oral phase dysphagia for those who have had radiation treatment to the head and neck. Without sufficient saliva in the oral cavity during chewing, there is poor bolus preparation and impaired bolus transportation over the tongue, and food sticks to the palate, teeth, tongue, or wall of the throat (Baum, 1986, 1989; Bertram, 1967; Caruso, Sonies, Fox, & Atkinson 1989; J. Scott, Flower, & Burns, 1987). Rapid decrease in salivary secretion may be an indication of a pathological condition or result from pharmacological interventions and medical interactions (Sonies, 1991b).

Smell   Decrement in smell is one of the first and most pervasive sensory changes noted during aging. Research suggests that changes in smell begin in the late fifties or early sixties, causing impairment in the ability to perceive and detect harmful odors (D.A. Leopold et al., 1989). Evidence points to active atrophy of the cells lining the nasopharynx as the major cause of odor misperception in the elderly. Cowart (1989) utilized threshold measures and detection of odorants above threshold measures to assess changes in smell. Results revealed age-related decrements in threshold detection where the elderly needed a stronger odorant than younger persons before it was perceived (Stevens & Cain, 1986).

Taste   The majority of the taste buds are found in the lining of the tongue, tongue tip, and dorsum as well as sprinkled throughout the oropharynx. There are several qualities of taste that are perceived by the taste buds: salty (NaCl), sweet (sucrose), bitter (quinine hydrochloride), sour (citric acid), and Umani (Japanese Savory). If taste is reduced or lost, it is defined as *dysgeusia* or *ageusia*. There is controversy as to whether taste is diminished with age, but it has been determined (Leopold et al., 1989;

Mistretta, 1984; Weiffenbach, 1984) that the threshold for detection of taste increases with age and that foods taste bland. Flavor enhancement appears to increase appetite and foster nutrition in the elderly.

GERD: Gastroesophageal Reflux Disease   Chronic gastroesophageal reflux disease (GERD) is a common complaint with advanced age and is often associated with a hiatal hernia. The person experiences discomfort after eating that is accompanied by regurgitation, heartburn, salty taste in the mouth, belching, burping, and acidity. As one ages, the muscles of the esophagus may become less contractile and the normal peristaltic activity is slowed, causing slower emptying of the stomach and backup of acid contents or partially digested food (Shaker et al., 1993; Shaw et al., 1995). There is another risk that aspiration will occur if there is backup into the pharynx and the refluxed material enters the open airway. When there is constant coughing or the voice becomes hoarse after meals, the probability of aspiration back into the pharynx is heightened (Koufman, 1991).

Abnormal Swallowing

Dysphagia, difficulty swallowing, is derived from the Greek *dys + phagein* "to eat" and is defined as difficulty moving food from the mouth to the stomach (*Dorland's,* 1988). Dysphagia is commonly associated with a variety of neurologic, neuromotor, systemic, immunologic, developmental, and iatrogenic conditions as well as infectious processes, surgical changes, and trauma. Dysphagia can occur in infants, children, adults, and the elderly. Conditions such as stroke, head and neck cancer, and Parkinson's disease are among the most common causes of dysphagia.

Aspiration and Penetration

One of the major symptoms of abnormal swallowing physiology, aspiration, can be determined from instrumental studies. Aspiration occurs when the individual directs the bolus into the respiratory system (trachea and lungs) instead of into the digestive system. When food or liquids enter the airway above the level of the vocal folds, it is called *penetration*, and when the material enters the airway below the vocal folds, it is termed *aspiration*. In normal persons, when swallowed material enters the airway, a protective cough is elicited to clear the material out of the laryngeal vestibule, just above the airway, and back into the pharynx, where it is then either swallowed or expelled orally. In persons with various conditions causing dysphagia, the reduced strength and coordination of the swallowing muscles, inadequacy of cranial nerve innervation, reduced oropharyngeal sensation, and structural abnormalities that accompany the conditions often promote aspiration. In some conditions such as Parkinson's disease, *silent aspiration* is found, where the individual is unaware of aspirated material and, therefore, does not clear the airway volitionally. Material can be aspirated from the mouth during or before a swallow, or it can back up from the esophagus and enter the airway after a swallow (reflux) (Koufman, 1991). In either case, once material enters the airway and passes into the trachea, it will enter the lungs, potentially causing infection and aspiration pneumonia or pneumonitis, which are serious medical complications and need aggressive medical treatment.

To adequately assess whether the person is safe for oral feeding or at risk of material entering the airway, results of instrumental studies must be carefully examined on a frame-by-frame, or moment-to-moment, basis. The two procedures that best examine whether the material is actually entering the airway or is cleared from the airway by coughing, clearing, or a subsequent swallow are the videofluoroscopy (VFS) and fiberoptic endoscopic evaluation of swallowing (FEES). From these instrumental studies, one can evaluate the amount, location, and type of material entering the airway above or below the level of the vocal folds. An objective eight-level measure, the Aspiration-Penetration Scale, was developed to provide an objective tool for following the effects of treatment or progression of symptoms in regard to airway protection (Rosenbek, Robbins, Roecker, Coyle, & Wood 1996).

Neurological Conditions Affecting Swallowing

The causes of neurogenic dysphagia can be vascular, infectious, traumatic, autoimmune, metabolic, neoplastic, or degenerative in etiology. Swallowing usually worsens over time in degenerative conditions, but for vascular, infectious, or trauma-induced swallowing, symptoms may be stable or improve as the condition itself improves (Table 16.3).

Stroke   Stroke, or cerebrovascular attack (CVA), is due to vascular dysfunction causing loss of oxygen to the brain and remains one of the primary causes of dysphagia. There is an annual incidence of 500,000 to 600,000 new cases of stroke per year and one-fourth to one-half result in dysphagia (Groher, 1997). Dysphagia caused by a stroke also results in death, as many patients become malnourished and experience respiratory complications and aspiration.

The effects of strokes can be caused by damage throughout the brain at the cortical or subcortical level. A common site of lesion for a stroke is in the left hemisphere in the frontal lobe, temporal lobe, or parietal lobe of the cortex. In most individuals, the left hemisphere is the site of dominance for language and many cognitive tasks; however, some individuals who are left-handed usually have right-hemisphere dominance. Left- and right-hemisphere strokes can occur from plaque buildup in the internal or middle carotid artery or from altered blood supply caused by an embolism, thrombosis, aneurysm, or hemorrhage. The severity of dysphagia is dependent on the size, depth, and exact location of the infarct. Patients experiencing dysphagia from a left-hemisphere stroke often exhibit milder oral or pharyngeal symptoms in comparison to patients with a right-hemisphere stroke (Levine, Robbins, & Maser, 1992; Robbins & Levine, 1988; Robbins et al., 1993). Studies indicate that when a stroke affects the right hemisphere, the symptoms of dysphagia are more severe, as the pharyngeal swallow is more impaired and aspiration is more common. About two-thirds of persons who suffered a stroke will recover, and of the third who do not fully recover, many will have swallowing problems ranging in severity from mild to severe.

Brain stem strokes usually cause dysphagia if the corticobulbar tracts, nucleus tract solitarius, trigeminal nuclear complexes, nucleus ambigus, hypoglossal nuclei, or medullary swallowing centers are involved (Groher, 1997). Brain stem strokes, first described in 1895 by Wallenberg, are referred to as the lateral medullary syndrome (Robbins & Levine, 1988). Bilateral brain stem strokes are severe in nature if the pons and medullary swallowing centers are affected and may cause total dysphagia with poor prognosis for recovery.

TABLE 16.3 Neurological Conditions Causing Dysphagia

Upper Motor Neuron Disorders

Cause	*Site*	*Neuropathology*
Vascular	Thromboembolism in any area of the brain (stroke)	Ischemia and infarction in affected area. Disconnection syndromes as manifested by blood flow/metabolic changes in areas remote from infarction
	Cerebral hemorrhage in any area of the brain	Degeneration of affected area; secondary ischemia and infarction in the tissue surrounding hemorrhagic lesion
Infectious	Meningitis	Bacterial, fungal, viral, or carcinogenic invasion of the meninges
	Encephalitis: Brain stem, cerebrum	Viral-induced inflammatory reaction and secondary degeneration of afflicted area
Traumatic	Closed head injury to the central nervous system (CNS)	Contusion, anoxia, hypoxic/ischemia, hemorrhage, or infarction of the affected area
	Neurosurgical intervention in the CNS	Cerebral edema, scarring, or loss of tissue in affected area
	Cerebral palsy (spastic, ataxic, choreoathetotic)	Static hypoxic/ischemic encephalopathy
Autoimmune	Multiple sclerosis: Central myelinated tracts	Demyelination with secondary inflammatory response in multiple areas of CNS
Metabolic	Wilson's disease: Basal ganglia, cerebellum	Deposition of copper in basal ganglia with secondary neuronal loss
Neoplastic	Intracranial tumors	Direct tissue disruption in affected areas; secondary affects of cerebral edema and increased intracranial pressure
Degenerative	Huntington's disease: Basal ganglia	Progressive neuronal loss in basal ganglia; diffuse strophic brain
	Parkinson's disease: Basal ganglia, substantia nigra of the midbrain	Progressive depletion of dopaminergic neurons
	Friedriech's ataxia: Widespread CNS involvement	Degeneration of cerebral, cellebellar, and brain stem systems
	Multisystem degenerations: ■ Progressive supranuclear palsy	■ Degeneration of autonomic pathways, nigrostriatal system, cerebellum, corticospinal tracts
Infectious	Poliomyelitis: Anterior horn cells in brain stem, spinal cord	Viral induced degeneration of motor neurons; secondary inflammatory responses

(Continued)

TABLE 16.3 (Continued)

Lower Motor Neuron Disorders

Cause	Site	Neuropathology
Traumatic	Closed head injury to peripheral nervous system (PNS)	Contusion, anoxia, hypoxic, hemorrhage, or infarction of brain stem motor neurons
	Neurosurgical intervention in PNS	Traction, scarring, or loss of tissue in infected area
Autoimmune	Guillain-Barré syndrome: PNS	Demyelination of peripheral and sensory nerves
	Myasthenia gravis: Myoneural junction	Inadequate number of acetycholine receptors on striated muscle
	Myasthenic syndrome: Motor neurons	Defective release of presynaptic acetycholine
	Inflammatory myopathies: Striated muscle	Multifocal muscle fiber loss; secondary replacement with connective tissue
Metabolic	Thyroid hypofunction	Myxedematous infiltration of mucosal tissue of vocal tract and/or oral cavity; muscle weakness
Degenerative	Muscular dystrophy: Striated muscle	Degeneration of muscle fibers
	Thoracic masses	Compression of recurrent laryngeal nerve

Upper and Lower Motor Neuron Disorders

Cause	Site	Neuropathology
Degnerative	Amyotrophic lateral sclerosis (ALS): Corticospinal tracts, anterior horn cells in brain stem and spinal cord, motor neurons	Demyelination and degeneration of both upper and lower motor neuron systems

Traumatic Brain Injury   Traumatic injury to the brain, brain stem, or spinal cord from an accident or blow to the head can cause dysphagia. Traumatic brain injury results in a more diffuse site of lesion, with cognitive impairments often co-occurring. Decreased cognitive functioning may complicate recovery as intervention techniques require a certain level of cognitive ability.

Amyotrophic Lateral Sclerosis   Amyotrophic lateral sclerosis (ALS) is a progressive disease resulting from the degeneration of both the upper and the lower motor neurons. The degeneration leads to flaccidity, spasticity, and atrophy in the cranial, spinal, and peripheral musculature. Degeneration of motor neurons in the brain stem results in overall weakness and incoordination, eventually leading to dysarthria, voice disorders, and dysphagia. All aspects of the swallow (oral, pharyngeal, and esophageal) are affected (Strand, Miller, Yorkston, & Hillel, 1996). As the disease progresses, a percutaneous endoscopic gastrostomy (PEG) tube will need to be inserted for nutrition and hydration. End-stage ALS is characterized by severe dysphagia and severe respiratory decompensation.

Parkinson's Disease   Parkinson's disease (PD) is a movement disorder caused by the progressive depletion and degeneration of dopaminergic neurons in the subcortical and brain stem regions. PD commonly presents as a combination of symptoms such as resting tremors, gait impairments, dysarthria, and dysphagia. It is estimated that dysphagia affects about 50 percent of PD patients. Many patients exhibit delayed initiation of the swallow secondary to tremor and/or spasticity of the tongue, velum, and pharynx. Due to tongue weakness and lack of coordination, some individuals exhibit impaired bolus formation and transport and also have changes in pharyngeal function. According to Robbins, Logemann, and Kirshner (1986), problems in oral transport are common, with lingual pumping and piecemeal deglutition. Common in PD is "silent aspiration," where food or liquid is aspirated without awareness of material entering the airway, so there is no cough or attempt to clear the throat to expel material. Silent aspiration may be caused by an underlying sensory condition. Many of the dysphagic symptoms of PD respond well to both behavioral and medical treatment.

Progressive Supranuclear Palsy   Progressive supranuclear palsy is a degenerative disease with Parkinson-like symptoms caused by the degeneration of the brain stem, diencephalon, cerebellum, and basal ganglia. Clinical characteristics include disturbed gait, impaired speech, ocular dysmotility, and impaired cognition (Litvan et al., 1996). Oropharyngeal dysphagia is a common symptom, though it does not appear at disease onset and may become progressively worse as the disease itself progresses (Sonies, 1992a).

In contrast to Parkinson's patients, who often have no awareness of material entering the airway, the patients studied by Sonies (1992a) all were aware of their swallowing difficulty, with many reporting coughing or choking following the swallow. Symptoms of oral phase problems, pharyngeal phase problems, delayed esophageal peristalsis, coughing, choking, and aspiration were observed.

Myasthenia Gravis   Myasthenia gravis (MG) is a disease process affecting the lower motor neurons, specifically at the myoneural junction, in which abnormal antibodies damage the acetylcholine receptors and cause defective neuromuscular transmission. There is a generalized weakness of muscles of the eyes, limbs, tongue, soft palate, and pharynx that worsens with activity or effort. MG can be treated by pharmacological intervention—specifically anticholinesterase medication and immunosuppressant agents—and by thymectomy, which surgically removes the source of antibody production (Groher, 1997).

Multiple Sclerosis   Multiple sclerosis (MS) is an autoimmune disorder affecting the central myelinated tracts of the brain and spinal cord. If the corticobulbar tracts or brain stem pathways that mediate swallowing are affected, dysphagia will result. The clinical profile of patients with MS may fluctuate with time, although it may be gradually progressive in nature. Dysphagia is rarely the primary presenting symptom in MS; rather, it may co-occur with dysfunction of the oral cavity and pharynx. Reports have also indicated changes in taste sensation in these patients (Groher, 1997).

Huntington's Disease   Huntington's disease (HD) is a progressive inherited autosomal dominant neurodegenerative movement disorder characterized by psychiatric disturbances, dementia, and involuntary movements. Its etiology results from a problem in recombinant DNA linked to the fourth chromosome. Dysphagia is a common clinical symptom, which oftentimes results in respiratory complications exacerbated by an impaired voluntary cough (Leopold & Kagel, 1985). The oral and pharyngeal phases of swallowing are most commonly affected by HD, but the esophageal phase also may be affected. Swallowing therapy using compensatory techniques and behavioral approaches to food presentation may be beneficial in the therapeutic intervention process.

Shy-Drager Syndrome   Shy-Drager syndrome is a multisystem degenerative disorder affecting the autonomic pathways, nigrostriatal system, cerebellum, and corticospinal tracts. It tends to develop in individuals between the ages of 35 and 75 and appears to be more common in males. Common clinical symptoms include postural hypotension accompanied by lightheadedness, fainting, dizziness, generalized weakness, slurred speech, and visual acuity problems. Sweating and thermoregulatory reflexes are commonly impaired. Dysphagia most commonly affects the pharyngeal phase of swallowing with delayed initiation of the swallow reflex.

Poliomyelitis and Post-Polio Syndrome   Poliomyelitis is a viral-induced degeneration predominantly of the lower motor neurons and may involve the brain stem (Groher, 1997). Dysphagia is a common result of this disorder and appears to worsen over time in the post-polio syndrome (Sonies & Dalakas, 1991, 1995). Major findings of videofluoroscopic swallowing studies in post-polio patients showed impairments in all phases of the swallow (Sonies, 1995; Sonies & Dalakas, 1991, 1995). Because of muscle weakness, oral exercises were only minimally effective, but postural and dietary treatment strategies were helpful in maintaining adequate nutrition.

Guillain-Barré Syndrome   Guillain-Barré syndrome is an autoimmune disorder affecting the peripheral nervous system. It results in demyelination of peripheral and cranial nerves, resulting in weakness and sensory loss involving structures of the oral cavity, pharynx, larynx, and limbs. During the acute phase of the disorder, a feeding gastrostomy tube is essential for many patients who may be totally unable to swallow. Spontaneous recovery of swallowing and other motor functions is a common feature of the disorder, and recovery rate may be accelerated by treatment with intravenous immunoglobulin.

Dementia   Dementia is a class of progressive diseases resulting from cortical impairment, such as Alzheimer's disease. Dysphagia is a well-documented feature of the disorder, commonly co-occurring with deterioration in cognitive abilities and personality changes. Persistent weight loss is often the first indicator of dysphagia; therefore, these patients are highly susceptible to nutritional and hydration deficiencies (Feinberg, Ekberg, Segall, & Tully, 1992). Reduced airway protection occurs because patients often do not swallow in direct response to food in the mouth; thus, because they are unaware of food, they are continually at risk for aspiration (Crary & Groher, 2003).

Head and Neck Cancer   Any cancer that affects the mouth, throat, tongue, larynx, pharynx, or esophagus will impact on the ability to swallow. In persons who smoke, drink, or are exposed to various airborne toxins, the incidence of head and neck cancer is increased. The specific treatment for these cancers—surgery, chemotherapy, and radiation therapy—all add to the likelihood that swallowing will be negatively impacted. This is because the potential side effects of the treatments cause swelling, disfigurement, numbness, pain, reduced saliva, mouth sores, taste loss, excess mucous, oral infections, and reduced motion and strength of oral, facial, laryngeal throat, and neck muscles, which combine to make swallowing, chewing, and speaking difficult (Crary & Groher, 2003; Logeman, 1998; McCulloch, Jaffe, & Hoffman 1997). Many persons who have had extensive surgery will be unable to eat orally and will need to receive nutrition by nonoral feeding tubes.

Diagnosis

Diagnosis of the physiology of swallowing is the first and an essential step in developing a treatment plan for persons who have dysphagia. An adequate diagnosis must be based upon a set of information including a patient's understanding of his own swallowing function. To assess this, a questionnaire that a patient or family member completes is often used. The Self-Assessment Questionnaire for Dysphagia (Sonies, 1988) has been used extensively with patients and will provide the clinician with a basis for determining how to proceed with an evaluation. The Self-Assessment Questionnaire (see Figure 16.3) is filled in by the person and the pattern of the complaints is used to interview the person and to plan treatment and follow progress in therapy. This can also be used to interview the person on the telephone to check on progress or to screen patients for follow-up appointments.

Detection of Aspiration

A major component of a swallowing study is to determine whether there is aspiration or whether the findings indicate that the individual is at risk for aspiration. Aspiration occurs when material enters the airway below the level of the vocal folds and cannot be ejected, thus putting the individual at risk for aspiration pneumonia (Rosenbek et al., 1996a). Aspirated material can come either from oral secretions or from partially

FIGURE 16.3   Self-assessment questionnaire for dysphagia (adapted from Sonies, 1998).

Ratings: Circle the rating that applies to you on the following scale.

1–normal   none   never
2–mild   a little   occasionally
3–moderate   a fair bit   often
4–severe   a lot   usually—always

1. Do you have difficulty swallowing?	1	2	3	4
2. Do you have pain when you swallow?	1	2	3	4
3. Do you have difficulty chewing hard foods?	1	2	3	4
4. Do you have a dry mouth?	1	2	3	4
5. Do you have excess saliva or drooling?	1	2	3	4
6. Do you cough or choke, before, during, or after swallowing?	1	2	3	4
7. Does your voice become hoarse after swallowing?	1	2	3	4
8. Do you notice food coming up into your nose?	1	2	3	4
9. Do you have heartburn or indigestion?	1	2	3	4
10. Do you have difficulty swallowing liquids?	1	2	3	4
11. Do you have difficulty swallowing solids?	1	2	3	4
12. Do you have difficulty swallowing pills?	1	2	3	4
13. Do you react to spicy foods?	1	2	3	4
14. Has your reaction to hot or cold food changed?	1	2	3	4
15. Have you had episodes of airway obstruction?	1	2	3	4
16. Have you had pneumonia or aspiration pneumonia?	1	2	3	4

digested material that is refluxed back up into the pharynx from the esophagus in persons with GERD.

Microsapiration of oral bacteria is a major cause of bacterial pneumonia. In those with decreased consciousness due to drugs, alcohol abuse, stroke, seizures, or neurologic diseases and in institutionalized elderly and hospitalized adults (Johnson & Hirsch, 2003), aspiration of gastric contents can cause pneumonitis (Marik, 2001). Aspiration can be detected radiographically or endoscopically (see the section on instrumental diagnostic procedures). Some of the signs that indicate risk of aspiration are listed in (Table 16.4).

Clinical Examination

A clinical or bedside examination of the oral sensory motor mechanism is another essential component of a complete swallowing evaluation that will yield important information on how the person swallows, the physiology of the oral mechanism, and the swallowing environment (Crary & Groher, 2003; Logemann, 1998a; Schulze-Delrieu & Miller, 1997; Sonies, 1994). From this evaluation, the clinician can determine if there is weakness, asymmetry, or incoordination of the oral pharyngeal muscles (lips, tongue, palate, larynx, jaw muscles) or oral sensory problems that may contribute to dysphagia. Signs and symptoms of aspiration or risk of aspiration can be determined

TABLE 16.4   Oropharyngeal Dysphagia

General Signs and Symptoms

- Patient reports feeling that something is stuck in her throat after eating
- Excessive coughing during eating
- Choking during eating
- Excessive drooling
- Wet, gurgling vocal quality after eating
- Poor lung sounds—rasping
- Dysphonia or loss of voice after meals
- Pocketing of food in the mouth
- Pills sticking in the throat
- Shortness of breath after swallowing
- Unexplained weight loss
- Fever or sweating following meals
- Pneumonia of unknown origin
- Voice changes (e.g., hoarseness)
- Heartburn or Indigestion

Risks in Compromised or Medically Fragile Patients

- Paralysis of pharynx or vocal cords
- Laryngeal trauma
- Oropharyngeal surgery
- Lung infections
- Prolonged intubation-nonoral feeding
- Infection near gastrostomy site
- Impaired lung function
- Leakage around a tracheostomy site
- Foreign material suctioned from a tracheostomy site

FIGURE 16.4
Oropharyngeal
dysphagia symptoms.

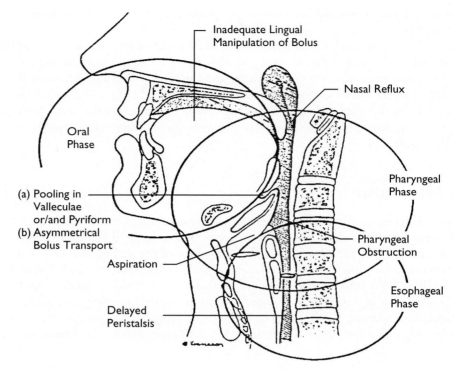

during the clinical examination. It will be important to observe actual eating or feeding, posture, dentition, mastication, and muscle tone; to determine the person's respiratory and cognitive status, memory, and language capacity; and to observe if she is independent or will need assistance to eat. The clinical examination should also test the function of the cranial nerves and determine if there is sufficient saliva to form a bolus. During this examination, the cough (Addington, Stephens & Gilliland, 1999; Addington, Stephens, Gilliland, & Rodriguez, 1999), gag, and voice quality should also be examined, as these functions give insight into whether there may be muscular, neurological, or structural problems as the cause for dysphagia. The person's medical and surgical history and medication intake must also be discussed as possible causes for difficulty swallowing or eating. Figure 16.4 shows oropharyngeal dysphagia symptoms.

Signs and Symptoms

Although many persons are only minimally aware of having difficulty swallowing until they have considerable problems, dysphagia can be detected if a variety of signs and symptoms are present. These signs and symptoms, listed in Table 16.4, can be used to determine if an instrumental examination of swallowing function is needed or if medical attention is required and to counsel patients and family. From the results of the clinical examination and the instrumental examination, a plan of care will be determined. For some individuals with severe dysphagia and frank aspiration, nonoral feeding will be recommended, and further medical attention and family counseling will be required.

Instrumental Diagnostic Procedures

In order to assess the physiological components of the swallowing mechanism and to determine what compensatory treatment procedures are appropriate for each person with dysphagia, it is essential that an instrumental swallowing study be conducted. The gold standard procedure for assessing the entire swallow is a radiographic procedure called videofluoroscopy or the modified barium swallow (Crary & Groher 2003; Logemann, 1986, 1998a). There are other effective procedures that assess specific or partial aspects of the swallow, including fiberoptic endoscopic imaging, ultrasound, electromyography, and manofluorography, which give information regarding major components of the swallow, useful during treatment. Newer technologies such as magnetic resonance imaging may be used to assess swallowing for research investigations.

In order to use each of the techniques appropriately, it is important to understand their advantages and limitations. For example, when conducting a swallowing study, the most complete technique must capture moving real-time images of the swallow from multiple imaging planes with real foods that represent the normal eating environment in the least invasive manner with minimal environmental effects. Each procedure will be discussed in the following sections to determine how it fits into the following general parameters: dynamic, complete, pictorial, multiple-plane images and level of invasiveness (Sonies, 1991a, 1994).

Videofluoroscopy   *Vidoefluoroscopic imaging of the swallow* (VFS), or the *modified barium swallow* (MBS), is the only dynamic, fully complete, pictorial, multiple-plane procedure used to examine the swallow (Logemann, 1986, 1998a). The entire swallow sequence can be viewed in real time from the moment food enters the mouth until it enters the stomach. VFS is a radiographic procedure that must be performed in an x-ray suite by radiologists and/or specially trained technologists in conjunction with the speech-language pathologist; obtained images are either recorded onto videotape or digitized for subsequent review and analysis. VFS gives a view of the entire swallow and provides the most thorough information on the physiology of the swallow process. In order to execute the radiographic study, the patient should be alert and should be able to take food orally (Logemann, 1986). Compensatory swallowing techniques and modified food textures can be studied. Drawbacks are that VFS exposes the person to radiation, which limits its ability to be used repeatedly, requires the use of a radiopaque substance (barium) to coat foods, and requires that the patient be transported to a facility with the equipment. For fragile and medically unstable patients who cannot sit unsupported, the examination can be uncomfortable. VFS is the most reliable way to image the oropharynx and provides us with the best information on how to plan treatment for most swallowing disorders. In addition, by adding timing information to the fluorographic image, subtle differences in airway protection and other abnormalities such as aspiration or penetration can be measured (Kendall, Leonard, & McKenzie, 2004a, 2004b; Logemann, 1986).

Because of the above-stated limitations and the cost of VFS, other procedures are sometimes used to assess swallowing. Since none of the other techniques gives a complete picture of the oropharyngeal and esophageal structures, they should not be used as a substitute for VFS during an initial assessement. In some clinical settings or institutions that do not have easy access to videofluoroscopy or where it is contraindicated, other procedures listed below can be used to examine the swallow.

Fiberoptic Endoscopic Examination of Swallowing (FEES) and FEEST   This procedure was first described in 1988 by Langmore, Schatz, and Olsen. In this procedure, while the patient is seated upright, a flexible endoscope with a light source is passed through the nasal passageway into the nasopharynx just below and posterior to the epiglottis, and studies are video-recorded (Langmore & McCulloch, 1997). Food is introduced, and after the patient has swallowed, the laryngopharynx is viewed to determine if material remains in the pharynx, penetrates into the laryngeal vestibule, or is aspirated into the airway with or without attempts to clear the throat. FEES is a partial procedure, obtaining a transverse view at the termination of the endoscopic light source. At the moment when the swallow occurs, there is a washout of the image as the epiglottis lowers. This procedure examines the movement of the vocal folds and the physical appearance of the pharyngeal and laryngeal structures. Many of the compensatory swallow maneuvers and postural adjustments that protect the airway and assist in safe bolus transport can be observed without the risk of radiation (Sonies, 1991a).

The sensitivity of the mucosa in the laryngeal region can also be assessed by puffs of air to determine if a cough or protective response is elicited and has been found to be effective in stroke patients. This procedure is called FEESST – fiberoptic endoscopic evaluation of swallowing with sensory testing (Aviv et al., 1998; Aviv, Liu, Parides, Kaplan, & Close, 2000; Aviv et al., 1999).

Ultrasound   Ultrasound imaging (US) of the swallow, first introduced in 1984 (Sonies et al., 1984), gives detail of the soft tissues and muscles of the oropharynx, especially the tongue, in real time during swallowing. Images can be obtained in 3D and 4D to give real-time assessment of the oral structures (Sonies, Fishman, & Miller, 2003). Ultrasound images give information on multiple anatomic planes during swallowing using any food materials, while the person is seated comfortably in any position or is lying down. A major use of ultrasound is to view the motion of the hyoid bone and to examine tongue/hyoid motion during single or sequential swallows and during swallowing of boluses of different sizes and textures (Sonies, 1991a, 1992a, 1994, 1997; Sonies et al., 2003). Power Doppler and Color US systems are used to study blood flow and can be applied to study vascularization in oral or lingual tumors. Since ultrasound is completely safe and has no biological effects, it is the most suitable technique to use when studying infant swallowing and for young children. Recent studies of fetal swallowing and oral laryngeal and pharyngeal development have been conducted using ultrasound (Macedonia, Miller, & Sonies, 2002; J. L. Miller, Sonies, & Macedonia, 2003). Ultrasound is an excellent technique to use for repeated studies and for biofeedback during dysphagia treatment.

Electromyography (EMG)   EMG, a procedure that has been useful in general muscle function research, is also being used in swallowing treatment and diagnosis (Palmer, 1989; Perlman, 1991; Sonies, 1991a; Vaiman, Eviatar, & Segal, 2004). EMG is a partial procedure to study swallowing, as it does not produce any visual images of the anatomy. Tracings of the electrical output of the timing and amplitude of signals are displayed; they are produced by output from surface electrodes placed on the skin over muscles presumed to be involved in swallowing activity. Because of a variety of physiological factors, the phases of the swallow can be examined only with surface EMG if the studies are conducted simultaneously with another procedure such as VFS (Vaiman et al., 2004). EMG output may provide visual feedback during swallowing that can be used as a biofeedback technique.

Manofluorography   Pairing of manometry, a procedure used by gastroenterologists to assess the pressure dynamics in the pharynx and upper esophageal sphincter (Castell, 1995), and VFS is called manofluorography (McConnel, 1988; McConnel,

Cerenko, & Mendelsohn, 1988). Solid-state catheters placed throughout the pharynx and esophagus record pressure changes associated with bolus passage, pharyngeal muscle contractions, and esophageal peristalsis at the same time as the actual oropharyngeal barium swallow is being captured on videotape during the fluoroscopic study. While the technique is complete and gives real-time images of the swallow, it is invasive due to the placement of the catheter and exposes the person to x-radiation; therefore, it is used primarily for research.

Evidence-Based Treatment

Recent emphasis has been placed on measuring outcomes of our treatment in regard to the efficacy and effectiveness of treatments provided. "*Treatment efficacy* involves the extent to which an intervention can be shown to be beneficial under optimal (or ideal) conditions; *treatment effectiveness* involves the extent to which services are shown to be beneficial under typical (or real-world) conditions" (Frattali, 1998, pp. 16–17). When measuring outcomes, the type of data gleaned depends on the levels of control obtained in the experimental study. Class I studies are the highest level and involve randomization, controlled clinical trials, and large data samples. Class II studies are deemed quasi-experimental, as they are typically nonrandom, with assignment to treatment groups or maybe case-control studies, whereas Class III studies are nonexperimental, with no clear grouping of subjects, and are mostly case studies, reports, or expert opinion (Frattali, 1998). For specific information on evidence-based practice and grants in this area go the website for the Agency for Healthcare Research and Quality, www.ahrq.gov.

Because of the nature of dysphagia and the health risks posed if patients were untreated (malnutrition, dehydration, aspiration), it would be harmful to deny treatment by randomization to a control, or nontreatment, group (Logemann, 1998c); therefore, the majority of the research in dysphagia is Class III, consisting of case reports, expert opinion, and no untreated control. Future well-planned experimental studies using evidence-based methodology will allow the clinician to better determine treatment options.

Compensatory Treatment Procedures

Treatment techniques can be either *direct,* where food is used, or *indirect,* where there is no food being introduced if the individual is felt to be at risk (Logemann, 1997; Logemann & Kahrilas, 1990). The various swallow maneuvers are designed to change swallow physiology by improving (1) range of motion of oral and pharyngeal structures, (2) sensory input prior to swallow, or (3) ability to take voluntary control over oropharyngeal movements during a swallow. These are not suitable for all cognitive levels, as they require the patient to follow directions and practice independently.

Postural Techniques

Postural techniques are used for a variety of patients with dysphagia. They are recommended to improve swallowing safety and reduce or eliminate aspiration. Postural techniques are primarily implemented to control the flow of food and eliminate the patient's symptoms without changing the physiology of the swallow. Furthermore, these can be used on patients of all cognitive levels. They involve little muscular effort and do not cause fatigue. There is no one posture to cure all swallowing problems; rather, many may be attempted during the instrumental evaluation and are widely used for treatment planning during the modified barium swallow procedure (adapted from Logemann, 1998a).

Chin Tuck, or Head Down, Posture   The chin tuck posture involves lowering the chin toward the neck area. With the chin down, the base of tongue and the epiglottis are in greater contact with the posterior pharyngeal wall, thereby reducing pooling in the throat and facilitating proper bolus flow through the pharynx. This maneuver is recommended for those patients with a delayed triggering of the pharyngeal swallow, reduced tongue-base posterior movement, or reduced laryngeal closure resulting in aspiration. The chin tuck maneuver widens the valleculae to prevent the bolus from entering the airway. It pushes the tongue base backward toward the pharyngeal wall and places the epiglottis in a more posterior position, thereby narrowing the laryngeal entrance (Robbins et al., 2008).

Head Rotation to the Weaker Side   Head rotation reduces the size of the hypopharynx and partially closes the damaged side of the pharynx so that food flows down the better side. This posture is utilized when the patient presents with unilateral vocal fold impairment, unilateral pharyngeal wall impairment, unilateral pharyngeal paresis, unilateral epiglottal dysfunction, and residue in the pyriform sinuses. This movement serves to narrow the laryngeal entrance to prohibit foreign substances from entering into the airway. Furthermore, it eliminates the damaged side of the pharynx from the bolus path, reducing the risk that residue in the pharynx will be aspirated after a swallow.

Swallow Maneuvers

Swallow maneuvers are used to place aspects of the pharyngeal stage of the swallow under voluntary control. In order to be utilized, the dysphagic patient must be able to follow directions, thereby excluding patients who have moderate to severe cognitive or language impairments.

Mendelsohn Maneuver   The Mendelsohn maneuver is intended to increase hyolaryngeal elevation and increase width and timing of the cricopharyngeal opening and relaxation/opening of the esophagus because of the increased pull by the hyoid bone. It is difficult to teach to cognitively impaired persons, as it requires ability to forcefully control the swallow (Cook et al., 1989; Logemann & Kahrilas, 1990).

Supraglottic Swallow   The supraglottic swallow closes off the vocal folds so that no foreign material can enter the airway. In order to accomplish this, the patient must be alert and must follow directions. Given instructions from the speech-language pathologist, the patient must take a deep breath and hold it while swallowing. Following the swallow, the patient is then instructed to cough to clear residue from the pharynx (Logemann, 1998a).

Effortful Swallow and Maneuver for Base of Tongue Retraction   Both of these maneuvers are designed to increase posterior motion of the tongue base during the pharyngeal swallow, thereby clearing vallecular residue. The patient is instructed to squeeze hard at the back of the throat during the swallow (Fuji & Logemann, 1996).

Thermal/Tactile Stimulation   Thermal/tactile stimulation involves circular rubbing of the anterior faucial arch with a cold laryngeal mirror. It is meant to alert the patient before bolus presentation and also heightens oral awareness to facilitate improved triggering of the pharyngeal swallow. This technique appears to be effective for patients who have suffered a stroke or those with reduced pharyngeal sensation and is even more successful when paired with other modalities (Rosenbek, Roecker, Wood, & Robbins, 1996; Sciortino, Liss, Case, Gerritsen, & Katz, 2003).

Tongue-Strengthening and Resistance Exercises   A series of studies has been completed investigating the effects of tongue-strengthening exercises on reducing risk of aspiration or penetration during swallowing in the elderly that has had positive results. Progressive resistance training using a tongue pressure device was used in an 8-week training program in a small group of patients. Training increased swallowing pressures during an effortful swallow and allowed the persons to use compensatory strategies more effectively and increase dietary intake (Clark, Hensen, Barber, Stierwalt, & Sherrill, 2003; Hind, Nicosia, Roecker, Carnes, & Robbins, 2001; Robbins et al., 2005).

Shaker Exercises   This simple-appearing exercise has proven to be quite effective in facilitating swallowing in elderly persons who have pharyngeal swallowing deficits resulting from impairment in upper esophageal opening/relaxation. The person lies flat and performs sustained head raising at a rate of three repetitions a minute with a rest of a minute for 30 trials, three times a day for 6 weeks (Shaker et al., 2002). The outcomes of this head-raising exercise revealed that the patients made significant improvements in opening of the UES and elevation of the larynx as well as positive changes in functional swallowing outcomes.

Biofeedback and Stimulation Techniques

Electromyography (EMG)   EMG has been used as a biofeedback technique during swallowing therapy to give the patient information on graphic output at the time of a swallow and compare it to nonswallowing movements (Hillel, Robinson, & Waugh, 1997). Surface electrodes are placed along the surface of the skin in order to stimulate activity in the geniohyoid, mylohyoid, digastric, and floor-of-mouth muscles. According to Logemann (1998a), EMG is most commonly used in conjunction with the Mendelsohn maneuver and may also be used as a biofeedback mechanism for the effortful swallow.

Electrical Stimulation   There are electrical devices that provide bursts of impulses to muscles that have been used by physical therapists and other rehabilitation professionals interested in muscle reeducation for many years. Electrodes can be placed on the skin to elicit a contraction of a muscle by a train of pulses that can be modulated to increase or decrease the strength of the contraction (Thresher & Popovic, 2004). Electrodes can be either implanted or placed on the skin, requiring different signal intensity levels to be effective. A technique used to assist patients with severe dysphagia combined with esophageal dilation, with electrodes placed on the neck in two positions that are repositioned until muscle contractions are felt/observed, and electrical stimulation may offer relief to some patients with dysphagia (Freed, Freed, Chatburn, & Christian, 2001). Research under way indicates that instead of elevating the hyoid as claimed, it may actually lower the hyoid and or have minimal effect on the swallow. This technology, however, is not currently supported by a scientific foundation and will require more research to understand its effects in treating persons with disordered swallowing (Coyle, 2002; Humbert et al., 2006).

Diet Modifications

Examination of the results of the modified barium swallow study will give insight regarding which textures are tolerated best and which textures may remain in the pharynx and be aspirated before, during, or after a swallow. The most common dietary modification is to thicken liquids, as many patients have impaired sensation in the oropharynx or do not have the oral control due to tongue and lip weakness to safely swallow thin liquids (Logemann, 1998a). It is difficult to eliminate all thin liquids from a diet, so thickeners can be used to change the consistency of the liquid. Such options are especially good for patients with neurological disorders. When thickeners are used, there is some concern that dehydration may occur, so the patient must be carefully monitored. Thickeners should not be used indiscriminately, and a complete swallow study and medical history are required to substantiate this modification.

The National Dysphagia Diet (NDD; National Dysphagia Diet Task Force, 2002) is a series of suggestions for dietary modifications based upon graded series of food consistencies from thin liquids to solids. Four levels of dietary intake were developed by a team of speech-language pathologists and dieticians with specific symptoms for each level. Each of the four levels lists foods that are recommended or should be avoided. An NDD Level 1 consists of pureed foods and liquids and contains a list of foods to be avoided such as chunky food, seeds, pulp, bread, dry cereals, coarse meats, and whole fruit. This diet also includes a seven-level rating system for determining who should be on which level by listing signs and symptoms that the person exhibits. For example, it states that persons with severe dysphagia who cannot be fed orally because they cannot clear material from the pharynx, who have no clearing cough, and who are aspirating on at least two consistencies are considered Level 1 (i.e., Severe dysphagia: NPO (nothing per oral): Unable to tolerate any food safely). This diet plan is being used in many institutions and hospitals where nutritionists and speech-language pathologists work in effective teams.

Most persons who have difficulty swallowing can be successfully treated to advance to a higher-level diet and to resume oral feeding by a combination of the compensatory strategies, stimulation techniques, and dietary modifications previously discussed. In all cases, follow-up examinations should be conducted.

There is always a group of patients whose medical condition is so severe that all attempts to remediate swallowing are futile. In these severe cases, the only option is often to limit or exclude oral feeding or recommend that they be NPO. Many NPO patients are able to sustain adequate nutrition and hydration and maintain a fair quality of life on tube feedings. The speech-language pathologist, along with the physician and nutritionist, is responsible for counseling the patient and the family on nonoral feeding and must exercise wise judgment and ethical behavior when interacting to discuss these issues.

Other Considerations in Treatment

One of the common causes of swallowing dysfunction, especially in persons with multiple illnesses or chronic medical conditions, is the use of polypharmacy—that is, multiple medications. It is a well-known fact that medications can cause dysphagia by drying the oral mucosa, changing oral sensation, or slowing down contractions of the muscles of the pharynx and esophagus. Therefore, it is essential that clinicians obtain a complete medication history of anyone they are treating.

case study

An 85-year-old woman recently had a stroke affecting the premotor cortex of the left hemisphere. She complained of dysphagia and unintentional weight loss of 20 pounds. She felt that food was sticking in the back of her throat and claimed that this was not cleared with a cough. She was on a complete oral diet. She lives alone and worries about her risk of choking. Medical records revealed a slight bilateral sensorineural hearing loss in the high frequencies (she does not use amplification). She is medicated for hypertension, high cholesterol, and gastroesophageal reflux. She has not undergone major surgery and has normal cognitive functioning. She received speech and language therapy for two years poststroke for imprecise articulation and expressive language problems, but was not treated for swallowing problems.

An oral motor function examination revealed right-sided facial weakness as a result of the stroke. She was unable to maintain a tight lip seal due to CN VII weakness. Her tongue deviated to the right upon protusion, and she had decreased range of motion due to CN XII weakness. Inspection of the oral cavity revealed decreased salivary function (xerostomia) due to a combination of medications and the normal effects of aging in women. Normal velar elevation and intact gag reflex were noted during the oral motor examination. She had no dentures and no missing teeth, and dentition was sufficient for mastication. Vocal quality was hoarse due to 30 years as a heavy smoker.

The modified barium swallow study was conducted consisting of multiple swallows of 5 and 10 cc thin liquids, 5 cc pudding consistencies, and a cracker coated with barium. Her swallow study revealed poor bolus formation, decreased hyolaryngeal elevation, delayed initiation of the swallow, and residue of pudding on the tongue and in the valleculae. No instances of aspiration or penetration were noted. After reviewing the videotaped swallow study, the clinician discussed the results with her patient and explained that the poor bolus formation could result from a number of factors, including tongue and lip weakness, poor control of tongue motion, and xerostomia. Furthermore, the residual pooled material in the valleculae could result from poor hyolaryngeal elevation due to tongue weakness

(CN XII) and weakness of the floor-of-the-mouth muscles (geniohyoid and mylohyoid). Reduced hyolaryngeal elevation also caused incomplete opening of the upper esophageal sphincter, making it difficult for the bolus to enter the esophagus. This caused the patient to feel like food was sticking in the back of her throat.

Recommendations for this patient included head turn to the right side (her weak side) to force the bolus to go down the strong side (her left side). The head turn facilitates the passage of the bolus so it will not pool in the pharyngeal cavities. In addition, it was recommended that the patient dilute thicker-consistency foods with milk or water (e.g., mashed potatoes with gravy), as the swallow study revealed no difficulty with thinner consistencies. Because of her dry mouth she was advised to always alternate sips of liquid with solids during all meals and to make sure she kept liquids available during the day to avoid dehydration.

QUESTIONS:

1. Which cranial nerves are affected based upon this case?
2. Why do you think she will continue to be an oral eater?
3. What other recommendations would you make?

SELECTED READINGS

Daniels, S. K., Foundas A. L. The role of the insular cortex in dysphagia. *Dysphagia* 1997; 12(3): 146–56.

McConnel FMS (1988). Analysis of pressure generation and bolus transit during pharyngeal swallowing. Dysphagia 2: 216–219.

Moxley, A., Mahendra, N. & Vega-Barachowitz, C. (2004, April 13). Cultural Competence in Health Care. The ASHA Leader.

Chapter SEVENTEEN

Hearing and Hearing Disorders

Frederick N. Martin
The University of Texas at Austin

Bart E. Noble
Austin VA Outpatient Clinic

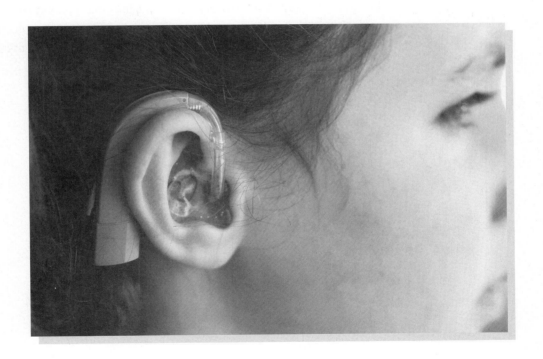

personal PERSPECTIVE

FREDERICK N. MARTIN

Being a less than stellar undergraduate student back in the early 1950s, I found myself, having lost my draft exemption, in the United States Air Force. Four years in this endeavor left me convinced that it was time to give college a new approach, one that included actually studying and a serious eye to the future. My problem was that I did not know what my major would be and how I wanted to spend my professional life. A veterans' counselor suggested the field of communication disorders, which was certainly one of the best pieces of advice I have ever received. In my first semester back in college, I met and became lifelong friends with the now renowned Dr. Mark Ross. We studied together, got interested in audiology together, and dreamed of one day making a professional contribution. There is no doubt that Mark has made his. My more than 50 years as a clinician, teacher, and researcher could not have been more rewarding, and I have missed it every day since my retirement from The University of Texas in 2005. While the profession of audiology faces many challenges and, like so many others, some uncertainties, it is one that brings joy through the discovery of new insights into hearing and hearing disorders and the knowledge that our efforts often have life altering results for our patients with hearing impairments and their significant others. That gratification is immeasurable, as any experienced audiologist can testify.

personal PERSPECTIVE

BART E. NOBLE

When asked how I decided to enter the field of audiology, I immediately think of my colleagues and dear friends Scott Haug and Ferman Wardell. Scott's family and mine both moved to the same small Texas town at about the same time. We immediately became friends and remained almost inseparable until Scott went off to college about a year later. Our paths were not to cross again until ten years later, when I was preparing to leave the Air Force. I was exploring audiology as a possible profession, before I knew that Scott had followed in the footsteps of his father, Olaf Haug, Ph.D., in becoming a clinical audiologist. In the process of visiting both of their clinics, I became impressed, not only with their professionalism and expertise, but also with the respect felt for them by both their patients and their colleagues. They showed me that audiologists had the privilege (not to mention the pleasure) of witnessing the immediate enhancement in the quality of their patients' lives as a result of their professional efforts.

Based largely on my experiences with Scott and his dad, I entered graduate school in audiology, where Ferman Wardell was one of my outstanding supervisors and, along with my coauthor of this chapter, one of my most influential mentors. I completed my coursework under their direction and subsequently my clinical fellowship under Scott's supervision. Both Scott's and Ferman's outstanding clinical careers ended prematurely, when Scott passed away of cancer at the age of 33 and Ferman later died suddenly at the age of 47. They had both dedicated their adult lives to the profession of audiology, to their patients, and to their friends and families, and they affected and inspired everyone with whom they came in contact. Their enthusiasm, professionalism, and dedication to helping people have greatly influenced my own career as a clinician, supervisor, and teacher. Over the years, I, too, have experienced the satisfaction and challenges that my mentors enjoyed so much, and, like them, I have remained excited about the future of the profession and still feel grateful about a career where I can truly help people every day.

If one were to ask a layperson how human beings communicate, "speech" would be the most likely response. Surely, when pointed out, it would be acknowledged that concepts of language and hearing must be involved as well, but communicative disorders are probably first thought of as speech disorders. It is because of the integral part played by hearing in the communicative process that a chapter on hearing and its disorders is included in this book.

Denes and Pinson (1963) coined the term *speech chain*. They acknowledged that the communicative process begins first with a thought or concept in the mind of the communicator on the "output" side of the communication process. For the thought to become a message, linguistic encoding is required, using words, grammar, syntax, and the like. This mechanism involves the use of specialized brain centers that allow for abstraction and symbolization.

The next step in the communicative chain of events involves articulation and phonation of the selected speech sounds. Because nature has not devised specialized organs for these functions, humans use those organs that have evolved for chewing, swallowing, and breathing. Vibrations from and the positioning of these organs set up perturbations in the air in the vocal tract, resulting in sound waves, which travel from the source.

The "input" process begins when sound waves reach a human ear. Reception of these waves involves the peripheral hearing apparatus, but it has been correctly stated that we do not hear with our ears, but with our brains. The auditory mechanism is a system that uses the sound waves around us to carry messages to our brains for decoding. The decoder must come up with the same message that the encoder intended (see Chapters 2 and 3). It is little wonder that "failure to communicate" is such a common explanation for why humans do not succeed in getting along with one another. (For details of the concepts of language and language disorders, see Chapters 11, 12, and 14).

Communication on the output side is adversely affected if a breakdown occurs in the generation of the message to be transmitted, in the production of linguistic coding, or in the articulation or phonation of the intended *phonemes* (speech sounds). Speech-language pathologists are the specialists who deal with such disorders. Any interference with the propagation of the waves from the speaker's lips to the listener's ears results in a distortion of and/or a reduction in the loudness of the signal. Abnormalities of the peripheral auditory system also result in degradations of the loudness or clarity of an acoustic message, and it is clinical audiologists, in concert with *otologists* (physicians who specialize in diseases of the ear), who serve to remediate such disorders. When disease or damage occurs in the specialized areas of the brain designed for decoding acoustic messages, speech-language pathologists and audiologists combine their skills in managing patients.

Audiologists and speech-language pathologists share common roots. Their basic educational tracks parallel each other, and it is not until graduate training that they separate into specialized advanced coursework. Specific interests and goals put them on similar tracks that converge when the needs of individuals with hearing loss present themselves. Each specialty shares a fundamental knowledge of the other's profession, along with specialized expertise in the rehabilitation of persons with hearing loss. (See Chapter 18 to learn about such therapeutic measures.)

The Nature of Sound

Humans live in a gaseous environment called air. The molecules in air are spread far apart, and as long as there is heat, they move about randomly, colliding, and retaining a certain amount of elasticity. Of course, similar molecular activity also exists in liquids

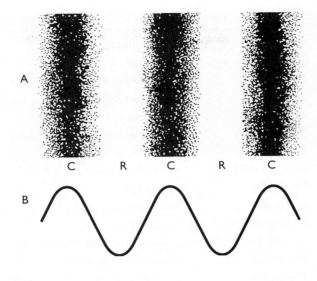

FIGURE 17.1
Simple wave motion in air. In part A, "C" represents areas of compression, where air molecules are packed closely together; "R" represents areas of rarefaction, where the molecules are farther apart. In part B, the pressure waves are displayed as they change over time (projected circular motion).
Source: From *Introduction to Audiology* (10th ed.), by F. N. Martin & J. G. Clark 2009. Reprinted with the permission of Allyn and Bacon.

and solids, but in those environments, the molecules are packed much more closely together than in air, resulting in a much faster rate of propagation.

When any vibration occurs in air, such as from a guitar string, a tuning fork, or human vocal cords, the result of that vibration is an impingement on the surrounding air molecules. These air molecules are then pushed more closely together than would normally be the case; they are *condensed*, or *compressed*, leaving behind them areas where the molecules are fewer in number. The result is a partial vacuum called a *rarefaction*. These alternate condensations and rarefactions are called pressure waves. An example of a simple pressure wave may be seen in Figure 17.1A.

The height of a wave—that is, the point of maximum displacement to which it moves—is called its *amplitude.* The amount of force or energy per unit volume of air is called *intensity.* The number of compressions and rarefactions in a given time period is referred to as *frequency.*

Intensity

A positive relationship exists between the physical property of intensity and its psychological correlate, *loudness.* That is, as the intensity of a sound is increased it is perceived as being louder. Special scales for rating loudness (known as phons) have been developed. Because of the extreme range of intensities that the human ear can hear (from barely audible to painfully loud), a linear system of intensity measurement is impractical. Therefore, the *decibel* (dB, one-tenth of a Bel, named for Alexander Graham Bell) is used, which expresses a ratio between two sound pressures or two sound powers. The decibel scale, therefore, is logarithmic rather than linear. A scale of intensities of some everyday sounds may be seen in Table 17.1.

Frequency

The frequency of a sound is the number of back-and-forth vibrations made during a single time period. It is convenient to use 1 second for this period. The number of complete compressions and rarefactions of a wave through 360 degrees is called the

TABLE 17.1   Scale of Intensities for Ordinary Environmental Sounds

0 dB SPL	Just audible sound
10 dB SPL	Soft rustle of leaves
20 dB SPL	A whisper at 4 feet
30 dB SPL	A quiet street in the evening with no traffic
40 dB SPL	Night noises in a city
50 dB SPL	A quiet automobile 10 feet away
60 dB SPL	Department store
60 to 70 dB SPL	Normal conversation at 3 feet
70 dB SPL	Busy traffic
80 dB SPL	Heavy traffic
80 to 90 dB SPL	Niagara Falls
90 dB SPL	A pneumatic drill 10 feet away
100 dB SPL	A riveter 35 feet away
110 dB SPL	Hi-fi phonograph with a 10-watt amplifier, 10 feet away
115 dB SPL	Hammering on a steel plate 2 feet away

The decibel reference is 20 µPa. (*threshold of human hearing*)

Source: Van Bergeijk, Pierce, & David, 1960.

frequency and is described in terms of the number *of cycles per second* (cps). Because of the major contributions of Heinrich Hertz, the 19th-century German physicist, his name is often used to denote cps. Therefore, if 1,000 complete cycles occur in 1 second, the frequency is said to be 1,000 cps, or 1,000 Hz (*hertz).* Because sound waves are a form of projected circular motion, a number of mathematical computations may be made about them. These waves are often called sine waves (see Figure 17.2).

Frequency has a relationship to pitch in the same way that intensity is related to loudness. As the frequency of a sound increases, so does its *pitch,* but once again, frequency is a physical measurement, and pitch is its perceptual counterpart. To say that a sound has a pitch of 1,000 Hz is as inaccurate as is the incorrect reference to loudness in decibels.

Like loudness, pitch scales have been developed that show the subjective highness (treble) and lowness (bass) of sounds. When a sound consists of only one frequency, it is said to be a *pure tone.* Equal multiples of the frequency of a pure tone are said to be overtones or *harmonics,* and the lowest frequency in a complex wave is called the first

FIGURE 17.2

Denotation of a sine wave in 360 degrees. *Source:* From *Introduction to Audiology* (10th ed.), by F.N. Martin & J. G. Clark, 2009. Reprinted with the permission of Allyn and Bacon.

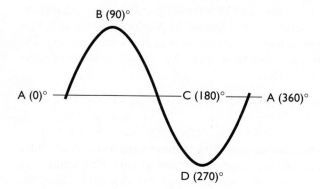

harmonic (*fundamental*) frequency. Given a composite wave including 100, 200, and 300 Hz, 100 Hz is the fundamental, 200 Hz is the second harmonic, 300 Hz is the third harmonic, and so forth.

Pure tones do not exist in nature. They can be generated by whistles, tuning forks, and electronic devices, but the closest human beings can come to generating a pure tone is to purse their lips and whistle. What we hear all around us is a series of complex tones. The complex sound that is of greatest interest to us acoustically is, of course, speech.

Acoustics of Speech

From an acoustic standpoint, speech is a complex wave that is constantly changing. The sounds of speech are divided into different classifications. Vowels, for example, are complex waves that tend to repeat their waveforms over time. A spectral analysis of vowel sounds shows that the fundamental frequency of the wave is determined by the lowest frequency of vibration of the talker's vocal folds. The length and cross-sectional area of the vocal tract (determined largely by the height and position of the tongue) act as filters. The peaks of energy at different harmonics, known as *formants*, are equal multiples of the fundamental frequency and determine the characteristics of specific vowel sounds. The first and second formants usually provide enough information to make each vowel recognizable. English vowels, as spoken, are not limited to the five vowels as written. Rather, they take on many different pronunciations, a fact that makes learning English as a second language quite formidable. Semivowels in English are shorter in duration and fewer in number than are vowels. They include the sounds /w/, /r/, /l/, and /y/.

The bulk of English sounds is made up of consonants. Each of the consonants varies to some degree in its production (and perception) based on the influence of other phonemes with which it is juxtaposed. For example, the phoneme /t/ is different in words like *too, hat, butter,* and *must.* Each of these variations is called an **allophone.**

Vowel sounds produce the bulk of the energy (intensity) of speech, while consonants provide most of its intelligibility. Persons with hearing difficulty in the higher frequencies who have normal low-frequency sensitivity often can hear the vowel components of speech, but miss many of the consonants. What results is the patient complaint heard by all audiologists, "I can hear, but I can't understand the words."

The production and ultimate perception of speech are influenced by elements of **prosody.** These include pitch, intonation, loudness, stress, duration, rhythm, tempo, and quality. Disorders of hearing may interfere with perception of the prosodic elements of speech, as well as with its articulation, which contributes to what has been called the *deaf speech* of persons with severe to profound hearing losses.

Disorders of Hearing

For the most part, disorders of hearing are examined in this chapter as a function of the time of onset in the patient's life: *prenatal* (before birth), *perinatal* (at the time of birth), and *postnatal* (following birth). We also discuss the most common disorders by progressing in the same way that an acoustic signal progresses, beginning at the outer ear and culminating in the brain. To begin, a cross-sectional drawing of the human ear is shown in Figure 17.3.

FIGURE 17.3
Cross section of the human ear showing the air-conduction and bone-conduction pathways.
Source: From *Introduction to Audiology* (10th ed.), by F. N. Martin & J. G. Clark, 2009. Reprinted with the permission of Allyn and Bacon.

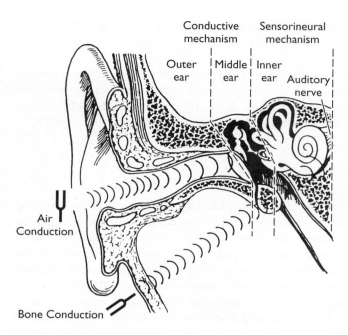

The Outer Ear

A simplified drawing of the outer ear is shown in Figure 17.4. It can be seen that the outer ear is composed of an external appendage called the *auricle* (pinna), whose function is to funnel sounds down the *external auditory canal* to the *tympanic membrane.* The tympanic membrane is commonly called the *eardrum,* which is technically incorrect because the "drum" is actually the entire middle ear, with the tympanic membrane serving as the drumhead. The external auditory canal is lined with skin, and its most lateral portion (that closest to the auricle) contains several glands, which produce *cerumen* (earwax).

Many of the disorders of the outer ear do not appear to affect hearing. Some people believe that damage to, or absence of, the pinna appears to be more of a cosmetic than an auditory problem. Indeed, measurement of hearing through earphones ignores the contribution of the pinna to human hearing. In actuality, the pinna is an excellent gatherer of high-frequency sounds from the environment, so that the sounds can be funneled into the external auditory canal. The absence of the pinna, therefore, can create significant difficulties in auditory localization, which is the ability to identify the direction of a sound source. Hearing losses resulting from problems in the outer ear are called *conductive losses* and are caused either by blockage of the canal or by damage to the tympanic membrane.

Prenatal Causes of Hearing Loss in the Outer Ear Pinnas may be missing or malformed because of the genetic influence of one or both parents or because of problems encountered during the gestational period of the fetus. The same is true of the external auditory canal, which may be totally or partially blocked, creating a condition known as *atresia* or *stenosis,* respectively. Illnesses or the ingestion of certain drugs (on the parts of fathers as well as mothers), sometimes before fertilization and sometimes after fertilization, may produce defects in the developing outer ear. (Chapter 9 discusses cleft palate, a major example of a congenital craniofacial abnormality.)

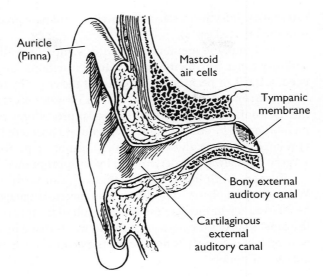

FIGURE 17.4

Cross section of the external ear.

Source: From *Introduction to Audiology* (10th ed.), by F. N. Martin & J. G. Clark, 2009. Reprinted with the permission of Allyn and Bacon.

Perinatal Causes of Hearing Loss in the Outer Ear   When the outer ear is affected at the time of birth, it is usually because of the trauma caused by violent uterine contractions. At times, during difficult deliveries, forceps may be used, which may inadvertently traumatize the external ear. Such trauma can cause atresias and/or malformed pinnas.

Postnatal Causes of Hearing Loss in the Outer Ear   Because they protrude from the sides of the head, pinnas are susceptible to damage from many sources. Included are burns, frostbite, and skin cancer, all of which can necessitate total or partial removal of a pinna. Trauma from a variety of sources can damage and deform a pinna. The "cauliflower ear," often seen on prizefighters, is a good example of the results of such trauma.

For reasons that have been debated, but not entirely agreed on, children are fond of putting small objects into their ears. Although less common, this is seen in adults as well. When the occluding object blocks the passage of sound in the external auditory canal, a conductive hearing loss results. Removal of such objects is imperative and is usually best performed by an otologist, who has the instrumentation and expertise required for such procedures. Improper techniques used in the simple removal of an object from a small child's ear can result in extreme damage and great pain.

Cerumen serves to keep insects and foreign substances from approaching the tympanic membrane. Typically, earwax migrates naturally toward the opening of the canal. When occlusion of the ear canal takes place as a result of excessive wax, it is often because the individual has packed it down while using an object like a cotton swab, which is very inadvisable. Cerumen removal is best left to nature or, if external auditory canal occlusion occurs, to an otologist, audiologist, or properly trained medical technician.

Infections of the external ear are common, especially in warm, damp climates. These are dermatologic disturbances that can usually be treated medically. If left untreated, however, these infections can result in the buildup of debris within the canal, and a great deal of pain (as well as hearing loss) can ensue. Audiologists frequently find that they cannot determine the extent of a hearing loss produced by an external ear infection because the swelling and pain preclude placing earphones into or over the infected ear(s).

The tympanic membrane vibrates sympathetically with sounds in the external auditory canal. The membrane's natural functions can be altered or lost if it is thickened, scarred, or perforated by disease of the ear or by trauma. Trauma can be inflicted by an instrument, sudden changes in air or water pressure, a blow to the head, or very intense sound. Several excellent surgical procedures are available to close tympanic membrane perforations, and they should be considered whenever possible. Under certain circumstances, these operations cannot be performed, but the indications for surgery must always be determined by an appropriately trained physician.

Tumors, both benign and malignant, can form in the external auditory canal. When they are observed by hearing or speech-language clinicians, the patient should be referred for immediate medical consultation. It is not until the size of a growth in the canal impedes the passage of sound waves that a hearing loss becomes evident, but hearing loss obviously is not the primary concern when medical referrals are made in the case of tumors.

The Middle Ear

The *middle ear* is a tiny air-filled space, the lining of which is mucous membrane, similar to that found in the lungs, nose, throat, and paranasal sinuses. Normally, the middle ear is separated from the external auditory canal by the tympanic membrane. Because any membrane vibrates best when the air pressure is the same on both of its sides, there must be a means to replenish the air in the middle-ear space that is constantly being absorbed by the mucous membrane that lines the middle ear. The *eustachian tube*, which connects the middle ear to the nasopharynx (where the nose and throat join), is normally closed, but it is opened by the pull of four sets of muscles during such actions as yawning and swallowing. When the tube is open, atmospheric pressure is restored to the middle-ear space, and the pressure on both sides of the tympanic membrane is equalized, which makes it maximally compliant, allowing for efficient transmission of vibrations through the middle ear to the inner ear.

Because the outer ear is filled with air and the inner ear is filled with fluid, the *impedances* (opposition to energy flow) of the two systems differ. Without the middle ear to match these impedances, many sounds that strike the tympanic membrane would bounce off or be distorted and attenuated (weakened) before they reached the inner ear. The matching of impedances is accomplished in two major ways. First, the area of the tympanic membrane is about 22 times larger than the area of the *oval window*, which is one of the two membranous entryways to the inner ear (with the *round window* being the other). This step-down ratio increases the pressure from the tympanic membrane to the oval window in much the same way that water pressure is increased in a garden hose when a thumb is placed over the end. Second, the architecture of the middle ear provides a system for matching impedances using leverage.

A diagram of the middle ear is shown in Figure 17.5. Each middle ear contains the three smallest bones in the human body, the *ossicles*. The ossicles in each middle ear are called the *malleus, incus,* and *stapes* (commonly known as the *hammer* or *mallet, anvil,* and *stirrup).* The fact that the malleus, the largest of the ossicles, moves like a lever on a fulcrum also increases the energy that passes through the middle ear. Therefore, whereas the outer ear is primarily a place of acoustic energy, the middle ear deals primarily with mechanical energy.

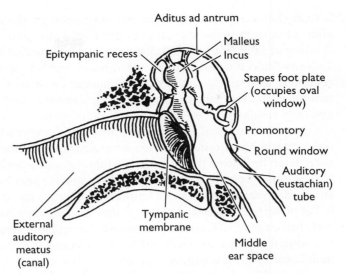

Aditus ad antrum

Malleus
Incus

Epitympanic recess

Stapes foot plate
(occupies oval
window)

Promontory

Round window

Auditory
(eustachian)
tube

External
auditory
meatus
(canal)

Tympanic
membrane

Middle
ear space

FIGURE 17.5

Cross section of the middle ear.
Source: From *Introduction to Audiology* (10th ed.), by F. N. Martin & J. G. Clark, 2009. Reprinted with the permission of Allyn and Bacon.

Prenatal Causes of Conductive Hearing Loss in the Middle Ear   Many genetic disorders have been associated with abnormalities of the middle ear. Sometimes a congenital malformation of the middle ear is seen with no other symptoms. At other times, middle-ear anomalies are part of a syndrome, such as craniofacial pathologies.

Perinatal Causes of Hearing Loss in the Middle Ear   Damage to the middle ear at the time of birth is relatively unusual. Severe trauma from violent uterine contractions or forceps, although they could conceivably damage the middle ear, would undoubtedly result in other severe damage to the fetus.

Postnatal Causes of Hearing Loss in the Middle Ear   One of the largest single causes of hearing loss—not only in the middle ear, but also in general—is **otitis media**, or infection of the middle-ear space. These infections are common in children as a result of upper respiratory infections, but they are often seen in adults as well. The infectious organisms may gain access to the middle-ear space through the eustachian tube, by way of the bloodstream, or through a perforation of the tympanic membrane. Before the advent of antibiotics, it was common for persistent otitis media to result in an infection of the mastoid bone (*mastoiditis*). This represented a serious threat to the patient's health because of the danger of infectious spread to the brain. In those earlier days, surgery was basically the only course of treatment for chronic otitis media, and it often resulted in disfigurement of the middle ear and permanent conductive hearing loss. Mastoiditis is still common in third-world countries and among people in lower socioeconomic groups in the United States who are not as likely to receive appropriate medical care.

Otitis media must be thought of primarily as a medical concern and secondarily from the point of view of hearing loss, with its concurrent communicative implications. Thus, medical treatment is primarily directed at alleviating the dangers of infection and secondarily at improving the hearing status. Surgery can be performed to close a perforation of the tympanic membrane, which can improve hearing sensitivity and, more importantly, provide protection from agents in the air or water that could irritate or infect the middle ear. Surgery is rarely performed to close a middle-ear system that is actively infected.

Although fluid in the middle ear is the hallmark of otitis media, there are times when the fluid itself is noninfectious. When eustachian-tube function is altered, the system that maintains equal air pressure between the outer and middle ears is affected. A drop in middle-ear pressure results in a partial vacuum that causes the drawing of fluid from the moist mucous membrane that lines the middle-ear walls. This condition is called *secretory otitis media,* and it is often the result of overgrown adenoids, allergy, or pathology of the muscles or nerves that would normally act to pull the eustachian tube open. Poor eustachian-tube function is common in infancy and early childhood.

A common surgical procedure performed on patients with fluid in the middle ear is *myringotomy.* The pressure and pain associated with secretory or infectious otitis media are relieved by lancing the tympanic membrane with a slender scalpel. Myringotomies are customarily performed on children in hospitals under light anesthesia or as part of an adenoidectomy–tonsillectomy procedure. Myringotomies are often done on adults in the physician's office, and although they can be somewhat painful, the procedure is quite brief, and relief from the discomfort is almost immediate for the patient.

After the tympanic membrane has been lanced and the fluid suctioned out of the middle-ear space, it is common practice to place a small ventilating tube or *pressure-equalizing (PE) tube* through the incision. This tube usually remains in place for several months or years. Although the patient must be careful to keep water out of the external ear because of the possibility of introducing infection into the middle ear, the tube usually does an excellent job functioning as an artificial eustachian tube in equalizing the pressure on either side of the tympanic membrane. The use of these PE tubes has been popular for many years, especially in the treatment of small children.

Because otitis media is so common in children, it is often discovered during routine hearing testing by speech-language pathologists while performing therapy on communicative disorders that ordinarily have nothing to do with hearing loss. In such situations, the clinician can become an advocate for the child by performing or requesting tests that may lead to the diagnosis of a middle-ear abnormality. Consequently, children often benefit from the eclectic training of their clinicians.

Otitis media in small children may have consequences beyond temporary hearing loss, pain, and discomfort. Northern and Downs (1991) discuss the possible effects of even very mild conductive hearing losses on the language development of small children. This condition is called *minimum auditory deprivation syndrome* (MADS), and it is of concern to many clinicians. During even temporary periods of mild hearing loss in babies, the developing brain cells may be adversely affected because of the lack of sensory stimulation. Conflicting research findings continue to fuel debate over this most important issue.

Otosclerosis, a condition seen primarily in adults, is caused by the growth of a new layer of bone over the oval window, which interferes with the vibrations of the stapes. Interestingly, this condition is more common in women than in men, and it is largely restricted to Caucasians. The development of the surgical microscope has led to several effective operative procedures for alleviating hearing loss that is due to otosclerosis.

Any condition that causes damage to the middle-ear system can produce a hearing loss. This includes burns, trauma, tumors, and a host of other pathologies. Whenever there is a suggestion of a middle-ear disorder, medical consultation becomes a critical priority.

The Inner Ear

The inner ear (Figure 17.6) is often called a *labyrinth* because of its resemblance to a winding and twisting cave. It is composed of two portions. The *vestibular* portion is responsible for balance and equilibrium. The *cochlear* portion functions as a transducer,

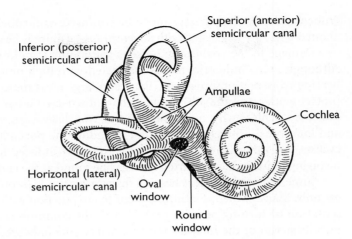

FIGURE 17.6
Diagram of the inner ear.
Source: From *Introduction to Audiology* (10th ed.), by F. N. Martin & J. G. Clark, 2009. Reprinted with the permission of Allyn and Bacon.

which converts the mechanical energy created by the middle ear into an electrochemical signal, which can then be sent to the brain for processing. The inner-ear fluids are called *endolymph* and *perilymph*, and while similar, they differ from each other chemically in important ways. The endolymph of the vestibule is continuous with the endolymph of the cochlea, just as the perilymph of the vestibule is continuous with the perilymph of the cochlea. The cochlea is a pressure-sensitive system, whereas the vestibule is a motion-sensitive system. And yet, with all its moving parts and complex functions, the inner ear is the size of a small pea.

Prenatal Causes of Inner-Ear Hearing Loss   Prenatal factors producing hearing loss in the inner ear are more common than those related to the outer or middle ears. Prenatal factors include genetic disorders in isolation or in conjunction with other abnormalities. Not all hereditary hearing losses are evident at the time of birth because some, called *hereditodegenerative losses,* are progressive and begin after birth.

Many of the factors that produce cochlear hearing loss, such as deprivation of oxygen to the fetus *(anoxia),* also produce damage to the central nervous system. Therefore, it is not uncommon to find hearing loss in association with such conditions as mental retardation and cerebral palsy. Other prenatal causes of hearing loss include maternal viral infections such as *cytomegalovirus* (one of the herpes viruses) and *rubella* (German measles), which can produce a variety of other abnormalities in such organs as the brain, heart, and eyes.

Along with many other causes of prenatal cochlear hearing loss are blood incompatibilities between the mother and fetus. Best known among these disorders is *Rh incompatibility.*

Perinatal Causes of Inner-Ear Hearing Loss   The birth process itself can be harmful to the inner ear. Children considered to be in medical distress may be placed on what has come to be called the *high-risk registry,* based on a number of contributing factors. Based on the more recent belief that the high-risk registry has failed to identify many children with hearing loss, a strong move toward universal hearing screening of all infants has developed nationally, which will be discussed in more detail in a subsequent part of this chapter (Joint Committee on Infant Hearing Screening, 2000.

Postnatal Causes of Inner-Ear Hearing Loss   Otitis media, usually associated with hearing loss in the middle ear, is also a common cause of cochlear hearing loss after birth. Bacterial meningitis and many viral infections such as mumps and measles (rubeola, the 10-day variety, not to be confused with rubella, which normally lasts about 3 days) are associated with adventitious (acquired) hearing loss.

Damage to the cochlea by noise is commonly seen in older children or adults. Although many industrial plants associated with high noise levels have established hearing conservation programs (thanks in large measure to federal laws designed to protect workers on the job), humans have discovered other ways to traumatize their sensitive cochleas with noise, such as firearms, lawn-care equipment, snowmobiles, and loud music. Stereo headphones, including the portable ones worn by runners, cyclists, and others, are often implicated in noise-induced hearing loss. A case study involving noise-induced hearing loss may be found at the end of this chapter.

Some acquired cochlear hearing losses are of sudden onset and are found in one ear only. Many of these conditions occur in conjunction with vertigo (an often violent sensation of turning or spinning). Two of the common causes of these conditions include spasm of the internal auditory artery (the only artery carrying blood to the inner ear) and *Ménière's disease*. These conditions are frequently very debilitating to the patient and require prompt medical attention when symptoms are first noticed, in hopes of averting a chronic condition.

As the world's population is achieving increased longevity, the incidence of hearing loss associated with aging can be expected to increase. Age-induced hearing loss is called *presbycusis*, which can usually be expected in males by their early sixties and females by their late sixties. With increased medical and sociological interest in the phenomena associated with aging, more is being learned about communicative disorders associated with elderly individuals. Age-related changes that occur in the central nervous system complicate the receptive communication problems of the elderly.

The Auditory Nerve and the Brain

Nerve impulses traveling from the cochlea reach the centers in the brain responsible for receptive auditory communication by way of the auditory nerve and a series of way stations leading to the brain. Damage to the auditory nerve usually produces pronounced difficulties in hearing and in discriminating among the sounds of speech. Interestingly, however, damage to the higher auditory centers affects processing of auditory information, but it does not always manifest a loss of hearing sensitivity to pure tones and speech stimuli.

Many of the neural centers beyond the auditory nerve that receive, process, and transmit impulses are duplicated on both sides of the brain. This redundancy is partially responsible for our specialized abilities to localize sound and to hear and understand speech in difficult listening situations, such as in noisy or reverberant backgrounds, or where there are competing messages. Often people's complaints about listening difficulties go unheeded because their hearing sensitivity remains essentially normal, while their speech recognition is impaired in subtle, but very detrimental ways.

Prenatal Causes of Hearing Loss in the Auditory Nerve and the Brain   As mentioned earlier in the discussion of prenatal causes of cochlear disorders, many of the causes of hearing loss also damage the central nervous system. Common causes include some of the maternal viral infections and genetic disorders. Evidence is growing about the adverse effects on the development of the fetus's central nervous systems resulting from substances ingested or inhaled by parents before and during pregnancy.

Perinatal Causes of Hearing Loss in the Auditory Nerve and the Brain
Trauma to the head during birth by uterine contractions or the use of forceps may produce damage to the brain. Other conditions that interrupt blood with its oxygen supply (e.g., umbilical strangulation) can also cause brain damage. As with prenatal causes, many of the perinatal causes of cochlear hearing disorders also manifest in abnormalities of the central nervous system, and they are not mutually exclusive.

Postnatal Causes of Hearing Loss in the Auditory Nerve and the Brain
Common causes of damage to the brain after birth include trauma (automobile accidents and gunshot wounds are frequently included in this category) and the formation of tumors. Many of the tumors, especially of the auditory nerve are benign and can be surgically removed. When these tumors are removed, it is common for the hearing to be completely lost on the affected side, even if only a mild loss was seen preoperatively. However hearing can sometimes be preserved.

The advent of the new imaging techniques, such as *computerized tomography* (CT) scans, *magnetic resonance imaging* (MRI), positron emission tomography (PET), and brain mapping, has objectified the diagnosis of brain lesions. Because these important and very expensive diagnostic tests must be ordered by a physician, it is the responsibility of the audiologist to identify audiologic test results that suggest a retrocochlear (beyond the cochlea) lesion.

Presbycusis was mentioned earlier as a result of cochlear dysfunction because many of the delicate inner-ear structures are destroyed and are not replaced during the aging process. Brain cells are also lost during this time, but this phenomenon is unique to each individual and may actually begin for some people as early as the third decade of life.

Erroneous Hearing Loss

A number of terms have been coined to describe the behaviors of patients who either fabricate a hearing loss deliberately or exaggerate a true loss. These include *nonorganic hearing loss, pseudohypacusis, functional hearing loss, psychogenic hearing loss, hysterical deafness, false or exaggerated hearing loss, factitious behavior,* and *malingering.* The term *malingering* is the most cause-specific of them all because it means that the patient is deliberately falsifying hearing test results for some financial or other gain. In other words, the patient is a liar, the kind of label that easily evokes litigious actions. The other terms leave room for some degree of psychological component, and that degree has always been hotly debated. The term we prefer is *erroneous hearing loss,* coined by Martin and Clark (2009).

Regardless of the term used, there are people, with differing motivations, who will present with symptoms of hearing loss that are greater than in actuality or totally feigned. The responsibility of the audiologist is not merely to unmask those people, who either consciously or unconsciously are feigning or exaggerating a hearing loss, but also to determine, often without patient cooperation, the nature and degree of the patient's true hearing status. To this end, a variety of special tests has been developed, some going back many years and some emerging at the time of this writing. The precise nature of these tests is beyond the purview of this book, but the interested reader is encouraged to pursue further knowledge on this subject by checking out the Selected Readings list.

The Measurement of Hearing

Early hearing tests took a variety of forms, such as the clicking of coins or the use of soft speech. The introduction of tuning-fork tests in the middle of the 19th century added a qualitative element. However, it was not until the development of the pure-tone *audiometer* that quantitative measurements of hearing could be made. The use of clinical audiometers allows for the comparison of *auditory thresholds* between patients and normal-hearing persons. Threshold may be defined as the level of a sound, measured in decibels, that is so soft that it can just barely be perceived approximately 50 percent of the time it is presented. The manufacturers of audiometers use data established by the American National Standards Institute (ANSI, 2004) to determine the sound-pressure levels required to reach a normal hearing level (0 dB HL). Thus, when an audiometer is set to 0 dB HL, the level of the sound that comes from the earphone is just intense enough to be at the hearing threshold of an average young adult with normal hearing.

Although some financial compensation regulations require reduction of hearing loss data to percentages, it is not a concept that is useful to people in understanding their hearing problems. Some clinicians still attempt to explain hearing loss as a percentage of hearing impairment, but this concept is not considered scientifically valid. Despite the fact that many people wish to know their percentage of hearing loss, the concept is virtually meaningless.

Pure-Tone Audiometry

Pure-tone audiometry is accomplished by instructing the patient to signal (pressing a response button or raising one hand is commonly used for this purpose) each time a tone is heard, even if the tone is barely audible. When working with special populations (e.g., children, the infirm, persons who are mentally challenged or who have multiple disabilities), voluntary responses are often difficult to obtain, and special techniques must be developed to elicit responses related to auditory threshold. Figure 17.7 shows a child signaling that he has heard a tone by raising his hand.

The results of pure-tone tests are customarily shown on a special graph called an *audiogram* (see Figures 17.9, 17.13, 17.14, and 17.15 later in this chapter). This type of graph is somewhat atypical, in that the decibel values are smaller at the top and grow larger toward the bottom. The auditory threshold for each frequency (shown in Hertz across the top of the graph) is indicated by the number of decibels (shown along the side of the graph) required to reach the threshold for that frequency. The intensity range on most audiograms is from −10 to 110 dB HL. The traditional frequency range, in octave and mid-octave points, is from 125 to 8,000 Hz. Although not shown on these audiograms, ultra-high-frequency audiometry allows for measurement of hearing sensitivity up to 20,000 Hz. There is a shaded area in the approximate center of the audiograms shown in this chapter. This is the range of intensities and frequencies within which most speech sounds are found. Because of its shape, this area is often called the *speech banana*.

Air Conduction

Tests by air conduction are accomplished by placing earphones over the pinnas of the outer ears or inserting receivers into the external auditory canals. Signals in the form of sound waves are carried through the outer ear and middle ear, converted to

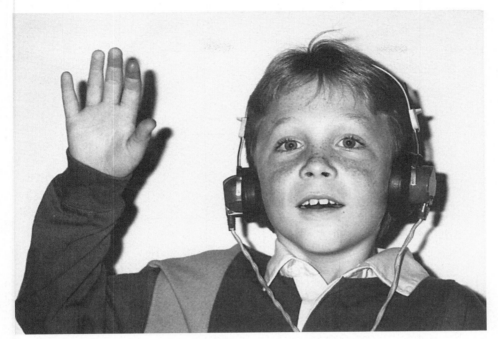

FIGURE 17.7
Photograph of a child signaling that he has heard a pure tone presented from an audiometer.
Source: Bart E. Noble.

electrochemical energy in the inner ear, and transmitted to the brain by the auditory nerve. The drawing of a cutaway of the ear in Figure 17.3 illustrates the air-conduction pathway. Test results are shown by placing a red circle for the right ear and a blue "X" for the left ear beneath the frequency being tested next to the number of decibels required to obtain threshold. Normal hearing is customarily represented by a range from −10 to 15 dB HL. Remember that 0 dB HL does not mean the absence of a sound, but rather the intensity at which people with normal hearing can barely hear that sound. Minus 10 dB HL, therefore, represents hearing sensitivity slightly better than what is normally expected. Any time numbers are averaged there are normal distributions around the means. There is, therefore, a range of intensities at which thresholds may be found for those with normal hearing.

Bone Conduction

Tests by bone conduction were designed to bypass the outer and middle ears and to measure only the sensitivity of the inner ear. Another look at Figure 17.3 illustrates this pathway. In actual practice, bone conduction is less simple than just stated, but it can be understood in this way for the beginner. Bone-conduction thresholds are obtained by placing a special oscillator on the head, usually on the mastoid process behind the pinna, although the forehead has been demonstrated to be a superior location. The bone-conduction oscillator stimulates the inner ear by literally distorting the skull slightly. Thresholds are obtained in the same manner for bone conduction as for air conduction and are usually graphed using a red "<" for the right ear and a blue ">" for the left ear. Persons interpreting test results should always consult the audiogram legend to be certain they are interpreting the symbols correctly. The symbols recommended by ASHA (1974) are shown in Figure 17.8. Persons with normal hearing

FIGURE 17.8

Symbols for use in pure-tone audiometry as recommended by the American Speech-Language-Hearing Association (1974).

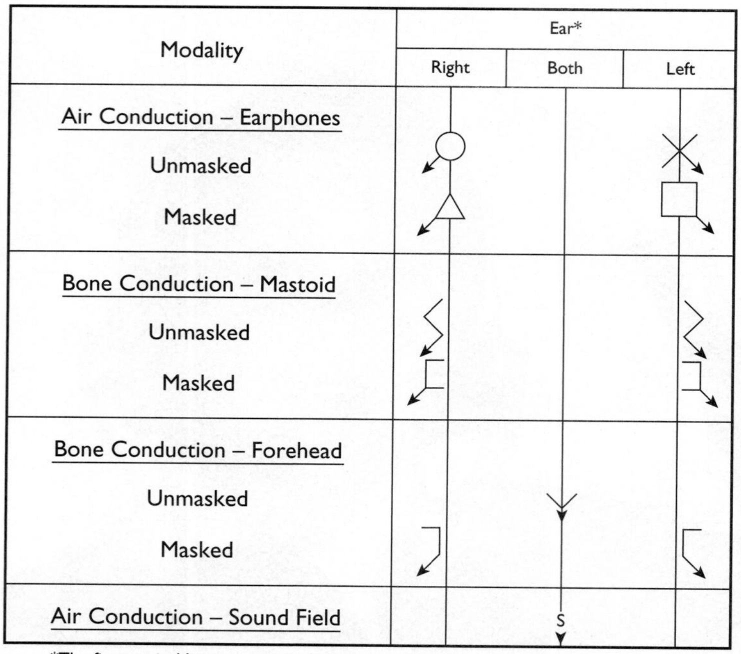

Modality	Ear*		
	Right	Both	Left
Air Conduction – Earphones Unmasked Masked			
Bone Conduction – Mastoid Unmasked Masked			
Bone Conduction – Forehead Unmasked Masked			
Air Conduction – Sound Field		S	

*The fine vertical lines represent the vertical axis of an audiogram.

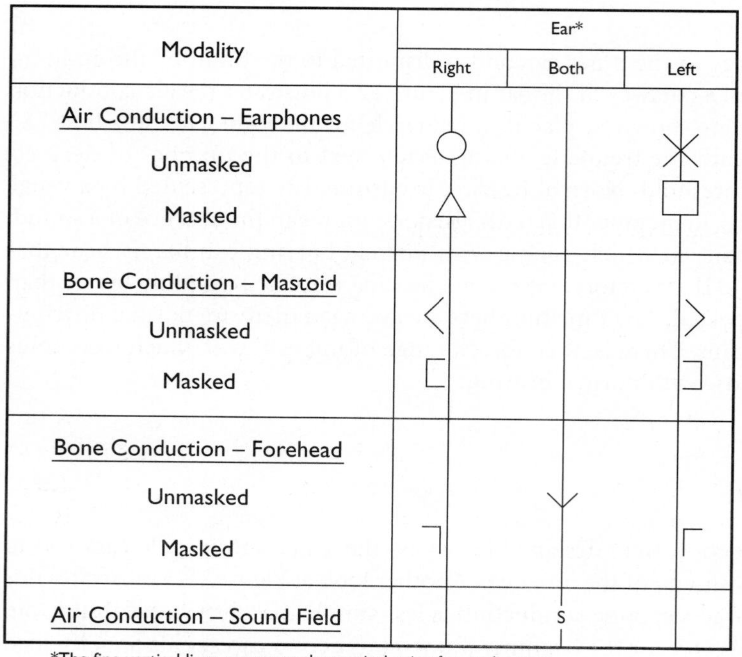

Modality	Ear*		
	Right	Both	Left
Air Conduction – Earphones Unmasked Masked			
Bone Conduction – Mastoid Unmasked Masked			
Bone Conduction – Forehead Unmasked Masked			
Air Conduction – Sound Field		S	

*The fine vertical lines represent the vertical axis of an audiogram.

will show hearing thresholds at 15 dB HL or lower at all frequencies for both air conduction and bone conduction. An example of an audiogram for a normal-hearing person may be seen in Figure 17.9.

Speech Audiometry   The development of speech audiometers was inevitable because pure tones do not exist in nature and because the most common complaint patients have about their hearing is that they have difficulty hearing and understanding speech.

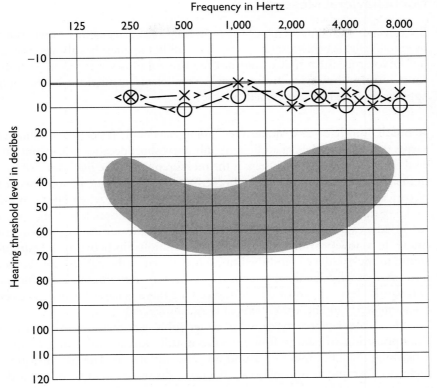

Frequency in Hertz

FIGURE 17.9
Audiogram illustrating normal hearing in both ears. *Note* that all thresholds are 10 dB HL or lower (better) for all frequencies in both ears.

Measurements Made with Speech Audiometers Several measurements of audition have been made possible through speech audiometry. The most common is the *speech recognition threshold* (SRT), which is the point at which speech can barely be heard and understood about 50 percent of the time. The SRT not only is a measurement of hearing loss for speech (a normal SRT is in the −10 to 15 dB HL range), but also typically approximates the *pure-tone average* (PTA) of the thresholds obtained at 500, 1000, and 2,000 Hz. Therefore, the SRT is often an excellent reliability check of pure-tone test results.

Another speech threshold sometimes measured in the diagnostic battery is the *speech detection threshold* (SDT), which is often called the *speech awareness threshold* (SAT). The SDT is the lowest level, in decibels, at which an individual can barely detect the presence of speech and recognize it as speech. SDTs usually require about 5–10 dB less intensity than do SRTs. SDTs are rarely measured today, but they also can be used to confirm pure-tone results.

Because, as mentioned, so many people complain that they can hear speech, but have difficulty understanding it, a routine audiologic examination includes tests of word recognition (discrimination) abilities. Many discrimination tests are available, but detailed descriptions of the stimuli and procedures are beyond the intended scope of this chapter. Suffice it to say, however, that each test leaves something to be desired in the determination of an individual's word-recognition abilities, although each can be useful in its own way. Word recognition is most commonly measured using special lists of monosyllabic words, and results are scored in terms of the percentage of the words correctly identified by verbal or written responses or, in the case of children, by pointing to pictures. These tests are customarily performed at levels well above threshold so that at least the loudness of the signal is at a comfortable listening level for the patient.

Nonbehavioral Measures

Because many patients seen for hearing evaluations either cannot or will not cooperate by giving reliable behavioral responses to sounds, the quest has always existed for more objective procedures that would not require voluntary responses. Throughout the short history of modern audiometry, several electroacoustic and electrophysiologic approaches have been developed.

Acoustic Immittance   Modern technology has made it possible to obtain measurements that the founders of audiology, only a few short decades ago, would have considered amazing. Chief among these is the measurement of the *impedance* of sound waves in the plane of the tympanic membrane. When the tympanic membrane, or the chain of ossicles in the middle ear, fails to function normally or when fluid is present in the middle ear, a conductive hearing loss exists. In this situation, less energy is admitted to the middle ear, and more sound is reflected from the surface of the tympanic membrane. It is now possible to determine the relationship between the *admittance* of a sound to the middle ear and the impedance placed in the pathway of that sound. The term used to describe these phenomena is *acoustic immittance,* a combination of the two words. Tests of acoustic immittance take three general forms: *static compliance, tympanometry,* and measurements of the *acoustic reflex.*

Static compliance is measured in either cubic centimeters (cm^3), when describing the opposition to energy flow into the middle ear, or millimhos (mmhos) when describing the admittance of sound into the middle ear. The two measurements are reciprocal because as one increases, the other decreases. Because of the wide range of individual variability, the overlap in immittance values between normal and abnormal ears has resulted in static immittance measures being somewhat less helpful in diagnosis than had earlier been hoped.

Tympanometry involves the measurement of a function that represents the compliance of the tympanic membrane as the air pressure placed against it is varied (Figure 17.10). The resulting plot is called a *tympanogram.* To perform this measurement, the examiner places the rubber or plastic tip of a probe assembly in the external auditory canal in the same manner as for static compliance measures. This assembly introduces a continuous "probe" tone to the tympanic membrane, and a microphone

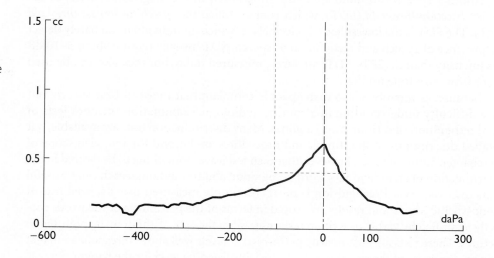

FIGURE 17.10
Tympanogram showing normal pressure/compliance function (Type A). *Note* that the peak of the curve (point of maximum compliance) is at 0 daPa (atmospheric pressure).
Source: Courtesy of Starkey Labs, Minneapolis, MN.

senses the amount of sound energy that is reflected from the membrane. An air-pressure pump then introduces positive air pressure against the membrane, which forces it gently in toward the middle ear, having the effect of partially clamping or stiffening the middle-ear system. The result of the positive pressure is a decrease in the compliance of the tympanic membrane, resulting in greater acoustic energy being reflected from it. The pressure is then gradually decreased until it reaches normal atmospheric pressure and is then further decreased until it becomes negative (forming a partial vacuum) in the external auditory canal.

Any vibrating membrane will be most compliant (mobile) when the air pressure is the same on both of its sides. This is also true of the tympanic membrane. Figure 17.10 illustrates the *tympanogram* (pressure compliance function) of a person's ear with normal middle-ear pressure. Dekapascals (10 Pascals, daPa) are customarily used as units of pressure. When the pressure in the outer ear is at 0 daPa, the normal tympanic membrane is maximally compliant. As both positive and negative changes in air pressure are made in the external auditory canal, the tympanic membrane becomes less compliant. Jerger (1970) has called this normal version the *type A* tympanogram.

A very common type of tympanogram is seen in persons whose middle-ear spaces are not properly ventilated by the eustachian tube. When this occurs, the pressure in the middle ear decreases, and the tympanic membrane becomes most compliant when the artificially induced pressure in the outer ear is negative. This is Jerger's (1970) *type C* tympanogram and can be seen in Figure 17.11.

When there is fluid in the normally air-filled middle-ear space, the pressure of this fluid against the tympanic membrane becomes greater than that which can be safely produced by the immittance device in the outer ear. In such cases, small or no changes in compliance of the tympanic membrane are found as air pressure from the immittance meter is varied from positive to negative. Jerger's (1970) *type B* tympanogram (Figure 17.12) is extremely accurate in diagnosing fluid in the middle ear.

The acoustic reflex results from the contraction of two small muscles in each middle ear, the *tensor tympani muscle* and the *stapedius muscle*. Although several kinds of stimuli are thought to cause these muscles to contract, the human stapedius muscle will normally contract in response to intense sounds. For most individuals with normal hearing, a sound about 85 dB SL (85 dB above the threshold at each frequency) in one ear will produce a stapedial reflex in both ears. It is possible to

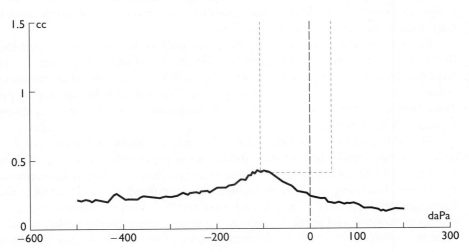

FIGURE 17.11

Tympanogram showing retracted tympanic membrane (Type C). *Note* that the peak of the curve is at −100 daPa (negative pressure). *Source:* Courtesy of Starkey Labs, Minneapolis, MN.

FIGURE 17.12
Tympanogram
suggesting fluid in
the middle ear (Type
B). *Note* that there
is no peak in this
curve and that the
compliance value is
very low.
Source: Courtesy of
Starkey Labs,
Minneapolis, MN.

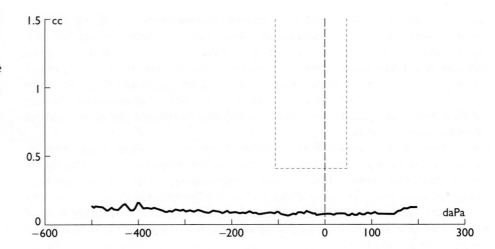

monitor the stapedial reflex using the same probe that is used to measure static compliance and tympanometry. When the stapedius muscle contracts in response to sound, observation of the acoustic immittance meter shows a decrease in the compliance of the tympanic membrane. Measurements of the *acoustic reflex threshold* (ART), which is the lowest intensity at which an acoustic reflex can be observed, often assist in the diagnosis of the type of hearing loss present and even, in many cases, the likely site of the pathology causing the loss.

The acoustic immittance battery has become an indispensable part of any diagnostic audiologic evaluation.

Auditory Evoked Potentials (AEPs)   For some time, emphasis has been placed on auditory evoked potentials as objective measures of auditory function and for site-of-lesion diagnosis. AEPs are elicited by introducing transient signals (tone bursts/pips or clicks) to patients via earphones or bone-conduction transducers. Electrode pickups placed on various locations (including but not limited to the scalp, forehead, earlobe, mastoid, external auditory canal, or medial wall of the middle ear) are then used to measure the electrical activity in the auditory system that is evoked by these sound stimuli. The rapid development of computer technology has allowed for amplification and signal averaging of the tiny microvoltages that emanate from the auditory system, so that the random ongoing electrical signals from the brain do not obscure the desired neurologic responses to the acoustic signals.

There are several types of AEP procedures, each evaluating different portions of the auditory nervous system. *Electrocochleography* (ECoG) measures electrical responses from the cochlea that take place 2–3 milliseconds (msec) after stimulus presentation. ECoG is used in the monitoring of cochlear function during surgical procedures (*intraoperative monitoring*) and in the diagnosis of certain inner-ear disorders such as Ménière's disease.

The AEP used most often clinically is the *auditory brainstem response* (ABR). The ABR occurs during the first 10 msec following the presentation of stimuli. This technique is employed for intraoperative monitoring and the estimation of hearing sensitivity of newborns, young children, and adults who are difficult to test. The ABR is also an important tool in the diagnosis of VIIIth nerve and brainstem disorders such as *acoustic neuromas* (tumors) and multiple sclerosis. A recent advance known as the *stacked ABR* measures activity from a broader frequency region of the cochlea than is possible with conventional ABR measures, which has allowed for more sensitive detection of even smaller tumors (less than 1 cm) (Don, 2003). The *middle latency response (MLR)* assesses neural activity from about 15 to 70 msec after stimulus onset. The MLR also allows for some degree of threshold estimation using frequency-specific tone bursts as well as diagnostic information in the region between the upper brain stem and the primary auditory cortex. The *late component response or slow vertex potential (SVP)* focuses on the recording of neural activities occurring more than 75 msec after stimulus onset and assesses higher-level auditory function. Unlike the earlier AEPs, the SVPs require the patient to pay attention to target stimuli, which has led to some of these measures being known as *event-related potentials (ERPs)*. As such, they are more affected by the patient's state of awareness during testing, but they also give a more detailed assessment of neurologic function and show promise in the diagnosis of auditory processing disorders. Another AEP measure known as the *auditory steady state response (ASSR)* allows for faster, more accurate, and more frequency-specific threshold estimations than have been previously possible with more traditional AEP tests (Burkard & McNerney, 2009).

Although these innovations in AEPs have led to significant improvements in estimating hearing sensitivity, even in babies, and in diagnosing lesion sites within the auditory system, they have some very real limitations. Experts in this area agree that AEPs should be viewed not as independent tests of hearing, but rather as measurements of synchronous neural activity in the auditory nervous system in response to a series of stimuli. Like all diagnostic procedures, the effectiveness of these measures must be viewed in proper perspective within the entire test battery. However, there is little doubt that these procedures will continue to serve as even more essential components of diagnostic audiology.

Otoacoustic Emissions (OAEs)   The cochlea had always been regarded as an organ whose activity was entirely involved in transducing and propagating signals from the middle ear to the auditory nerve. However, in 1978, Kemp reported that in many cases sounds are actually produced by the cochlea that can be detected by tiny, sensitive microphones placed in the external auditory canal. These sounds can occur without stimulation of the ears as *spontaneous otoacoustic emissions* (SOAEs). They may also be elicited by clicks or tone bursts presented to the external ear, in which case they are known as *evoked otoacoustic emissions* (EOAEs). The EOAEs are present in most normal auditory systems and are obtained quickly and with minimal patient involvement. However, they are not measurable when a conductive loss exists or when a cochlear hearing loss is present that is of a moderate degree or greater. Several subcategories of EOAEs have been developed for testing patients to determine site of lesion, presence of auditory neuropathy (to be discussed later in this chapter), and effects of ototoxic drugs and noise exposure. OAEs (the more widely used term for EOAEs) are also useful in the evaluation of those whose hearing sensitivity might not otherwise be measurable, including neonates and those who feign a hearing loss. The development of OAE measures has also allowed for better diagnostic differentiation among the types of hearing losses which are described in the next section (Prieve & Fitzgerald, 2009).

Types of Hearing Loss

Hearing loss is usually divided into three general types: conductive, sensorineural, and mixed, which will be discussed in more detail below.

TABLE 17.2   Degree of Hearing Impairment Based on the Average Thresholds Obtained at 500, 1000, and 2000 Hz

Pure-Tone Average (dB)	Degree of Impairment
−10 to 15	None
16 to 25	Slight
26 to 40	Mild
41 to 65	Moderate
66 to 80	Moderately severe
81 to 95	Severe
>95	Profound

Hearing levels are with reference to the ANSI 1996 standard.

Complete agreement does not exist among experts regarding the functional effects of different degrees of hearing loss (Martin & Champlin, 2000). Table 17.2 reflects our view. Many people consider 25 dB HL to be the lower limit of normal hearing. However, many years of seeing patients with hearing losses of 20 or 25 dB have led us to conclude that this much hearing loss should be considered a significant impairment and may very well have disabling effects. Indeed, there are people whose hearing levels are close to the 15 dB level, shown in Table 17.2 as representing the lower limit of normal hearing, who complain of a hearing impairment. The wise clinician is guided more by the social, emotional, and educational implications of the patient's hearing loss than by any arbitrary rules of thumb that relate threshold levels to functional ability.

General rules in interpreting audiograms follow:

1. Air-conduction thresholds show the total amount of hearing loss present (the difference, in decibels, between 0 dB HL and the patient's air-conduction threshold at each frequency).

2. Bone-conduction thresholds show the amount of the hearing loss that is sensory/neural (the difference, in decibels, between 0 dB HL and the patient's bone-conduction threshold at each frequency).

3. The air-bone gap (the difference, in decibels, between the patient's thresholds by air conduction and bone conduction in the same ear at each frequency) shows the portion of the hearing loss that is conductive at each frequency. In conductive hearing losses, word-recognition scores are usually quite high, regardless of the degree of loss, because the primary problem lies in the loss of the intensity of sound and not in its clarity. In sensorineural hearing losses, there is usually some degree of distortion and discrimination difficulty, and often it is directly related to the amount of hearing loss.

Conductive Hearing Loss

Conductive hearing losses are those that result from the blockage or obstruction of sound that prevents vibrations from passing normally through the outer ear and middle ear. These can be in the form of obstructions to sound, fluid (either infected or

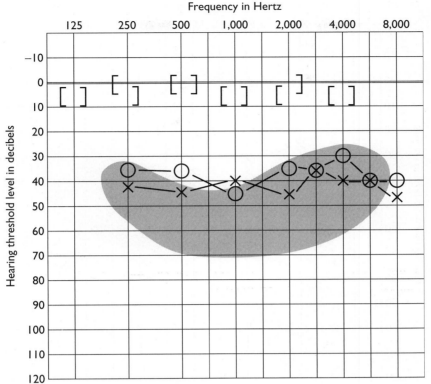

FIGURE 17.13

Audiogram illustrating a mild to moderate conductive hearing loss in both ears. *Note* that, while the thresholds are above normal (poorer hearing—lower on the graph) for air conduction, they are normal for bone conduction.

sterile) in the middle-ear space, or abnormalities of the tympanic membrane or ossicular chain. Conductive hearing losses usually result in an audiogram similar to the one in Figure 17.13, in which the air-conduction thresholds are elevated (made poorer) in direct proportion to the amount of hearing loss found. Because the inner ear and pathways beyond are unaffected in conductive hearing losses, the bone-conduction thresholds should theoretically remain normal.

Sensory/neural Hearing Loss

Hearing losses caused by damage to the inner ear or the auditory nerve are called *sensorineural*. The term is rather nonspecific because one cannot tell from looking at an audiogram whether the problem is in the sensory or the neural portions of the auditory system. In sensorineural hearing losses, the amount of hearing loss by air conduction is approximately the same (within 10 dB) as the amount of loss by bone conduction. An example of a sensorineural hearing loss is seen in Figure 17.14.

Persons with sensorineural hearing losses usually evidence some distortion of the sounds they hear, even if those sounds are amplified to comfortably loud levels. As a general rule, the greater the amount of sensorineural hearing loss, the greater the speech distortion, although the extent of hearing loss as shown on an audiogram is not always a good predictor of word-recognition ability. Because of this distortion of sound, word-recognition scores are usually adversely affected, and many patients have great difficulty in discriminating among the sounds of speech, even when those sounds are sufficiently loud.

FIGURE 17.14
Audiogram illustrating a mild to severe sensorineural hearing loss in both ears. *Note* that the thresholds for all frequencies show the same degree of hearing loss for air conduction as they do for bone conduction.

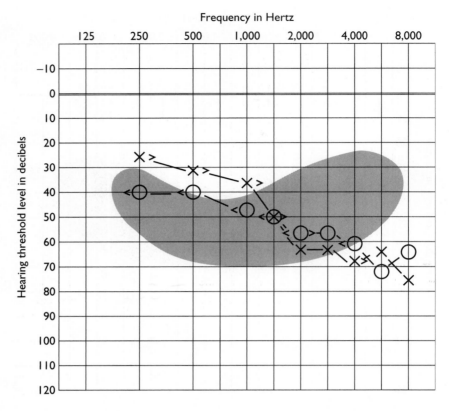

Mixed Hearing Loss

Conductive and sensorineural hearing losses are not mutually exclusive. Often patients exhibit symptoms of both types of losses. When this occurs, the term applied is *mixed hearing loss.* The causes of the sensorineural and conductive components of a mixed hearing loss may be the same, or each component may be caused by completely different factors. For example, a person may have a conductive hearing loss from wax accumulation in the external auditory canal and may have damage to the inner ear from noise exposure. A mixed hearing loss is illustrated in Figure 17.15.

The amount of word-recognition difficulty in a mixed hearing loss cannot be predicted based on the total amount of hearing loss present. Rather, it is the sensorineural component of a mixed hearing loss that represents the amount of distortion of speech sounds that will be present. Therefore, the bone-conduction audiogram is often the best predictor of how a patient might perform on a word-recognition test. Experienced clinicians do not rely on the audiogram alone in estimating how much difficulty a person may have in discriminating speech. Word-recognition tests should be carried out whenever possible.

Implications of Hearing Loss

The implications of a hearing loss for any individual are determined by several factors. Chief among these are the type and degree of loss and the age of onset. Combinations of these factors make for varying degrees of optimism when prognostic statements are made about any individual with a hearing impairment.

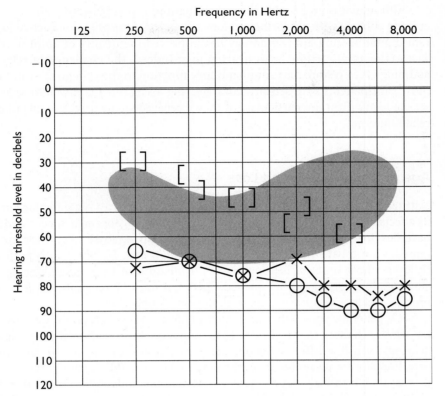

FIGURE 17.15
Audiogram illustrating severe mixed hearing loss in both ears. Note that there is a greater loss of hearing for air conduction than there is for bone conduction, although both are abnormal.

Type and Degree of Hearing Loss

If one had to have a hearing loss, a conductive (rather than a sensorineural) loss would be preferred. Many conductive hearing losses are reversible through medical or surgical means. Even if the loss is permanent, word recognition is still usually quite good, making the patient an excellent candidate for amplification using hearing aids.

The ability to discriminate among speech sounds is not affected by the degree of hearing impairment in cases of conductive hearing loss. The problems associated with communication in such cases are largely because the sounds of speech are not sufficiently loud. This is not true of sensory/neural hearing losses, in which some degree of distortion is almost always present in speech signals. Usually, with sensorineural hearing losses, the greater the degree of loss, the greater the distortion and the more difficulty experienced in discriminating speech sounds.

Except in unusual circumstances, persons with sensorineural hearing losses have irreversible hearing problems. Their impaired speech recognition causes them difficulty in communicating, especially in noisy background situations or when several people talk simultaneously. These patients are sometimes reluctant to use amplification, particularly if they find that simply making speech louder does not make it clearer. In some cases, it is likely that disappointment results if unrealistic expectations of hearing-aid benefit exist. In fact, years ago there was a notion among some physicians and audiologists that persons with sensorineural hearing losses should not wear hearing aids at all because the distortion they already hear would be made even more pronounced with amplification. Fortunately for the patients involved, this view has changed.

Although it is unarguable that rehabilitation involving hearing aids is more difficult for persons with sensorineural losses than for those with conductive losses, current digital hearing-aid technology has improved the quality of amplification for a vast majority of persons with hearing loss. Indeed, the challenge of rehabilitative audiology is to restore maximum auditory function to those in greatest need. For the most part, patients with sensorineural hearing losses can adapt well to appropriately selected amplification, particularly if they receive adequate professional guidance and rehabilitation.

Age of Onset of Hearing Loss

Naturally, the age at which a hearing loss begins can make a big difference in terms of its effects on the individual. Those who develop hearing loss after speech and language have developed are said to have *postlinguistic* hearing losses. For such individuals, remediation must come in the form of *rehabilitation. Habilitation* is performed on children whose onset of hearing loss is *prelinguistic,* or beginning before speech and language concepts have been formed. Speech, it must be remembered, is an imitative process, which is best learned through the sense of hearing.

It is generally agreed that the earlier in life a hearing loss can be detected, the better are the chances that a child can be taught communication through speech and hearing. Even if a different avenue of communication is chosen for the child, early detection almost always increases the potential for a child's learning. Having said this, it must then be asked which kinds of screening methods should be used and at what point in a child's life should they be attempted. There is no earlier time than when a child is in the hospital immediately after birth.

The concept of *universal newborn hearing screening* certainly appears justified because it has been estimated that one neonate in 1,000 will have a profound hearing impairment at birth (Northern & Downs, 1991). The yield of identifying children with hearing impairments using modern screening procedures may well be greater than that found in the routine screening performed for other medically significant conditions. This movement culminated in the Joint Committee on Infant Hearing Screening's Year 2000 Position Statement, which stated that "all infants' hearing should be screened using objective, physiologic measures in order to identify those with congenital or neonatal onset hearing loss," and it endorsed "the development of family-centered, community-based early hearing detection and intervention (EHDI) systems...available to all infants." (2000, pp. 8-9).

The use of ABR measures has become increasingly popular in the hearing screening of infants. When using ABR in young children, the clinic's equipment must be normed for responses based on the age of the child because the relative maturity of the central auditory nervous system can affect the interpretation of responses. Because premature babies are more "at risk" for hearing loss than are full-term babies, the audiologist must consider not only the chronological ages of children being tested (referenced to the date of birth), but also their gestational ages (referenced to the date of conception). OAEs have also found a place in the armamentarium of those interested in screening for hearing loss in neonates, and they show a high success rate in identifying the type and degree of hearing impairment in infants and toddlers. Commercial devices for measuring OAEs have become plentiful, less expensive, easier to operate, and more accurate (Prieve & Fitzgerald, 2009).

Other Auditory Disorders

Other categories of auditory dysfunction have also been investigated and should be mentioned briefly. One of the more recently emphasized areas is *auditory neuropathy (AN)* (sometimes know as *auditory dys-synchrony [AD]*), which is a disorder of the inner ear and/or auditory nerve that typically results in hearing loss with poorer-than-expected speech discrimination, absent acoustic reflexes, abnormal ABR waveforms, and normal OAEs and tympanograms (Hood, 2007).

Auditory processing disorders (APDs) refer to more diffuse lesions in the brain that produce real, but sometimes subtle symptoms. Often central disorders do not show up on routine hearing tests, but are suspected by alert clinicians during the taking of a patient's case history. Both AN/AD and APDs may prevent many patients from taking full advantage of amplification and thus their full hearing potential, and various diagnostic measures and management programs have been developed to address these problems.

Summary

No person professionally involved with people who have speech and language problems can escape dealing with patients who have hearing impairments. The purpose of this chapter has been to introduce concepts associated with hearing and its disorders to those persons interested in the processes of communication and their breakdown. The concentration here has been on the fundamentals of hearing leading up to the diagnostic aspects of clinical audiology. Diagnosis without treatment is useless, and it is to the issues of patient and family counseling, auditory (re)habilitation (including amplification systems) and general hearing-health care that this chapter is devoted.

case study VIOLET

About 20 years ago I was halfway through my introductory audiology class at The University of Texas. I had taught that class many times before and always especially enjoyed student participation. A student in the class, with a severe hearing loss of which I was unaware, asked if she could tell her story when we were on the topic of the dangers of accepting false-positive responses during hearing tests. Neither the students, nor I, will forget the terrible injustice done to Violet by a careless clinician—and the magnificent way she overcame an early misdiagnosis. This young woman, and others with tales of audiologic mistakes, can serve as beacons to keep audiologists ever alert to the seriousness of their profession.

Violet was a bright, affectionate child, born to a family with no known history of hearing loss, but her parents wondered about the fact that her language skills were developing more slowly than had been anticipated, based on her other areas of development. Additionally, her speech and voice lacked the precision of other children her age.

When she was 3 years of age, Violet's parents asked her pediatrician whether there might be something wrong with the child. They were made to feel that she was just a little slower than normal in her speech development, but that she would be fine. Her hearing was judged to be normal when she turned around on hearing the pediatrician clap his hands behind her back. Her excellent use of visual information and her motivation to please her parents and be accepted by others allowed Violet to compensate enough to convince everyone around her that she had normal hearing. Indeed, she had no way of knowing that it was not; she had always heard imperfectly and knew no other way. It was not until she was 12 years old that her hearing loss was correctly diagnosed. She was found to have normal hearing for low-pitched sounds, but a severe loss of hearing for high-pitched sounds, a condition that she had probably had her entire life. Because the energy of most environmental sounds is in the low-pitch range, Violet gave normal responses to such things as handclaps, door slams, and even the vowel sounds of speech. She could not hear high-pitched sounds well, which caused her to miss many of the consonants that make speech intelligible.

Violet's first-grade teacher wondered about the possibility of a hearing loss, based on her behavior in class. Her parents were notified, and she was taken to have her hearing tested. Testing suggested the possibility of a hearing loss, and a conference was held between the clinician and Violet's father. The clinician explained that Violet had been inconsistent in her responses and that the test results could not be considered valid. Violet was reprimanded by her father for what was perceived as her inattention, and she was returned to the sound suite for retesting.

Violet felt that she had disappointed her father by not responding each time a tone was presented to her. To succeed the second time, she watched the face and movements of the tester very carefully to search for any clue that a stimulus might be presented, even though she heard very few of them. Violet had had years to practice taking advantage of visual clues. At the end of a short time, the second test was concluded, and Violet's father was told that she had done much better, that her hearing was normal, and that there was nothing to worry about.

Because Violet had been told when she was young that her hearing was normal, she simply assumed this to be the case. She wondered why students paid attention in class to teachers who just seemed to move their lips, but make little or no sound, but she assumed that this was somehow normal. When she did not understand things, she assumed that it was her own fault. She blamed all of her scholastic and communication difficulties on herself.

At age 12, Violet was finally correctly diagnosed and fitted with hearing aids, and her life changed dramatically. She realized for the first time what she had been missing. Today she wears two hearing aids and is a successful advocate for the deaf community. The hearing aids opened a whole new world of environmental sounds and drastically improved her ability to communicate. Her hearing aids are now among her most treasured possessions.

Because of her intelligence and motivation, Violet now has very good communicative skills, but her speech and voice are not as clear as someone with normal hearing. The reader should realize that Violet's story is the exception rather than the rule. Violet bears no ill will against the people who failed to make the appropriate diagnosis earlier in her life. She does, however, vow to see that these kinds of oversights do not happen in any circumstances over which she has control.

QUESTIONS

1. How does the story of Violet illustrate problems with accepting false-positive responses?
2. What are the implications of delayed identification of hearing loss in children in terms of the speech and language development?
3. Violet was allowed to face the audiologist during her pure-tone examination. In what ways did that contribute to the erroneous diagnosis of normal hearing?

case study MR. HUNTER

Mr. Hunter was first seen in the audiology clinic at age 25 with a complaint of a constant high-pitched ringing noise, which was more pronounced in his left ear than in his right. He denied any difficulty in hearing and initially declined to have a hearing evaluation. His history revealed that he had been a hunter since his teenage years, but he did not associate that type of noise exposure with the ringing in his ears. Subsequent examinations over a period of years revealed that his hearing sensitivity continued to deteriorate, more in his left ear than in his right ear. The ringing sound was found to be in the high pitch range, corresponding to his high-frequency hearing loss. While he initially declined to wear hearing protection, he eventually acceded to this recommendation. Eventually, when his hearing loss became moderately severe, he gave up shooting entirely. He subsequently returned to the clinic complaining, "I can hear people talking to me, but I have trouble understanding what they are saying." Some ten years after his first visit to the clinic, he was finally fitted with hearing aids in both ears, which he wears with moderately good success. It seems obvious that Mr. Hunter's irreversible hearing loss was caused entirely or at least partially by the gunfire. This case exemplifies some of the frustration felt by audiologists when they are unable to convince a patient to avoid the almost inevitable consequences of prolonged exposure to high levels of noise.

QUESTIONS

1. Why does Mr. Hunter say that he can hear but he can't understand the words people are saying"
2. Why are Mr. Hunter's SRTs and SDTs within normal limits despite the fact that he has a documented hearing loss?
3. What tympanogram type would you expect to find in Mr. Hunter's case? Explain why.

STUDY QUESTIONS

1. What is minimal auditory deprivation syndrome *(MADS)*, and how does it relate conductive hearing loss in small children to language learning disorders?

2. What are the main causes of middle-ear infections?

3. List as many causes of hearing loss as you can. Divide them into categories of prenatal, perinatal, and postnatal onset and conductive, mixed, and sensorineural losses.

4. Sketch an audiogram illustrating a mild conductive hearing loss. Try to predict the probable speech recognition threshold and word-recognition scores.

5. What are the advantages and disadvantages of neonatal hearing screening?

SELECTED READINGS

Clark, J. G., & English, K. E. (2004). *Audiologic counseling: Helping patients and families adjust to hearing loss.* Boston, MA: Allyn & Bacon.

Clark, J. G., & Martin, F. N. (Eds.) (1994). *Effective counseling in audiology.* Boston, MA: Allyn & Bacon.

Luterman, D. M. (1991). *Counseling the communicatively disordered and their families* (2nd ed.). Austin, TX: Pro-Ed.

Martin, F. N., Clark, J. G. (2009). *Introduction to audiology* (10th ed.) Boston, MA: Allyn & Bacon.

Martin, F. N., & Clark, J. G. (Eds.) (1996). *Hearing care for children.* Boston, MA: Allyn & Bacon.

Northern, J. L., & Downs, M. P. (1991). *Hearing in children* (4th ed.). Baltimore, MD: Williams & Wilkins.

Chapter EIGHTEEN

Audiologic Rehabilitation

Alice E. Holmes
University of Florida

Shawna M. Dell
University of Florida

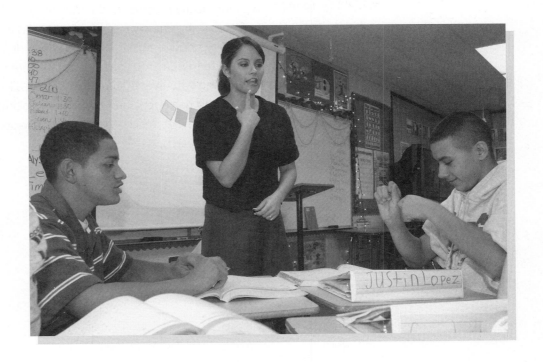

personal PERSPECTIVE

ALICE E. HOLMES

When I started out in college, I was a dual major in chemistry and physics destined to spend my life working in a laboratory, or so I thought. During the summer of my freshman year, I worked as a counselor at the Texas Lions Camp for Crippled Children, and I realized how much I loved working with children with disabilities. Still unsure of my calling, I switched my major to pre-medicine, but after a year realized I did not want to deal with the life-and-death issues of medicine. With my continuing summer experiences at the Lions Camp, I gravitated to children with hearing loss and switched my major again to deaf education. It was in my senior year that I took my first introductory course in audiology. It changed my life. I finally found a helping profession with a scientific basis that worked with persons with hearing loss. Graduating with my undergraduate degree in deaf education, I went on to graduate school in audiology and never looked back. I worked as an educational audiologist and then went to Penn State University for my Ph.D. in Communication Disorders with a minor in Human Development and Family Studies. In the mid-1980s, as a junior faculty member at the University of Florida, I was fortunate to be a part of one of the first cochlear implant teams in the country. I have had the opportunity to see how cochlear implants and audiologic rehabilitation provide improved quality of life to numerous patients with severe to profound hearing loss. Even after working with over 800 implant patients, I still get a chill the first time my patients are able to perceive sound from their implants. My career as a rehabilitative audiologist has been extremely rewarding. I love working with patients and students as well as doing research.

personal PERSPECTIVE

SHAWNA M. DELL

Like every other college freshman, excitement and high hopes of making a difference in the world filled every part of me. I started out my college career majoring in forestry to become an advocate for conserving and protecting our natural resources. However, after realizing that I craved human interaction and wanted to become a better influence on others' lives, I changed my major to communication sciences and disorders. After taking a few audiology courses and observing numerous audiologists, I knew audiology was for me. As an audiologist, I am a teacher, a supporter, and a champion for those individuals living with hearing loss. Audiology allows me to help those that experience the daily difficulties associated with living with hearing loss. Also, audiology is an exciting, constantly changing field that encourages me to never stop learning, listening, and loving my profession. I love audiology so much that I decided to pursue a doctor of philosophy in audiology, so that health disparities among Americans will become history.

Introduction

Audiologic rehabilitation (AR) is defined as "those professional efforts designed to help a person with hearing loss (including) services and procedures for lessening or compensating for a hearing impairment and specifically involve facilitating adequate receptive and expressive communication" (Schow & Nerbonne, 2002, p. 4). AR incorporates the diagnosis and quantification of the hearing loss as well as the provision of appropriate listening devices (Tye-Murray, 1998). AR has had many names including aural and auditory rehabilitation. The term *rehabilitation* suggests the reteaching of a skill. Children who are born with hearing loss or who develop hearing loss prior to learning speech and language have no auditory skills to *re*-habilitate. For this reason, often you will find *habilitation* used when referring to AR with children who have prelingual hearing impairment. For the purposes of this chapter, audiologic rehabilitation will be used as a general, all-encompassing term.

This chapter describes the major components of AR with both children and adults. The primary tools of AR are hearing aids, but they are by no means the final step in the rehabilitation process (Bess, Lichtenstein, & Logan, 1990). Hearing aids and other amplification devices can significantly improve the communication abilities of those with hearing loss, but they do not restore hearing to normal. Thus, other AR techniques are necessary to help compensate for the hearing loss. This chapter will cover amplification devices, assistive listening devices, speechreading, and AR therapy approaches for both children and adults. The goal of this chapter is to familiarize the reader with the different faces of AR and develop an appreciation of the audiologist's role in AR.

Amplification Devices

Hearing Aids

Hearing aids are appropriate for individuals with hearing loss that cannot be medically corrected. These losses are typically sensorineural in nature (inner-ear damage/nerve loss). The goal of hearing aids is provide the impaired ear with an amplified signal to improve the perception of speech.

All hearing aids contain three primary components: the microphone, the amplifier, and the receiver. The microphone picks up the acoustical signal from the environment and converts it into an electrical signal. The amplifier then takes the signal and increases it. Finally, the amplified signal is sent to the receiver, where it is changed back to an acoustic signal and delivered to the external ear canal. Audiologists classify hearing aids by their style (physical appearance or size; see Figure 18.1) and by the circuitry used to amplify the signal.

Style

Most current-generation hearing aids are worn at ear level. All components are placed on or in the ear. The patient and audiologist determine style by the level and type of hearing loss and cosmetic preferences.

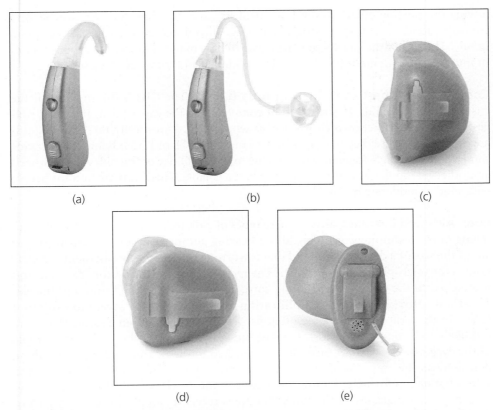

(a)   (b)   (c)

(d)   (e)

Behind-the-Ear Hearing Aids (BTEs)   The BTE is a curved hearing aid that sits on top of the external ear. Various components lie within the hearing aid. The BTE, connected via a short tube to a custom earmold, delivers the amplified signal to the ear. These aids tend to be the largest ear-level instruments and can be equipped with more circuitry. BTEs fit a broad range of hearing losses and are appropriate for any degree of hearing loss or configuration making BTEs the most flexible aid.

Open-Fit Behind-the-Ear Hearing Aids (Open-Fit BTEs)   Open-fit BTEs are similar to conventional BTEs except that open-fit BTEs do not use a custom earmold. Instead, a slim, small sound tube delivers the amplified signal to the ear, leaving the ear canal open. Open-fit BTEs address the problem of the occlusion effect, which is often present with conventional hearing aids. This style of hearing aid can accommodate mild to moderate hearing losses. Also, this style is very cosmetically appealing.

In-the-Ear Hearing Aids (ITEs)   The ITE is a custom-fit hearing aid that is placed directly into the external ear, filling the entire concha. The components are housed in the concha portion of the aid, and, therefore, there are no parts that hang over the ear or that are worn on the body. An ITE accommodates most hearing losses except for the most severe. This aid, like the BTE, is usually large enough to include optional components such as a **telecoil**, direct audio input to assistive devices, and directional microphones, which will be discussed later in the chapter.

In-the-Canal Hearing Aids (ITCs)   The ITC is also a custom-fit aid; however, the ITC fits in the external ear canal and fills only a very small portion of the concha. This design allows for the natural resonances and diffraction effects of the external ear by leaving this portion open. However, its small size may not allow for user switches and controls and other additional components (e.g., directional microphones, direct audio input). The size of the canal also plays a role in how many additional components can fit into the aid. This aid is best for mild to moderate and some severe losses.

Completely-in-the-Canal Hearing Aids (CICs)   The CIC is the smallest of the custom-fit hearing aids. It is made to fit completely in the ear canal, as the name suggests. Its biggest attraction is clearly its cosmetic appeal. Acoustically, these hearing aids are desirable because they fit deeper in the canal than ITE or ITC aids and may provide some additional high-frequency boost. Due to the small size of this aid, volume wheels and other manipulative controls are often not available. These aids are best for people with mild to moderate hearing losses.

Body Aids and Eyeglass Aids   These types of aids are rarely used due to advancements in the technology. A body aid is a hearing aid made up of a casement that is about the size of a deck of cards and that is worn on the torso. The casement typically houses the microphone and amplifier. The receiver, which has a custom earmold and is attached to the casement via a long cord, delivers the amplified sound to the ear. These aids provide powerful amplification and are useful for severe to profound losses. In the past, body aids were often used with young children because they were less likely to be damaged or lost. Eyeglass aid components are housed in the temple of the eyeglasses. A custom earmold is connected to the hearing aid through tubing that delivers the amplified signal to the earmold. These aids tend to be heavy and somewhat uncomfortable. Another downside to the eyeglass aid is that, if the person does not require glasses all the time, then he is receiving amplification only part of the time.

Circuitry or Signal Processing

The more important means of classifying hearing aids is based on the circuitry used to amplify the signal. Signal processing represents the way the acoustic signal entering the hearing aid is manipulated. The three types of circuitry currently used in hearing aids are analog, digitally programmable, and digital.

In an analog hearing aid, the processor takes the acoustic signal; turns it into an electrical signal, which it amplifies; returns the signal to an acoustical signal; and then delivers that signal to the external ear canal. The amplified signal can be filtered or shaped so that more amplification is provided in the frequency range with the most hearing loss. The audiologist is able to make limited adjustments, depending on the options available and the size limitations of the instruments, using physical controls in the form of dials or screw adjustments.

Analog hearing aids can also be digitally programmable. Programmable simply means that the device's acoustic parameters are adjusted using a computer, handheld device, or remote control. Each hearing aid manufacturer has its own unique software for programming its products with various options, allowing the audiologist to more accurately make adjustments.

In contrast, digital signal processors take the acoustic signal; change it to an electrical signal and then to a numerical code, which is manipulated via algorithms to achieve a desired target; and finally convert it back to an acoustic signal that is sent into the external ear canal. Digital processing provides an easier and more efficient way to manipulate the acoustic signal, often resulting in clearer, better quality, and more specific amplified sound. As with digitally programmable devices, the manufacturer provides the software and programming options.

Other Aids

Bone-Conduction Hearing Aids   For some people, traditional hearing aids that utilize air-conduction receivers are not appropriate. These people may have no external ear canal or may have middle-ear disorders that make it impossible to use a traditional hearing aid. In these cases, a bone-conduction hearing aid can provide the amplification they need.

Traditional bone-conduction devices deliver the amplified signal to the ear via a vibrator that is placed on the mastoid bone behind the pinna. A metal headband holds the vibrator in place against the mastoid bone. The rest of the components are housed in either a BTE or a body aid. The microphone picks up the signal, which is then amplified and causes the device against the mastoid bone to vibrate. These vibrations then set the skull into vibration and transmit the sound to the cochleas. These devices are made to fit snugly and can be very uncomfortable, leading to soreness and headaches; oftentimes they do not stay in place.

Bone-Anchored Hearing Aids   The bone-anchored hearing aid (BAHA) is a type of bone-conduction hearing aid that is attached to the skull. The hearing aid consists of a surgically implanted titanium fixture and an abutment to which a detachable sound processor attaches. The surgery to implant the fixture is done under local or general anesthesia by an otolaryngologist. After implantation, the patient must wait approximately three months before being fitted with the sound processor to allow the titanium implant to integrate with the bone tissue. The BAHA works exactly like the bone-conduction hearing aid, but without the discomfort of the headband.

Vibrotactile Aids   A vibrotactile aid is not really hearing aid; it is a vibrator that sends information about the acoustic environment to the user via the sense of touch. The vibrator is usually placed on the sternum. Vibrotactile aids are designed for persons who receive little or no benefit from conventional hearing aids. The vibrotactile aid is designed to support speechreading by providing tactile information on those parts of the speech signal that are not highly visible on the lips.

Middle Ear Implants (MEIs)   The MEI, a device approved by the U.S. Food and Drug Administration (FDA), is partially or completely implanted within the middle-ear space by a surgeon. Unlike the BAHA, which is designed for individuals with maximum conductive losses, the MEI's main application is for those with sensorineural losses and those with residual hearing. Because the MEI is implanted, it does not require the use of an external earmold, which users may see as an advantage. Earmolds can encourage cerumen or ear wax impaction, cause discomfort, and hold moisture inside the ear canal, which can lead to external ear infections. MEI users may not experience the feedback that some conventional hearing aid users may experience. Feedback is the "whistling" noise you may hear coming from an improperly seated/fit hearing aid. Feedback occurs when any amplified sound being put into the ear by the receiver leaks out of the ear and is picked up by the external microphone, where it becomes reamplified and creates an oscillation, causing a feedback loop to occur.

Cochlear Implants (CIs)   Unfortunately, for persons with little or no residual hearing, traditional hearing aids offer only limited or no assistance in communication. Even the most powerful devices are unable to provide enough meaningful information for environmental sound awareness or speech perception for these individuals. CI technology offers them an alternative means to receive some important information from their impaired auditory systems.

The CI is not an amplifier. It is a surgically implanted device that electrically stimulates the auditory nerve of patients with severe to profound hearing loss to provide them with sound and speech information. The CI does not restore normal hearing. CI recipients experience varying amounts of benefit from the device. For some individuals, the CI provides only auditory awareness, detection of environmental sounds, and improvement in their speechreading abilities, while other patients are able to achieve open-set speech perception without visual cues. Many patients are able to conduct conversations over the telephone.

Successful CI programs have a multidisciplinary team to work with the patients. These team members should be involved in the entire process from the evaluation for candidacy through the AR process. The team must include both an otolaryngologist/otologist and an audiologist who serve as team leaders. The otolaryngologist/otologist makes medical decisions and performs the surgery. The audiologist determines audiologic candidacy, programs the speech processor, and develops the AR plan in conjunction with the other team members, which may include speech-language pathologists, psychologists, teachers of the hearing impaired, social workers, and parents.

During the surgery, the otologist makes an incision behind the ear and drills a small space in the mastoid bone for the placement of the receiver stimulator and the insertion of the electrode array. The otologist then threads the electrode through the mastoid and the middle-ear cavity and inserts it in the scala tympani of the cochlea.

All CI systems commonly in use consist of an externally worn headset connected to a speech processor, with a battery source and a surgically implanted internal receiver stimulator attached to the electrode array (Figure 18.2). Sound is picked up by the microphone and sent to a speech processor (microcomputer) that codes the information into electrical impulses. These impulses are then sent to a transmitting coil, placed on the head via a magnet over the skin where the internal receiver is located. Impulses are sent through the skin via radio frequency waves to the internal receiver stimulator, which sends them to the electrodes in the cochlea, where the auditory (VIII) nerve is stimulated and information is sent to brain, resulting in a sound stimulation.

Auditory Brain Stem Implants (ABIs)   ABIs have been developed for persons who do not have functioning auditory (VIII) nerves. The FDA has approved the use of ABIs for individuals over 12 years of age with neurofibromatosis who are deafened from bilateral VIII nerve tumors. This implant is placed on the cochlear nucleus of the brain stem during the surgery to remove the tumor. Results with this implant are similar to those of early generation multielectrode implants and show promise for those who cannot benefit from CIs because they lack functioning VIII nerves.

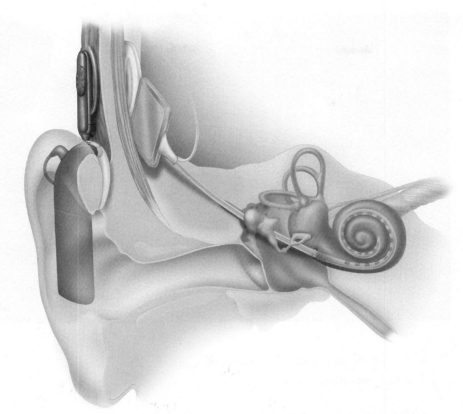

FIGURE 18.2
Diagram of a cochlear implant. The microphone and speech processor are worn behind the ear and attached to the transmitting coil worn over the skin. The internal receiver is just below the skin and imbedded in the mastoid bone, and the electrode array is placed in the cochlear.
Source: Courtesy of Cochlear Americas.

Counseling

Successful amplification and CI procedures depend heavily on the counseling skills of the audiologist, the appropriate use of communication strategies, and the patient's level of motivation. Unlike eyeglasses, hearing aids and CIs are not perfect instruments. They do not "restore normal hearing"; they simply amplify the signal in the case of hearing aids or provide an auditory sensation in the case of CIs. The expectation of normal hearing leads many first-time hearing aid users to reject their instruments. No matter how appropriately amplified and processed the acoustic signal is, the damaged ear cannot perceive it as it would with normal hearing. Audiologists must, therefore, be excellent counselors and prepare their patients and their significant others to have realistic expectations of the hearing aids (Figure 18.3). Good counseling skills are critical for successful fittings. Audiologists must also train and encourage both patients and their significant others to use communication strategies to facilitate ease of communication:

- Watching the speaker when she talks
- Getting the person's attention before speaking
- Talking face to face from the same room
- Asking for repetition when necessary
- Summarizing what is heard so the person can fill in the blanks

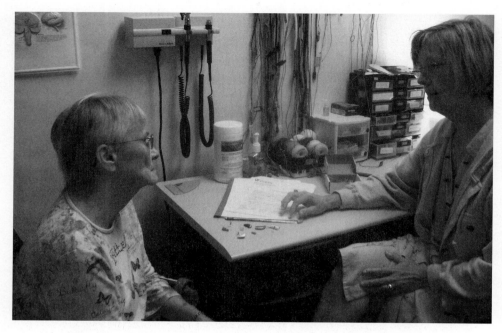

- Stating the topic before beginning the conversation
- Paying attention to key words

These strategies make communication easier for both communication partners and reduce their stress and frustration levels. Role playing is an excellent tool for practicing these strategies in the audiologist's office.

Assistive Listening Devices

Assistive listening devices (ALD), shown in Figure 18.4, are designed to improve communication in circumstances where hearing aids alone are not providing adequate signal-to-noise ratios. They can improve distance listening, assist group conversation, and provide individuals with hearing loss independence from friends and family. Most ALDs were originally developed for use in classrooms for children with hearing impairment. While they are still widely used in education, ALDs are now commonly used in many situations for both children and adults. The Americans with Disabilities Act of 1990 require the availability of ALDs in many public places.

The primary goals of ALDs are to maintain favorable signal-to-noise ratios, to allow individuals to adjust the acoustic signal, to provide mobility for the speakers and listeners, and to allow individuals with hearing loss to hear the primary speaker and other speakers as well as their own voice.

Hardwired Devices

Hardwired ALDs use a wire to connect the microphone to the amplifier, much like body hearing aids. The amplifier then sends the signal to the receiver, which is worn by the listener. The amplifier is small enough to be placed in a pocket or carried in the hand.

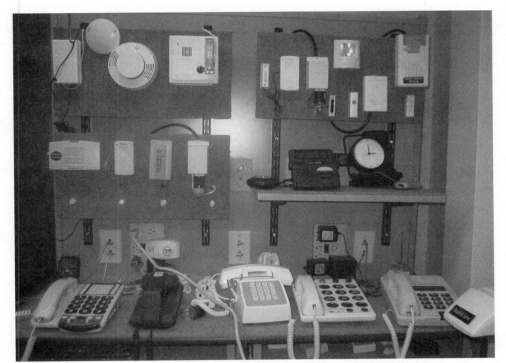

FIGURE 18.4
Display of assistive listening devices. *Source:* Shawna M. Dell.

The person using the ALD can be "self-wired" or give the microphone to the speaker they wish to hear. It can be very helpful in one-on-one situations where the speaker and the person with hearing loss are in close proximity. Disadvantages include size and connecting wires. Large-group hardwired devices are available in some churches and classrooms. In these cases, the microphone is generally part of the facility's amplifying system, and the receivers are hardwired into headsets at selected desks or pews.

Sometimes an external microphone can be plugged into a hearing aid via a wire, adding a hardwire option to the device. The user can hand the microphone to a speaker in difficult listening situations so he can receive a more direct signal. This hearing aid feature is called direct audio input (DIA).

Wireless Devices

A personal **frequency-modulating (FM) system** is a type of wireless system that picks up the speaker's voice through a wireless FM microphone that is located 3–4 inches from the speaker's mouth. The acoustic signal is changed to electrical energy and transmitted via an FM radio signal to a radio receiver worn by the person with hearing loss. The signal is then amplified, converted back to an acoustic signal, and sent to the ear-worn receiver (Figure 18.5). It is possible to couple a receiver to earbuds, to earphones, or directly to the hearing aid through DAI.

A **sound field FM system** uses loudspeakers to transmit the speaker's voice to all individuals in an area. These systems are very helpful in large-group settings such as meetings, churches, theaters, and classrooms. FM systems have many positive attributes, including little to no electrical interference and ease of use. The drawback to these systems is that they are vulnerable to FM interference from other sources on similar frequency bands.

Another wireless option, the infrared light wave system, is made up of a wireless microphone, infrared converter, and infrared receiver. The microphone changes the acoustic signal to an electrical signal, which is transmitted to a converter. The converter then transduces the electrical signal to an infrared light signal and transmits it to the receiver worn by the listener. Receivers come in a variety of styles, including headphones, insert earphones, and DAI. The listener must be in a direct line of sight with the transmitter to properly receive the signal. One drawback to these systems is that they are vulnerable to interference from direct sunlight because it contains infrared light rays.

The induction loop system consists of a microphone connected via hardwire or FM transmitter to an amplifier, which is then connected to a loop of wire that encircles the room or seating area. A personal induction loop wire can also be worn around the neck of the listener. An electrical current flows through the loop, creating a magnetic field, which can be picked up by hearing aids with telecoils. The hearing aid user simply sets the hearing aid to the telecoil setting to pick up the magnetic signal rather than the acoustic signal from the microphone.

Telephone Listening Devices

Listening over the telephone is one of the hardest listening situations for individuals with hearing loss because there are no visual cues and the person must rely solely on audition. Telephone listening devices can lessen some difficulties experienced when using the telephone.

Telecoils   The hearing aid telecoil can detect electromagnetic leakage from the telephone receiver, amplify that signal, transduce it into an acoustic signal, and deliver it to the person's hearing aid. Telecoil technology is available in most modern hearing aids as long as size permits. Not all telephones have enough electromagnetic leakage for telecoil use; therefore, patients must use hearing-aid-compatible phones.

Amplifiers   Telephone amplifiers allow the individual to increase volume of the incoming signal. These devices either are built into the telephone or are small, portable amplifiers that simply snap onto the phone handset. A volume control allows the person to adjust the level of the amplifier. In addition to the volume control, many phones include tone controls, and some allow the individual to choose a low-frequency or high-intensity ringer. Severely hearing impaired individuals may also choose to use a visual signaling device for the telephone, such as a flashing light to alert the person when the telephone is ringing.

Keyboard Devices for Telephone Users

Individuals with little or no residual hearing can use Telecommunication Devices for the Deaf (TDDs) or Teletypewriters (TTYs) to type messages through the phone lines. These systems require the people at both ends to have a TTY and a modem. Each person can type a message on her keyboard, which is then transmitted from the modem through the telephone line to the receiver's keyboard, where it appears on the receiver's screen. Telephone relay services (TRSs) provide a relay between TYY users and non-TYY users. When a TYY user wants to communicate with a hearing person, he can call a relay station, and a relay operator will transmit the message in the appropriate form for the receiver. Captel devices use voice recognition technology to provide a typed message to the hearing-impaired listener without a relay service.

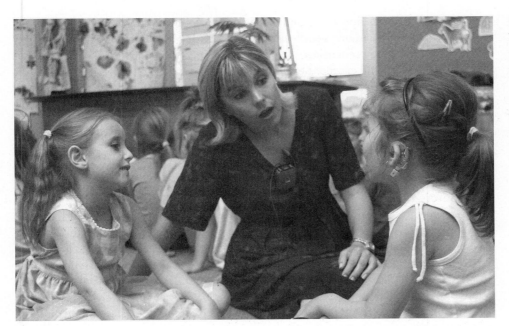

FIGURE 18.5
Teacher and child using an FM system that uses direct audio input into the child's hearing aids.
Source: Photo courtesy of Phonak Hearing Systems.

Television-Compatible Devices

Several forms of ALDs can be used in conjunction with the television. These systems take the form of earphones/headphones that plug directly into the television; wireless infrared listening systems; FM systems; closed captioning, where text appears onscreen as the speaker is talking; and reflective captioning. Reflective captioning uses a light emitting diode (LED) screen that follows the auditory signal by flashing captions of what is being said. An LED wall is situated behind the viewer and is a mirror image of normal text.

Alerting Systems

Alerting systems use alternate sensory input, such as visual, olfactory, or vibrotactile input, to alert the individual with hearing loss when something has happened. Some examples include alarm clocks that use a flashing light, bed vibrator, or pillow vibrator; multipurpose alarms; multipurpose light-flashing systems; and vibrotactile systems for the doorbell, smoke alarm, and/or baby monitor.

Therapy Approaches for Persons with Hearing Impairment

Speechreading

Visual cues play a huge role in the comprehension of speech and environmental sounds for individuals with both normal and impaired hearing. Lipreading involves watching the mouth for visual cues to determine what sounds are produced. The term *speechreading* includes lipreading and all other visual cues available to the listener. In noisy environments, many people living with and without hearing loss rely on speechreading for comprehension.

Speechreading is an excellent tool for individuals with hearing loss because it provides additional cues, increasing message redundancy. Many speech sounds are highly visible on the lips and, when combined with body language, facial expressions, and gestures, can be easily determined by the speechreader. However, visemes are phonemes that look alike on the lips, but sound different i.e. /p/, /b/ (Table 18.1). When speechreading without any auditory cues, visemes can often be confused, leading to a meaning very different from the intended one. When a person with hearing loss combines her residual hearing with speechreading, she can often more accurately comprehend conversation.

Because each person forms sounds on the lips slightly differently, speechreading clarity varies from speaker to speaker. Certain speakers are easier to speechread than others. Factors that influence the visual intelligibility of speech include articulation, the amount of mouth opening when speaking, and the use of nonverbal communication. As a general rule, women are easier to speechread than men are. Daly, Bench, & Chappell (1997) listed three primary reasons for this: Female talkers use more of the factors shown to positively influence the ease of speechreading (stated above), their visual speech factors are strongly correlated with visual speech intelligibility, and their visual speech follows a more standard pattern than does that of male talkers.

One method for teaching speechreading uses practice with short, simple stimuli (e.g., ma, fa, la). As speechreading skills improve, longer and more-complex stimuli are used. This method of analyzing speech into its basic parts is called the analytic method (Alpiner & McCarthy, 2000). The analytic method is highly structured and simple for the speechreader to learn. The counterpart to the analytic method uses a more holistic approach known as the synthetic method. Unlike the analytic method, the synthetic

TABLE 18.1   Examples of Viseme Groups as Determined by Various Research Groups

Woodward & Barber (1960)	*Fisher (1968)*		*Binnie et al., (1976)*	*Erber (1972)*	*Lesner, Sandridge, & Kricos (1987)*
	Initial	*Final*			
/f,v/ labiodentals	/f,v/	/f,v/	/f,v/	/p,b,m/	/p,b,m/
/p,b,m/ bilabials	/p,b,m,d/	/p,b/	/p,b,m/	/f,v/	/f,v/
/w,r/ rounded labials	/hw ,w, r/	ʃ,ʒ,ʤ,tʃ	/w/	/θ,ð/	/θ,ð/
/t,d,n,θ,ʃ,ʤ,h,s, z,k,g,ŋ,ʒ/ nonlabials			/l,n/	/ð,ʒ/	/ð,ʒ,ʤ,tʃ/
	/ʃ,t,n,l,s,z,ʤ,j,h/	/t,d,n,θ,ð,s,z,r,l/	/ʃ,ʒ/	/w,r/	/w,r/
	/k,g/	/k,g,ŋ,m/	/r/	/l/	/l/
			/θ,ð/	/n,d,t,s,z/	/t,d,s,z,n,k,g,j/
			/t,d,s,z/	/k,g/	
			/k,g/	/h/	

method uses phrases, sentences, and real-life situations as opposed to phonemes or individual words. Complex stimuli are used to motivate individuals to bring speech components together into larger elements of meaning.

Auditory Training

Both analytic and synthetic methods are used in **auditory training**. Auditory training involves teaching a child or adult with hearing impairment to develop speech recognition abilities using the auditory signal and taking full advantage of available cues (Schow & Nerbonne, 2002; Tye-Murray, 1998). Auditory training teaches the individual to maximize both his residual hearing and environmental cues to comprehend speech. Traditionally, auditory training does not encourage the individual to speechread, and therapists may cover their mouths to prevent it. Before beginning an auditory training program, individuals should be fit with appropriate amplification.

Historical Approaches   In 1960, Raymond Carhardt described an auditory training program for children based on normal language developmental stages. His program involved four major skill development stages: (1) sound awareness, (2) gross discriminations, (3) broad discriminations among simple speech sounds, and (4) fine speech discriminations (Tye-Murray, 1998). The sound awareness development stage involves teaching the child to acknowledge sound's presence. The gross discriminations stage involves showing the child that sounds differ from one another. The next stage focuses on the discrimination of sounds that vary in frequency, intensity, and duration. When the child has mastered all of these stages, then Carhardt suggests introducing tasks that are centered on learning gross speech-sound discriminations. In the last stage, the child works on developing fine speech-sound discriminations and integrating of vocabulary for conversational speech.

Erber (1982) developed a similar auditory training program focusing on four major auditory skills: sound awareness or detection, sound discrimination, identification, and comprehension. Training should not progress to the next skill until the child has mastered the one before.

Sound awareness or detection is defined as acknowledging the presence and absence of sound. The goal is to have the child pay attention to sound. Without sound awareness, perception is impossible.

The next stage, sound discrimination, involves the ability to determine differences between environmental sounds or phonemes and phoneme patterns in word form. When working on discrimination with a child, the therapist may use a toy like an airplane and say "aaah" to the child as it is pushed through the air. Next, the therapist may take a rabbit and say "h-h-h" as he bounces the rabbit. The goal is to train the child to listen to the differences between the sound patterns and the /a/ sound and the /h/ sound. The child will then associate the toy with the sound and attempt to produce the sound. When these sounds are mastered, the therapist will move on to new sounds.

The third stage, identification, is essentially the ability to identify a word with an object. During this stage, the therapist must be sure the child is identifying the stimuli and not just imitating. The therapist may have toys on the table and tell the child to show her a dog; the child would then point to or pick up the dog.

The final skill, comprehension, is a higher-level skill and involves listening and understanding speech. The child must have a significant vocabulary to reach this stage.

When working with a child on comprehension, the therapist might read a story aloud and then ask the child questions about the story.

Individual Adult AR

In the past, AR focused heavily on speechreading, but today AR provided on an individual basis can take the form of several types of interactions. AR includes selecting, fitting, and adjusting the amplification device as well as incorporating the use of ALDs when needed. Throughout this process, the audiologist counsels the patient on mean to cope with and accept hearing loss, realistic expectations of amplification devices, and use of communication strategies. The counseling during the initial fitting of the hearing aid is typically referred to as the *hearing aid orientation* (HAO). The audiologist does the majority of the talking during the orientation, covering the devices function, use, and care as well as its limitations. Follow-up visits include discussion of the patient's experiences with the device, troubleshooting, and device adjustments. The patient can also be scheduled for one-on-one therapy sessions either before or after being fit with amplification to work on speechreading, auditory training, communication strategies, or counseling on personal adjustment issues (Alpiner & McCarthy, 2000).

Group Adult AR

Group AR is an excellent tool for individuals with hearing loss. Abrams, Chisolm, and McArdle (2002) found that hearing aid fittings paired with short-term group AR is more cost effective than hearing aid fittings without AR. The ideal AR group is made up of no more than 8 to 10 people. Spouses, family members, and close friends are encouraged to attend to learn what the individual with hearing loss is experiencing. The group also provides the family members and friends with an outlet to discuss their experiences and frustrations as communication partners. Preminger (2003) found that participation in an AR group significantly reduces self-perceived hearing disability, especially in subjects whose significant others accompany them. Hearing loss can provoke feelings of isolation from the normal hearing world. The group provides a safe environment where members can speak openly about personal difficulties and provides the opportunity to practice communication skills in a real-world setting (Israelite & Jennings, 1995). Group AR can be extremely cathartic, allowing members to learn from one another and to serve as a support network (Israelite & Jennings, 1995).

Hearing Aid Orientation Group   Similar to an individual HAO, a group format can be implemented to instruct hearing aid users how to appropriately wear, use, and maintain hearing aids as well as to provide information on how to improve communication. These groups, which can include significant others, usually meet weekly for 1–2 hours for about a month. HAO programs provide information slowly, allowing group members to retain more of what they have learned. Studies have shown that new hearing aids users who attend HAO groups are more satisfied with their hearing aids, return them less often, and retain information longer than do those who attend only individual HAO (Abrams, Hnath-Chisolm, Guerreiro, & Ritterman, 1992).

Living with Hearing Loss (LWHL) Group   An LWHL program is similar to the HAO; however, it involves more input from the group members. The goal is to provide group members with information regarding hearing, hearing aids, ALDs, communication strategies, and consumer groups. The audiologist or group leader acts as a facilitator, speaking less than 30 percent of the time and encouraging group members to share experiences, questions, and advice. The LWHL program should include written resources as well as some formal information on given topics of interest to the group (e.g., hearing loss and its effects, ALDs, communication strategies, consumer organizations; Alpiner & McCarthy, 2000). The leader must be flexible and not thrown off by the group's ineritable tangents—they are part of the fun!

AR with Children

The goal of pediatric AR is to develop auditory and language skills as the audiologist assesses and manages the impairment. The parents play a vital role and must be committed for the program to be successful. The type of AR the child receives depends to a great extent on the developmental age of the child, the severity of the hearing loss, any comorbidities, and the choice of the parents. The child may be taught speechreading, receive auditory training using auditory stimulation through hearing aids or CIs, and/or learn the use of sign language (see Figure 18.6). The earlier the child is identified and treated, the better the prognosis for language development.

AR providers are members of multidisciplinary teams that may include audiologists, speech-language pathologists, otolaryngologists, educators, psychologists, social workers, and the child's primary guardian(s). The team members' cooperation is vital to the success of the child. A primary goal of the team is to help parents choose the educational/communication approach that will be used with their child, ranging from those that exclusively use the auditory channel to those that exclusively use sign language. No one best method is appropriate for every child with hearing loss. Individual strengths and differences must be considered. One of the major goals of the rehabilitative audiologist and the rest of the team is to educate the parents on the various options available. The parents have the right to choose the method used with their

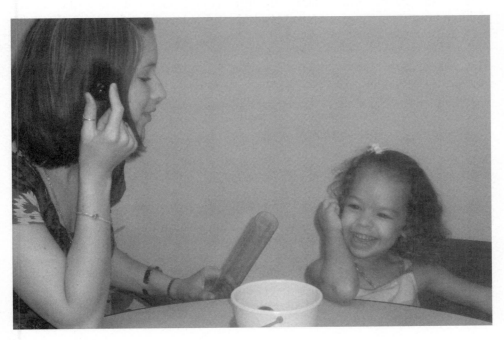

FIGURE 18.6 Child with a cochlear implant receiving AR therapy.
Source: Shawna M. Dell.

child. Our duty is to provide the information so that they can make an informed decision and to help design and implement the therapy/educational program.

Auditory Verbal Approach   The **auditory verbal** (AV) method is an early intervention program that emphasizes audition or learning to listen to develop spoken language. This approach focuses on residual hearing and spoken language as the primary mode of communication. The term *unisensory approach* or *acupedics* is sometimes used to describe this method. The AR therapist's goal is to teach the child to develop her auditory system with directed listening practice without emphasis on visual cues. At times, the therapist may partially cover his face to force the child to use her auditory channel rather than her visual channel to comprehend speech stimuli. Appropriate amplification, through hearing aids, CIs, and assistive devices, is critical for the success of this method. Speechreading is used only as a secondary teaching strategy in this method (Schow & Nerbonne, 2002). According to the Learning to Listen Foundation, (http://www.welisteninternational.com/) the auditory verbal approach encourages

- Early detection and diagnosis of hearing impairment, ideally in the newborn nursery
- Consistent use of bilateral amplification or cochlear implants for maximum detection of all sounds and speech understanding
- Individualized therapy and learning environments where listening and spoken language are the expected communication modes

Oral Approach   The oral approach is based on the principle that most deaf and hard-of-hearing children have some residual hearing and can be taught to develop their auditory and speech skills with early intervention and consistent training. Like the auditory verbal approach, the oral approach emphasizes the use of residual hearing and speech as the primary form of communication, but unlike the auditory verbal approach, the child is also encouraged to speechread. The use of amplification and/or other assistive devices is important in the success of this approach. The goal is to teach children how to use their vision and residual hearing for spoken language. Generally, manual communication is not used, although natural gestures can be used. The education goal of the oral approach is placement of the child in a mainstreamed classroom. The proponents behind both the oral and the AV approaches feel that the child will have fewer restrictions on his daily life and greater educational and vocational opportunities because most of the world uses auditory/oral speech and language (Alpiner & McCarthy, 2000). Others argue that this method is too difficult and may not allow the child to develop critical language skills.

Total Communication   The philosophy behind total communication (TC) is the use of all means available to communicate. TC combines signing, finger spelling, audition, and speechreading, as well as nonverbal communication, to maximize language comprehension. The child may or may not use amplification in this approach. Many TC approaches use simultaneous spoken and manual communication. Signing Exact English (SEE), a type of sign language often used for the simultaneous approaches, is a manually represented form of spoken English with a one-to-one ratio for sign to word. Advocates of TC emphasize that inclusion of manual communication allows for easier language development, while also developing spoken language. Others feel that the child will revert to the easier mode of manual communication to the detriment of speech.

American Sign Language (ASL) ASL is the form of manual communication, independent of oral languages, established by the Deaf (Schow & Nerbonne, 2002). ASL is a language with its own grammatical structure. It comprises over 6,000 signs and does not have a sign to correlate with each English word. Some children are taught ASL, to the on exclusion of oral language, using a manual approach. ASL does not have a written form, so as the child learns to read he or she will be exposed to written English.

Many persons with severe to profound hearing loss identify themselves as part of Deaf culture. The Deaf community defines Deafness with a capital "D" as a culture, rather than a disability, characterized by its own language, ASL. Some individuals within the Deaf community have expressed strong opinions against educating children with hearing impairments to communicate orally. Some feel that the use of hearing aids and CIs and the emphasis on speech therapy are not best for the overall development of the child whose "natural language" is sign. Some are opposed to the use of CIs, especially in children, because this is a procedure that tries to "fix the child." Many of their feelings may stem from years of professionals forcing oral programming on all children with hearing loss and from their own frustrations with traditional amplification.

The Commission on the Education of the Deaf has recommended a bilingual/bicultural approach when using ASL (Schow & Nerbonne, 2002). The premise of this approach is to teach ASL as the deaf child's primary language and, once it is mastered, to introduce written English as a second language.

AR with Infants and Preschool-Age Children The advent of Universal Newborn Hearing Screening has allowed identification of hearing loss or the risk of hearing loss at a very early age. The primary goal of early identification and intervention is to introduce language and/or auditory stimulation during the critical period of language development in infancy. Studies have shown that children who are identified and receive intervention by the age of 6 months will outperform children who were identified later with hearing loss on language measures through age 3 (Yoshinaga-Itano, 2003). The children who receive intervention, regardless of the method or approach, at or before 6 months of age also have been shown to have near-normal rates of language development through age 3.

Many early intervention programs today focus on the family. Parents are critical in the intervention program. Their decisions on the mode of communication and type of amplification to use determine the type of AR appropriate for their child's communication needs. Home-based therapy programs involve visits to the home by an audiologist, speech-language pathologist, or deaf educator. The therapist guides the family through the child's language learning process, providing insight into the child's prelinguistic and linguistic communication attempts. The home is an ideal therapy location because of the many natural opportunities to expose the child to sound. The goal is to help the family encourage the child to rely on her residual hearing.

SKI-HI is a family-centered, home-based program designed for infants, toddlers, and preschool-age children with hearing impairment (www.skihi.org). This program works on auditory skills and speech and language development with a parent resource manual that includes instructional materials.

Center-based programs are also available for infants and preschool-age children. In these programs, the children attend therapy at a center/clinic for a designated number of hours each week. Parents are still strongly encouraged to participate in these programs to incorporate the skills their children are learning.

AR with School-Age Children   Once a child reaches school age, parents must make several decisions about his intervention plan, including whether to send him to a day or residential school program. Intervention in a public school system can take place in a self-contained classroom that includes only children who are deaf or hard of hearing or in a mainstream classroom. In a mainstreamed program, both children with normal hearing and children with hearing impairments attend the same classes together. In some instances, the deaf or hard of hearing child may spend part of the day in a self-contained class or resource room for therapy. Programs are also available where the child is completely mainstreamed.

A primary goal of AR with school-age children is to facilitate successful academic performance (Alpiner & McCarthy, 2000). Typically, these children need speech and language intervention as well as educational intervention such as the use of ALDs, note takers, interpreters, or captioning.

Educational Audiologists   Educational audiologists work within school systems to provide audiologic services. They play a vital role in the hearing health care of children. According to the regulation implementing the individuals with Disabilities Education Act, educational audiologists' responsibilities include

i. Identification of children with hearing loss:

ii. Determination of the range, nature, and degree of hearing loss, including referral for medical or other professional attention for the habilitation of hearing:

iii. Provision of habilitative activities, such as language habilitation, auditory training, speech reading (lip-reading), hearing evaluation, and speech conservation:

iv. Creation and administration of programs for prevention of hearing loss:

v. Counseling and guidance of children, parents, and teachers regarding hearing loss: and

vi. Determination of children's needs for group and individual amplification, selecting and fitting an appropriate aid, and evaluating the effectiveness of the amplification. [34 C.F.R. $ 300.34(c) (2009)]

Outcome Measures

Outcome measures evaluate the effect therapy is having on the individual's physiological or emotional disability. The authors of this chapter define disability as any chronic physical problem that limits one's activity. An example of a disability would be a child who is unable to hear their teacher's instructions in class. Furthermore, the authors define handicap as anything that restricts one's participation in activities. An example of a handicap would be when hearing loss restricts an adult from playing cards with their friends because they have difficulty hearing what is being said. Outcome measures allow the AR provider to compare his goals for the patient to what the patient has actually accomplished as a result of rehabilitation. Outcome measures are becoming increasingly more important in this age of third-party payers because audiologists must demonstrate that the treatment provided helps to reduce the patient's disability. They are also an excellent tool for demonstrating to the patient the impact AR is having on her personal perception of her disability. Outcome measures are also available to measure the perception of the disability from the points of view of significant others, teachers, and parents/guardians.

Subjective Measures

Subjective outcome measures used with adults (Table 18.2) often involve the use of self-inventories to determine the level of disability adults experience or to indicate areas where they feel they need improvement. With children (Table 18.3), these assessments usually come in the form of parent or teacher checklists. These checklists help to identify and measure the child's hearing problems as well as providing a way to monitor progress.

TABLE 18.2   Examples of Subjective Adult Outcome Measures

Outcome Measure	Developers	Appropriate Population in Years	Number of Items
Abbreviated Profile for Hearing Aid Benefit (APHAB)	Cox and Alexander (1995)	18+	24 (4 subscales)
Communication Profile for the Hearing Impaired (CPHI)	Demorest and Erdman (1987)	18+	145
Client-Oriented Scale of Improvement (COSI)	Dillon, James, and Ginis (1997)	18+	5
Hearing Handicap Inventory for the Elderly	Newman, Weinstein, Jacobson, and Hug (1990)	65+	25
Hearing Handicap Inventory for Adults	Ventry and Weinstein (1982)	18–64	25
Glasgow Hearing Aid Benefit Profile (GHABP)	Gatehouse (1999)	18+	Up to 8 situations with 7 dimensions each

TABLE 18.3   Examples of Subjective Pediatric Outcome Measures

Outcome Measure	Developers	Appropriate Population in Years	Number of Items	Measurement
Fisher's Auditory Problems Checklist	L. I. Fisher (1985)	5–12	25	Screening for hearing loss
Screening Instrument for Targeting Educational Risk (SIFTER)	K. Anderson (1989)	5+	15	Implications of hearing status for education
Listening Inventory for Education: An Efficacy Tool	K. Anderson & Smaldino (1996)	5–12	15	Efficacy of amplification systems

Objective Measures

Objective outcome measures are used to assess speech perception with and without hearing instruments (Tables 18.4 and 18.5). These measures can be influenced by several factors, including internal variables such as vocabulary, cognitive abilities, and chronological age; external variables such as response mode, appropriate use of reinforcement, and memory load; and methodological variables such as presentation mode and open or closed set (C. E. Johnson & Danhauer, 2002). Objective outcome measures provide proof of benefit to third-party payers and administrators as well as to patients and families.

TABLE 18.4 Objective Adult Outcome Measures

Outcome Measure	Developers	Appropriate Population in Years	Number of Items	Measurement
Speech Perception in Noise (SPIN)	Kalikow, Stevens, & Elliott (1977)	18+	8 sets of 50 sentences	Speech perception when listening in noise
Hearing in Noise Test (HINT)	Nilsson, Soil, & Sulliran, (1994)	18+	25 lists of 10 sentences	Sentence speech reception thresholds in quiet or in noise

TABLE 18.5 Objective Children's Outcome Measures

Outcome Measure	Developers	Appropriate Population in Years	Number of Items	Measurement
PBK-50 Word List	Haskins (1949)	6	3 lists of 50 words	
Monosyllable-Trochee-Spondee Test (MTS)	Erber & Alencewicz (1976)	Level A: 4–5 Level B: 6	60 items per level	Effectiveness of hearing instrument
Word Intelligibility by Picture Identification (WIPI)	Ross & Lermann (1970)	5–6 with moderate hearing losses 7–8 with severe hearing losses	4 lists of 25	Speech perception Ross & Lermann (1970) Northwestern University Children's Perceptions of Speech Number of Items: 2 books, 67 words
Northwestern University Children's Perceptions of Speech	Elliott & Katz (1980)	3+	2 books, 67 words	Speech perception
Early Speech Perception Test (ESP)	Moog & Geers	6	36 words (3 subsets of 12)	Auditory perception

Summary

AR is defined as professional efforts that are designed to help persons with hearing loss lessen or compensate for a hearing impairment and, specifically, that involve facilitating adequate receptive and expressive communication. Hearing aids, the primary tool of AR, contain three primary components: the microphone, the amplifier, and the receiver. Hearing aids are classified by their style and by the type of circuitry or signal processing used. Basic contemporary styles of hearing aids included BTE, open-fit BTE, ITE, ITC, and CIC. Signal processing is the way the acoustic signals entering the hearing aid are manipulated. The three classifications of signal processing are analog, digitally programmable, and digital. Other types of amplification are available for people who cannot wear conventional hearing aids.

The CI is a surgically implanted device that electrically stimulates the auditory nerve of patients with severe to profound hearing loss to provide them with sound and speech information. Unlike hearing aids, CIs bypass the peripheral auditory system and directly stimulate the auditory nerve. The CI does not restore "normal" hearing, and users receive varying amounts of benefit from the device.

ALDs are designed to improve communication of the hearing impaired when hearing aids alone are not providing adequate signal-to-noise ratios. They improve distance listening, assist group conversation, and provide individuals with hearing loss independence from friends and family. ALDs can be hardwired devices, wireless devices, telephone listening devices, keyboard devices for telephone users, television-compatible devices, or alerting systems.

AR combines the assessment and the management of the hearing impairment and can include programs for speechreading, auditory training, and communication strategies. Interventions are given throughout the life span, from early invention programs for infants with hearing loss to Living with Hearing Loss programs for the elderly. Counseling patients and families on the effects of hearing loss and treatment options is critical for the AR provider. The goal of pediatric AR is to develop auditory and language skills, whereas the goal for older children and adults who develop hearing loss is to maintain their communication. AR provides the patients and those around them the opportunity to function with their hearing loss to their best capacity.

case study ADULT

Mr. T is a 72-year-old male patient with a moderate to severe sensorineural hearing loss bilaterally. He is experiencing increasing difficulty conversing with his grandchildren and other members of his family. However, he is extremely nervous about going through the hearing instrument evaluation process as well as pursuing amplification. The audiologist can tell that Mr. T wants to pursue amplification, but he is very tentative. The audiologist is faced with the task of encouraging the pursuit in a sensitive manner. How can this be done?

case study PEDIATRIC

Amy is a 16-year-old female with normal sloping to moderate hearing loss bilaterally. Amy wears BTE hearing aids and reports that she has ear discomfort due to excessive buildup of ear wax. She further reports that she no longer wants to wear her aids and feels that they are no longer a benefit to her. Thus, Amy's parents scheduled an audiologic evaluation with her pediatric audiologist. What hearing aid options should the audiologist give Amy, and how can she measure Amy's benefit from hearing aids?

STUDY QUESTIONS

1. Compare and contrast the five different types of traditional hearing aids.

2. What is a cochlear implant? How does it differ from a hearing aid?

3. What are assistive listening devices and when are they appropriate? Briefly describe the different types.

4. What are some of the benefits to group AR versus individual AR?

5. Describe the different signed approaches to language.

6. Why is counseling so important to recipients of amplifications devices?

SELECTED READINGS

Cooper, H., & Craddock, L. (2006). *Cochlear implants: A practical guide* (2nd ed.). Hoboken, NJ: Wiley.

Gordan-Salant, S., & Callahan, J. S. (2009). The benefits of hearing aids and closed captioning for television viewing by older adults with hearing loss. *Ear and Hearing, 30* (4), 458–465.

Niparko, J. K. (2009). *Cochlear implants: Principles & practices* (2nd ed.). Philadelphia, PA: Lippincott, Williams & Wilkins.

Saunders, G. H., Lewis, M. S., & Forsline, A. (2009). Expectations, prefitting counseling, and hearing aid outcome. *Journal of American Academy of Audiology, 20*(5), 320–334.

Schow, R. L., & Nerbonne, M. A. (2007). *Introduction to audiologic rehabilitation* (5th ed.). Boston, MA: Allyn & Bacon.

Tye-Murray, N. (2009). *Foundations of aural rehabilitation: Children, adults, and their family members* (3rd ed.). San Diego, CA: Singular Publishing Group.

Yoshinaga-Itano, C. (2003). Early intervention after universal neonatal hearing screening: Impact on outcomes. *Mental Retardation and Developmental Disabilities Research Reviews, 9*(4), 252–266.

WEBSITES OF INTEREST

www.agbell.org
   AG Bell Foundation
www.audiology.org
   American Academy of Audiology
www.audrehab.org
   American Academy of Rehabilitative Audiology
www.ata.org
   American Tinnitus Association
www.betterhearing.org
   Better Hearing Institute
www.hearingloss.org
   Hearing Loss Association of America

www.lhh.org
   League for the Hard of Hearing
www.hearingconservation.org
   National Hearing Conservation Association
www.nidcd.nih.gov/health/hearing/coch.asp
   National Institute on Deafness and Other Communication Disorders Information on Cochlear Implants
www.nidcd.nih.gov/health/hearing/hearingaid.asp
   National Institute on Deafness and Other Communication Disorders Information on Hearing Aids

Glossary

accent The phonological, prosodic, and vocal characteristics or habits of spoken language influenced by the geographical region and/or first language of the speaker.

acquired disability A disability not present at birth—that is, not congenital—that usually occurs as a result of disease or injury.

additions Speech errors involving the production of an added sound not normally present in a word.

Aerodynamic instrumentation Equipment that can be used to assess airflow and air pressure changes with velopharyngeal opening and closure.

aerodynamics The study of air and other gases in motion, forces setting them in motion, and results of such motion. In speech, aerodynamics refers especially to the air pressures and flows involved in speech production.

affricate A complete blockage of the airway followed by a slow release of the impounded air.

African American Vernacular English (AAVE) A dialectal variety of Standard American English (SAE) spoken by many, but not all, African Americans in informal and familiar social situations. However, for many children, particularly those from working-class environments, it is the major home language and singular medium of communication. AAVE is a creole derived from a mixture of African and European languages and is a survival from the preslavery era. Its maintenance today is due mainly to the important roles it serves for group identity and cultural pride, in addition to social isolation of its speakers. While there are more similarities than differences between AAVE and SAE, there are recognizable features that characterize AAVE in phonology, morphology, syntax, lexicon, idiom, and pragmatics. It is most important to note that AAVE is not a misuse or corruption of SAE, but a legitimate, logical, rule-governed, fully comprehensible variant of the English language.

age-referenced norms Ages at which a certain percentage (50% or more) of typically developing children produce a sound correctly.

agrammatism The omission of small grammatical words and word endings.

aided communication technique Any communication technique that uses an external aid or assistive device.

air pressure and flow techniques Warren and DuBois (1964) described this technique for measuring intra-oral pressure and nasal airflow during speech. The measurements of intra-oral pressure and nasal airflow are subjected to a hydrokinetic equation that translates the data into an estimate of the size of the velopharyngeal orifice.

alerting systems Warning systems that use alternate sensory input, such as the visual, olfactory, or vibrotactile input, to help alert the individual with hearing loss when something has happened.

allophone A speech sound that is accepted as a variant of a phoneme, but is not used to differentiate two words in a language. A perceptual grouping of phones or similar speech sounds.

alveolus/alveoli (plural) A small hollow or pit.

American Sign Language (ASL) The form of manual communication, independent of oral languages, established by the Deaf that uses its own grammatical structure.

analog signal processing A type of signal processing that takes the acoustic signal, turns it into an electrical signal, amplifies it, returns it to an acoustical signal, and then puts that signal into the external ear canal.

antonym A pair of gradable word opposites such as *hot–cold*.

Apert syndrome (Acrocephalosyndactyly Type I) Caused by a mutation of a gene located on chromosome 10; is characterized by multiple anomalies of the skull, face, hands, feet, and joints. The nose may appear "beak-shaped." There may also be stenosis, or closing, of the posterior part of the nose (termed *choanal atresia*), which compromises the nasal airway. Many of the skull and facial differences are caused by premature closure of one or more sutures of the skull. Syndactyly, in which the fingers and toes appear to be fused or "mitten-like," is a striking feature of the syndrome. Mental retardation is common, but not universal. This syndrome shares the facial features of Crouzon syndrome.

aphasia An acquired language disorder caused by brain damage and resulting in partial or complete impairment of language comprehension, formulation, and use for communication.

aphonia The complete loss of voice.

apraxia of speech A disturbance in the selection and sequencing of speech sounds that is due to brain damage. A neurologic, phonologic disorder resulting from sensorimotor impairment of the capacity to select, program, or execute, in coordinated and normally timed sequences, the positioning of the speech muscles for the volitional production of speech sounds; involuntary movements remain intact. Sometimes considered a form of aphasia.

articulation (1) Use of the articulators (teeth, tongue, etc.) to produce speech sounds. (2) The motor movements involved in the production of speech.

articulators Those structures responsible for the modification of the vocal tract: tongue, lips, soft and hard palates, and teeth.

artificial larynx An electronic or pneumatic sound source that substitutes for the larynx after it has been surgically removed.

arytenoid Pitcher-shaped.

assistive listening devices (ALDs) Devices designed to improve communication of persons with hearing impairment in circumstances where hearing aids alone are not providing adequate signal-to-noise ratios.

audiologic rehabilitation (AR) Those professional efforts that are designed to help a person with hearing loss, including services and procedures for lessening or compensating for a hearing impairment, and that specifically involve facilitating adequate receptive and expressive communication.

auditory brain stem implant (ABI) An implanted device that is placed on the cochlear nucleus of the brain stem of individuals who do not have functioning auditory (VIII) nerves.

auditory scanning A message transmission technique: Selections are offered by listening through the earphones or in the free field, and the user interrupts the auditory scan when appropriate selections are offered.

auditory training A process of teaching the child or adult with hearing impairment to develop his or her abilities to recognize speech using the auditory signal by taking full advantage of available auditory clues.

auditory verbal (AV) method An early intervention program that emphasizes audition, learning to listen in order to develop spoken language. This approach focuses on use of residual hearing and spoken language as the primary mode of communication.

autism A condition characterized by a failure to develop normal verbal and nonverbal communication behaviors and responsivity to other persons, a failure to use objects appropriately, and a generalized overreaction to certain sensory stimuli or a notable lack of response to other sensory stimuli.

autosomal Referring to chromosomes other than sex chromosomes.

babbling Long strings of sounds that children begin to produce at 4 months of age.

base pair Two bases that form a "rung of the DNA ladder." A DNA nucleotide is made of a molecule of sugar, a molecule of phosphoric acid, and a molecule called a base. The bases are the "letters" that spell out the genetic code. In DNA, the code letters are A, T, G, and C, which stand for the chemicals adenine, thymine, guanine, and cytosine, respectively. In base pairing, adenine always pairs with thymine, and guanine always pairs with cytosine.

baseline The pretreatment level of a target behavior, which, when quantified, can be used as a basis against which to measure progress.

behind-the-ear hearing aid (BTE) A curved hearing aid that sits on top of the external ear and houses all the functional components within the body of the hearing aid. The BTE is coupled via a short tube to a custom earmold that delivers the amplified signal to the ear.

Bernoulli effect A drawing inward of the walls of a narrowed section of a flexible tube, such as at the vocal folds in the larynx, when the velocity of the airflow is increased.

bidialectal Having linguistic competence in two or more variations of a language and the ability to code-switch appropriately for use of each.

bilingualism Refers to individuals with various levels of proficiency in English plus one or more other languages. However, for this text, bilingual is used in the context of *bilingual education* to refer to individuals whose first language is not English, particularly children whose families are recent immigrants to the United States.

body aid A hearing aid worn on the body made up of a casement that is worn on the torso and houses the microphone and amplifier. The receiver with a custom earmold is attached to the casement via a long cord and delivers the amplified sound to the ear.

bone-anchored hearing aid (BAHA) A type of bone-conduction hearing aid that is attached to the skull via a surgically implanted titanium fixture called an abutment.

bone-conduction hearing aid A type of hearing aid that sends the amplified signal to the ear via a vibrator that is placed on the mastoid bone behind the pinna. The vibrator is placed on a metal headband that holds the vibrator against the mastoid bone. The rest of the components are housed in either a BTE or a body aid.

bootstrapping The process of learning language in which children use what they know to decode more mature language. For example, children may use semantic knowledge to aid in decoding and learning syntax.

breath group The series of syllables or words produced on one exhalation.

breathiness A perceived voice quality when there is incomplete glottal closure, resulting in air escape between the vocal folds.

Broca's area A region of the frontal lobe of the brain (typically the left hemisphere) that is classically thought to be important for the production of speech. Named after the French physician and anthropologist Pierre Broca (1824–1880).

bronchial tubes The large windpipes that permit air passage into and out of the lungs.

central auditory processing disorder (CAPD) An impairment in a child's ability to perceive or understand speech and language in the absence of a hearing impairment. Some clinicians and researchers believe this is a subtype of language impairment.

central nervous system (CNS) The portion of the nervous system that includes the brain and spinal cord.

cerebral palsy A nonprogressive neuromotor disorder due to an insult or malformation of the brain that occurred before, at, or shortly after the time of birth that may be accompanied by a variety of associated disorders due to the brain damage.

circumlocution In attempts to avoid stuttering, the person may rearrange words and insert additional words in a sentence. For example, he may wish to say, "Sarah and I are going to the movie this evening," but may end up saying something like, "You know, Sarah and me, we want to um you know this evening go to the movie."

clause A unit of language consisting of both a noun and a verb. Clauses may be independent and a sentence—as in *Mommy threw the ball*—or dependent and attached to an independent clause—as in *that we found at the beach* in the sentence *Mommy threw the ball **that we found at the beach.***

cluttering Rapid, often unintelligible speech characterized by omission of speech sounds or entire words.

coarticulation (1) Co-occurrence of the characteristics of two or more phonemes as one phoneme influences another in perception or in production: may be forward (anticipatory) or backward (carryover). (2) Movement of the articulators to a target sound before the sound is produced.

cochlear implant A surgically implanted device that electrically stimulates the auditory nerve of patients with severe-to-profound hearing loss to provide them with sound and speech information.

coda In syllable structure, a consonant or consonant sequence that follows the nucleus.

code-switching The act of shifting from one language or one dialect of a language to another, usually under the control of the social situation or context.

cognates A pair of constant phonemes that have the same place and manner of articulation and that differ only in voicing.

communication The process of encoding, transmitting, and decoding signals to exchange information and ideas between the participants.

compensatory errors Articulation gestures that are the individual's response to velopharyngeal dysfunction (or dental malocclusion) rather than the direct result of velopharyngeal dysfunction; also known as *active speech characteristics.*

completely-in-the-canal hearing aid The smallest of the custom-fit hearing aids that is made to fit completely in the ear canal.

complexity The physical complexity of a symbol or a manual sign. (For example, the variable of strokes and semantic elements may be identified as the best predictors of perceived complexity for Blissymbols.)

conjoining The process of joining or combining two or more clauses into larger units or sentences.

conjunction A word used to join or combine two or more clauses into larger units or sentences.

consonant A speech sound that is formed with an obstruction or narrowing at one or more points in the vocal tract. Consonants can be voiced or voiceless speech sounds.

contralateral innervation The general pattern of neural control in which one side of the body is controlled by the opposite side of the brain.

control goals Therapy goals that are not immediately addressed by intervention activities, but are monitored to reveal the change due to maturation. Control goals may eventually become target goals.

cortex The outer layer of an organ.

counterconditioning reciprocal inhibition Learning a response that competes with an undesirable response.

creole A language formed on the basis of the phonology and grammar of a dominant language, but using vocabulary of a nondominant language.

cricoid laryngeal cartilage.

criterion A requirement set by a clinician (e.g., percent correct) that a child must achieve before intervention proceeds to a new level or intervention may be terminated.

Crouzon syndrome (craniofacial dysostosis) Persons with Crouzon syndrome have premature fusion of one or more sutures of the skull. As a result, there is ocular proptosis (bulging eyes) and midface deficiency. Patients resemble persons with Apert syndrome, but do not exhibit limb deformities. The severity of this syndrome varies widely, as does its impact upon speech and development. The primary etiology is thought to be an autosomal-dominant mutation.

cul-de-sac resonance Abnormal resonance during speech that occurs when the transmission of acoustic energy is trapped in a blind pouch in the vocal tract with only one outlet; the speech is perceived as muffled due to the fact that the sound is contained in a cavity with no direct means of escape.

cul-de-sac resonance Resonance created by a faulty velopharyngeal valve and nasal passages that are obstructed.

culture The set of values, perceptions, beliefs, institutions, technologies, and survival systems used by members of a specified group to ensure the acquisition and perpetuation of what they consider to be a high quality of life.

decode The act of interpreting spoken and written symbols.

dedicated communication device A computerized device designed specifically for communication. It is often portable and allows a variety of input methods. Some function as keyboard emulators.

deep structure The basic structure or meaning that underlies a sentence; generated through the use of phrase structure rules; Chomskyan concept.

deictic terms Words or phrases that can be interpreted only from the physical location of the speaker.

dentition The teeth and their alignment.

developmental apraxia of speech (DAS) A disorder affecting the motor planning for speech production.

developmental disfluency A normally occurring increase in the effortless repetitions of syllables and words; usually appears for a short time between the ages of 2 and 3 years and then disappears.

developmental verbal apraxia Synonymous with DAS. A disorder affecting the motor planning for speech production.

diadochokinesis Rapidly alternating movements by articulators.

diagnosis   A determination of the precise nature or extent of a communication disorder, the prognosis, and the recommended approach and sequence of intervention.

dialect   A variety within a given language derived from historical, social, regional, and cultural influences and inclusive of surface and deep structure and the rules for language use.

diaphragm   A large dome-shaped muscle of respiration that separates the thoracic cavity from the abdominal cavity.

digital signal processor   A type of signal processing that takes the acoustic signal and changes it to an electrical signal and then to a numerical code that is manipulated via algorithms to achieve a desired target; then it is converted back to an acoustic signal and put into the external ear canal.

digitized speech   Speech based on copy synthesis. The human voice is recorded, digitized, and then played back. The quality of digitized speech is excellent.

diphthong   A vowel sound made by gliding from one vowel position to another. For example, the word *boy* consists of a consonant and a vowel sound, but if you say the word slowly and lengthen the vowel sound, two vowel sounds become obvious.

direct selection   An augmentative and alternative communication technique. The user points to objects, pictographs, and/or symbols to transmit a message. Direct selection methods include pointing (e.g., with finger or light beam), activating keys on a keyboard, and using eye gaze.

discourse   An orderly exchange of ideas; extended expressions of thought on a subject; connected speech or writing.

disfluencies   Properties in speech that interrupt the smooth, forward flow of an utterance; usually refers to pauses, hesitations, interjections, prolongations, and repetitions.

distinctive features   The articulatory and/or acoustic characteristics of speech sounds.

distortion   (1) Production of a speech sound in a substandard manner. (2) A speech error involving the production of a sound that differs from the target yet is not identifiable as any other sound in the language.

DNA (deoxyribonucleic acid)   The molecule that encodes genetic information. DNA is a double-stranded molecule held together by weak bonds between base pairs of nucleotides. The four nucleotides in DNA contain the bases adenine (A), guanine (G), cytosine (C), and thymine (T). In nature, base pairs form only between A and T and between G and C; thus, the base sequence of each single strand can be deduced from that of its partner.

dominant   Refers to a gene that almost always results in a specific physical characteristic—for example, a disease—even though the patient's genome possesses only one copy. With a dominant gene, the chance of passing on the gene (and therefore the disease) to children is 50-50 in each pregnancy.

Down syndrome   A specific syndrome caused by chromosomal abnormality, occurring in approximately 1 in 700 births. It is often characterized by wideset, Oriental- looking eyes; mild to moderate mental retardation; a simian or single crease across the palm; and a wide range of other birth defects.

dysarthrias   A group of motor speech disorders characterized by various forms of articulatory inaccuracy and poor intelligibility with generally consistent errors.

dyslexia   A specific learning disability involving the failure to master reading at a normal age level.

echolalia   An involuntary, parrotlike imitation of words and phrases spoken by others, often accompanied by the twitching of muscles; frequently seen in persons with autism and schizophrenia.

educational audiologist   An audiologist who works within the school system to provide audiologic services for the children in a designated area.

EEC syndrome (ectrodactyly-ectodermal dysplasia-clefting)   This autosomal-dominant syndrome is characterized by absent or hypoplastic nails; ectrodactyly ("lobster claw" deformity of the hands and/or feet); nasolacrimal duct obstruction, resulting in dryness of the eyes; sparse hair; dry skin; missing or abnormal teeth (e.g., hypoplasia of the enamel); urogenital abnormalities; and cleft palate with or without cleft lip. Cognitive impairment is common, as is conductive hearing loss, hoarse voice quality, and the speech characteristics of cleft palate.

electronic scanning   An electronic device such as a microswitch is used to select an item while the items in a display are systematically scanned.

embedding   The process or result of placing a word, phrase, or clause in an existing sentence.

encoding   The act of transforming an idea into a message that is conveyed by vocal or nonvocal communication.

establishment   The elicitation of initial correct productions of a sound, syllable, or word.

eustachian tube   The tube that connects the middle ear with the nasopharynx. It allows ventilation of the middle ear and drainage of fluids.

Evidence-based practice   The systematic use of evidence in making clinical decisions such as what intervention method to use. The three sources of evidence are research, the clinician, and the client.

facial grimace   A ticlike movement of the nostrils or adjacent facial muscles, used in an attempt to reduce nasal airflow.

fast mapping   The quick assumption of word meaning based on limited exposure. Fast mapping enables an individual to increase his or her vocabulary rapidly. Fuller meanings take longer to develop.

faucial pillars   Bilateral curtainlike structures in the posterior portion of the oral cavity; the anterior faucial pillar is formed as the velum curves downward toward the tongue, and the posterior faucial pillar is just behind the anterior pillar.

figurative language   Expressions that use words or phrases to represent an abstract concept. Such expressions cannot be interpreted literally. For example, *Father hit the roof* cannot be explained at a syntactic level. Types of figurative language include idioms, metaphors, similes, and proverbs.

final common pathway   The terminal portion of diverging nerves that transmit neural commands to the muscles.

fistula   An abnormal channel in the body connecting two spaces or extending from a space or abscess in the body.

fistula   (pl. fistulae or fistulas) An abnormal hole or passage from one epithelialized cavity to another. This can be due to surgical breakdown.

formant (bands)   Regions of prominent energy distribution in a speech sound.

frequency-modulating (FM) system   A type of wireless system that picks up the speaker's voice through a wireless FM microphone and transmits it by the FM radio signal to a radio receiver worn by the person with hearing loss.

fricative   A speech sound generated by the friction of air passing through a constriction.

functional   Refers to a disorder with no identifiable physical or organic cause.

functional communication   Expressive and receptive language that is related to being successful in conducting one's activities of daily living.

Furlow Z plasty   A surgical procedure that can be used as a primary palate repair or as a secondary procedure. Its purpose is to lengthen the velum.

gene   The fundamental physical and functional unit of heredity. A gene is an ordered sequence of nucleotides located in a particular position on a particular chromosome that encodes a specific functional product (i.e., a protein or RNA molecule).

gene expression   The process by which a gene's coded information is converted into the structures present and operating in the cell. Expressed genes include those that are transcribed into mRNA and then translated into protein and those that are transcribed into RNA but not translated into protein (e.g., transfer and ribosomal RNAs).

generalization goal   A selected improvement in the child's speech that is not expected to result directly from intervention.

genetics   The study of inheritance patterns of specific traits.

genome   The genome is an organism's complete set of DNA. Genomes vary widely in size: The smallest known genome for a free-living organism (a bacterium) contains about 600,000 DNA base pairs, while human and mouse genomes have some 3 billion. Except for mature red blood cells, all human cells contain a complete genome.

genomics   The study of genes and their function in humans.

genotype   The genetic constitution of an organism, as distinguished from its physical appearance (its phenotype).

gerund   A noun-like word or phrase made by adding *ing* to a verb, as in *Fishing for trout is enjoyable.*

glide   A consonant produced while gliding from one vowel position to another.

glissando   Gliding up or down a musical scale.

glottis   The space between the vocal folds.

hard palate   The hard, front part of the roof of the mouth and the floor of the nose, composed of bone and covered by mucous membrane.

hard palate   The bony structure that forms the roof of the mouth. It separates the oral cavity from the nasal cavity.

hardwired device   A type of assistive listening device that uses a wire to connect the microphone to the amplifier much like a body hearing aid. The amplifier then sends the signal to the receiver that is used by the listener.

hemianopsia (hemianopia)   Defective vision in one half of the visual field of one eye. Homonymous hemianopsia indicates a corresponding visual field loss in both eyes.

hemifacial microsomia (HFM)   The second most common facial birth defect, next to cleft lip and palate, is sporadic (although there have been some reports of familial cases). The primary manifestations (in widely varying severity) are microphthalmia, underdevelopment of the lower jaw (mandible), external- and middle-ear anomalies, nerve involvement, and soft tissue deficiency (Vento, La Brie, & Mallisen, 1991). A third to half of all children with HFM have velopharyngeal insufficiency (VPI) (Luce, Mcgibbon, & Hoopes, 1977). The etiological basis of the VPI is more commonly associated with underdevelopment of the pharyngeal muscles rather than a cleft palate. The oral opening can sometimes be larger on the affected side (macrostomia). This craniofacial condition goes by a number of other syndromic names, including ocular-auricular-vertebral, Goldenhar, and first and second branchial arch.

hemiparesis   Weakness of one lateral half of the body.

hemiplegia   Paralysis of one lateral half of the body.

high-back   An articulatory description of vowel production in which the tongue has a high and back position (example: the vowel in the word *who*).

high-front   An articulatory description of vowel production in which the tongue has a high and front position (example: the vowel in the word *he*).

hoarseness   A perceived voice quality when there is noise (aperiodicity) in the voice.

homonymous   Having the same meaning.

hypernasality   A resonance disorder that occurs when sound enters the nasal cavity inappropriately during speech; the perceptual quality of speech is often described as just "nasal," muffled, or characterized by mumbling; is particularly perceptible on vowels.

hypo-hypernasality   Speech that has excessive nasal resonance of vowels, but loss of some nasal characteristics of the nasal phonemes.

hyponasality   A type of abnormal resonance that occurs when there is a reduction in nasal resonance during speech due to blockage in the nasopharynx or in the entrance to the nasal cavity; particularly affects the production of the nasal consonants (/m/, /n/, and /ng/).

identification   The use of tests or procedures to determine whether a communication disorder is present.

ideogram   The graphic representation that suggests the idea of the referent it represents, but does not depict the referent directly.

in-the-canal hearing aid   A custom-fit aid that fits in the external ear canal and only fills a very small portion of the concha.

in-the-ear hearing aid   A custom-fit hearing aid that is placed directly into the external ear, filling the entire concha.

incisive foramen   A hole in the bone that is located in the alveolar ridge area of the maxillary arch, just behind the central incisors, and that forms the tip of the premaxilla.

incisive suture lines   Embryological suture lines in the hard palate that go between the lateral incisors and canines and meet posteriorly at the area of the incisive foramen; the suture lines that separate the premaxilla.

independent analysis   A phonological analysis that examines the child's speech without reference to the intended adult targets.

indirect request   A request for action that is stated indirectly, as in *Shouldn't someone check the cookies?* to indicate they are burning and should be taken out of the oven.

infantile reflexes   A number of behaviors that may be observed in newborns and infants that are reflex in nature and that disappear as a normal infant develops.

intelligibility   The extent to which a listener can understand the speaker's message.

jargon   Fluent, well-articulated, phonologically correct utterances that make little sense.

language   A socially shared code or conventional system for representing concepts through the use of arbitrary symbols and rule-governed combinations of those symbols.

laryngectomee   An individual who has had the larynx removed.

lateral   A speech sound made with a midline closure of the vocal tract, but with lateral openings that direct the air stream through the oral cavity along the sides of the tongue (e.g., the consonant in the word *law*).

lateralization   The representation or control of a function to one side (hemisphere) or the other of the brain. Also referred to as cerebral dominance.

lexicon   The inventory of words stored in memory and available for use in communication.

linear scanning   A technique in which all items to be scanned are presented one at a time. This is the simplest scanning technique.

linguistic competence   (1) A native speaker's underlying knowledge of the rules for generating and understanding conventional linguistic forms. (2) Knowledge of the rules of syntax, semantics, and phonology of a language necessary to produce and understand an unlimited number of grammatical utterances of a language.

linguistic performance   Actual language use, reflecting linguistic competence and the communication constraints.

liquid   Refers to consonants with the vowel-like quality of little air turbulence.

localization   The assignment of a function to a discrete region of the brain.

low-back   An articulatory description of vowel production in which the tongue has a low and back position (example: the vowel in the word *pot*).

low-front   An articulatory description of vowel production in which the tongue has a low and front position (example: the vowel in the word *had*).

lung   The organ of respiration or breathing. The lungs are paired organs that occupy the thoracic cavity and effect the aeration of the blood.

maintenance   The continued production of a target sound after training has been completed.

manner of articulation   A phonetic feature of speech sounds that specifies the way in which a particular sound is formed, such as the degree of narrowing of the vocal tract (e.g., stop, fricative, glide) or the path of energy transmission (e.g., oral vs. nasal).

medial compression force   The force developed between the vocal folds as they meet at midline.

median palatine suture line   The embryological suture line that begins at the incisive foramen and ends at the posterior nasal spine; separates the paired palatine processes of the maxilla and the horizontal plates of the palatine bones; also known as the *intermaxillary palatine suture line*.

metalinguistics (metalinguistic cues)   Linguistic intuitions on the acceptability of communication.

metaphonological abilities   General knowledge and skills that permit a child to talk and make judgments about the sounds and structures of phonology, play phonological word games, and correct errors.

middle-ear implant (MEI)   A partially or completely implanted amplification device within the middle-ear space that is used for sensorineural hearing losses.

mixed nasality   A combination of hypernasality, hyponasality, or cul-de-sac resonance during connected speech.

morpheme   The smallest unit of meaning: indivisible (*dog*) without violating the meaning or producing meaningless units (*do, g*). There are two types of morphemes, free and bound.

morphology   The aspect of language concerned with rules governing change in meaning at the intraword level.

multilingual   Being able to speak and to understand more than one language. The term can also be extended to include being able to also read and write in more than one language. The use of the term does not necessarily suggest proficiency in the languages.

multimodal communication   The use of different channels or forms of communication such as speech, gestures, graphic symbols, and writing.

multisensory stimulation   Perceiving or sending information using more than one faculty (e.g., listening to a story and looking at pictures, looking at a grapheme of a speech sound while hearing the phoneme produced while writing the grapheme).

muscles of the rib cage   A set of muscles that run from one rib to another or connect the ribs to other bony structures, such as the vertebrae. The muscles work in groups to permit the lungs to expand and contract.

myasthenia   Overall condition of muscular weakness.

myelination   The process by which neuronal axons are coated with myelin (a fatty substance that insulates the neuron).

nasal air emission   An inappropriate flow of the airstream through the nose during speech, causing distortion of the speech; usually caused by velopharyngeal dysfunction; also called *nasal escape*.

nasal cavity   The air cavity system of the nose; the space between the nostrils and the velopharynx.

nasal escape   The loss of air through the nasal passages on phonemes that normally require oral production.

nasal rustle   A fricative sound that occurs as air pressure is formed through a partially opened velopharyngeal valve, causing the airflow to become turbulent and resulting in a bubbling of secretions above the opening; also called *nasal turbulence.*

nasalance score   Represents the relative amount of nasal acoustic energy in the person's speech as determined by the Nasometer; the ratio of nasal acoustic energy over total (oral plus nasal) acoustic energy during speech as determined through the use of the Nasometer; the score represents the mean of the percentage points that are calculated for an entire speech passage.

nasality   A perceived deviation in voice quality when there is inappropriate or incomplete velopharyngeal closure causing increased nasal resonance.

nasals   Oral cavity blocks exiting air, but the velum is lowered to allow breath to exit via the nasal cavity.

nasometry   Assessment using a computer-based instrument, the Nasometer (Kay Elemetrics, Inc., Pinehurst, NJ), that measures the relative amount of nasal acoustic energy in a patient's speech.

nasopharyngoscopy   A minimally invasive endoscopic procedure that allows visual observation and analysis of the velopharyngeal mechanism or larynx during speech through the use of a scope (nasopharyngoscope) that is inserted through the nose until it reaches the nasopharynx; can be used to evaluate velopharyngeal function, phonation, or swallowing; also called *nasendoscopy* or video *endoscopy.*

neighborhood density   Determined by the number of possible words that differ by one phoneme. Important for perception and production of early language.

neurogenic   Arising from the nervous system.

neurons   Those cells of the nervous system that transmit an electrical impulse.

new information   Topics or meanings that are known to the speaker, but not to the listener (i.e., not already stated or obvious from the context).

nonlinguistics (nonlinguistic cues)   Coding devices that contribute to communication, but are not a part of speech. Examples include gestures, body posture, eye contact, head and body movement, facial expression (kinesics), and physical distance (proxemics).

nucleotide   One of the structural components, or building blocks, of DNA and RNA. A nucleotide consists of a base (one of four chemicals: adenine, thymine, guanine, and cytosine) plus a molecule of sugar and one of phosphoric acid.

nucleus   The sonorant peak of a syllable, usually a vowel.

objective outcome measures   Measures used to assess speech perception with and without the hearing instrument. These are often used as proof of benefit to third-party payers.

obligatory errors   Speech characteristics that are the product of structural abnormality or dysfunction; include hypernasality, nasal air emission, weak consonants, and short utterance length; also known as passive speech characteristics where the articulation placement (the function) is normal, but the abnormality of the structure causes distortion of speech.

occlusion   Dental occlusion is also referred to as bite type. It refers to the relationship or contact of the mandibular teeth to the maxillary teeth.

occult submucous cleft   A defect in the velum that is under the mucous membrane and not visible on the oral surface; this defect can usually be viewed on the nasal surface of the velum through nasopharyngoscopy.

old information   Topics or meanings that are known to the speaker and the listener (i.e., previously stated or obvious from context).

omissions   (1) Not producing one or more sounds in a word. (2) Errors in which sounds normally present in a target word are not produced.

onset   In syllable structure, a consonant or consonant sequence that precedes the nucleus (vowel) of a syllable.

operational competence   The ability to efficiently and independently operate a communication device.

optimum pitch   That vocal pitch at which the voice is produced with maximum efficiency. It is usually about five musical tones above the low end of the individual's range.

oral approach   intervention based on the principle that most children identified as deaf or hard-of-hearing have some residual hearing and can be taught to listen and speak with early intervention and consistent training to develop their auditory and speech skills.

oral apraxia (or oral buccal apraxia)   A disorder in which an individual makes erroneous movements of the oral structures when requested to make such movements.

oral cavity   The mouth; a space bordered anteriorly by the lips and posteriorly by the palate.

organic   Refers to a disorder with an identifiable physical cause.

otitis media   An infection of the middle-ear space, often accompanied by accumulation of fluid (called effusions).

outcome measures   Measures used to evaluate the effect a particular therapy is having on an individual's physiological or emotional disability or handicap.

overt submucous cleft   A submucous cleft that can be identified on the nasal surface of the velum based on features such as a zona pellucida, bifid or hypoplastic uvula, or apparent diastasis of the levator muscle that particularly apparent during phonation.

palatal lift   A prosthetic appliance that can be used to raise the velum for speech in cases where the velum is long enough to achieve velpharyngeal closure, but does not move well, often due to neurological impairment.

palatal obturator   A prosthetic appliance that can be used to cover an open palatal defect, such as an unrepaired cleft palate or a palatal fistual; this device can be used to improve an infant's ability to achieve compression of the nipple for suction or to close a palatal defect for speech.

paralinguistics (paralinguistic codes)   Vocal and nonvocal codes that are superimposed on a linguistic code to signal the speaker's attitude or emotion or to clarify or provide additional meaning.

partner-assisted scanning   A message transmission technique in which the scanning is provided by a person with whom the user wishes to communicate.

peripheral nervous system (PNS)   The portion of the nervous system that includes the cranial and spinal nerves.

pharyngeal augmentation   An injection of a filler substance (i.e., collagen or hydroxyl apetit) that is placed in the posterior pharyngeal wall to help close a small velopharyngeal opening.

pharyngeal cavity   Throat; a respiratory and digestive passageway bordered inferiorly by the esophagus and superiorly by the nasal cavities.

pharyngeal flap   A surgical procedure to correct velopharyngeal dysfunction by elevating a flap from the posterior pharyngeal wall and suturing it into the velum to partially close the nasopharynx in middline.

pharynx   (adj. pharyngeal) The walls of the throat between the esophagus and nasal cavity.

phenotype   The observable traits or characteristics of an organism—for example, hair color, weight, or the presence or absence of a disease. Phenotypic traits are not necessarily genetic.

philtral ridges   The raised lines on either side of the philtrum, which are embryological suture lines that are formed as the segments of the upper lip fuse.

philtrum   (adj. philtral) A long dimple or indentation that courses from the columella down to the upper lip and is bordered by the philtral ridges on each side.

phonation   The production of sound by the vibration of the vocal folds.

phoneme   The smallest linguistic unit of sound that can signal a difference in meaning when modified; each phoneme has distinctive features.

phoneme awareness   Understanding that words are made up of sounds and that sounds can be blended into words; the ability to analyze words into component sounds and represent sounds with orthographic letters.

phonetic   The physical realizations of speech in the acoustic characteristics of speech sounds or the motor movements involved in saying them.

phonetic level   The component of the speech-sound system that includes the physical mechanisms of audition and speech production as well as their associated neuromotor and neurosensory systems.

phonological awareness   This is a another term used to describe metaphonological abilities.

phonological level   The component of the speech-sound system that includes representations and rules.

phonology   That aspect of language concerned with units such as features, segments, syllables, words, and phrases; the representation of these units; and the rules that govern their combination and form.

pidgin   A simplified linguistic system consisting of words, phrases, and gestures developed to facilitate verbal interaction between speakers of different languages, especially for the purpose of trade.

place of articulation   A phonetic feature of speech sounds that specifies the location in the vocal tract of the major constriction for a particular sound (e.g., sounds made with lip closure have a bilabial place of articulation).

polymerase chain reaction (PCR)   A fast, inexpensive technique for making an unlimited number of copies of any piece of DNA. Sometimes called *molecular photocopying*, PCR has had an immense impact on biology and medicine, especially genetic research.

pragmatics   The aspect of language concerned with language use within a communication context.

presupposition   The process of estimating the knowledge of the listener and the amount of information needed for comprehension.

premaxilla   A triangular-shaped bone that is bordered on either side by the incisive suture lines; this bony segment normally contains the central and lateral maxillary incisors.

prognosis   The anticipated speed and extent of recovery from a disorder.

prosody   Aspects of language that convey meaning and mood and give melody to the speech act by changes in rate, rhythm, or stress.

psycholinguistics; psycholinguistic theory   The study of the psychological aspects of language, especially as they apply to the psychological processes involved in learning, processing, and using language.

reauditorization   The process of reconstructing spoken and heard words, phrases, sentences, or digits to oneself, in "one's head" or "one's mind's ear."

recessive   Refers to a genetic disorder that appears only in patients who have received two copies of a mutant gene, one from each parent.

referent   The event or object to which a symbol refers.

relapse   A return to a pretherapy state. It may also refer to substitution of new undesirable behaviors for the old ones.

relational phonological analyses   Direct comparisons of a child's productions to the intended adult targets.

resonance   (1) An acoustical phenomenon; the vibratory response of a body or air-filled cavity to a frequency imposed on it. (2) As related to voice, the process of increasing the prominence of certain tones or overtones by adjusting the cavities of the respiratory tract to respond to the frequency of particular partials (to resonate). (3) The selective absorption and radiation of acoustic energy at specific wavelengths or frequencies.

rhotic   A speech sound that has an *r*-like quality.

Robin sequence   An isolated palatal cleft combined with a small mandible that allows the tongue to occlude and compromise the airway. It is hypothized that children with Robin sequence are born with cleft palate because of a series of prenatal events during which an abnormally small mandible (lower jaw) prevents the tongue from lowering during fetal development so that the palatal shelves can fuse.

row-column scanning   A message transmission technique in which selections are offered by scanning down the rows until the user interrupts the scan and then selections are offered by scanning across the columns until the user interrupts the scan at the desired location.

scanning   A message transmission technique with a variety of modes. In a linear scanning mode, item choices are presented one at a time until the desired item is selected by the individual. The scanning array may be presented by a communication partner via an electronic communication aid. In row-column scanning, selections are offered by scanning down the rows until the user interrupts the scan, and then selections are offered by scanning across the columns until the user interrupts the scan at the desired location. Directed scanning requires the user to activate multiple switches or a joystick to direct the scanning cursor to the desired location.

schwa   The ultimate vowel /ə/, which is unstressed, lax or short, and midcentral. It can achieve the minimal duration for a vowel sound.

screening   The use of tests or procedures to determine whether a child needs to be tested further to then determine whether a communication disorder is present.

semantics   The aspect of language concerned with word-meaning or word-content rules and grammatical rules.

sequence   The occurrence of a pattern of multiple anomalies within an individual that arise from a single known or presumed prior anomaly or mechanical factor; where one anomaly leads to the development of the other anomalies, as in Pierre Robin sequence.

sequencing errors   Speech errors that involve the exchange, addition, or deletion of phonetic segments (e.g., when a speaker says, "I hissed my mystery lesson" for "I missed my history lesson").

shunt   As used in this book, a surgically created tracheoesophageal fistula or channel extending from the back wall of the trachea to the esophagus. Produced in laryngectomized persons to divert pulmonary air to the esophagus for voice production.

signal processing   The way the acoustic signal entering the hearing aid is manipulated. There are three classifications of circuitry currently used in hearing aids: analog, digitally programmable, and digital.

social competence   The ability by the user of alternative and augmentative communication to appropriately use the pragmatic aspects of communication such as when to speak and what to talk about.

sociolinguistics   The study of the sociological influences, especially cultural and situational variables, on language learning and use, including dialects, bilingualism, and parent–child interactions.

soft palate   (also referred to as velum) The fleshy or muscular part of the palate that helps to close the velopharyngeal opening during swallowing and the production of non-nasal speech sounds.

sound field FM system   An amplification system that uses loudspeakers to transmit the speaker's voice to all individuals in an area.

source-filter theory of speech acoustics   A theory of the acoustic production of speech that states that sound energy (such as that produced by the vibrating vocal folds) is filtered by the resonances of the vocal tract. This theory was formulated especially by Gunnar Fant.

Southern White Nonstandard English   A dialect of American English spoken by working-class Southern Caucasians.

spastic   An adjective describing muscle that is affected by the condition of spasticity.

spasticity   A condition in which muscles tend to have too much tone, with that tone increasing even more abnormally when a muscle is stretched. There is also an abnormally strong reaction of the affected muscles to certain reflexes.

spectrogram   A graphic sound analysis containing information on frequency, time, and intensity, usually in the form of a three-dimensional diagram in which frequency is represented on the vertical axis, time on the horizontal axis, and intensity as variations in darkness (gray scale).

spectrum   A graph showing the distribution of signal energy as a function of frequency.

speech   The dynamic neuromuscular process of producing speech sounds for communication; a verbal means of communicating or conveying meaning.

speech bulb obturator   A prosthetic device that can be considered when the velum is too short to close completely against the posterior pharyngeal wall; this device consists of a retaining appliance and a bulb (usually of acrylic) that fills in the pharyngeal space for speech; also known as a *speech aid appliance*.

speech community   A group of individuals sharing a common set of linguistic and communication rules, values, and experiences.

speech-generating device   Any AAC device that includes speech output as a transmission method. Speech output may be digitized or synthesized.

speechreading   The process of watching the lips and any other visual cues available to the listener to determine what the speaker is saying.

sphincter pharyngoplasty   A surgical procedure to correct velopharyngeal dysfunction by releasing and elevating the posterior faucial pillars, including their internal muscles, and rotating them back to be sutured together on the posterior pharyngeal wall. This forms a type of sphincter to further close the pharyngeal port around the sides.

spontaneous recovery   (1) The period that reflects the natural resolution of impairments that were incurred as the result of stroke. (2) The tendency for people who stutter to stop stuttering on their own, usually without intervention.

Standard African American English   English spoken by formally educated people of African descent throughout the world; used especially in formal situations.

standardized test   A test that has been given to a large number of individuals who are representative of the age levels, cultural groups, and so on of students for whom the test is to be used.

starters   In reference to stuttering, these are a form of trick or avoidance used in attempts to slide into or out of a sound or word the person expects to stutter or is stuttering.

stereotypys   The small number of (often meaningless) utterances in the speech of aphasic individuals who have poor comprehension and extremely limited verbal output. These utterances are used when verbal behavior is called for, independent of their appropriateness.

Stickler syndrome   Often associated with Robin sequence. This autosomal—dominantly inherited syndrome includes severe myopia, a high incidence of retinal detachments, cataracts, joint laxity, a round face, micrognathia (small lower jaw), cleft palate and associated hypernasality, and/or hyponasality resulting in a small nasal airway.

stimulability   The child's ability to produce error sounds or syllables correctly when provided with instructions or when imitating an adult model.

stop   A consonant produced by a complete blockage of airflow.

strategic competence   The acquisition of compensatory strategies by users of alternative and augmentative communication (AAC) to communicate effectively within the restrictions imposed by AAC systems.

strength   The component of movement that contributes to differential ability in the velocity or amount of muscle contractibility and load shift.

stuttering   A fluency disorder characterized by repetitions, prolongations, and blocks often referred to as core behaviors. Accompanying these are associated learned behaviors in the form of vocal and nonvocal behaviors. These learned patterns are used in attempts to hide or disguise the core behaviors.

subglottal air pressure   The air pressure developed below the vocal folds (glottis). Generally, this air pressure is nearly equal to that developed in the lungs and is an energy source for sound production (e.g., subglottal air pressure provides the energy for vocal fold vibration during voiced sounds).

subjective outcome measures   In adults, they are measures that involve the use of self-inventories to determine the level of disability the person is experiencing or to indicate areas where one feels she or he needs improvement. In children, they are parent and/or teacher checklists that determine how the child is performing with an amplification device or other intervention and/or areas where the child needs improvement.

submucous cleft palate   A congenital defect that affects the underlying structures of the palate, while the structures on the oral surface are intact; can involve the muscles of the velum and also the bony structure of the hard palate.

submucous cleft palate   A cleft in underlying muscle, and often of the bony palate, with a thin mucous covering that may obscure the condition.

substitutions   (1) Replacing one speech sound (phoneme), word, phrase, or clause with another. (2) Speech errors that involve the production of another phone of the language in place of the target segment.

successive approximations   A therapy approach for articulation or phonological disorders in which correct production is approached in a series of gradual steps. For example, an intermediate step between the production of /t/ and /s/ for a child who substitutes /t/ for /s/ might be /st/.

symbol   A unit in oral or written expression used to represent an object, event, or idea.

symbol set   A defined, closed set of symbols. It can be expanded, but it does not have clearly defined rules for expansion.

symbol system   A set of symbols designed to work together for maximum communication; includes rules or logic for the development of additional symbols.

synaptogenesis   The process by which synapses (functional contacts between neurons) are formed.

syndrome   A pattern of multiple anomalies or malformations that regularly occur together and are pathogenically related and, therefore, have a common known or suspected cause; craniofacial syndromes involving the head and face (e.g., Down syndrome) cause affected individuals to look alike, even when there is no family relationship.

synonym   A word that can be used as a substitute for another word and that shares essential meanings with the word for which it can stand.

syntagmatic-paradigmatic shift   A change in word-associated behavior from a syntactic to a semantic basis; occurs during school-age years.

syntax   Organizational rules for ordering words in a sentence and for specifying word order, sentence organization, and word relationships.

synthesized speech   Speech generated by computer using a program of mathematical and phonological rules that model human speech production.

target goals   Therapy goals that are the direct focus of intervention.

telecoil   An optional component within a hearing aid that will pick up the electromagnetic leakage from the telephone receiver, amplify the signal, transduce it into an acoustic signal, and deliver it to the person's hearing aid.

telegraphic speech   Communication that sounds like a spoken telegram because of the omission of grammatical words and word endings.

text   A passage or group of connected utterances.

thyroid   The largest of the cartilages that form the anterior wall of the larynx. It consists of two plates that are joined at an angle to form a v-shape.

timing   Accuracy in the onset and termination of muscular contraction.

tone   The relatively constant background state of muscular contraction characteristic of normal muscle.

tongue thrust   A condition in which the pattern of swallowing involves a protrusion of the tongue rather than an upward and backward motion.

tonsils   Lymphoid tissue that is located on either side of the mouth between the anterior and posterior faucial pillars.

trachea   The cylindrical tube of cartilage extending from the larynx to the bronchial tubes.

transfer   Used synonymously with generalization. The extension of correct productions of sounds, syllables, or words to new contexts.

translational research   The bridge of basic science research conducted in a laboratory to application in clinical settings with actual individuals.

Treacher Collins syndrome   Results from a mutation of the treacle gene on the long arm of the 5th chromosome (5q32-33.1) and is also an autosomal dominant disorder (Dixon, 1996). Craniofacial features include underdevelopment of the cheekbones (zygomas), maxilla, and mandible. The eyes slant downwards, and there is often a notching (colobomas) in the lower eyelids and absent eyelashes in the medial third of the lower lids. Bilateral conductive hearing loss necessitating bone conduction hearing aids is most always seen. Cleft palate is present in about one-third of all patients. The anterior-posterior airway is typically small because of the maxillary hypoplasia. As such, there is often cul-de-sac type resonance. In addition, the small airway results in very few children requiring a secondary surgical procedure to correct velopharyngeal insufficiency following the primary palate repair. Intelligence is normal.

turnabout   A conversational device used by a parent or caregiver with a preschooler to maintain the conversation and aid the child in making on-topic comments. In its usual form, the turnabout consists of a comment or reply to the child's utterance followed by a cue, such as a question, for the child to reply.

tympanometry   Measurement, on an acoustic immitance meter, of the movement of the eardrum caused by various degrees of positive and negative air pressure.

unaided communication technique   Does not require a physical aid for transmission. Examples are gesture, manual sign, facial expression, and natural speech.

unilateral neglect   The inability to attend and/or respond to stimuli on the side opposite the brain damage.

uvula   A teardrop-shaped structure that is typically long and slender and hangs freely from the back or free edge of the velum; it has no known function.

velocardiofacial syndrome   This highly variable autosomal syndrome includes cleft palate or congenital velopharyngeal incompetence, heart anomalies, and a characteristic facial appearance, including a long nose with a prominent nasal root. Speech is marked by severe hypernasality and glottal stops. Learning disabilities are common, and psychiatric illnesses may occur in adolescence or later in life.

velopharyngeal dysfunction (VPD)   One of the generic terms that is used to describe abnormal veloparyngeal function, regardless of the cause.

velopharyngeal incompetence (VPI)   A neuromotor or physiological disorder that results in poor movement of the velopharyngeal structures.

velopharyngeal insufficiency (VPI)   An anatomical or structural defect that precludes adequate velopharyngeal closure by causing the velum to be short relative to the posterior pharyngeal wall.

velopharyngeal mislearning   Inadequate velopharyngeal closure due to faulty learning of appropriate articulation patterns.

velum   The part of the palate that is located in the back of the mouth and consists of muscles that are covered by the same mucous membrane as the hard palate; frequently referred to as the *soft palate.*

vernacular   The common mode of expression in a speech community; especially used for informal exchanges among members of that community.

vibrotactile aid   A vibrator that is placed on the sternum, which sends information about the acoustic environment to the user via the sense of touch.

videofluoroscopy   A radiological procedure that can be used for the evaluation of the structures and function of the velopharyngeal mechanism and swallowing.

visual scanning   The ability to search for and to voluntarily stop and select a graphic symbol or a sign or a word presented visually.

vocal fold   A laryngeal structure formed of muscle and connective tissue that vibrates to produce the sound of voice. The vocal folds are paired structures that attach anteriorly to the thyroid cartilage and posteriorly to the arytenoid cartilages.

vocal tract   That part of the vocal mechanism lying above the vocal folds. It includes the pharynx, oral, and nasal cavities.

voiced   Sound produced with vibration of the vocal folds; includes some consonants and all vowels.

voiced speech   Speech that is produced with voicing as an energy source (i.e., sounds produced with vibration of the vocal folds).

voicing   A phonetic feature of speech sounds that specifies the activity of the vocal folds—that is, whether they are vibrating or not.

vowel   A speech sound that is made with an open vocal tract and typically has the greatest energy of a syllable in which it is contained. Vowels are normally voiced except in whispered speech.

vowel quadrilateral   A four-sided diagram that represents the articulatory or acoustic dimensions of vowel production. Different vowels can be represented as points in the diagram. In articulatory terms, the vowel quadrilateral represents the relative position of the tongue in the oral cavity (high vs. low and front vs. back). In acoustic terms, the diagram represents the values of the first and second formants.

Wernicke's area   A region of the temporal lobe of the brain (typically the left hemisphere) thought to be important for the comprehension of spoken language. Named after the German neurologist Karl Wernicke (1848–1905).

References

Abbeduto, L., & Hagerman, R. J. (1997). Language and communication in fragile X syndrome. *Mental Retardation and Developmental Disabilities Research Reviews, 3*, 313–322.

Abbott, J. A. (1947). Repressed hostility as a factor in adult stuttering. *Journal of Speech Disorders, 12*, 428–430.

Abedi, J. (2002). Standardized achievement tests and English language learners: Psychometric issues. *Educational Assessment, 8*, 231–257.

Abrahamsen, A., Cavallo, M. M., & McCluer, J. A. (1985). Is the sign advantage a robust phenomenon? From gesture to language in two modalities. *Merrill-Palmer Quarterly, 31*, 177–209.

Abrams, H., Chisolm, T. H., & McArdle, R. (2002). A cost-utility analysis of adult group audiologic rehabilitation: Are the benefits worth the cost? *Journal of Rehabilitation Research and Development, 39*, 549–558.

Abrams, H. B., Hnath-Chisolm, T., Guerreiro, S. M., & Ritterman, S. I. (1992). The effects of intervention strategy on self-perception of hearing handicap. *Ear and Hearing, 13*, 371–377.

Abramson, D. L., Marrinan, E. M., & Mulliken, J. B. (1997). Robin sequence: Obstructive sleep apnea following pharyngeal flap. *Cleft Palate Craniofacial Journal, 34*(3), 256–260.

Adams, M. J. (1990). *Beginning to read: Thinking and learning about print.* Cambridge, MA: MIT Press.

Adams, M. R. (1978). Further analysis of stuttering as a phonetic transition defect. *Journal of Fluency Disorders, 3*(4), 265–271.

Adams, M. R. (1980). The young stutterer: Diagnosis, treatment and assessment of progress. In W. Perkins (Ed.), *Seminars in speech-language-hearing: Strategies in stuttering therapy* (pp. 289–299). New York, NY: Thieme-Stratton.

Adams, M. R., & Ramig, P. R. (1980). Vocal characteristics of normal speakers and stutterers during choral reading. *Journal of Speech and Hearing Research, 23*, 457–469.

Adams, M. R., Sears, R. L., & Ramig, P. R. (1982). Vocal changes in stutterers and nonstutterers during monotoned speech. *Journal of Fluency Disorders, 7*, 21–25.

Addington, W. R., Stephens, R. E., & Gilliland, K. (1999). Assessing the laryngeal cough reflex and the risk of developing pneumonia after stroke: An inter-hospital comparison. *Stroke, 30*, 1203–1207.

Addington, W. R., Stephens, R. E., Gilliland, K., & Rodriguez, M. (1999). Assessing the laryngeal cough reflex and the risk of developing pneumonia after stroke. *Archives of Physical and Medical Rehabilitation, 80*, 150–154.

Ainsworth, S. (1945). Integrating theories of stuttering. *Journal of Speech Disorders, 10*, 205–210.

Ainsworth, S. H. (1960). Profession devoted to speech and hearing problems. *ASHA, 2*, 399–402.

Akshoomoff, N. (2000). Neurological underpinnings of autism. In A. Wetherby & B. Prizant (Eds.), *Autism spectrum disorders: A transactional developmental perspective* (pp. 167–190). Baltimore, MD: Paul H. Brookes.

Alberts, M. J., Bennett, C. A., & Rutledge, V. R. (1996). Hospital charges for stroke patients. *Stroke, 27*, 1825–1828.

Alberts, M. J., Horner, J., Gray, L., & Brazer, S. R. (1992). Aspiration after stroke: Lesion analysis by brain MRI. *Dysphagia, 7*, 170–173.

Albrecht, K., & Miller, L. G. (2001). *Innovations: Infant and toddler development.* Beltsville, MD: Gryphon House.

Alm, P. A. (2004). Stuttering, emotions, and heart rate during anticipatory anxiety: A critical review. *Journal of Fluency Disorders, 290*, 123–133.

Alpiner, J. G., & McCarthy, P. A. (2000). *Rehabilitative audiology: Children and adults.* Baltimore, MD: Lippincott Williams & Wilkins.

Amayreh, M. M., & Dyson, A. T. (1998). The acquisition of Arabic consonants. *Journal of Speech, Language, and Hearing Research, 41*, 642–653.

American Cleft Palate–Craniofacial Association. (1993). Parameters for the evaluation and treatment of patients with cleft lip/palate or other craniofacial anomalies. *Cleft Palate–Craniofacial Journal, 30*(Suppl. 1), 512.

American Educational Research Association, American Psychological Association, & National Council on Measurement in Education. (1999). *Standards for educational and psychological testing.* Washington, DC: American Educational Research Association.

American National Standards Institute (ANSI). (2004). *American National Standard specification for audiometers* (ANSI S3. 6-2004). New York, NY: Author.

American Psychiatric Association. (1994). *Diagnostic and statistical manual of mental disorders* (DSM-IV) (4th ed.). Washington, DC: Author.

American Psychiatric Association. (2000). *Diagnostic and statistical manual of mental disorders* (4th ed., Text revision). Washington, DC: Author.

American Speech and Hearing Association. (1974). Guidelines for audiometric symbols. *ASHA, 16*, 260–264.

American Speech-Language-Hearing Association. (1982). Definitions: Communicative disorders and variations. *ASHA, 24*, 949–950.

American Speech-Language-Hearing Association. (1983). *How does your child hear and talk?* Rockville, MD: National Association for Hearing and Speech Action.

American Speech-Language-Hearing Association. (1993). Definitions of communication disorders and variations (relevant paper). Available from www.asha.org/policy

American Speech-Language-Hearing Association. (1998). *Exciting opportunities in science and research.* Rockville, MD: Author.

American Speech-Language-Hearing Association. (2001a). *Scope of practice in audiology.* Rockville, MD: Author.

American Speech-Language-Hearing Association. (2001b). Roles and responsibilities of speech-language pathologists with respect to reading and writing in children and adolescents (position statement, executive summary of guidelines, technical report). *ASHA, 21*(Suppl.), 17–27. Rockville, MD: Author.

American Speech-Language-Hearing Association. (2002). *American English dialects: Technical report.* Rockville, MD: Author.

American Speech-Language-Hearing Association. (2004a). *Background information and standards and implementation for the certificate of clinical competence in speech language pathology.* Retrieved November 1, 2004, from www.asha.org/about/membership-certification/handbooks/slp/slp_standards_new.htm

American Speech-Language-Hearing Association. (2004b). *Evidence-based practice in communication disorders: An introduction* (technical report). Accessed from www.asha.org/members/deskref-journals/deskref/default.

American Speech-Language-Hearing Association. (2004c). Knowledge and skills needed by speech-language pathologists and audiologists to provide culturally and linguistically appropriate services. *ASHA, 24* (Suppl.),.

American Speech-Language-Hearing Association. (2004d). Scope of practice in audiology. *ASHA, 24* (Suppl.),.

American Speech-Language-Hearing Association. (2005a). Audiologists providing clinical services via telepractice: Position statement. *ASHA, 25* (Suppl.),.

American Speech-Language-Hearing Association. (2005b). *Evidence-based practice in communication disorders* (position statement). Accessed from www.asha.org/members/deskref-journals/deskref/default

American Speech-Language-Hearing Association. (2005c). Speech-language pathologists providing clinical services via telepractice: Position statement. *ASHA, 25* (Suppl.),.

Americans with Disabilities Act (1990). P. L. 101–336. Retrieved March 2, 2004, from www.usdoj.gov/crt/ada/pubs/ada.txt

Anderson, A. H., Clark, A., & Mullin, J. (1994). Interactive communication between children: Learning how to make language work in dialogue. *Journal of Child Language, 21,* 439–463.

Anderson, K. (1989). *Screening Instrument for Targeting Educational Risk.* Austin, TX: Pro-Ed.

Anderson, K., & Smaldino, J. (1996). Listening inventories for education: A classroom measurement tool. *The Hearing Journal, 52,* 75–76.

Andreasson, M. L., Leeper, H. A., & MacRae, D. L. (1991). Changes in vocal resonance and nasalization following adenoidectomy in normal children: Preliminary findings. *Journal of Otolaryngology, 20*(4), 237–242.

Andrews, M. L. (1994). *Manual of voice treatment: Pediatrics through geriatrics.* San Diego, CA: Singular Publishing Group.

Anglin, J. M. (1995, April). *Word knowledge and the growth of potentially knowable vocabulary.* Paper presented at the biennial meeting of the Society for Research in Child Development, Indianapolis, IN.

Apel, K., & Masterson, J. (2001). Theory-guided spelling assessment and intervention: A case study. *Language, Speech, and Hearing Services in Schools, 32,* 182–194.

Applebee, A. N. (1978). *The child's concept of story.* Chicago, IL: University of Chicago Press.

Aronson, A. E. (1990). *Clinical voice disorders* (3rd ed.). New York, NY: Thieme.

Arvedson, J. (2004). *Treatment efficacy summary: Pediatric feeding and swallowing disorders.* Retrieved July 2004, from www.asha.org/members/slp/healthcare/efficacy.htm

Arvedson, J., & Brodsky, L. (Eds.). (1993). *Pediatric swallowing and feeding: Assessment and management.* San Diego, CA: Singular Publishing Group.

Arvedson, J. C., & Rogers, B. T. (1998). Dysphagia in children. In A. F. Johnson & B. H. Jacobson (Eds.), *Medical speech-language pathology: A practitioner's guide.* New York, NY: Thieme.

Ashcraft, M. (1994). *Human memory and cognition* (2nd ed.). New York, NY: HarperCollins.

Ashford, J. R., Logemann, J. A., & McCullough, G. (2004). *Treatment efficacy summary: Swallowing disorders (dysphagia).* Retrieved July 2004, from www.asha.org/members/slp/healthcare/efficacy.htm

Atchison, B. J. (2007). Sensory modulation disorders among children with a history of trauma: A frame of reference for speech-language pathologists. *Language, Speech, and hearing Services in Schools, 38,* 109–116.

Au, K. (1990). Children's use of information in word learning. *Journal of Child Language, 17,* 393–416.

Aviv, J. E., Kim, T., Sacco, R. L., Kaplan, S., Goodhart, K., Diamond, B., & Close, L. G. (1998, May). FEEST: A new bedside endoscopic test of the motor and sensory components of swallowing. *Annals of Otology, Rhinology, and Laryngology, 107*(5 Pt. 1), 378–87.

Aviv, J. E., Liu, H., Parides, M., Kaplan, S. T., & Close, L. G. (2000). Laryngopharyngeal sensory deficits in patients with laryngopharyngeal reflux and dysphagia. *Annals of Otology, Rhinology, and Laryngology, 109*(11), 1000–1006.

Aviv, J. E., Martin, J. H., Martin, J. H., Kim, T., Sacco, R. L., Thomson, J. E., Diamond, B., & Close, L. G. (1999). Laryngopharyngeal sensory discrimination testing and the laryngeal adductor reflex. *Annals of Otology, Rhinology, and Laryngology, 108*(8), 725–730.

Backus, A. (1999). Mixed native languages: A challenge to the monolithic view of language. *Topics in Language Disorders, 19*(4), 11–22.

Bagnato, S. J., Neisworth, J. T., & Munson, S. M. (1997). *Linking assessment and early intervention: An authentic curriculum-based approach.* Baltimore, MD: Paul H. Brookes.

Bailey, D. B., Hatton, D. D., & Skinner, M. (1998). Early developmental trajectories of males with fragile X syndrome. *American Journal on Mental Retardation, 103,* 29–39.

Baken, R. J. (1987). *Clinical measurement of speech and voice.* Boston, MA: College-Hill Press.

Barbara, D. (1954). *Stuttering: A psychodynamic approach to its understanding and treatment.* New York, NY: Julian Press.

Barczi, S. R., Sullivan, P. A., & Robbins, J. (2000). How should dysphagia care of older adults differ? Establishing optimal practice patterns. *Seminars in Speech and Language, 21,* 347–361.

Barlow, J. (2001–2002). Clinical forum: Recent advances in phonology: Theory and treatment: Parts I and II. *Language, Speech, and Hearing Services in Schools, 32–33.*

Barlow, J., & Giarut, J. (1999). Optimality theory in phonological acquisition. *Journal of Speech, Language, and Hearing Research, 42,* 1482–1498.

Barlow, S. M., Finan, D. S., Andretta, R. D., & Boliek, C. (2009). Kinematic measurement of speech and early orofacial movements. In M. R. McNeil (Ed.), *Clinical management of sensorimotor speech disorders* (2nd ed.). New York, NY: Thieme.

Barnett, S. (2001). Preschool education for economically disadvantaged children: Effects on reading achievement and related outcomes. In S. B. Neuman & D. K. Dickinson (Eds.), *Handbook of early literacy* (pp. 421–443). New York, NY: Guilford Press.

Bartlette, D. (1995). Seize the day. *ASHA, 37*(5), 34.

Barton, J. (1996). Interpreting character emotions for literature comprehension. *Journal of Adolescent and Adult Literacy, 40,* 22–28.

Bashir, A., Conte, B. M., & Heerde, S. M. (1998). Language and school success: Collaborative challenges and choices. In D. Merritt & B. Culatta (Eds.), *Language intervention in the classroom.* San Diego, CA: Singular Publishing Group.

Bashir, A. S., Wiig, E. H., & Abrams, J. C. (1987). Language disorders in childhood and adolescence: Implications for learning and socialization. *Pediatric Annals, 16,* 145–158.

Bass, N. H. (1997). Neurologic disorders of swallowing. In M. E. Groher (Ed.), *Dysphagia: Diagnosis and management.* Boston, MA: Butterworth-Heinemann.

Bates, E., Marchman, V., Thal, D., Fenson, L., Dale, P., Reznick, J. S., . . . Hurtung, J. (1994). Developmental and stylistic variation in the composition of early vocabulary. *Journal of Child Language, 21,* 85–123.

Bates, E. A. (2004). Explaining and interpreting deficits in language development across clinical groups: Where do we go from here? *Brain and Language, 88,* 248–253.

Battle, D. E. (1998). *Communication disorders in multicultural populations.* Boston, MA: Butterworth-Heinemann.

Bauer, D. J., Goldfield, B. A., & Reznick, J. S. (2002). Alternative approaches to analyzing individual differences in the rate of early vocabulary development. *Applied Psycholinguistics, 23,* 313–335.

Baum, B. J. (1986). Salivary gland function during aging. *Gerodontics, 2,* 61–64.

Baum, B. J. (1989). Salivary gland function secretion during aging. *Journal of the American Geriatric Society, 37,* 453–458.

Baumann, J. F., & Kameenui, E. J. (1991). Research on vocabulary instruction: Ode to Voltaire. In J. Flood, J. D. Lapp, & J. R. Squire (Eds.), *Handbook of research on teaching the English language arts* (pp. 604–632). New York, NY: Macmillan.

Baumgart, D., Johnson, J., & Helmstetter, E. (1990). *Augmentative and alternative communication systems for persons with moderate and severe disabilities.* Baltimore, MD: Paul H. Brookes.

Baxendale, J., & Hesketh, A. (2003). Comparison of the effectiveness of the Hanen Parent Programme and traditional clinic therapy. *International Journal of Language and Communication Disorders, 38,* 397–415.

Beals, D. E., DeTemple, J. M., & Dickinson, D. K. (1994). Talking and listening that support early literacy development of children from low-income families. In D. K. Dickinson (Ed.), *Bridges to literacy: Children, families, and schools* (pp. 1–15). Cambridge, MA: Blackwell.

Bear, D., & Templeton, S. (1998). Explorations in spelling: Foundations for learning and teaching phonics, spelling, and vocabulary. *Reading Teacher, 52,* 222–242.

Beck, I. L., & McKeown, M. G. (1991). Conditions of vocabulary acquisition. In R. Barr, M. Kamil, P. Mosenthalt, & P. D. Pearson (Eds.), *Handbook of reading research* (pp. 789–824). New York, NY: Longman.

Beck, I. L., McKeown, M. G., & Kucan, L. (2002). *Bringing words to life: Robust vocabulary instruction.* New York, NY: Guilford Press.

Beckman, M., & Edwards, J. (2000). The ontogeny of phonological categories and the primacy of lexical learning in linguistic development. *Child Development, 71,* 240–249.

Bedore, L. M., & Leonard, L. B. (1998). Specific language impairment and grammatical morphology: A discriminant function analysis. *Journal of Speech, Language, and Hearing Research, 41,* 1185–1192.

Beeson, P., Rising, K., & Volk, J. (2003). Writing treatment for severe aphasia: Who benefits? *Journal of Speech, Language, and Hearing Research, 46,* 1038–1050.

Beeson, P. M., & Robey, R. R. (2006). Evaluating single-subject treatment research: Lessons learned from the aphasia literature. *Neuropsychology Review, 16,* 161–169.

Beeson, P. M., & Robey, R. R. (2008, May). *Meta-analyses of aphasia treatment outcomes: Examining the evidence.* Invited platform presentation at the Annual Clinical Aphasiology Conference, Jackson Hole, WY.

Bellinger, D. (1980). Consistency in the pattern of change in mother's speech: Some discriminant analysis. *Journal of Child Language, 22,* 89–106.

Bello, J. (1995). *Communication facts.* Rockville, MD: ASHA.

Benelli, B., Belacchi, C., Gini, G., & Lucanggeli, D. (2006). "To define means to say what you know about things": The development of definitions skills as metalinguistic acquisition. *Journal of Child Language, 33,* 71–97.

Bennett, A. T. (1982). Discourses of power, the dialects of understanding the power of literacy. *Journal of Education, 165,* 53–74.

Bennett-Kaster, T. (1986). Cohesion and predication in child narrative. *Journal of Child Language, 13,* 353–370.

Berglund, E., Eriksson, M., & Johansson, I. (2001). Parental reports of spoken language skills in children with Down syndrome. *Journal of Speech and Hearing Research, 44,* 179–191.

Berliss, J., Borden, P., & Vanderheiden, G. (1989). *Trace resource book: Assistive technologies for communication, control, and computer access.* Madison, WI: Trace Research & Development Center.

Berman, R. (1986). A crosslinguistic perspective: Morphology and syntax. In P. Fletcher & M. Garman (Eds.), *Language acquisition* (2nd ed.). New York, NY: Cambridge University Press.

Bernhardt, B., & Stoel-Gammon, C. (1994). Nonlinear phonology: Introduction and clinical application. *Journal of Speech, Language, and Hearing Research, 37,* 123–143.

Bernstein, D. K., & Tiegerman-Farber, E. (2009). *Language and communication disorders in children* (6th ed.). Boston, MA: Pearson.

Bernstein Ratner, N., & Benitez, M. (1985). Linguistic analysis of a bilingual stutterer. *Journal of Fluency Disorders, 10,* 211–219.

Bernthal, J. E., & Bankson, N. W. (1988). *Articulation disorders* (2nd ed.). Englewood Cliffs, NJ: Prentice-Hall.

Bernthal, J. E., & Bankson, N. W. (1998). *Articulation disorders* (4th ed.). Englewood Cliffs, NJ: Prentice-Hall.

Bernthal, J. E., & Beukelman, D. R. (1977). The effect of changes in velopharyngeal orifice area on vowel intensity. *Cleft Palate Journal, 14,* 63–77.

Bertram, U. (1967). Saliva, xerostomia, clinical aspects pathology and pathogenesis. *Acta Odon of Scandinavia, 25* (Suppl. 49), 1–126.

Bess, F., Lichtenstein, M., & Logan, S. (1990). Audiologic assessment of the hearing-impaired elderly. In W. B. Rintelmann (Ed.), *Hearing assessment* (pp. 511–548). Austin, TX: Pro-Ed.

Beukelman, D. R., & Ansel, B. M. (1995). Research priorities in augmentative and alternative communication. *AAC, 11,* 131–134.

Beukelman, D. R., & Garrett, K. L. (1988). Augmentative and alternative communication for adults with acquired severe communication disorders. *Augmentative and Alternative Communication, 4,* 104–121.

Beukelman, D. R., & Mirenda, P. (1992). *Augmentative and alternative communication: Management of severe communication disorders in children and adults.* Baltimore, MD: Paul H. Brookes.

Beukelman, D. R., & Mirenda, P. (1998). *Augmentative and alternative communication: Management of severe communication disorders in children and adults* (2nd ed.). Baltimore, MD: Paul H. Brookes.

Beukelman, D. R., & Yorkston, K. M. (1989). Augmentative and alternative communication application for persons with severe acquired communication disorders: An introduction. *Augmentative and Alternative Communication, 5,* 42–48.

Beukelman, D. R., Yorkston, K. M., & Reichle, J. (Eds.). (2000). *Augmentative alternative communication for adults with acquired neurologic disorders.* Baltimore, MD: Paul H. Brookes.

Bialystok, E., Luk, G., & Kwan, E. (2005). Bilingualism, language proficiency, and learning to read in two writing systems. *Journal of Educational Psychology, 97,* (580–590).

Bird, J., Bishop, D. V. M., & Freeman, N. H. (1995). Phonological awareness and literacy development in children with expressive phonological impairments. *Journal of Speech and Hearing Research, 38,* 446–462.

Bishop, D. V. M., & Adams, C. (1990). A prospective study of the relationship between specific language impairment, phonological disorders and reading retardation. *Journal of Child Psychology and Psychiatry, 31,* 1027–1050.

Blachman, B. A. (1989). Phonological awareness and word recognition: Assessment and intervention. In A. G. Kamhi & H. W. Catts (Eds.), *Reading disabilities: A developmental language perspective* (pp. 133–158). Boston, MA: College-Hill Press.

Blachman, B. A. (1994). Early literacy acquisition: The role of phonological awareness. In G. P. Wallach & K. G. Butler (Eds.), *Language learning disabilities in school-age children and adolescents* (pp. 253–274). Boston, MA: Allyn & Bacon.

Blackman, J. A. (1990). *Medical aspects of developmental disabilities in children birth to three* (2nd ed.). Rockville, MD: Aspen.

Blank, M., Marquis, M. A., & Klimovitch, M. O. (1994). *Directing school discourse.* Tucson, AZ: Communication Skill Builders.

Bless, D. M., & Hicks, D. M. (1996). Diagnosis and measurement: Assessing the "WHs" of voice function. In W. S. Brown, B. Vinson, & M. Crary (Eds.), *Organic voice disorders: Assessment and treatment.* San Diego, CA: Singular Publishing Group.

Blischak, D. M., Gorman, A., & Lombardino, L. J. (2003). Application of current literacy theory, efficacy research, and clinical practice to AAC users. In R. W. Schlosser (Ed.), *The efficacy of augmentative and alternative communication: Toward evidence-based practice* (pp. 427–448). San Diego, CA: Academic Press.

Blischak, D. M., & Lloyd, L. L. (1996). Multimodal augmentative and alternative communication: Case study. *Augmentative and Alternative Communication, 12,* 37–46.

Bliss, C. (1965). *Semantography.* Sydney, Australia: Semantography Publications.

Blom, E. D. (1995). Tracheoesophageal speech. *Seminars in Speech and Language, 16*(3), 191–204.

Blom, E. D., Singer, M. I., & Hamaker, R. C. (1998). *Tracheoesophageal voice restoration following total laryngectomy.* Florence, KY: Thompson Learning.

Bloodstein, O. (1960a). The development of stuttering: I. Changes in nine basis features. *Journal of Speech and Hearing Disorders, 25,* 219–237.

Bloodstein, O. (1960b). The development of stuttering: II. Development phases. *Journal of Speech and Hearing Disorders, 25,* 366–376.

Bloodstein, O. (1975). *A handbook on stuttering.* Chicago, IL: National Easter Seal Society for Crippled Children and Adults.

Bloodstein, O. (1995). *A handbook on stuttering.* San Diego, CA: Singular Publishing Group.

Bloodstein, O., & Bernstein Ratner, N. (October 25, 2007). *A handbook on stuttering* (6'th ed.). New York, NY: Delmar Cengage Learning.

Bloom, L. (1970). *Language development: Form and function of merging grammars.* Cambridge, MA: MIT Press.

Bloom, L. (1973). *One word at a time: The use of single-word utterances before syntax.* The Hague, Netherlands: Mouton.

Bloom, L., & Lahey, M. (1978). *Language development and language disorders.* New York, NY: Wiley.

Bloom, L., Lahey, P., Hood, L., Lifter, K., & Fiess, K. (1980). Complex sentences: Acquisition of syntactic connectors and the semantic relations they encode. *Journal of Child Language, 7,* 235–262.

Bloomberg, K. (1985). *Compics: Computer pictographs for communication.* Presented on behalf of the Victorian Symbol Standardization Committee at the Australian Group on Severe Communication Impairment Study Day, Melbourne, Australia.

Boone, D. R., & McFarlane, S. C. (1994). *The voice and voice therapy* (5th ed.). Englewood Cliffs, NJ: Prentice-Hall.

Boone, D. R., & McFarlane, S. C. (2000). *The voice and voice therapy* (6th ed.). Boston: Allyn & Bacon.

Bornstein, M. H., Cote, L. R., Maital, S., Painter, K., Park, S., Pascual, L., . . . Vyt, A. (2004). Cross-linguistic analysis of vocabulary in young children: Spanish, Dutch, French, Hebrew, Italian, Korean, and American English. *Child Development, 75,* 1115–1139.

Bosch, L., & Sebastián-Gallés, N. (1997). Native-language recognition abilities in 4-month-old infants from monolingual and bilingual envirinment. *Cognition, 65*(2), 33–69.

Botting, N., Simkin, Z., & Conti-Ramsden, G. (2006). Associated reading skills in children with a history of Specific Language Impairment (SLI). *Reading and writing, 19,* 77–98.

Boudreau, D. M., & Chapman, R. S. (2000). The relationship between event representation and linguistic skill in narratives of children and adolescents with Down syndrome. *Journal of Speech, Language, and Hearing Research, 43,* 1146–1159.

Bowerman, M. (1974). Discussion summary—Development of concepts underlying language. In R. Schiefelbusch & L. Lloyd (Eds.), *Language perspectives: Acquisition, retardation and intervention.* Baltimore, MD: University Park Press.

Brazelton, T. B., & Greenspan, S. I. (2000). *The irreducible needs of children: What every child must have to grow, learn and flourish.* Cambridge, MA: Perseus.

Bredekamp, S., & Copple, C. (Eds.). (1997). *Developmentally appropriate practice in early childhood programs* (Rev. ed.). Washington, DC: National Association for the Education of Young Children.

Brice, A. E. (2002). *The Hispanic child: Speech, language, culture and education.* Boston, MA: Allyn & Bacon.

Bricker, D., & Squires, J. (1999). *Ages and stages questionnaires: A parent-completed, child-monitoring system* (2nd ed.). Baltimore, MD: Paul H. Brookes.

Bridges, S. J. (2004). Multicultural issues in augmentative and alternative communication and language: Research to practice. *Topics in Language Disorders, 24,* 62–75.

Bridges, S., Funk, J., Kovach, T. M., Lykes, A., Stuart, S., & Zangari, C. (1994). Communicating diversity: "The essence of life"—Five case studies. (Short course at ASHA, New Orleans, Nov. 20.)

Brinton, B., & Fujiki, M. (1984). Development of topic manipulation skills in discourse. *Journal of Speech and Hearing Research, 27,* 350–358.

Brinton, B., & Fujiki, M. (1989). *Conversational management with language-impaired children: Pragmatic assessment and intervention.* Rockville, MD: Aspen.

Brinton, B., & Fujiki, M. (1993). Language, social skills, and socioemotional behavior. *Language, Speech, and Hearing Services in Schools, 24,* 194–198.

Brinton, B., & Fujiki, M. (2004). Social and affective factors in language impairments and literacy learning. In C. A. Stone, E. R. Silliman, B. J. Ehren, & K. Apel (Eds.), *Handbook of language and literacy: Development and disorders* (pp. 130–153). New York, NY: Guilford Press.

Brinton, B., & Fujiki, M. (2005). Social competence in children with language impairment: Making connections. *Seminars in Speech and Language, 26*(3), 151–159.

Brinton, B., Fujiki, M., & Higbee, L. M. (1998). Participation in cooperative learning activities by children with specific language impairment. *Journal of Speech, Language, and Hearing Research, 41,* 1193–1206.

Brinton, B., Fujiki, M., & McKee, L. (1998). Negotiation skills of children with specific language impairment. *Journal of Speech, Language, and Hearing Research, 41,* 927–940.

Brinton, B., Robinson, L. A., & Fujiki, M. (2004). Description of a program for social language intervention: "If you can have a conversation, you can have a relationship." *Language, Speech, and Hearing Services in Schools, 35,* 283–290.

Brinton, B., Spackman, M. P., Fujiki, M., & Ricks, J. (2007). What should Chris say? The ability of children with specific language impairment to recognize the need to dissemble emotions in social situations. *Journal of Speech, Language, and Hearing Research, 50,* 798-811.

Bristol, M. M. (1984). Family resources and successful adaptation to autistic children. In E. Schopler & G. B. Mesibov (Eds.), *The effects of autism on the family* (pp. 289–310). New York, NY: Plenum.

Britto, P. R., & Brooks-Gunn, J. (2001). Beyong shared book reading: Dimensions of home literacy and low-income African American preschoolers' skills. In P. Britto & J. Brooks-Gunn (Eds.), *The role of family literacy environments in promoting young children's emergent literacy skill* (pp. 73–90). San Francisco, CA: Jossey-Bass.

Britton, J. (1990). Talking to learn. In D. Barnes, J. Britton, & M. Tobe (Eds.), *Language, the learner, and the school* (4th ed.). Portsmouth, NH: Heinemann.

Britton, J. (1993). *Language and learning* (2nd ed.). Portsmouth, NH: Boynton/Cook Publishers.

Broen, P. A., Devers, M. C., Doyle, S. S., Prouty, J. M., & Moller, K. T. (1998, June). Acquisition of linguistic and cognitive skills by children with cleft palate. *Journal of Speech, Language, and Hearing Research, 41*(3), 676–687.

Brown, R. (1973). *A first language: The early stages.* Cambridge, MA: Harvard University Press.

Bruestedt, A. (1983). Age-induced changes in the oral mucosa and their therapeutic consequences. *International Dental Journal, 33*(3), 272–280.

Brutten, E. J., & Shoemaker, D. J. (1967). *The modification of stuttering.* Englewood Cliffs, NJ: Prentice-Hall.

Bryngelson, B. (1955). Voluntary stuttering. In C. Van Riper (Ed.), *Speech therapy: A book of readings.* Englewood Cliffs, NJ: Prentice-Hall.

Bryson, S. (1996). Brief report: Epidemiology of autism. *Journal of Autism and Developmental Disorders, 26,* 165–168.

Burkard, R., & McNerney, K. (2009). Introduction to auditory evoked potentials. In J. Katz, L. Medwetsky, R. Burkard, & L. Hood (Eds.), *Handbook of clinical audiology,* (pp. 222–241). Baltimore, MD: Lippincott Williams & Wilkins.

Burlingame, G. (2007). *Wedding evidence-based practice with practice-based evidence: Methods for maximizing patients' outcomes.* Invited address at annual conference of Michigan Association of Community Mental Health Boards, Lansing, MI.

Burns, M. S., Griffin, P., & Snow, C. (Eds.). (1999). *Starting out right: A guide to promoting children's reading success.* Washington. DC: National Academy Press.

Burns, M. S., Halper, A. S., & Mogil, S. I. (1985). *Clinical management of right hemisphere dysfunction.* Gaithersburg, MD: Aspen.

Buzolich, M. J., & Lunger, J. (1995). Empowering system users in peer training. *Augmentative and Alternative Communication, 11,* 37–48.

Byrne, B., & Fielding-Barnsley, R. (1991). *Sound foundations.* Sydney, Australia: Peter Leyden Educational.

Cain, K., Patson, N., & Andrews, L. (2005). Age- and ability-related differences in young readers' use of conjunctions. *Journal of Child Language, 32,* 877–892.

Calandrella, A. M., & Wilcox, M. J. (2000). Predicting language outcomes for prelinguisitc children with developmental delay. *Journal of Speech, Language, and Hearing Research, 43,* 1061–1071.

Calnan, J. S. (1954). Submucous cleft palate. *British Journal of Plastic Surgery, 6,* 164–168.

Camarata, S., & Nelson, K. E. (2006). Conversational recast intervention with preschool and older children. In R. McCauley & M. Fey (Eds.), *Treatment of language disorders in children* (pp. 237–264). Baltimore, MD: Paul H. Brookes.

Canale, M. (1983). From communicative competence to communicative language pedagogy. In J. C. Richards & R. W. Schmit (Eds.), *Language and communication* (pp. 2–27). White Plains, NY: Longman.

Capone, N. C., & McGregor, K. K. (2004). Gesture development: A review for clinical and research practices. *Journal of Speech, Language, and Hearing Research, 47,* 173–186.

Carlson, F. (1984). *Picsyms categorical dictionary.* Lawrence, KS: Baggeboda Press.

Carr, E. G., & Durand, V. M. (1985). Reducing behavior problems through functional communication training. *Journal of Applied Behavior Analysis, 18,* 111–126.

Carroll, D. (2008). *Psychology of language* (5th ed.). Pacific Grove, CA: Brooks/Cole.

Caruso, A. J., Sonies, B. C., Fox, P. C., & Atkinson, J. (1989). Objective measures of swallowing in patients with primary Sjogren's syndrome. *Dysphagia 4*(2), 101–105.

Carvill, S. (2001). Sensory impairments, intellectual disability and psychiatry. *Journal of Intellectual Disability Research, 45,* 467–483.

Caselli, M. C., Vicari, S., Longobardi, E., Lami, L., Pizzoli, C., & Stella, G. (1998). Gestures and words in early development of children with Down syndrome. *Journal of Speech, Language, and Hearing Research, 41,* 1125–1135.

Casper, J. K., & Colton, R. H. (1998). *Clinical manual for laryngectomy and head and neck cancer rehabilitation.* San Diego, CA: Singular Publishing Group.

Castell, J. A. (1995). Esophageal manometry. In D. O. Castell (Ed.), *The esophagus* (2nd ed.). Boston, MA: Little, Brown.

Catts, H. W. (1997). The early identification of language-based reading disabilities. *Language, Speech, and Hearing Services in Schools, 28,* 86–87.

Catts, H. W., Fey, M. E., Tomblin, J. B., & Zhang, X. (2002). A longitudinal investigation of reading outcomes in children with language impairments. *Journal of Speech, Language, and Hearing Research, 45,* 1142–1157.

Catts, H. W., Fey, M., Zhang, X., & Tomblin, J. B. (1999). Language basis of reading and reading disabilities: Evidence from a longitudinal investigation. *Scientific Studies of Reading, 3,* 331–361.

Catts, H. W., Fey, M., Zhang, X., & Tomblin, J. B. (2001). Estimating the risk of future reading difficulties in kindergarten children: A research-based model and its clinical instrumentation. *Language, Speech, and Hearing Services in Schools, 32,* 38–50.

Catts, H. W., & Kamhi, A. G. (2005). Causes of reading disabilities. In H. W. Catts & A. G. Kamhi (Eds.), *Language and reading disabilities.* Boston, MA: Allyn & Bacon.

Cazden, C. (1988). *Classroom discourse: The language of teaching and learning.* Portsmouth, NH: Heinemann.

Chang, J., Lai, A. Y., & Shimizu, W. (1995). LEP parents as resources: Generating opportunity to learn beyond schools through parental involvement. In L. L. Cheng (Ed.), *Integrating language and learning for inclusion: An Asian-Pacific focus* (pp. 265–290). San Diego, CA: Singular Publishing Group.

Chang, S. E., Erickson, K. I., Ambrose, N. G., Hasegowa-Johnson, M. A., & Ludlow, C. L. (2008). Brain anatomy differences in childhood stuttering. *Neuro Image, 39,* 1333–1344.

Chapman, K. L., Hardin-Jones, M. A., Schulte, J., & Halter, K. A. (2001). Vocal development of 9-month-old babies with cleft palate. *Journal of Speech, Language, and Hearing Research, 44*(6), 1268.

Chapman, R. (1992). *Childtalk: Processes in child language acquisition.* St. Louis, MO: Mosby.

Chapman, R. S., Hesketh, L. J., & Kistler, D. J. (2002). Predicting longitudinal change in language production and comprehension in individuals with Down syndrome: Hierarchical linear modeling. *Journal of Speech, Language, and Hearing Research, 45,* 902–915.

Chapman, R., & Miller, J. (1980). Analyzing language and communication in the child. In R. C. Schiefelbusch (Ed.), *Nonspeech language and communication: Acquisition and intervention* (pp. 159–196) Baltimore, MD: University Park Press.

Chapman, R. S., Seung, H. K., Schwartz, S. E., & Kay-Raining Bird, E. (1998). Language skills of children and adolescents with Down syndrome: II. Production deficits. *Journal of Speech, Language, and Hearing Research, 41,* 861–873.

Chen, K. T., Wu, J., & Noordhoff, S. M. (1994). Submucous cleft palate. *Chang Keng I Hsueh, 17*(2), 131–137.

Chen, P. K., Wu, J., Hung, K. F., Chen, Y. R., & Noordhoff, M. S. (1996). Surgical correction of submucous cleft palate with Furlow palatoplasty. *Plastic and Reconstructive Surgery, 97*(6), 1136–46; discussion 1147–1149.

Chenery, H. J. (1998). Perceptual analysis of dysarthric speech. In B. E. Murdock (Ed.), *Dysarthria: A physiological approach to assessment and treatment* (pp. 36–37). Cheltenham, England: Stanley-Thornes.

Cheng, L. (1987). Cross-cultural and linguistic considerations in working with Asian populations. *ASHA, 29*(6), 33–37.

Cheng, L. (Ed.). (1991). *Assessing Asian language performance: Guidelines for evaluating LEP students.* Oceanside, CA: Academic Communication Associates.

Cheng, L. L. (2007, May 29). Codes and contexts: Exploring linguistic, cultural, and social intelligence. *The ASHA Leader,* pp. 8–9, 32–33.

Cheng, L., & Chang, J. (1995). Asian/Pacific Islander students in need of effective services. In H. Kayser (Ed.), *Bilingual speech-language pathology: A Hispanic focus.* San Diego, CA: Singular Publishing Group.

Cherney, L., Halper, A., Holland, A., & Cole, R. (2008). Computerized script training for aphasia: Preliminary finding. *American Journal of Speech-Language Pathology, 17,* 19–34.

Cherney, L., Patterson, J., Raymer, A., Frymark, T., & Schooling, T. (2008). Evidence-based systematic review: Effects of intensity of treatment and constraint-induced language therapy for individuals with stroke-induced aphasia. *Journal of Speech, Language, and Hearing Research, 51,* 1282–1229.

Cherry, J., & Margulies, S. (1968). Contact ulcer of the larynx. *Laryngoscope, 78,* 1937–1940.

Chodosh, P. L. (1977). Gastro-esophagopharyngeal reflux. *Laryngoscope, 87,* 418–427.

Chomsky, N. (1965). *Aspects of the theory of syntax.* Cambridge, MA: MIT Press.

Chouinard, M. M., & Clark, E. V. (2003). Adult reformulations of child errors as negative evidence. *Journal of Child Language, 30,* 637–669.

Cirrin, F. M. (1994). Assessing language in the classroom and the curriculum. In J. B. Tomblin, H. L. Morris, & R. D. C.

Spriesterback (Eds.), *Diagnosis in speech-language pathology.* San Diego, CA: Singular Publishing group.

Clark, E. (1990). On the pragmatics of contrast. *Journal of Child Language, 17,* 417–431.

Clark, H., Hensen, P., Barber, W. D., Stierwalt, J., & Sherrill, M. (2003). Relationships among subjective and objective measures of tongue strength and oral phase swallowing impairments. *American Journal of Speech-Language Pathology, 12,* 40–50.

Cleave, P., & Rice, M. (1997). An examination of the morpheme BE in children with specific language impairment: The role of contractibility and grammatical form class. *Journal of Speech, Language, and Hearing Research, 40,* 480–492.

Coady, J. A., & Aslin, R. N. (2003). Phonological neighbour-hoods in the developing lexicon. *Journal of Child Language, 30,* 441–469.

Code of Fair Testing Practices in Education. (1988). Washington, DC: Joint Committee on Testing Practices.

Coggins, T. (1998). Clinical assessment of emerging language: How to gather evidence and make informed decisions. In A. M. Wetherby, S. F. Warren, & J. Reichle (Eds.), *Transitions in prelinguistic communication.* Baltimore, MD: Paul H. Brookes.

Cohen, C. G., & Palin, M. W. (1986). Speech syntheses and speech recognition devices. In M. L. Grossfeld & C. A. Grossfeld (Eds.), *Microcomputer application in rehabilitation of communication disorders* (pp. 183–211). Rockville, MD: Aspen.

Cohen, D. J., Klin, A., McSweeny, J. L., Paul, R., Shriberg, L. D., & Volkmar, F. R. (2001). Speech and prosody characteristics of adolescents and adults with high-functioning autism and Asperger syndrome. *Journal of Speech, Language, and Hearing Research, 44,* 1097–1115.

Cohen, M., Polley, J. W., & Figueroa, A. A. (1993). Secondary (intermediate) alveolar bone grafting. *Clinical Plastic Surgery, 20*(4), 691–705.

Coleman, M. A., Roth, F. P., & West, T. (2009). Roadmap to pre-K RTI: Applying response to intervention to preschool settings. New York, NY: National Center for Learning Disabilities.

Coleman, T. J. (2000). *Clinical management of communication disorders in culturally diverse children.* Boston, MA: Allyn & Bacon.

Colton, R. H., & Casper, J. K. (1990). *Understanding voice problems: A physiological perspective for diagnosis and treatment.* Baltimore, MD: Williams & Wilkins.

Compher, C., Kim, J. N., & Bader, J. G. (1998). Nutritional requirements of an aging population with emphasis on subacute care patients, *AAN Clinical Issues, 9*(3), 441–450.

Cone-Wesson, B., Dowell, R. C., Tomlin, D., Rance, G., & Ming, W. J. (2002) The auditory steady-state response: Comparisons with the auditory brainstem response. *Journal of the American Academy of Audiology, 13*(4), 173–187.

Conte, B. M. (1993). *The effect of genre, vocabulary, and syntax on the comprehension of expository text in language impaired and non-impaired adolescents* (Unpublished doctoral dissertation). Boston University, MA.

Conti-Ramsden, G., Botting, N., & Faragher, B. (2001). Psycholinguistic markers for specific language impairment (SLI). *Journal of Child Psychology and Psychiatry, 42,* 741–748.

Conture, E. G., & Curlee, R. F. (2007). *Stuttering and related disorders of fluency* (3rd ed.). New York, NY: Thieme.

Conture, E. G., McCall, G., & Brewer, D. W. (1977). Laryngeal behavior during stuttering. *Journal of Speech and Hearing Research, 20,* 661–668.

Conture, E. G., & Yaruss, J. S. (2004). *Treatment efficacy summary: Stuttering.* Retrieved July 2004, from www.asha.org/members/slp/healthcare/efficacy.htm

Cook, I. J., Dodds, W. J., Dantas, R. O., Massey, B., Kern, M. K., Lang, I. M., . . . Hogan, W. J. (1989). Opening mechanisms of the human upper esophageal sphincter. *American Journal of Physiology, 257,* G748–G759.

Cooper, D. H., Roth, F. P., Speece, D. L., & Schatschneider, C. (2002). The contribution of oral language skills to the development of phonological awareness. *Applied Psycholinguistics, 23,* 399–416.

Cooper, E. B., & Cooper, C. S. (1985). *Personalized fluency control therapy.* Allen, TX: DLM.

Cooper, E. B., & Cooper, C. S. (1998). Multicultural considerations in the assessment and treatment of stuttering. In D. E. Battle (Ed.), *Communication disorders in multicultural populations* (pp. 247–274). Boston, MA: Butterworth-Heinemann.

Cowart, B. J. (1989). Relationship between taste and smell across the adult life span. In C. Murphy, W. S. Cain, & D. M. Hegsted (Eds.), *Nutrition and the chemical senses in aging: Recent advances and current research needs* (pp. 39–55). New York, NY: Annals of the New York Academy of Sciences.

Cox, R., & Alexander, G. (1995). The abbreviated profile of hearing aid benefit. *Ear and Hearing, 16,* 176–186.

Coyle, J. L. (2002). Critical appraisal of a treatment publication: Electrical stimulation for the treatment of dysphagia. *Perspectives on Swallowing and Swallowing Disorders, ASHA Division 13 Newsletter, 11*(4), 12–15.

Crago, M. (1990). Development of communicative competence in Inuit children: Implications for speech-language pathology. *Journal of Childhood Communication Disorders, 13,* 73–83.

Craig, H. (1993). Social skills of children with specific language impairment: Peer relationships. *Language, Speech, and Hearing Services in Schools, 24,* 206–215.

Craig, H. K., Washington, J. A., & Thompson-Porter, C. (1998). Average c-unit lengths in the discourse of African American children from low-income, urban homes. *Journal of Speech, Language, and Hearing Research, 41,* 433–444.

Crais, E. R. (1995). Expanding the repertoire of tools and techniques for assessing the communication skills of infants and toddlers. *American Journal of Speech-Language Pathology, 4,* 47–58.

Crary, M. A., & Groher, M. E. (2003). *Introduction to adult swallowing disorders.* St. Louis, MO: Butterworth-Heinemann.

Creaghead, N., Newman, P., & Secord, W. (1989). *Assessment and remediation of articulatory and phonological disorders* (2nd ed.). Columbus, OH: Merrill.

Creaghead, N. A., & Tattershall, S. S. (1991). Observation and assessment of classroom language skills. In C. S. Simon (Ed.), *Communication skills and classroom success: Assessment and therapy methodologies for language and learning disabled students* (pp. 106–124). Eau Claire, WI: Thinking Publications.

Cregan, A. (1980). *Sigsymbols* [Videotape]. Watford, England: Chiltern Consortium.

Cregan, A., & Lloyd, L. L. (1990). *Sigsymbols: American edition.* Wauconda, IL: Don Johnston Developmental Equipment.

Cress, C. J., & Marvin, C. A. (2003). Common questions about AAC services in early intervention. *Augmentative and Alternative Communication, 19,* 254–272.

Croft, C. B., Shprintzen, R. J., Daniller, A. I., & Lewin, M. L. (1978). The occult submucous cleft palate and the musculus uvuli. *Cleft Palate Journal, 15,* 150–154.

Croft, C. B., Shprintzen, R. J., & Rakoff, S. J. (1981). Patterns of velopharyngeal valving in normal and cleft palate subjects: A multi-view videofluoroscopic and nasendoscopic study. *Laryngoscope, 91,* 265–271.

Croft, C. B., Shprintzen, R. J., & Ruben, R. J. (1981). Hypernasal speech following adenotonsillectomy. *Otolaryngology—Head and Neck Surgery, 89,* 179–188.

Crone, D. A., & Whitehurst, G. J. (1999). Age and schooling effects on emergent literacy and early reading skills. *Journal of Educational Psychology, 91,* 604–614.

Crown, C. L., Feldstein, S., Jasnow, M. D., Beebe, B., & Jaffe, J. (2002). The cross-modal coordination of interpersonal timing: Six-week-old infants' gaze with adults' vocal behavior. *Journal of Psycholinguistic Research, 31,* 1–23.

Culatta, B., & Hall, K. (2006). Phonological awareness instruction in early childhood settings. In L. M. Justice (Ed.), *Clinical approaches to emergent literacy intervention.* San Diego, CA: Plural.

Culatta, B., & Kovarsky, D. (2003). Quantitative and qualitative documentation of early rhyme instruction. *American Journal of Speech-Language Pathology, 12,* 172–188.

Culp, D. M., & Carlisle, M. (1988). *Partners in augmentative training: A resource guide for interaction facilitation training for children.* Tucson, AZ: Communication Skills Builders.

Culton, G. L., & Gerwin, J. M. (1998). Current trends in laryngectomy rehabilitation: A summary of speech-language pathologists. *Otolaryngology—Head and Neck Surgery, 118,* 458–463.

Cummings, M. (1997). *Human heredity* (4th ed.). Eagan, MD: West/Wadsworth.

Cummins, J. (1984). *Bilingualism and special education: Issues in assessment and pedagogy.* Austin, TX: Pro-Ed.

Cunningham, E. T., & Jones, B. (2003). Anatomical and physiological overview. In B. Jones (Ed.), *Normal and abnormal swallowing* (pp. 11–34). New York, NY: Springer-Verlag.

Curlee, R. F. (1980). A case selection strategy for young disfluent children. In W. Perkins (Ed.), *Seminars in speech-language-hearing: Strategies in stuttering therapy* (pp. 277–287). New York, NY: Thieme-Stratton.

Czeizel, A. E., & Dudás, V. (1992). Prevention of the first occurrence of neural-tube defects by periconceptional vitamin supplementation. *New England Journal of Medicine, 327*(26), 1832–1835.

D'Antonio, L. L., Eichenberg, B. J., Zimmerman, G. J., Patel, S., Riski, J. E., Herber, S. C., & Hardesty, R. A. (2000). Radiographic and aerodynamic measures of velopharyngeal anatomy and function following Furlow Z-plasty. *Plastic and Reconstructive Surgery, 106*(3), 539–549; discussion 550–553.

D'Antonio, L. L., Snyder, L. S., & Samadani, S. (1996). Tonsillectomy in children with or at risk for velopharyngeal insufficiency: Effects on speech. *Otolaryngology—Head and Neck Surgery, 115,* 319–323.

D'Odorico, L., Cassibba, R., & Salerni, N. (1997). Temporal relationships between gaze and vocal behavior in prelinguistic and linguistic communication. *Journal of Psycholinguistic Research, 26,* 539–556.

D'Odorico, L., & Franco, F. (1985). The determinants of baby talk: Relationship to context. *Journal of Child Language, 12,* 567–586.

Dale, P. S. (1991). The validity of a parent report measure of vocabulary and syntax at 24 months. *Journal of Speech and Hearing Sciences, 34,* 565–571.

Daly, D. A. (1992). Helping the clutterer: Therapy considerations. In F. Myers & K. St. Louis (Eds.), *Cluttering: A clinical perspective.* Leicester, England: FAR Communications.

Daly, N., Bench, J., & Chappell, H. (1997). Gender differences in visual speech variables. *Journal of the Academy of Rehabilitative Audiology, 30,* 62–76.

Damico, J. S. (1991a). Clinical discourse analysis: A functional approach to language assessment. In C. S. Simon (Ed.), *Communication skills and classroom success: Assessment and therapy methodologies for language and learning disabled students* (pp. 125–148). Eau Claire, WI: Thinking Publications.

Damico, J. S. (1991b). Descriptive assessment of communicative ability in limited English proficient students. In E. Hamayan & J. Damico (Eds.), *Limiting bias in the assessment of bilingual students.* Austin, TX: Pro-Ed.

Damico, J. S. (1992). Systematic observation of communicative interaction: A valid and practical descriptive assessment technique. *Best Practices in School Speech-Language Pathology, 3,* 133–143.

Damico, J. S., & Hamayan, E. V. (1992). *Multicultural language intervention.* Buffalo, NY: Educom.

Daniels, S. K. (2004). *Neurological disorders and dysphagia.* Presented at the Charleston Swallowing Conference: State of the Science in Practice, Charleston, SC.

Daniels, S. K., & Foundas, A. L. (1997). The role of the insular cortex in dysphagia. *Dysphagia, 12,* 146–156.

Daniels, S. K., Foundas, A. L., Iglesia, G. C., & Sullivan, M. A. (1996). Lesion site in unilateral stroke patients with dysphagia. *Journal of Stroke and Cerebrovascular Disorders, 6,* 30–34.

Darley, F. L. (1982). *Aphasia.* Philadelphia, PA: W. B. Saunders.

Darley, F. L., Aronson, A. E., & Brown, J. R. (1969a). Differential diagnostic patterns of clysarthria. *Journal of Speech and Hearing Research, 12,* 246–269.

Darley, F. L., Aronson, A. E., & Brown, J. R. (1969b). Clusters of deviant speech dimensions in the dysarthrias. *Journal of Speech and Hearing Research, 12,* 462–496.

Darley, F. L., Aronson, A. R., & Brown, J. R. (1975). *Motor speech disorders.* Philadelphia, PA: W. B. Saunders.

Davis, D. M. (1939). The relation of repetitions in the speech of young children to certain measures of language maturity and situational factors. Part I. *Journal of Speech and Hearing Disorders, 4,* 303–318.

Davis, D. M. (1940). The relation of repetitions in the speech of young children to certain measures of language maturity and situational factors. Parts II and III. *Journal of Speech and Hearing Disorders, 5,* 235–246.

Davis, G. A., & Wilcox, M. J. (1981). Incorporating parameters of natural conversation in aphasia treatment. In R. Chapey (Ed.), *Language intervention strategies in adult aphasia.* Baltimore, MD: Williams & Wilkins.

Davis, G. A., & Wilcox, M. J. (1985). *Adult aphasia rehabilitation.* San Diego, CA: College-Hill Press.

Dawson, G., Hill, D., Spencer, A., Galpert, L., & Watson, L. (1990). Affective exchanges between young autistic children and their mothers. *Journal of Autism and Developmental Disorders, 28,* 479–485.

Dawson, G., & Osterling, J. (1997). Early intervention in autism. In M. Guralnick (Ed.), *The effectiveness of early intervention* (pp. 307–326). Baltimore, MD: Paul H. Brookes.

de Villiers, J., & de Villiers, P. (1973). Development of the use of word order in comprehension. *Journal of Psycholinguistic Research, 2,* 331–341.

Dean Qualls, C., O'Brien, R. M., Blood, G. W., & Scheffner Hammer, C. (2003). Contextual variation, familiarity, academic literacy, and rural adolescents' idiom knowledge. *Language, Speech, and Hearing Services in Schools, 34,* 69–79.

Deevy, P., & Leonard, L. (2004). The comprehension of wh-questions in children with specific language impairment. *Journal of Speech, Language, and Hearing Research, 47,* 802–815.

DeHart, G., & Maratsos, M. (1984). Children's acquisition of presuppositional usages. In R. Schiefelbusch & J. Pickar (Eds.), *The acquisition of communication process.* Baltimore, MD: University Park Press.

Dejaeger, E., Pelemans, W., Ponette, E., & Joosten, E. (1997). Mechanisms involved in postdeglutition retention in the elderly. *Dysphagia, 12*(2), 63–67.

Delahunty, J. E., & Cherry, J. (1968). Experimentally produced vocal cord granulomas. *Laryngoscope, 78,* 1941–1947.

Dell, C. W., Jr. (1996). *Treating the school age stutterer.* Memphis, TN: Stuttering Foundation of America.

DeLuke, D. M., Marchand, A., Robeles, E. C., & Fox, P. (1997). Facial growth and the need for orthognathic surgery after cleft palate repair: Literature review and report of 28 cases. *Journal of Oral and Maxillofacial Surgery, 55*(7), 694–697.

DeMeo, J. H. (1998). Collaborative partnerships and decision making. In D. Merritt & B. Culatta (Eds.), *Language intervention in the classroom.* San Diego, CA: Singular Publishing Group.

Demorest, M., & Erdman, S. (1986). Scale composition and item analysis for the communication profile for the hearing impaired. *Journal of Speech and Hearing Research, 29,* 226–240.

Denckla, M. B., & Rudel, R. (1976). Rapid "automatized" naming (R. A. N.): Dyslexia differentiated from other learning disabilities. *Neuropsychologia, 14,* 471–479.

Denes, P. B., & Pinson, E. N. (1963). *The speech chain.* New York, NY: Bell Telephone Laboratories.

Diamond, K., & Squires, J. (1993). The role of parental report in the screening and assessment of young children. *Journal of Early Intervention, 17,* 107–115.

Dickinson, D. K., & Tabors, P. O. (2001). *Young children learning at home and school: Beginning literacy with language.* Baltimore, MD: Paul H. Brookes.

Diefendorf, A. (2004). *Treatment efficacy summary: Hearing loss in children.* Retrieved July 2004, from www.asha.org/members/slp/healthcare/efficacy.htm

Dillon, H., James, A., & Ginis, J. (1997). Client Oriented Scale of Improvement (COSI) and its relationship to several other measures of benefit and satisfaction provided by hearing aids. *Journal of the American Academy of Audiology, 8,* 27–43.

DiMeo, J. H., Merritt, D., & Culatta, B. (1998). Collaborative partnerships and decision making. In D. Merritt & B. Culatta (Eds.), *Languages intervention in the classroom.* San Diego, CA: Singular Publishing Group.

Dimitrijevic, A., John, M. S., Van Roon, P., Purcell, D. W., Adamonis, J., Ostroff, J., . . . Picton, T. W. (2002), *Journal of the American Academy of Audiology, 13*(4), 205–224.

Dinkins, E. L., Norris, J. A., & Hoffman, P. R. (2006, November). Teaching language arts skills in context. *ADVANCE for Speech-Language Pathologists and Audiologists, 16*(47), 10–11.

Dixon, M. J. (1996). Treacher Collins syndrome. *Human Molecular Genetics,* 1996;5. 1391–1396.

Dodd, B., & Thompson, L. (2001). Speech disorder in children with Down's syndrome. *Journal of Intellectual Disability Research, 45,* 308–316.

Dodici, B. J., Draper, D. C., & Peterson, C. A. (2003). Early parent–child interactions and early literacy development. *Topics in Early Childhood Special Education, 23,* 27–47.

Dollaghan, C. (1994). Children's phonological neighborhoods: Half empty or half full. *Journal of Child Language, 21,* 257–271.

Dollaghan, C. (2004, April 13). Evidence-based practice myths and realities. *The ASHA Leader,* p. 12.

Domingue, B., Cutler, B., & McTarnaghan, J. (2000). The experience of autism in the lives of families. In A. Wetherby & B. Prizant (Eds.), *Autism spectrum disorders: A transactional developmental perspective* (pp. 369–393). Baltimore, MD: Paul H. Brookes.

Don, M. (2003). *Stacked ABR: Fundamentals and use in small tumor screening.* Paper presented at the 2003 American Academy of Audiology Convention, San Antonio, TX.

Don, M., & Kwong, B. (2009). Auditory brainsten response: Differential diagnosis. In J. Katz, L. Medwetsky, R. Burkard, & L. Hood (Eds.), *Handbook of clinical audiology* (pp. 265–292). Baltimore, MD: Lippincott Williams & Wilkins.

Donahue, M. L. (1994). Differences in classroom discourse styles of students with learning disabilities. In D. Ripich & N. Creaghead (Eds.), *School discourse problems* (2nd ed.). San Diego, CA: Singular Publishing Group.

Donahue, M. L., & Pidek, C. M. (1993). Listening comprehension and paraphrasing in content-area classrooms. *Journal of Childhood Communication Disorders, 15,* 35–42.

Donnellan, A. M., Mirenda, P. L., Mesaros, R. A., & Fassbender, L. L. (1984). Analyzing the communicative functions of aberrant behavior. *Journal of the Association for Persons with Severe Handicaps, 9*(3), 201–212.

Donnelly, M. J. (1994). Hypernasality following adenoid removal. *Irish Journal of Medical Science, 163*(5), 225–227.

Dore, J. (1979). Conversational acts and the acquisition of language. In E. Ochs & B. Schieffelin (Eds.), *Developmental pragmatics.* New York, NY: Academic Press.

Dore, J. (1986). The development of conversational competence. In R. L. Schiefelbusch (Ed.), *Language competence: Assessment and intervention* (pp. 3–60). San Diego, CA: College-Hill.

Dorland's Illustrated Medical Dictionary. (27th ed.). (1988). Philadelphia, PA: W. B. Saunders.

Doss, L. S., & Reichle, J. (1989). Establishing communicative alternatives to the emission of socially motivated excess behavior: A review. *Journal of the Association for Persons with Severe Handicaps, 14*(2), 101–112.

Dowden, P. A., & Marriner, N. A. (1995). Augmentative and alternative communication: Treatment principles and strategies. *Seminars in Speech and Language, 16,* 140–158.

Doyle, P. C. (1994). *Foundations of voice and speech rehabilitation following laryngeal cancer.* Florence, KY: Thomson Learning.

Doyle, P. J. (2002). Measuring health outcomes in stroke survivors. *Archives of Physical Medicine and Rehabilitation, 83,* (12 Suppl. 2), S39–S43.

Dunlap, K. (1932). *Habits: Their making and unmaking.* New York, NY: Liveright.

Dunlap, W. R. (1985). A functional classification system for the deaf-blind. *American Annals for Deaf, 130,* 236–243.

Duquette, C., Stodel, E., Fullarton, S., & Hagglund, K. (2006). Persistence in high school: Experiences of adolescents and young adults with fetal alcohol spectrum disorders. *Journal of Intellectual and Developmental Disability, 31,* 219–231.

Durand, V. M. (1990). *Severe behavior problems: A functional communication training approach.* New York, NY: Guilford Press.

Dziewas, R., Soros, P., Ishii, R., Chau, W., Henningsen, H., Ringelstein, E. B., . . . Pantev, C. (2003). Neuroimaging evidence for cortical involvement in the preparation and in the act of swallowing. *Neuroimage, 20,* 135–144.

Eadie, P. A., Fey, M. E., Douglas, J. M., & Parsons, C. L. (2002). Profiles of grammatical morphology and sentence imitation in children with specific language impairment and Down syndrome. *Journal of Speech, Language, and Hearing Research, 45,* 720–732.

Echols, C. H., Crowhurst, M. J., & Childers, J. B. (1997). Perception of rhythmic units in speech by infants and adults. *Journal of Memory and Language, 36,* 202–225.

Edmonds, L., & Kiran, S. (2006). Effect of semantic naming on cross-linguistic generalization in bilingual aphasia. *Journal of Speech, Language, and Hearing Research, 49,* 729–748.

Education for All Handicapped Children Act. (1975). P. L. 94–142, 20 U. S. C. §1400 *et seq.*

Education of the Handicapped Act. (1986). P. L. 99–457, 20 U. S. C. §1400 *et seq.*

Edmonds, L. D., & James, L. M. (1990). Temporal trends in the prevalence of congenital malformations at birth based on the birth defects monitoring program, United States, 1979–1987. *Morbidity and Mortality Weekly Report, 39*(4), 19–23.

Educational Audiology Association. (2001). *What do educational audiologist do?* Retrieved February 22, 2004, from www.edaud.org

Ehren, B. J. (2000, July). Views of cognitive referencing from the pragmatist's lens. *Language Learning and Education, ASHA Division 1 Newsletter,* 3–8.

Ehri, L. C. (1987). Learning to read and spell words. *Journal of Reading Behavior, 19,* 5–31.

Ehri, L. C. (1989). Movement into word reading and spelling: How spelling contributes to reading. In. J. M. Mason (Ed.), *Reading and writing connections* (pp. 65–81). Boston, MA: Allyn & Bacon.

Elbert, M., Rockman, B., & Saltzman, D. (1980). *Contrasts: The use of minimal pairs in articulation training.* Austin, TX: Exceptional Books.

Elliott, L. L., & Katz, J. (1980). *Northwestern University Children's Perception of Speech (NU-CHIPS).* St. Louis, MO: Auditec.

Ellis Weismer, S. (2007). Typical talkers, late talkers, and children with specific language impairment: A language endowment spectrum? In R. Paul (Ed.), *Language disorders from a developmental perspective* (pp. 83–101). Mahwah, NJ: Lawrence Erlbaum.

Ellis Weismer, S., Plante, E., Jones, M., & Tomblin, J. B. (2005). A functional magnetic resonance imaging investigation of verbal working memory in adolescents with specific language impairment. *Journal of Speech, Language, and Hearing Research, 48,* 405–425.

Elman, R., & Bernstein-Ellis, R. (1999). The efficacy of group communication treatment in adults with chronic aphasia. *Journal of Speech, Language, and Hearing Research, 42,* 411–419.

Erber, N., & Alencewicz, C. (1976). Audiological evaluation of deaf children. *Journal of Speech and Hearing Disorders, 41,* 256–267.

Erber, N. P. (1982). *Auditory training.* Washington, DC: Alexander Graham Bell Association for the Deaf.

Ervin, S. (1961). Changes with age in the verbal determinants of word-association. *American Journal of Psychology, 74,* 361–372.

Ervin-Tripp, S. (1980, May 14). Lecture, University of Minnesota.

Estivill, X., Govea, N., Barcelo, E., Badenas, C., Romero, E., Moral, L., . . . Torroni, A. (1998). Familial progressive sensorineural deafness is mainly due to the mtDNA A1555G mutation and is enhanced by treatment of aminoglycosides. *American Journal of Medical Genetics, 62,* 27–35.

Evans, W. J. (1995). What is sarcopenia? *Journal of Gerontology, 50A,* 5–8.

Ezell, H., & Goldstein, H. (1991). Comparison of idiom comprehension of normal children and children with mental retardation. *Journal of Speech and Hearing Research, 34,* 812–819.

Fabbro, F. (2001). The bilingual brain: Bilingual aphasia. *Brain and Language, 79,* 201–210.

Fasold, R. (1984). *The sociolinguistics of society.* London, England: Basil Blackwell.

Fawcett, A. J., & Nicolson, R. I. (2000). Systematic screening and intervention for reading disability. In N. Badian (Ed.), *Prediction and prevention of reading failure* (pp. 57–85). Timonium, MD: York Press.

Fawcus, B. (1986). Persistent puberphonia. In M. Fawcus (Ed.), *Voice disorders and their management.* Dover, NJ: Croom Helm.

Feinberg, M. J., Ekberg, O., Segall, L., & Tully, J. (1992). Deglutition in elderly patients with dementia: Findings of video-fluorographic evaluation and impact on staging and management. *Radiology, 183*(3), 811–814.

Felsenfeld, S. (1997). Epidemiology and genetics of stuttering. In Curlee, R., and Siegel, G (Eds.), *Nature and treatment of stuttering: New directions* (2nd ed.). Boston, MA: Allyn & Bacon.

Fernandes, D. B., Grobbelaar, A. O., Hudson, D. A., & Lentin, R. (1996). Velopharyngeal incompetence after adenotonsillectomy in non-cleft patients. *British Journal of Oral and Maxillofacial Surgery, 34*(5), 364–367.

Fewell, R. R., & Rich, J. S. (1987). Play assessment for examining cognitive, communication and social skills in multihandicapped children. *Journal of Psychoeducational Assessment, 2,* 107–118.

Fey, M. (1986). *Language intervention with young children.* Austin, TX: Pro-Ed.

Fey, M. E., Cleave, P. L., Long, S. H., & Ravida, A. I. (1994). Effects of grammar facilitation on the phonological performance of children with speech and language impairments. *Journal of Speech and Hearing Research, 37,* 594–607.

Fey, M., Edwards, M. L., Elbert, M., Hodson, B., Hoffman, P., Kamhi, A., & Schwartz, R. (1992). Clinical forum: Issues in phonological assessment and treatment. *Language Speech and Hearing in Schools, 23,* 224–282.

Fey, M. E., & Loeb, D. F. (2002). An evaluation of the facilitative effects of inverted yes-no questions on the acquisition of auxiliary verbs. *Journal of Speech and Hearing Research, 45,* 160–174.

Fey, M. E., Long, S. H., & Finestack, L. H. (2003). Ten principles of grammar facilitation for children with specific language impairments. *American Journal of Speech-Language Pathology, 12,* 3–15.

Field, J. (2004). *Psycholinguistics: The key concepts.* London, England: Routledge.

Filipek, P., Accardo, P., Baranek, G., Cook, E., Dawson, G., Gordon, B., . . . Volkmar, F. (1999). The screening and diagnosis of autistic spectrum disorders. *Journal of Autism and Developmental Disorders, 29,* 439–484.

Fisher, H. B. (1966). *Improving voice and articulation.* Boston, MA: Houghton Mifflin.

Fisher, H. B., & Logemann, J. A. (1971). *The Fisher-Logemann test of articulation competence.* Boston Houghton Mifflin.

Fisher, J., Schumaker, J., & Deshler, D. (2002). Improving the reading comprehension of at-risk adolescents. In C. C. Block & M. Presley (Eds.), *Comprehension instruction: Research-based best practices* (pp. 351–364). New York, NY: Guilford Press.

Fisher, L. I. (1985). Learning disabilities and auditory processing. In R. J. Van Hattum (Ed.), *Administration of speech and language services in schools: A manual* (pp. 231–290). San Diego, CA: College-Hill Press.

Flanagan, B., Goldiamond, I., & Azrin, N. (1958). Operant stuttering: The control of stuttering behavior through response-contingent consequences. *Journal of the Experimental Analysis of Behavior, 1,* 173–177.

Fodor, J. D., Ni, W., Crain, S., & Shankweiler, D. (1996). Tasks and timing in the perception of linguistic anomaly. *Journal of Psycholinguistic Research, 25,* 25–57.

Fombonne, E. (2007). Epidemiology of pervasive development disorders, In J. M. Perez, P. M. Gonzales, M. L. Comi, & C. Nieto (Eds.), *New developments in autism: The future is today* (pp. 14–32). London, England: Jessica Kingsley.

Fordham, S. (1988). Racelessness as a factor in black students' school success: Pragmatic strategy or pyrrhic victory? *Harvard Educational Review, 58*(1), 54–83.

Foster, S. (1986). Learning topic management in the preschool years. *Journal of Child Language, 13,* 231–250.

Fowler, W., Ogston, K., Roberts-Fiati, G., & Swenson, A. (1997). The effects of enriching language in infancy on early and later development of competence. *Early Childhood Development and Care, 125,* 41–77.

Fox, L., Long, S. H., & Langlois, A. (1988). Patterns of language comprehension deficits in abused and neglected children. *Journal of Speech and Hearing Disorders, 53,* 239–244.

Fox, R. A., & Nissen, S. L. (2005). Sex-related acoustic changes in voiceless English fricatives. *Journal of Speech, Language, and Hearing Research, 48,* 753–765.

Foy, J. G., & Mann, V. (2003). Home literacy environment and phonological awareness in preschool children: Differential effects for rhyme and phoneme awareness. *Applied Psycholinguistics, 24,* 59–88.

Frattali, C. M. (1998). *Measuring outcomes in speech-language pathology.* New York, NY: Theime.

Frattali, C. M., Thompson, C. K., Holland, A. L., Wohl, C. B., & Ferketic, M. M. (1995). *Functional Assessment of Communicative Skills for Adults.* Rockville, MD: ASHA.

Freed, M. L., Freed, L., Chatburn, R. L., & Christian, M. (2001). Electrical stimulation for swallowing disorders caused by stroke. *Respiratory Care, 46*(5), 466–474.

Freeman, F., & Ushijima, T. (1978). Laryngeal muscle activity during stuttering. *Journal of Speech and Hearing Research, 21,* 538–562.

Fried-Oken, M., Howard, J. M., & Stewart, S. R. (1991). Feedback on AAC intervention from adults who are temporarily unable to speak. *Augmentative and Alternative Communication, 7,* 43–50.

Fried-Oken, M., & Tarry, E. (1985). Development of an auditory scanning communication system with multiple voice output for severely disabled users. In C. Brubaker (Ed.), *Proceedings of the eighth annual conference on rehabilitation technology.* Washington, DC: RESNA.

Frijters, J. C., Barron, R. W., & Brunello, M. (2000). Direct and mediated influences of home literacy on prereaders' oral vocabulary and early written language skill. *Journal of Educational Psychology, 92,* 466–477.

Fristoe, M., & Lloyd, L. (1979). Non-speech communication. In N. Ellis (Ed.), *Handbook of mental deficiency.* New York, NY: Lawrence Erlbaum.

Froeschels, E. (1952). Chewing method as therapy. *Archives of Otolaryngology, 56,* 427–434.

Fucile, S., & Wright, P. M., (1998). Functional oral-motor skills: Do they change with age? *Dysphagia, 13,* 195–201.

Fudala, J. (1970). *Arizona Articulation Proficiency Scale: Revised.* Los Angeles, CA: Western Psychological Services.

Fuji, M., & Logemann, J. A. (1996). The effect of a tongue-holding maneuver on posterior pharyngeal wall movement during deglutition. *American Journal of Speech-Language Pathology, 5*(1), 23–30.

Fujiki, M., Brinton, B., Hart, C. H., & Fitzgerald, A. H. (1999). Peer acceptance and friendship in children with specific language impairment. *Topics in Language Disorders, 19,* 34–48.

Fujiki, M., Brinton, B., Morgan, M., & Hart, C. H. (1999). Withdrawn and social behavior of children with language impairment. *Language, Speech, and Hearing Services in Schools, 30,* 183–195.

Fujiki, M., Spackman, M., Brinton, B., & Illig, T. (2008). The ability of children with language impairment to understand emotion conveyed by prosody in a narrative passage. *International Journal of Language and Communication Disorders, 43,* 330–345.

Fuller, D. R., & Lloyd, L. L. (1987). A study of physical and semantic characteristics of a graphic symbol system as predictors of perceived complexity. *Augmentative and Alternative Communication, 3,* 26–35.

Fuller, D. R., Lloyd, L. L., & Schlosser, R. W. (1992). The further development of an augmentative and alternative communication symbol taxonomy. *Augmentative and Alternative Communication, 8,* 67–74.

Gallagher, A., Frith, U., & Snowling, M. J. (2000). Precursors of literacy-delay among children at genetic risk of dyslexia. *Journal of Child Psychology and Psychiatry, 4,* 203–213.

Garber, S. F., & Martin, R. R. (1977). Effects of noise and increased vocal intensity on stuttering. *Journal of Speech and Hearing Research, 20,* 233–240.

Garcia, S. B., & Ortiz, A. A. (2006). New directions in research: Cultural considerations with respect to international models. *Reading Research Quarterly.*

Garcia Velasco, M., Ysunza, A., Hernandez, X., & Marquez, C. (1988). Diagnosis and treatment of submucous cleft palate: A review of 108 cases. *Cleft Palate Journal, 25*(2), 171–173.

Gardner, H. (1975). *The shattered mind.* New York, NY: Knopf.

Garrett, K., & Beukelman, D. R. (1992). Augmentative communication approaches for persons with severe aphasia. In K. M. Yorkston (Ed.), *Augmentative communication in medical settings* (pp. 245–338). Tucson, AZ: Communication Skills Builders.

Garrett, K., Beukelman, K., & Low-Morrow, D. (1989). A comprehensive augmentative communication system for an adult with Broca's aphasia. *Augmentative and Alternative Communication, 5,* 55–61.

Gatehouse, S. (1999). A self-report outcome measure for the evaluation of hearing aid fittings and services. *Health Bulletin, 57,* 424–436.

Gates, G., Ryan, W., Cantu, E., & Hearne, E. (1982). Current status of laryngectomy rehabilitation: I. Results of therapy. *American Journal of Otolaryngology, 3,* 8–14.

Gathercole, V. (1989). Contrast: A semantic instrument? *Journal of Child Language, 16,* 685–702.

Gauger, L. M., Lombardino, I. J., & Leonard, C. M. (1997). Brain morphology in children with specific language impairment. *Journal of Speech, Language, and Hearing Research. 40,* 1272–1284.

Genesee, F., Paradis, J., & Crago, M. (2003). *Dual language development and disorders: A handbook for professionals.* Baltimore, MD: Paul H. Brookes.

Gentry, J. R. (2000). A retrospective on invented spelling and a look forward. *The Reading Teacher, 54,* 318–332.

Geraghty, J. A., Wenig, B. L., Smith, B. E., & Portugal, L. G. (1996). Long-term follow-up of tracheoesophageal puncture results. *Annals of Otology, Rhinology, and Laryngology, 105,* 501–503.

Gereau, S. A., & Shprintzen, R. J. (1988). The role of adenoids in the development of normal speech following palate repair. *Laryngoscope, 98,* 99–303.

German, D., & Newman, R. (2004). The impact of lexical factors on children's word finding errors. *Journal of Speech, Language, and Hearing Research, 47,* 624–636.

German, D., & Simon, E. (1991). Analysis of children's word-finding skills in discourse. *Journal of Speech and Hearing Research, 34,* 309–316.

Gertner, B., Rice, M., & Hadley, P. (1994). The influence of communicative competence on peer preference in a preschool classroom. *Journal of Speech and Hearing Research, 37,* 913–923.

Gethen, M. (1981). *Communicaid.* Available from author, 173 Old Bath Road, Cheltenham, Gloucestershire GL 53 7DW England.

Gierut, J. (1998). Treatment efficacy: Functional phonological disorders in children. *Journal of Speech, Language, and Hearing Sciences, 41,* 85–100.

Gierut, J. (2001). Complexity in phonological treatment: Clinical factors. *Language, Speech, and Hearing Services in Schools, 32,* 229–241.

Gierut, J. (2004). *Treatment efficacy summary: Phonological disorders in children.* Retrieved July 2004, from www.asha.org/members/slp/healthcare/efficacy.htm

Gierut, J. (2005), Phonological intervention: The how or the what? In A. Kamhi & K. Pollock (Eds.), *Phonological disorders in children: Clinical decision making in assessment and intervention* (pp. 201–210). Baltimore, MD: Paul H. Brookes.

Gierut, J., Elbert, M., & Dinnsen, D. (1987). Functional analysis of phonological knowledge and generalization learning in misarticulating children. *Journal of Speech and Hearing Research, 30,* 462–479.

Gilger, J. W., & Wise, S. E. (2004). Genetic correlates of language and literacy impairments. In C. A. Stone, E. R. Silliman, B. J. Ehren, & K. Apel (Eds.), *Handbook of language and literacy: Development and disorders* (pp. 25–48). New York, NY: Guilford Press.

Gillam, R. B. (1998). *Memory and language impairment in children and adults: New perspectives.* Frederick, MD: Pro-Ed.

Gillam, R. B., & Gorman, B. K. (2004). Language and discourse contributions to word recognition and text interpretation. In E. R. Silliman & L. C. Wilkinson (Eds.), *Language and literacy learning in schools* (pp. 63–97). New York, NY: Guilford Press.

Giolas, T. G. (1982). *Hearing-handicapped adults.* Englewood Cliffs, NJ: Prentice-Hall.

Girolametto, L., & Weitzman, E. (2006). It takes two to talk—The Hanen Program for Parents: Early language intervention through caregiver training. In R. J. McCauley & M. E. Fey (Eds.), *Treatment of language disorders in children* (pp. 77–101). Baltimore, MD: Paul H.

Girolametto, L., Weitzman, E., & Greenberg, J. (2003). Training day care staff to facilitate children's language. *American Journal of Speech-Language Pathology, 12,* 299–311.

Girolametto, L., Wiigs, M., Smyth, R., Weitzman, E., & Pearce, P. S. (2001). Children with a history of expressive vocabulary delay: Outcomes at 5 years of age. *American Journal of Speech-Language Pathology, 10,* 358–369.

Gladstone, V. (2000). From the chief staff officer for audiology. In E. Cherow & H. Ilecki (Eds.), *Audiology in ASHA: Our year 2000 in review* (pp. 4–7). Rockville, MD: ASHA.

Gleitman, L. (1993). The structural sources of verb meanings. In P. Bloom (Ed.), *Language acquisition: Core readings.* Cambridge, MA: MIT Press.

Glennen, S. L. (1997). Appendix A: Product directory. In S. L. Glennen & D. C. DeCoste (Eds.), *Handbook of augmentative and alternative communication* (pp. 681–717). San Diego, CA: Singular Publishing Group.

Goeke, J. L. (2009). *Explicit instruction: A framework for meaningful direct teaching.* Upper Saddle River, NJ: Merrill.

Golding-Kushner, K. J. (2001). *Therapy techniques for cleft palate speech and related disorders.* San Diego, CA: Singular Publishing Group.

Golding-Kushner, K. J., Argamaso, R. V., Cotton, R. T., Grames, L. M., Henningsson, G., Jones, D. L., … Skolnick, L. (1990). Standardization for the reporting of nasopharyngoscopy and multi-view videofluoroscopy: A report from an international working group. *Cleft Palate Journal, 27,* 337–347.

Goldman, R. (1967). Cultural influences on the sex ratio in the incidence of stuttering. *American Anthropologist, 69,* 78–81.

Goldman, R., & Fristoe, M. (2000). *Goldman-Fristoe Test of Articulation–2.* Circle Pines, MN: American Guidance Service.

Goldstein, B. (2000). *Cultural and linguistic diversity resource guide for speech-language pathologists.* San Diego, CA: Singular Publishing Group.

Goldstein, B. A., & Iglesias, A. (1996). Phonological patterns in normally developing Spanish-speaking 3- and 4-year-olds of Puerto Rican descent. *Language, Speech, and Hearing Services in Schools, 27,* 82–89.

Goldstein, H., & Prelock, P. (2004). *Treatment efficacy summary: Child language disorders.* Retrieved July 2004, www.asha.org/members/slp/healthcare/efficacy.htm

Golinkoff, R. M., Mervis, C. B., & Hirsh-Pasek, K. (1994). Early object labels: The case for a developmental lexical principles framework. *Journal of Child Language, 21,* 135–155.

Goodglass, H., & Kaplan, E. (1983). *The assessment of aphasia and related disorders* (2nd ed.). Philadelphia, PA: Lea & Febiger.

Goodglass, H., Kaplan, E., & Barresi, B. (2001). *The Boston Diagnostic Aphasia Examination* (3rd ed.). Philadelphia, PA: Lippincott, Williams & Wilkins.

Goossens, C., & Crain, S. S. (1987). Overview of nonelectronic eye-gaze communication techniques. *Augmentative and Alternative Communication, 3,* 77–89.

Gorlin, R., Cohen, M. J., & Hennekam, R. C. M. (2001). *Syndromes of the head and neck* (4th ed.). New York, NY: Oxford University Press.

Gosain, A. K., Conley, S. F., Marks, S., & Larson, D. L. (1996). Submucous cleft palate: Diagnostic methods and outcomes of surgical treatment. *Plastic and Reconstructive Surgery, 97*(7), 1497–1509.

Gosain, A. K., Conley, S. F., Santoro, T. D., & Denny, A. D. (1999). A prospective evaluation of the prevalence of submucous cleft palate in patients with isolated cleft lip versus controls. *Plastic and Reconstructive Surgery, 103*(7), 1857–1863.

Graham, M. S. (1997). *A clinician's guide to alaryngeal speech therapy.* Woburn, MA: Butterworth-Heinemann.

Grice, H. P. (1975). Logic and conversation. In P. Cole & J. L. Morgan (Eds.), *Syntax and semantics: Speech acts* (pp. 41–58). New York, NY: Academic Press.

Groher, M. E. (1997). *Dysphagia: Diagnosis and management.* Boston, MA: Butterworth-Heinemann.

Grolman, W., Schowenburg, P. F., deBoer, M. F., Kegt, P. P., Spoelstra, H. A., & Meeuwis, C. A. (1995). First results with the Blom-Singer Adjustable Tracheostoma Valve. *ORL-Journal of Otorhinolaryngology and Its Related Specialties, 57,* 165–170.

Gruenewald, L. J., & Pollack, S. A. (1990). *Language interaction in curriculum and instruction* (2nd ed.). Austin, TX: Pro-Ed.

Grunwell, P. (1985). *Phonological Assessment of Child Speech (PACS).* San Diego, CA: College-Hill Press.

Guitar, B. (2006). *Stuttering: An integrated approach to its nature and treatment.* Baltimore, MD: Williams & Wilkins.

Guneren, E., & Uysal, O. A. (2004). The quantitative evaluation of palatal elongation after Furlow palatoplasty. *Journal of Oral and Maxillofacial Surgery, 62*(4), 446–450.

Guralnick, M. J. (1997). *The effectiveness of early intervention.* Baltimore, MD: Brookes.

Gutierrez-Clennen, V. F., & Pena, E. (2002). Dynamic assessment of diverse children: A tutorial. *Language, Speech, and Hearing Services in Schools, 33,* 212–233.

Hadley, P. (1998). Early verb-related vulnerability among children with specific language impairment. *Journal of Speech, Language, and Hearing Research, 41,* 1384–1397.

Hadley, P., & Rice, M. (1991). Conversational responsiveness of speech and language impaired preschoolers. *Journal of Speech and Hearing Research, 34,* 1308–1317.

Hagen, C. (1981). Language disorders secondary to closed head injury: Diagnosis and treatment. *Topics in Language Disorders, 1,* 73–87.

Hagerman, R. (1993). Clinical overview of fragile X syndrome. *Neurogenetic Advances, 2,* 1–2.

Hall, K., Bingham, G., & Culatta, B. (in press). playful practice: A model for differentiated instruction. *Communication Disorders Quarterly.*

Hall, S., & Moats, L. (1999). *Straight talk about reading.* Chicago, IL: Contemporary Books.

Hamayan, E. V., & Damico, J. S. (Eds.). (1991). *Limiting bias in assessment of bilingual students.* Austin, TX: Pro-Ed.

Hamdy, S., Mikulis, D. J., Crawley, A., Xue, S., Lau, H., Henry, S., & Diamant, N. E. (1999). Cortical activation during human volitional swallowing: An event-related fMRI study. *American Journal of Physiology, 277*(1), G219–G255.

Hammer, C. S., Lawrence, F. R., & Miccio, A. W. (2007). Bilingual children's language abilities and reading outcomes in Head Start and kindergarten. *Language, Speech, and Hearing Services in Schools, 38,* 237–248.

Hammer, C. S., & Weiss, A. L. (1999). Guiding language development: How African American mothers and their infants structure play interactions. *Journal of Speech, Language, and Hearing Research, 42,* 1219–1233.

Hamming, K. K., Finkelstein, M., & Sidman, J. D. (2009). Hoarseness in children with cleft palate. *Otolaryngology—Head and Neck Surgery, 140*(6), 902–906.

Hampson, J., & Nelson, K. (1993). The relation of maternal language to variation in rate and style of language acquisition. *Journal of Child Language, 20,* 313–342.

Hane, A. A., Feldstein, S., & Dernetz, V. H. (2003). The relation between coordinated interpersonal timing and maternal sensitivity in four-months-olds. *Journal of Psycholinguistic Research, 32,* 525–539.

Hardin-Jones, M. A., & Jones, D. L. (2005). Speech production in preschoolers with cleft palate. *Cleft Palate–Craniofacial Journal, 42,* 7–13.

Harding, A., & Grunwell, P. (1996). Characteristics of cleft palate speech. *European journal of Disorders of Communication, 31*(4), 331–357.

Harris, J. L. (1997). Reminiscence: A culturally and developmentally appropiate language intervention for older adults. *American Journal of Speech-Language Pathology, 6,* 19–24.

Harris, M., Yeeles, C., Chasin, J., & Oakley, Y. (1995). Symmetries and asymmetries in early lexical comprehension and production. *Journal of Child Language, 22,* 1–18.

Harry, B. (2002). Trends and issues in serving culturally diverse families of children with disabilities. *The Journal of Special Education, 36,* 131–138.

Hart, B., & Risley, T. R. (1995). *Meaningful differences in the everyday experience of young American children.* Baltimore, MD: Paul H. Brookes.

Harvey, E., Secker, D., Brai, B., Picone, G., & Balfe, J. W. (1996). The team approach to the management of children on chronic peritoneal dialysis. *Advances in Renal Replacement Therapy, 3,* 13.

Haskins, J. (1949). *Kindergarten phonetically balanced word lists* (PBK). St. Louis, MO: Auditec.

Havkin, N., Tatum, S. A., III, & Shprintzen, R. J. (2000). Velopharyngeal insufficiency and articulation impairment in velo-cardio-facial syndrome: The influence of adenoids on phonemic development. *International Journal of Pediatric Otorhinolaryngology, 54,* 103–110.

Heath, S. B. (1982). What no bedtime story means: Narrative skills at home and school. *Language in Society, 11,* 49–76.

Helm-Estabrooks, N. (1992). *Aphasia Diagnostic Profile (ADP).* Chicago, IL: Riverside Press.

Helm-Estabrooks, N., Fitzpatrick, P. F., & Barresi, B. A. (1982). Visual action therapy for global aphasia. *Journal of Speech and Hearing Disorders, 47,* 385–389.

Henningsson, G., & Isberg, A. (1988). Influence of tonsils on velopharyngeal movements in children with craniofacial anomalies and hypernasality. *American Journal of Orthodontics and Dentofacial Orthopedics, 94,* 253–61.

Henry, J., Sloane, M., & Black-Pond, C. (2007). Neurobiology and neurodevelopment impact of childhood traumatic stress and prenatal alcohol exposure. *Language, Speech, and Hearing Service in Schools, 38,* 99–108.

Henry, J. A., Jastreboff, M. M., Jastreboff, P. J., Schechter, M. A., & Fausti, S. A. (2002). Assessment of Patients for Treatment with Tinnitus Retraining Therapy. *Journal of the American Academy of Audiology, 13*(10), 523–544.

Hetzroni, O. E., & Harris, O. L. (1996). Cultural aspects in the development of AAC users. *AAC, 12,* 52–58.

Hickey, T. (1993). Identifying formulas in first language acquisition. *Journal of Child Language, 20,* 27–41.

Hillel, A. D., Robinson, L. R., & Waugh, P. (1997). Laryngeal electromyography for the diagnosis and management of swallowing disorders. *Otolaryngology—Head and Neck Surgery, 116*(3), 344–348.

Hind, J. A., Nicosia, M., Roecker, E., Carnes, M., & Robbins, J. (2001). Comparison of effortful and non-effortful swallows in healthy middle-aged and older adults. *Archives of Physical Medicine and Rehabilitation, 82,* 1661–1665.

Hirano, M. (1981). Clinical examination of voice. In G. E. Arnold, F. Winckel, & B. D. Wyke (Eds.), *Disorders of human communication* (Vol. 5). New York, NY: Springer-Verlag.

Hodson, B. W. (1986a). *The assessment of phonological processes* (Rev. ed.). Danville, IL: Interstate Printers & Publishers.

Hodson, B. W. (1986b). *Computer Analysis of Phonological Processes(CAPP).* Stonington, IL: Phono-Comp.

Hodson, B. W., & Paden, E. (1991). *Targeting intelligible speech.* Austin, TX: Pro-Ed.

Hoff-Ginsberg, E. (1990). Maternal speech and the child's development of syntax: A further look. *Journal of Child Language, 17,* 85–99.

Hoffman, P. (1990). Spelling, phonology, and the speech-language pathologist: A whole language perspective. *Language, Speech, and Hearing Services in Schools, 21,* 238–243.

Hogikyan, N. D., & Sethurman, G. (1999). Validation of an instrument to measure voice-related quality of life (V-RQOL). *Journal of Voice, 13*(4), 555–569.

Holland, A., Frattali, C., & Fromm, D. (1999). *Communicative Activities of Daily Living (CADL-2).* Austin, TX: Pro-Ed.

Hood, L. J. (2002). Auditory neuropathy/auditory dys-synchrony: New insights. *The Hearing Journal, 55*(2), 10–18.

Hood, L. J. (2007). Auditory neuropathy and dys-synchrony. In R. F. Burkard & D. M. Eggermont (Eds.), *Auditory evoked potentials: Basic principles and clinical applications.* Baltimore: Lippincott Williams & Wilkins.

Hopper, T., & Holland, A. (1998). Situation-specific training for adults with aphasia: An example. *Aphasiology, 12,* 933–944.

Hopper, T., Holland, A., & Rewega, M. (2002). Conversational coaching: Treatment outcomes and future directions. *Aphasiology, 16,* 745–762.

Horner, R. H., & Budd, C. M. (1985). Acquisition of manual sign use: Collateral reduction of maladaptive behavior, and factors delimiting generalization. *Education and Training of the Mentally Retarded, 20,* 39–47.

Houston-Price, C., Plunkett, K., & Haris, P. (2005). Word-learning wizardry at 1;6. *Journal of Child Language, 32,* 175–189.

Howard, V., Williams, B., & Lepper, C. (2010). *Very young children with special needs: A foundation for educators, families, and service providers.* Pearson, (4).

Howell, J., & Dean, E. (1994). *Phonological disorders in children: Metaphon—theory to practice.* London, England: Whurr.

Huer, M. B. (2000). Examining perceptions of graphic symbols across cultures: Preliminary study of the impact of culture/ethnicity. *AAC, 16,* 180–185.

Huer, M. B., & Lloyd, L. L. (1988a). Parents' perspectives of AAC users. *Exceptional Parent, 18*(4), 32–33.

Huer, M. B., & Lloyd, L. L. (1988b). Perspectives of AAC users. *Communication Outlook, 9*(3), 10–18.

Hughes, C., & Leekam, S. (2004). What are the links between theory of mind and social relations? Review, reflections and new direction for studies of typical and atypical development. *Social Development, 13,* 590–619.

Hull, R. (1998). *Aural rehabilitation: Serving children and adults.* San Diego, CA: Singular Publishing Group.

Humbert, I., Poletto, C., Saxon, K., Kearney, P., Crujido, L., Wright-Harp, W., . . . Ludlow, C. (2006). Effect of surface electrical stimulation on hyolaryngeal movement in normal individuals at rest and during swallowing. *Journal of Applied Physiologist, 101,* 1657–1653.

Hwang, B., & Hughes, C. (2000). The effects of social interactive training on early social communication skills of children with autism. *Journal of Autism and Developmental Disorders, 30,* 331–344.

Hymes, D. (1971). Competence and performance in linguistic theory. In R. Huxley & E. Ingram (Eds.), *Language acquisition: Models and methods.* London, England: Academic Press.

Hymes, D. (1981). In vain I tried to tell you. In *Essays in Native American ethnopoetics.* Philadelphia, PA: University of Pennsylvania Press.

Hyter, Y. D. (2008, January 22). Considering conceptual frameworks in communication sciences and disorders. *The ASHA Leader,* pp. 30–31.

Im-Bolter, N., Johnson, J., & Pascual-Leone, J. (2006). Processing limitations in children with specific language impairment: The role of executive function. *Child Development, 77,* 1822–1841.

Individuals with Disabilities Education Improvement Act. (2004). P. L. 108-446, Stat. 2647.

Ingram, D. (1976). *Phonological disability in children.* New York, NY: American Elsevier.

Ingram, D. (1981). *Procedures for the phonological analysis of children's language.* Baltimore, MD: University Park Press.

Ingram, D. (1995). The cultural basis of prosodic modifications to infants and children: A response to Fernald's universalist theory. *Journal of Child Language, 22,* 223–233.

Israelite, N. K., & Jennings, M. B. (1995). Participant perspectives on group aural rehabilitation: A qualitative inquiry. *Journal of the Academy of Rehabilitative Audiology, 28,* 26–36.

Jackson-Maldonado, D., Thal, D., Marchman, V., Bates, E., & Gutierrez-Clennan, V. (1993). Early lexical development in Spanish-speaking infants and toddlers. *Journal of Child Language, 20,* 523–549.

Jacobson, B. H., Johnson, A., Grywalski, C., Silbergleit, A., Jacobson, G., Beuninger, M. S., & Newman, C. W (1997). The Voice Handicap Index (VHI): Development and validation. *American Journal of Speech-Language Pathology, 6,* 66–70.

Jacobson, E. (1976). *You must relax* (5th ed.). New York, NY: McGraw-Hill.

Jaffe, J., Beebe, B., Feldstein, S., Crown, C. L., & Jasnow, M. D. (2001). Rhythms of dialogue in infancy. *Monographs of the Society for Research in Child Development,* Serial No. 265, 66, No. 2.

Jerger, J. (1970). Clinical experience with impedance audiometry. *Archives of Otolaryngology, 92,* 311–324.

Jernigan, T., Hesselink, J., Sowell, E., & Tallal, P. (1991). Cerebral structure on magnetic resonance imaging in language and learning-impaired children. *Archives of Neurology, 48,* 539–545.

Johnson, C. E., & Danhauer, J. L. (2002). *Handbook of outcome measures in audiology.* Clifton Park, NY: Thompson Delmar Learning.

Johnson, C. J., & Anglin, J. M. (1995). Qualitative developments in the content and form of children's definitions. *Journal of Speech and Hearing Research, 38,* 612–629.

Johnson, J. L., & Hirsch, C. S. (2003). Aspiration pneumonia. *Postgraduate Medicine, 113*(3), 99–112.

Johnson, R. (1981). *The picture communication symbols.* Solana Beach, CA: Mayer-Johnson.

Johnson, R. (1985). *The picture communication symbols—Book II.* Solana Beach, CA: Mayer-Johnson.

Johnson, W. (1938). The role of evaluation in stuttering behavior. *Journal of Speech Disorders, 3,* 85–89.

Johnson, W. (1942). A study of the onset and development of stuttering. *Journal of Speech Disorders, 7,* 251–257.

Johnson, W. (1944). The Indians have no word for it. 1. Stuttering in children. *Quarterly Journal of Speech, 30,* 330–337.

Johnson, W. (1961). *Stuttering and what you can do about it.* Minneapolis, MN: University of Minnesota Press.

Johnson, W., & Rosen, L. (1937). Studies in the psychology of stuttering: 7. Effect of certain changes in the speech pattern upon frequency of stuttering. *Journal of Speech Disorders, 2,* 105–110.

Joint Committee on Infant Hearing Screening. (2000, August). Year 2000 position statement. *Audiology Today* (Special Issue), 6–27.

Jones, D. L. (2005). Perceptual aspects of nasality. *Perspectives on Speech Science and Orofacial Disorders, 15*(1), 9–14.

Jones, E., Southern, W. T., & Brigham, F. (1998, March). Curriculum-based assessment: Testing what is taught and teaching what is tested. *Intervention in School and Clinic, 33*(4), 239–249.

Jones, K. L. (2006). *Smith's recognizable patterns of human malformation* (5th ed.), Philadelphia, PA: Elsevier.

Jones, M. C. (1988). Etiology of facial clefts: Prospective evaluation of 428 patients. *Cleft Palate Journal, 25,* 16–20.

Juel, C. (1988). Learning to read and write: A longitudinal study of 54 children from first through fourth grades. *Journal of Educational Psychology, 80,* 437–447.

Jusczyk, P. W. (1999, September 30). *Making sense of sounds: Foundations of language acquisition.* Presentation at State University of New York, Geneseo.

Jusczyk, P. W., & Hohne, E. A. (1997). Infants' memory for spoken words. *Science, 277,* 1984–1986.

Jusczyk, P. W., Houston, D., & Newsome, M. (1999). The beginning of word segmentation in English-learning infants. *Cognition Psychology, 39,* 159–207.

Justice, L., & Ezell, H. (2002). Use of storybook reading to increase print awareness in at risk children. *American Journal of Speech-Language Pathology, 11,* 17–29.

Justice, L., Invernizzi, M. A., & Meier, J. D. (2002). Designing and implementing an early literacy screening protocol: Suggestions for the speech-language pathologist. *Language, Speech, and Hearing Services in Schools, 33,* 84–101.

Justice, L. M. (2006). Evidence-based practice, response to intervention and prevention of reading difficulties. *Language, Speech, and Hearing Services in Schools, 37,* 284–297.

Justice, L. M., Kaderavek, J. N., Fan, X., Sofka, A., & Hunt, A. (2009). Accelerating preschoolers' early literacy development through classroom-based teacher–child storybook reading and explicit print referencing. *Language, Speech, and Hearing Services in Schools, 40,* 67–85.

Justice, L., M., & Pullen, P. C. (2003). Promising interventions for promoting emergent literacy skills: Three evidence-based approaches. *Topics in Early Childhood Special Education, 23*(3), 99–113.

Kagan, A. (1998). Supported conversation for aphasia: Methods and resources for training conversational partners. *Aphasiology, 12,* 816–830.

Kalikow, D., Stevens, K., & Elliott, L. (1977). Development of a test of speech intelligibility in noise using sentence materials with controlled word predictability. *Journal of the Acoustical Society of America, 61,* 1337–1351.

Kamhi, A., & Lee, R. (1988). Cognition. In M. Nippold (Ed.), *Later language development, ages nine through nineteen.* Boston, MA: College-Hill.

Kamhi, A. G. (1981). Developmental vs. difference theories of mental retardation: A new look. *American Journal of Mental Deficiency, 86,* 1–7.

Kamhi, A. G. (2006). Treatment decisions for children with speech-sound disorders. *Language, Speech, and Hearing Services in Schools, 37,* 271–279.

Kamhi, A. G., & Catts, H. W. (2005). Language and reading: Convergences and divergences. In H. W. Catts & A. G. Kamhi (Eds.), *Language and reading disabilities* (2nd ed., pp. 1–25). Boston, MA: Allyn & Bacon.

Kamhi, A. G., Pollock, K. E., & Harris, J. L. (1996). *Communication development and disorders in African American children.* Baltimore, MD: Paul H. Brookes.

Kangas, K. A., & Allen, G. D. (1990). Intelligibility of synthetic speech for normal-hearing and hearing-impaired listeners. *Journal of Speech and Hearing Disorders, 55,* 751–755.

Kangas, K. A., & Lloyd, L. L. (1988). Early cognitive prerequisites to augmentative and alternative communication use: What are we waiting for? *Augmentative and Alternative Communication, 4,* 211–221.

Kao, W. W., Mohr, R. M., Kimmel, C. A., Getch, C., & Silverman, C. (1994). The outcome and technique of primary and secondary tracheoesophageal puncture. *Archives of Otolaryngology—Head and Neck Surgery, 120,* 301–307.

Kaplan, E. N. (1975). The occult submucous cleft palate. *Cleft Palate Journal 12,* 356–368.

Karling, J., Larson, O., & Henningsson, G. (1993). Oronasal fistulas in cleft palate patients and their influence on speech. *Scandinavian Journal of Plastic and Reconstructive Surgery, 27,* 193–201.

Karniol, R. (1992). Stuttering out of bilingualism. *First Language, 12,* 255–283.

Karrass, J., Braungart-Rieker, J. M., Mullins, J., & Lefever, J. B. (2002). Processes in language acquisition: The roles of gender, attention, and maternal encouragement of attention over time. *Journal of Child Language, 29,* 519–543.

Kaufman, B. A., Terbrock, A., Winters, N., Ito, J., Klosterman, A., & Park, T. S. (1994). Disbanding a multidisciplinary clinic: Effects on the health care of myelomeningocele patients. *Pediatric Neurosurgery, 21,* 36.

Kaufman, F. R., Halvorson, M., & Carpenter, S. (1999). Association between diabetes control and visits to a multidisciplinary pediatric diabetes clinic. *Pediatrics, 103,* 948–951.

Kay, J., Lesser, R., & Coltheart, M. (1992). *Psycholinguistic Assessment of Language Processing in Aphasia (PALPA).* East Sussex, England: Erlbaum.

Kayser, H. (1995a). Bilingualism, myths, and language impairments. In H. Kayser (Ed.), *Bilingual speech-language pathology: An Hispanic focus.* San Diego, CA: Singular Publishing Group.

Kayser, H. (Ed.). (1995b). *Bilingual speech-language pathology: An Hispanic focus.* San Diego, CA: Singular Publishing Group.

Kayser, H., & Restrepo, M. A. (1995). Language samples: Elicitation and analysis. In H. Kayser (Ed.), *Bilingual speech-language pathology: An Hispanic focus* (pp. 265–286). San Diego, CA: Singular Publishing Group.

Kemp, D. T. (1978). Stimulated acoustic emissions from within the human auditory system. *Journal of the Acoustical Society of America, 64,* 1386–1391.

Kemper, S., Thompson, M., & Marquis, J. (2001). Longitudinal change in language production: Effects of aging and dementia on grammatical complexity and prepositional content. *Psychology and Aging, 16,* 600–614.

Kendall, K. A., Leonard, R. J., & McKenzie, S. (2004a). Airway protection: Evaluation with videofluoroscopy. *Dysphagia, 19,* 65–70.

Kendall, K. A., Leonard, R. J., & McKenzie, S. (2004b). Common medical conditions in the elderly: Impact on pharyngeal bolus transit. *Dysphagia, 19,* 71–77.

Kent, R. D. (1998). *The speech sciences.* San Diego, CA: Singular Publishing Group.

Kent, R. D. (2009). Perceptual sensorimotor speech examination for motor speech disorders In M. R. McNeil (Ed.), *Clinical management of sensorimotor speech disorders* (2nd ed.). New York, NY: Thieme.

Kertesz, A. (1982). *The Western Aphasia Battery.* New York, NY: Grune & Stratton.

Khan, L., & Lewis, N. (1986). *Khan-Lewis Phonological Analysis.* Circle Pines, MN: American Guidance Service.

Kidd, K. K. (1977). A genetic perspective on stuttering. *Journal of Fluency Disorders, 2,* 259–269.

Killion, M., & Villchur, E. (1993). Kessler was right—partly: But SIN test shows some aids improve hearing in noise. *The Hearing Journal, 46*(9), 31–35.

Kim, W. S., Buchholz, D., Kumar, A. J., Donner, M. W., & Rosenbaum, A. E. (1987). Magnetic resonance imaging for evaluating neurogenic dysphagia. *Dysphagia, 2,* 40–45.

Kimmel, E. (1994). *The gingerbread man.* New York, NY: Holiday House.

Kimmel, E. (2000). *The runaway tortilla.* New York, NY: Winslow Press.

Kintsch, W. (1998). *Comprehension: A Paradigm for cognition.* New York, NY: Cambridge University Press.

Kiran, S., & Edmonds, L. (2004). Effect of semantic naming treatment on cross-linguistic generalization in bilingual aphasia. *Brain and Language, 91*(1), 75–77.

Kiran, S., & Thompson, C. (2003). The role of semantic complexity in treatment of naming deficits: Training semantic categories in fluent aphasia by controlling exemplar typicality. *Journal of Speech, Language, and Hearing Research, 46,* 773–787.

Kirstein, I. (Compiler), & Bernstein, C. (Illustrator). (1981). *Oakland schools picture dictionary.* Pontiac, MI: Oakland Schools Communication Enhancement Center.

Klima, E., & Bellugi, U. (1966). Syntactic regularities in the speech of children. In J. Lyons & R. Wales (Eds.), *Psycholinguistic papers.* Edinburgh, Scotland: Edinburgh University Press.

Klink, M., Gerstman, L., Raphael, L., Schlanger, B., & Newsome, L. (1986). Phonological process usage by young EMR children and nonretarded preschool children. *American Journal of Mental Deficiency, 91,* 190–195.

Kloth, S. A. M., Janssen, P., Kraaimaat, F. W., & Brutten G. J. (1995). Communicative behavior of mothers of stuttering and non stuttering high-risk children prior to the onset of stuttering. *Journal of fluency Disorders, 20,* 365–378.

Koegel, L. (1995). Communication and language intervention. In R. Koegel & L. Koegel (Eds.), *Teaching children with autism* (pp. 17–32). Baltimore, MD: Paul H. Brookes.

Koegel, R., Camarata, S., Koegel, L., Ben-Tall, A., & Smith, A. (1998). Increasing speech intelligibility in children with autism. *Journal of Autism and Developmental Disorders, 28,* 241–251.

Kohnert, K. J., & Bates, E. (2002). Balancing bilinguals II: Lexical comprehension and cognitive processing in children learning Spanish and English. *Journal of Speech, Language, and Hearing Research, 45,* 347–359.

Kohnert, K. J., Bates, E., & Hernandez, A. E. (1999). Balancing bilinguals: Lexical-semantic production and cognitive processing in children learning Spanish and English. *Journal of Speech, Language, and Hearing Research, 42,* 1400–1413.

Kopit, A. (1978). *Wings.* New York, NY: Hill & Wang.

Koppenhaver, D. A., Coleman, P. P., Kalman, S. L., & Yoder, D. E. (1991, September). The implications of emergent literacy research for children with development disabilities. *American Journal of Speech-Language Pathology, 1* (1), 38–44.

Koppenhaver, D. A., & Erickson, K. A. (2003). Natural emergent literacy supports for preschoolers with autism and severe communication impairments. *Topics in Language Disorders, 23,* 283–292

Koufman, J. A. (1991). The otolaryngologic manifestations of gastroesophageal reflux disease (GERD): A clinical investigation of 225 patients using ambulatory 24-hour pH monitoring and an experimental investigation of the role of acid and pepsin in the development of laryngeal injury. *Laryngoscope, 101* (Suppl. 53), 1–78.

Koul, R. K., & Corwin, M. (2003). Efficacy of AAC intervention in individuals with chronic severe aphasia. In R. W. Schlosser (Ed.), *The efficacy of augmentative and alternative communication: Toward evidence-based practice* (pp. 449–470). San Diego, CA: Academic Press.

Kovarsky, D., & Maxwell, M. (1997). Rethinking the context of language in schools. *Language, Speech, and Hearing Services in Schools, 28,* 219–230.

Krassowski, E., & Plante, E. (1997). IQ variability in children with SLI: Implications for use of cognitive referencing in determining SLI. *Journal of Communication Disorders, 30,* 1–9.

Kreiborg, S., & Cohen, M. M., Jr. (1992). The oral manifestations of Apert syndrome. *Journal of Craniofacial Genetics and Developmental Biology, 12*(1), 41–48.

Kummer, A. W. (2005). *The MacKay-Kummer SNAP Test–R: Simplified nasometric assessment procedures.* Accessed from www.kaypentax.com/snaptestr.htm

Kummer, A. W. (2008). *Cleft palate and craniofacial anomalies: The effects on speech and resonance,* (2nd ed.). New Albany, NY: Delmar Cengage Learning.

Kummer, A. W., Myer, C. M. I., Smith, M. E., & Shott, S. R. (1993). Changes in nasal resonance secondary to adenotonsillectomy. *American Journal of Otolaryngology, 14*(4), 285–290.

Kurland, B. F., & Snow, C. E. (1997). Longitudinal measurement of growth in definitional skill. *Journal of Child Language, 24,* 603–625.

Laganaro, M., & Oveton Venet, M. (2001). Acquired alexia in multilingual aphasia and computer-assisted treatment in both languages: Issues of generalization and transfer. *Folia phoniatrica et Logopedia, 53,* 135–144.

Lahey, M., & Bloom, L. (1994). Variability and language learning disabilities. In G. Wallach & K. Butler (Eds.), *Language learning disabilities in school-age children and adolescents.* New York, NY: Macmillan.

Lander, E. S., & Shrock, N. J. (1994). Genetic dissection of complex traits. *Science, 266,* 2037–2048.

Langdon, H. (1992). Language communication and sociocultural patterns in Hispanic families. In H. Langdon & L. Cheng (Eds.), *Hispanic children and adults with communication disorders: Assessment and intervention* (pp. 99–131). Rockville, MD: Aspen.

Langdon, H. W. (1996a). Assessment instruments for Spanish-speaking students. In H. W. Langdon & T. I. Saenz (Eds.), *Language assessment and intervention with multicultural students: A guide for speech-language-hearing professionals* (pp. 75–82). Oceanside, CA: Academic Communication Associates.

Langdon, H. W. (1996b). Assessment and intervention for Hispanic/Latino students. In H. W. Langdon & T. I. Saenz (Eds.), *Language assessment and intervention with multicultural students: A guide for speech-language-hearing professionals* (pp. 71–74). Oceanside, CA: Academic Communication Associates.

Langmore, S. E., & McCulloch, T. M. (1997). Examination of the pharynx and larynx and endoscopic examination of pharyngeal swallowing. In A. L. Perlmann & K. Shultze-Delrieu (Eds.), *Deglutition and its disorders: Anatomy, physiology, clinical diagnosis and management* (pp. 201–226). San Diego, CA: Singular Publishing Group.

Langmore, S. E., Schatz, K., & Olsen, N. (1988). Fiberoptic endoscopic examination of swallowing safety: A new procedure. *Dysphagia, 2,* 216–219.

Langmore, S. E., Skarupski, K. A., Park, P. S., & Fries, B. E. (2002). Predictors of aspiration pneumonia in nursing home residents. *Dysphagia, 17,* 298–307.

LaParo, K. M., Justice, L., Skibbe, L. E., & Pianta, R. C. (2004). Relations among maternal, child, and demographic factors and the persistence of preschool language impairment. *American Journal of Speech-Language Pathology, 13,* 291–303.

LaRossa, D., Jackson, O. H., Kirschner, R. E., Low, D. W., Solot, C. B., Cohen, M. A., . . . Randall, P. (2004, April). The Children's Hospital of Philadelphia modification of the Furlow double-opposing z-palatoplasty: Long-term speech and growth results. *Clinical Plastic Surgery, 31*(2), 243–249.

Lass, N. J., Ruscello, D. M., Pannbacker, M. D., Middleton, G. F., Schmitt, J. F., & Scheuerle, J. F. (1995). Career selection and satisfaction in the professions. *ASHA, 35*(4), 48–51.

Learning to read and write. (1998). Joint Position Statement of International Reading Association and National Association for the Education of Young Children. Washington, DC.

Lee, S., Potamianos, A., & Naryanan, S. (1999). Acoustics of children's speech: Developmental changes of temporal and spectral parameters. *Journal of the Acoustical Society of America, 105,* 1455–1468.

Leith, W. R., & Mims, H. A. (1975). Cultural influences in the development and treatment of stuttering: A preliminary report on the black stutterer. *Journal of Speech and Hearing Research, 40*(4), 459–466.

Lemoncello, R., & Fanning, J. L. (2008, October). *Practice-based evidence: Strategies for generating your own evidence.* Presentation at the Oregon Speech-Language-Hearing Convention, Salem, OR.

Lenneberg, E. H. (1967). *Biological foundations of language.* New York, NY: Wiley.

Leonard, L. (1985). Unusual and subtle phonological behavior in the speech of phonologically disordered children. *Journal of Speech and Hearing Disorders, 50,* 4–13.

Leonard, L. (1998). Children with specific language impairment. Cambridge, MA: MIT Press.

Leonard, L. B. (1991). Specific language impairment as a clinical category. *Language, Speech, and Hearing Services in Schools, 22,* 66–68.

Leonard, L. B. (2009). Is expressive language disorder an accurate diagnostic category? *American Journal of Speech-Language Pathology,18,* 115–123.

Leonard, L. B., Camarata, S., Pawlowska, M., Brown, B., & Camarata, M. (2008). The acquisition of tense and agreement morphemes by children with specific language impairment during intervention: Phase 3. *Journal of Speech, Language, and Hearing Research, 51,* 120–125.

Leonard, L. B., Deevy, P., Miller, C. A., Rauf, L., Charest, M., & Kurtz, R. (2003). Surface forms and grammatical function: Past tense and passive participle use by children with specific language impairment. *Journal of Speech and Hearing Research, 46,* 43–55.

Leopold, D. A., Bartoshuk, L., Doty, R. L., Jafek, B., Smith, D. V., & Snow, J. B. (1989). Aging of the upper airway and the senses of taste and smell. *Otolaryngology—Head and Neck Surgery, 100*(4), 287–289.

Leopold, N. A., & Kagel, M. C. (1985). Dysphagia in Huntington's disease. *Archives of Neurology, 42,* 57–63.

Levelt, W. J. M., & Wheeldon, L. (1994). Do speakers have access to a mental syllabary? *Cognition, 50,* 239–269.

Levine, R. L., Robbins, J. A., & Maser, A. (1992). Periventricular white matter changes & oropharyngeal swallowing in normal individuals. *Dysphagia, 7,* 142–147.

Levy, E., & Nelson, K. (1994). Words in discourse: A dialectal approach to the acquisition of meaning and use. *Journal of Child Language, 21,* 367–389.

Lewin, M. L., Croft, C. B., & Shprintzen, R. J. (1980). Velopharyngeal insufficiency due to hypoplasia of the musculus uvulae and occult submucous cleft palate. *Plastic and Reconstructive Surgery, 65,* 585–591.

Liao, Y. F., Chuang, M. L., Chen, P. K., Chen, N. H., Yun, C., & Huang, C. S. (2002). Incidence and severity of obstructive sleep apnea following pharyngeal flap surgery in patients with cleft palate. *Cleft Palate–Craniofacial Journal, 39*(3), 312–316.

Liberman, I. Y., & Shankweiler, D. (1985). Phonology and the problems of learning to read and write. *Remedial and Special Education, 6,* 8–17.

Lidral, A. C., & Moreno, L. M. (2005). Progress toward discerning the genetics cleft lip. *Current Opinion in Pediatrics, 17,* 731–739.

Lidz, C. S. (Ed.). (1987). *Dynamic assessment: An interactional approach to evaluating learning potential.* New York, NY: Guilford Press.

Lidz, C. S. (1991). *Practitioner's guide to dynamic assessment.* New York, NY: Guilford Press.

Lidz, C. S. (2005). Dynamic assessment with young children: We've come a long way baby. *Journal of Early Childhood and Infant Psychology, 1,* 99–112.

Lidz, C. S., & Pena, E. D. (1996). Dynamic assessment: The model, its relevance as a nonbiased approach, and its application to Latino American preschool children. *Language, Speech, and Hearing Services in Schools, 27,* 367–372.

Lieven, E., Behrens, H., Speares, J., & Tomasello, M. (2003). Early syntactic creativity: A usage-based approach. *Journal of Child Language, 30,* 333–370

Light, J. (1989). Toward a definition of communicative competence for individuals using augmentative and alternative communication systems. *Augmentative and Alternative Communication, 5,* 137–144.

Light, J. C., Beukelman, D., & Reichle, J. (2003). *Communicative competence for indidivuals who use AAC: From research to effective practice.* Baltimore, MD: Paul H. Brookes.

Light, J. C., & Kent-Walsh, J. (2003). Fostering emergent literacy for children who require AAC. *ASHA Leader, 27,* 4–8.

Light, J., Stoltz, B., & McNaughton, D. (1996). Community based employment: Experiences of adults who use AAC. *AAC, 12,* 215–228.

Liles, B. (1987). Episode organization and cohesive conjunctions in narratives of children with and without language disorders. *Journal of Speech and Hearing Research, 30,* 185–196.

Linan-Thompson, S., & Ortiz, A. A. (2009). Response to intervention and English-language learners: Instructional and assessment considerations. *Seminars in Speech and Language, 30,* 105–120.

Lindamood, C. H., & Lindamood, P. C. (1998). *Lindamood Phoneme Sequencing Program (LIPS).* Austin, TX: Pro-Ed.

LIPP 2.1. (2001). Miami, FL: Intelligent Hearing Systems.

Litvan, I., Mangone, C. A., McKee, A., Verry, M., Parsa, A., Jellinger, K., . . . Pearce, R. K. (1996). Natural history of progressive supranuclear palsy (Steele-Richardson-Olszewski syndrome) and clinical predictors of survival: A clinicopathological study. *Journal of Neurology, Neurosurgery, and Psychiatry, 60*(6), 615–620.

Lloyd, L. L., & Fuller, D. R. (1986). Toward an augmentative and alternative communication symbol taxonomy: A proposed superordinate classification. *Augmentative and Alternative Communication, 2,* 165–171.

Lloyd, L. L., & Fuller, D. R. (1990). The role of iconicity in augmentative and alternative communication symbol learning. In W. I. Fraser (Ed.), *Key issues in mental retardation research* (pp. 295–306). London, England: Routledge.

Lloyd, L. L., Fuller, D. R., Loncke, F., & Bos, H. (1997). Introduction to AAC symbols. In L. L. Lloyd, D. R. Fuller, & H. H. Arvidson (Eds.), *Augmentative and alternative communication: A handbook of principles and practices.* Boston, MA: Allyn & Bacon.

Lloyd, L. L., & Karlan, G. R. (1984). Nonspeech communication and symbols: Where have we been and where are we going? *Journal of Mental Deficiency Research, 28,* 3–20.

Lloyd, L. L., Quist, R. W., & Windsor, J. (1990). A proposed augmentative and alternative communication model. *Augmentative and Alternative Communication, 6,* 172–183.

Lloyd, L. L., Taylor, O. L., Buzolich, M., Harris, O., & Soto, G. (1994, November 19). *Multicultural issues in augmentative and alternative communication.* Presentation at ASHA, New Orleans, LA).

Lobel, A. (1976). *Frog and toad all year.* New York, NY: Harper Trophy.

Locke, J. (1980a). The inference of speech perception in the phonologically disordered child. Part I: A rationale, some criteria, the conventional tests. *Journal of Speech and Hearing Disorders, 45,* 431–444.

Locke, J. (1980b). The inference of speech perception in the phonologically disordered child. Part II: Some clinically novel procedures their use, some findings. *Journal of Speech and Hearing Disorders, 45,* 445–468.

Logan, K. J. (2003). Language and fluency characteristic of preschoolers' multiple-utterance conversational turns. *Journal of Speech, Language, and Hearing Research, 46,* 178–188.

Logemann, J. A. (1986). *Manual for the videofluorographic study of swallowing* (2nd ed.). Austin, TX: Pro-Ed.

Logemann, J. A. (1997). Therapy for oropharyngeal swallowing disorders. In A. L. Perlmann & K. Shultze-Delrieu (Eds.), *Deglutition and its disorders: Anatomy, physiology, clinical diagnosis and management* (pp. 449–462). San Diego, CA: Singular Publishing Group.

Logemann, J. A. (1998a). Differential diagnosis of swallowing disorders. In B. J. Phillips & D. Ruscello (Eds.), *Differential diagnosis in speech-language pathology* (pp. 337–352). Boston, MA: Butterworth-Heinemann.

Logemann, J. A. (1998b). *Evaluation and treatment of swallowing disorders.* Austin, TX: Pro-Ed.

Logemann, J. A. (1998c). Efficacy, outcomes and cost effectiveness in dysphagia. In C. M. Frattali (Ed.), *Measuring outcomes in speech-language pathology.* New York, NY: Thieme.

Logemann, J. A., & Kahrilas, P. J. (1990). Relearning to swallow post CVA: Application of maneuvers and indirect biofeedback: A case study. *Neurology, 40,* 1136–1138.

Long, S., & Fey, M. (2000). *Computerized Profiling.* Available from www.cwru.edu/artsci/cosi/faculty/long/research/cp.htm

Long, S. H. (2006). Language and linguistically-culturally diverse children. In V. A. Reed (Ed.), *An introduction to children with language disorders* (3rd ed., pp. 301–334). Boston, MA: Allyn & Bacon.

Lonigan, C. J., Bloomfield, B. G., Anthony, J. L., Bacon, K. D., Phillips, B. M., & Samwel, C. S. (1999). Relations among emergent literacy skills, behavior problems, and social competence in preschool children from low- and middle-income households. *Topics in Early Childhood Special Education, 19,* 40–53.

Lonigan, C. J., Burgess, S. R., & Anthony, J. L. (2000). Development of emergent literacy and early reading skills in preschool children: Evidence from a latent-variable longitudinal study. *Development Psychology, 36,* 596–613.

Lord, C., & Paul, R. (1997). Language and communication in autism. In D. Cohen & F. Volkmar (Eds.), *Handbook of autism and pervasive developmental disorders* (2nd ed., pp. 195–225). New York, NY: Wiley.

Lorenzen, B., & Murray, L. (2008). Bilingual aphasia: A theoretical and clinical review. *American Journal of Speech-Language Pathology, 17,* 299–317.

Losken, A., Williams, J. K., Burstein, F. D., Malick, D., & Riski, J. E. (2003). An outcome evaluation of sphincter pharyngoplasty for the management of velopharyngeal insufficiency. *Plastic and Reconstructive Surgery, 112*(7), 1755–1761.

Lubinski, R., & Frattali, C. (2001). *Professional issues in speech-language pathology and audiology* (2nd ed.). San Diego, CA: Singular Publishing Group.

Luce, E. A., McGibbon, B., & Hoopes, J. E. (1977, October). Velopharyngeal insufficiency in hemifacial microsomia. *Plastic and Reconstructive Surgery, 60*(4), 602–606.

Luschei, E. S., & Finnegan, E. M. (2009). Electromyographic techniques for the assessment of motor speech disorders. In M. R. McNeil (Ed.), *Clinical management of sensorimotor speech disorders* (2nd ed.). New York, NY: Thieme.

Luterman, D. M. (1987). Counseling parents of hearing-impaired children. In F. N. Martin (Ed.), *Hearing disorders in children* (pp. 303–319). Austin, TX: Pro-Ed.

Lutke, J. (1997). Spider web walking: Hope for children with FAS through understanding. In A. Streissguth & J. Kanter (Eds.), *The challenge of fetal alcohol syndrome: Overcoming secondary disabilities* (pp. 177–184). Seattle, WA: University of Washington Press.

Lynch, W., & Hanson, M. (2004). *Developing cross-cultural competence: A guide for working with young children and their families* (3rd ed.). Baltimore, MD: Paul H. Brookes.

Lyytinen, H., Erskine, J., Tolvanen, A., Torppa, M., Poikkeus, A-M., & Lyytinen, P. (2006). Trajectories of reading development: A follow-up from birth to school age of children with and without risk for dyslexia. *Merrill-Palmer Quarterly, 52,* 514–546.

MacDonald, J. D. (1989). *Becoming partners with children: From play to conversation.* Chicago, IL: Riverside.

MacDonald, J. D., & Carroll, J. (1992). Communicating with young children: An ecological model for clinicians, parents, and collaborative professionals. *American Journal of Speech-Language Pathology, 1,* 39–48.

Macedonia, C., Miller, J. L., & Sonies, B. C. (2002). Power Doppler imaging of the fetal upper aerodigestive tract using a 4-point standardized evaluation: A preliminary report. *Journal of Ultrasound Medicine, 21,* 869–878.

MacKenzie-Stepner, K., Wiltzel, M. A., Stringer, D. A., Lindsay, W. K., Munro, I. R., & Hughs, H. (1987). Velopharyngeal insufficiency due to hypertrophic tonsils: A report of two cases. *International Journal of Pediatric Otorhinolaryngology, 14,* 57–63.

Maher, L.M., Kendall, D., Swearengin, J. A., Rodriguez, A., Leon, S. A., Pingel, K., . . . Gonzalez Rothi, L. J. (2006). A pilot study of use-dependent learning in the context of constraint induced language therapy. *Journal of the International Neuropsychological Society, 12,* 843–852.

Mange, E., & Mange, A. (1999). Basic human genetics (2nd ed.) Sunderland MA: Sinauer Associates.

Manning, W. H. (2000). *Clinical decision making in fluency disorders* (2nd ed.). San Diago, CA: Singular Publishing group.

Marchman, V. A., & Martinez-Sussmann, C. (2002). Concurrent validity of caregiver/parent report measures of language for children who are learning both English and Spanish. *Journal of Speech, Language, and Hearing Research, 45,* 983–997.

Marcus, G. F. (2001). *The algebraic mind.* Cambridge, MA: MIT Press.

Marik, P. E. (2001). Aspiration pneumonitis and aspiration pneumonia. *New England journal of Medicine, 34*(9), 665–671.

Marik, P. E., & Kaplan, D. (2003). Aspiration pneumonia and dysphagia in the elderly. *Chest, 124,* 328–346.

Marrinan, E. M., LaBrie, R. A., & Mulliken, J. B. (1998). Velopharyngeal function in nonsyndromic cleft palate: Relevance of surgical technique, age at repair, and cleft type. *Cleft Palate–Craniofacial Journal, 35,* 95–100.

Martin, B. J., Logemann, J. A., Shaker, R., & Dodds, W. J. (1994). Coordination between respiration and swallowing: Respiratory phase relationships and temporal integration. *Journal of Applied Physiology, 76*(2), 714–723.

Martin, F. N., & Champlin, C. A. (2000). Reconsidering the limits of normal hearing. *Journal of the American Academy of Audiology, 11,* 64–66.

Martin, F. N., & Clark, J. G. (2009). *Introduction to audiology* (10th ed.). Boston, MA: Allyn & Bacon.

Martin, F. N., George, K. A., O'Neal, J., & Daly, J. A. (1987). Audiologists' and parents' attitudes regarding counseling of families of hearing-impaired children. *ASHA, 29*(2), 27–33.

Martin, F. N., Krall, L., & O'Neal, J. (1989). The diagnosis of acquired hearing loss: Patient reactions. *ASHA, 31,* 47–50.

Martin, R. E., & Sessle, B. J. (1993). The role of the cerebral cortex in swallowing. *Dysphagia, 8,* 195–202.

Martin-Harris, B., Brodsky, M. B., Price, C. C., Michel, Y., & Walters, B. (2003). Temporal coordination of pharyngeal and laryngeal dynamics with breathing during swallowing: Single liquid swallows. *Journal of Applied Physiology, 94,* 1735–1743.

Marton, K., & Schwartz, R. G. (2003). Working memory capacity and language processes in children with specific language impairment. *Journal of Speech, Language, and Hearing Research, 46,* 1138–1153.

Marton, K., Schwartz, R. G., & Braun, A. (2005). The effect of age and language stucture in working memory performance. In B. G. Bara, L. Barsalou, & M. Bucciarelli (Eds.), *Proceedings of the XXVII annual meeting of the Cognitive Science Society* (pp. 1413–1418). Mahwah, NJ: Lawrence Erlbaum.

Masataka, N. (1995). The relation between index-finger extension and the acoustic quality of cooing in three-month-old infants. *Journal of Child Language, 22,* 247–257.

Mason, R. M., & Warren, D. W. (1980). Adenoid involution and developing hypernasality in cleft palate. *Journal of Speech and Hearing Disorders, 45,* 469–80.

Masur, E. F. (1997). Maternal labelling of novel and familiar objects: Implications for children's development of lexical constraints. *Journal of Child Language, 24,* 427–439.

Mattes, L. J., & Omark, D. R. (Eds.). (1991). *Speech and language assessment for the bilingual handicapped* (2nd ed.). Oceanside, CA: Academic Communication Associates.

Mayo, W. J. (1933). *The value of the imponderables in clinical medicine.* Proceedings of the Interstate Post-Graduate Medical Assembly of North America.

McCabe, A. (1995). Evaluating narrative discourse skills. In K. Cole, P. Dale, & D. Thal (Eds.), *Assessment of communication and language* (pp. 121–141). Baltimore, MD: Paul H. Brookes.

McCabe, A., & Bliss, L. S. (2003). *Patterns of narrative discourse: A multicultural, life span approach.* Boston, MA: Allyn & Bacon.

McCabe, R., & Bradley, D. (1975). Systematic multiple phonemic approach to articulation therapy. *Acta Symbolica, 6,* 1–18.

McCardle, P., & Chhabra, V. 2004. *The voice of evidence in reading research.* Baltimore, MD: Paul H. Brookes.

McCathren, R. B., Warren, S. F., & Yoder, P. J. (1996). Prelinguistic predictors of later language development. In K. N. Cole, P. S. Dale, & D. J. Thal (Eds.), *Communication and Language Intervention Series: Vol. 6. Advances in assessment of communication and language* (pp. 55–76). Baltimore, MD: Paul H. Brookes.

McCathren, R. B., Warren, S. F., & Yoder, P. J. (1999). The relationship between prelinguistic vocalization and later expressive language in young children with developmental delay. *Journal of Speech, Language, and Hearing Research, 42,* 915–924.

McConnel, F. M. S., Cerenko, D., & Mendelsohn, M. S. (1988). Manofluorographic analysis of swallowing. *Otolaryngology Clinics of North America, 21*(4), 625–637.

McCormick, L., & Wegner, J. (2003). Supporting augmentative and alternative communication. In L. McCormick, D. F. Loeb, & R. L. Schiefelbusch (Eds.), *Supporting children with communication difficulties in inclusive settings: School-based language intervention* (2nd ed., pp. 438–459). Boston, MA: Allyn & Bacon.

McCulloch, T. M., Jaffe, D. M., & Hoffman, H. T. (1997). Diseases and operation of head and neck structures affecting swallowing. In A. L. Perlmann & K. Shultze-Delrieu (Eds.), *Deglutition and its disorders: Anatomy, physiology, clinical diagnosis and management* (pp. 343–382). San Diego, CA: Singular Publishing Group.

McEachem, D., & Haynes, W. O. (2004). Gesture–speech combinations as a transition to multiword utterances. *American Journal of Speech-Language Pathology, 13,* 227–235.

Mc Gregor, C., Newman, R., Reilly, R., & Capone, N. (2002). Semantic representation and naming in children with specific language impairment. *Journal of Speech, Language, and Hearing Research, 45,* 998–1014.

McGregor, K. K. (2004). Developmental dependencies between lexical semantics and reading. In C. A. Stone, E. R. Silliman, B. J. Ehren, & K. Apel (Eds.), *Handbook of language and literacy: Development and disorders* (pp. 302–317). New York, NY: Guilford Press.

McGregor, K., & Schwartz, R. (1992) . Converging evidence for underlying phonologial representation in a misarticulating child. *Journal of Speech and Hearing Research, 35,* 596–603.

McGregor, K. K., Sheng, L., & Smith, B. (2005). The precocious two-year-old: Status of the lexicon and links to the grammar. *Journal of Child Language, 32,* 563–585.

McHale, S., Simeonson, R., Marcus, L., & Olley, J. (1980). The social and symbolic quality of autistic children's communication. *Journal of Autism and Developmental Disorders, 10,* 299–310.

McLaughlin, S. (2006). *Second Language Acquisition in Childhood: Vol. 1. Preschool children* (2nd ed.). NJ: Lawrence Erlbaum.

McLean, J., Raymore, S., Long, L., & Brown, K. (1976). *Stimulus shift articulation program.* Bellevue, WA: Edmark Associates.

McLean, J., & Snyder-McLean, L. S. (1999). *How children learn language.* San Diego, CA: Singular Publishing Group.

McNaughton, D., Light, J., & Gulla, S. (2003). Opening up a "whole new world": Employer and co-worker perspectives on working with individuals who use augmentative and alternative communication. *Augmentative and Alternative Communication, 19,* 235–253.

McNaughton, S. (1985). *Communicating with Blissymbolics.* Toronto, Canada: Blissymbolics Communication Institute.

McNaughton, S. (1990). Gaining the most from AAC's growing years. *Augmentative and Alternative Communication, 6,* 2–14.

McNeilly, L. (2001). *Infusion of genomics into speech language pathology curricula.* The Health Resources and Services Administration (HRSA), Bureau of Health Professions [CD-ROM].

McNeilly, L., & Coleman, T. J. (2000). Language disorders in culturally diverse populations: Intervention issues and strategies. In T. J. Coleman (Ed.), *Clinical management of communication disorders in culturally diverse children* (pp. 157–172). Boston, MA: Allyn & Bacon.

McReynolds, L. V., & Bennett, S. (1972). Distinctive feature generalization in articulation training. *Journal of Speech and Hearing Disorders, 37,* 462–470.

McWilliams, B. J., Glaser, E. R., Philips, B. J., Lawrence, C., Lavorato, A. S., Beery, Q. C., & Skolnick, M. L. (1981). A comparative study of four methods of evaluating velopharyngeal adequacy. *Plastic and Reconstructive Surgery, 68,* 1–9.

McWilliams, R. A. (Ed.). (1996). *Rethinking pull-out services in early intervention: A professional resource.* Baltimore, MD: Paul H. Brookes.

Meadows, D., Elias, G., & Bain, J. (2000). Mothers' ability to identify infants' communicative acts consistently. *Journal of Child Language, 27,* 393–406.

Mehler, J., Jusczyk, P. W., Lambertz, G., Halsted, N., Bertoncini, J., & Amiel-Tison, C. (1998). A precursor of language acquisition in young infants. *Cognition, 29,* 144–178.

Meisels, S. (1996). Charting the continuum of assessment and intervention. In S. Meisels & E. Fenichel (Eds.), *New visions for the developmental assessment of infants and young children* (pp. 27–52). Washington, DC: Zero to Three/National Center for Infants, Toddlers, and Families.

Meisels, S., & Fenichel, E. (1996). *New visions for the developmental assessment of infants and young children.* Washington, DC: Zero to Three.

Meltzer, L. (Ed.). (2007). *Executive function in education: From theory to practice.* New York, NY: Guilford Press.

Merritt, D. D., & Culatta, B. (1998). *Language intervention in the classroom.* San Diego, CA: Singular Publishing group.

Merritt, D. D., & Culatta, B., & Trostle, S. (1998). Narratives: Implementing a discourse framework. In D. D. Merritt & B. Culatta (Eds.), *Language intervention in the classroom* (pp. 277–330). San Diego, CA: Singular Publishing group.

Merritt, D. D., & Liles, B. (1987). Story grammar ability in children with and without language disorder: Story generation, story retelling, and story comprehension. *Journal of Speech and Hearing Research, 30,* 539–552.

Mervis, C. B., & Bertrand, J. (1995). Early lexical acquisition and the vocabulary spurt: A response to Goldfield & Reznick. *Journal of Child Language, 22,* 461–468.

Michaels, S. (1981). "Sharing time": Children's narrative styles and differential access to literacy. *Language in Society, 10,* 423–442.

Michaels, S., & Collins, J. (1984). Oral discourse styles: Classroom interaction and the acquisition of literacy. In D. Tannen (Ed.), *Coherence in spoken and written discourse.* Norwood, NJ: Ablex.

Miles, S., & Chapman, R. S. (2002). Narrative content as described by individuals with Down syndrome and typically developing children. *Journal of Speech, Language, and Hearing Research, 45,* 175–189.

Miller, C. A., & Leonard, L. B, (1998). Deficits in finite verb morphology: Some assumptions in recent accounts of specific language impairment. *Journal of Speech, Language, and Hearing Research, 41,* 701–707.

Miller, D., Light, J., & Schlosser, R. (2000). The impact of AAC on natural speech development: A meta-analysis. In *Conference Proceedings, Ninth Biennial Conference, Aug. 2–6, Washington, D.C.* Toronto, Canada: ISAAC.

Miller, G. A., & Gildea, P. M. (1987). How children learn words. *Scientific American, 257,* 94–99.

Miller, J. F. (1991). Quantitative productive language disorders. In J. Miller (Ed.), *Research on child language disorders: A decade of progress.* Austin, TX: Pro-Ed.

Miller, J. F., & Chapman, R. (1984). Disorders of communication: Investigating the development of language of mentally retarded children. *American Journal of Mental Deficiency, 88,* 536–545.

Miller, J. L., Sonies, B. C., & Macedonia, C. (2003). Emergence of oropharyngeal, laryngeal and swallowing activity in the developing fetal upper aerodigestive tract: An ultrasound evaluation. *Early Human Development, 71,* 61–87.

Miller, L., Gilliam, R., & Peña, E. (2001). *Dynamic assessment and intervention: Improving children's narrative abilities.* Austin, TX: Pro-Ed.

Milosky, L. M. (1994). Nonliteral language abilities: Seeing the forest for the trees. In G. P. Wallach, & K. G. Butler (Eds.), *Language learning disabilities in school-age children and adolescents: Some principles and applications.* Boston, MA: Allyn & Bacon.

Mirenda, P. (1997). Supporting individuals with challenging behavior through functional communication training and AAC: Research review. *AAC, 13,* 207–225.

Mirenda, P. (2001). Autism, augmentative communication, and assistive technology: What do we really know? *Focus on Autism and Other Developmental Disabilities, 16,* 141–151.

Mirenda, P. (2003). Toward functional augmentative and alternative communication for students with autism: Manual signs, graphic symbols and voice output communication aids. *Language, Speech, and Hearing Services in Schools, 34,* 203–216.

Mirenda, P., & Erickson, K. A. (2000). Augmentative communication and literacy. In A. M. Wetherby & B. M. Prizant (Eds.), *Autism spectrum disorders: A transactional developmental perspective.* Baltimore, MD: Paul H. Brookes.

Mirenda, P., & Iacono, T. (1990). Communication options for persons with severe and profound disabilities: State of the art and future directions. *Journal of the Association for Persons with Severe Handicaps, 15,* 3–22.

Mirenda, P., & Mathy-Laikko, P. (1989). Augmentative and alternative communication applications for persons with severe congenital communication disorders: An introduction. *Augmentative and Alternative Communication, 5,* 3–13.

Mirrett, P. L., Roberts, J. E., & Price, J. (2003). Early intervention practices and communication intervention strategies for young males with fragile X syndrome. *Language, Speech, and Hearing Services in Schools, 34,* 320–331.

Mistretta, C. M. (1984). Aging effects on anatomy and neurophysiology of taste and smell. *Gerodontology, 3*(2), 131–136.

Miyazaki, T., Matsuya, T., & Yamaoka, M. (1975). Fiberscopic methods for assessment of velopharyngeal closure during various activities. *Cleft Palate Journal, 12,* 107–114.

Moersch, M. (1977). Training deaf-blind. *The American Journal of Occupational Therapy, 3,* 425–431.

Moog, J., & Geers, A. (1975). *Scales of early communication skills for hearing impaired children.* St. Louis, MO: Central Institute for the Deaf.

Moon, C., Bever, T. G., & Fifer, W. P. (1992). Canonical and non-canonical syllable discrimination by two-day-old infants. *Journal of Child Language, 19,* 1–17.

Moon, J. B., & Kuehn, D. P. (1996). Anatomy and physiology of normal and disordered velopharyngeal function for speech. The National Center for Voice and Speech, Status and Progress Report No. 9, 143–158

Moon, J. B., Kuehn, D. P. (2004). Anatomy and physiology of normal and disordered velopharyngeal function for speech. In K. R. Bzoch (Ed.), *Communicative disorders related to cleft lip and palate* (5th ed.). Austin, TX: Pro-Ed.

Moore, C. A., & Ruark, J. L. (1996). Does speech emerge from earlier appearing oral motor behaviors? *Journal of Speech and Hearing Research, 39,* 1034–1047.

Morgan, J. L. (1994). Converging measures of speech segmentation in prelingual infants. *Infant Behavior and Development, 17,* 389–403.

Morgan, J. L., & Saffran, J. R. (1995). Emerging integration of sequential and suprasegmental information in preverbal speech segmentation. *Child Development, 66,* 911–936.

Mulliken, J. B. (1985, April). Principles and techniques of bilateral complete cleft lip repair. *Plastic and Reconstructive Surgery, 75*(4), 477–487.

Mundy, P. (1995). Joint attention, social-emotional approach in children with autism. *Development and Psychopathology, 7,* 63–82.

Mundy, P., Kasari, C., Sigman, M., & Ruskin, E. (1995). Nonverbal communication and early language acquisition in children with Down syndrome and in normally developing children. *Journal of Speech and Hearing Research, 38,* 157–167.

Mundy, P., & Markus, J. (1997). On the nature of communication and language impairment in autism. *Mental Retardation and Developmental Disabilities Research Reviews, 3,* 343–349.

Mundy, P., Sigman, M., & Kasari, C. (1990). A longitudinal study of joint attention and language development in autistic children. *Journal of Autism and Developmental Disorders, 20,* 115–128.

Mundy, P., & Stella, J. (2000). Joint attention, social orienting and nonverbal communication in autism. In A. Wetherby & B. Prizant (Eds.), *Autism spectrum disorders: A transactional developmental perspective* (pp. 55–77). Baltimore, MD: Paul H. Brookes.

Munoz-Sandoval, A. F., Cummins, J., Alvarado, C. G., & Ruef, M. L. (1998). *Bilingual Verbal Ability Tests, comprehensive manual.* Itasca, IL: Riverside.

Munson, B., Edwards, J., & Beckman, M. E. (2005). Relationships between nonword repetition accuracy and other measures of linguistic development in children with phonological disorders. *Journal of Speech, Language, and Hearing Research, 48,* 61–78.

Murdoch, B. E. (2009). Acquired speech and language disorders: A neuroanatomical and functional neurological approach (2nd ed.). Oxford, England: Wiley-Blackwell.

Murdoch, B. E., Ozanne, A. E., & Cross, J. A. (1990). Acquired childhood speech disorders: Dysarthria and dyspraxia. In B. E. Murdock (Ed.), *Acquired neurological speech/ language disorders in childhood.* London England: Taylor & Francis.

Murray, J. C. (2002). Gene/environment causes of cleft lip and/or palate. *Clinical Genetics, 61,* 248–256.

Myers-Jennings, C. C. (2000). Phonological disorders in culturally diverse populations: Intervention issues and strategies. In T. J. Coleman (Ed.), *Clinical management of communication disorders in culturally diverse children* (pp. 173–196). Boston, MA: Allyn & Bacon.

Naigles, L. (1990). Children use syntax to learn verb meanings. *Journal of Child Language, 17,* 357–374.

Nakamura, K., Newell, A. F., Alm, N., & Waller, A. (1998). How do members of different language communities compose sentences with a picture-based communication system? A cross-cultural study of picture-based sentences constructed by English and Japanese speakers. *AAC, 14,* 71–79.

Nail-Chiwetalu, B. J., & Bernstein-Ratner, N. (2006). Information literacy for speech-language pathologists: A key to evidence-based practice. *Language, Speech, and Hearing Services in Schools, 37,* 157.

Namy, L. L., & Waxman, S. R. (1998). Words and gestures: Infants' interpretations of different forms of symbolic reference. *Child Development, 69,* 295–308.

Nathan, L., Stackhouse, J., Goulandris, N., & Snowling, M. J. (2004). The development of early literacy skills among children with speech difficulties: A test of the "critical age hypothesis." *Journal of Speech, Language, and Hearing Research, 47,* 377–391.

Nathan, L., Wells, B., & Donlan, C. (1998). Can children with speech difficulties process an unfamiliar accent? *Applied Psycholinguistics, 22,* 343–361.

Nation, K., & Hulme, C. (1997). Phonemic segmentation, not onset-rime segmentation, predicts early reading and spelling skills. *Reading Research Quarterly, 32,* 154–167.

National Dysphagia Diet Task Force. (2002). *National Dysphagia Diet: Standardization for optimal care.* Washington, DC: American Dietetic Association.

National Human Genome Research Institute (NHGRI). (2000). *Genetics: The future in medicine.* NIH Publication no. 00-4873.

National Institute on Alcohol Abuse and Alcoholism (NIAAA). (1990, January). *Seventh special report to the U.S. Congress on alcohol and health.* From the Secretary of Health and Human Services, U.S. Department of Health and Human Services, DHHS Publication No. [ADM] 90-1656. Washington, DC: U.S. Government Printing Office.

National Institutes of Health (NIH). (1979). *National research strategy for neurological and communicative disorders* (No. 79-1910). Washington, DC: National Institutes of Health.

National Institutes of Health (NIH). (2000). News release on National Reading Panel Report on Effective Reading Instruction, April 13.

National Joint Committee on Learning Disabilities (NJCLD). (1994). Position paper. Reprinted in *Topics in Language Disorders, 16*(1996), 69–73.

National Reading Panel. (2000). *Report of the National Reading Panel: Teaching children to read.* Washington, DC: National Institute of Child Health and Human Development.

Natvig, K. (1983). The laryngectomees in Norway: Study no. 3: Pre- and postoperative factors of significance to esophageal speech acquisition. *Journal of Otolaryngology, 12,* 322–328.

Nazzi, T., Bertoncini, J., & Mehler, J. (1998). Language discrimination by newborns: Towards an understanding of the role of rhythm. *Journal of Experimental Psychology: Human Perception and Performance, 24,* 756–766.

Nazzi, T., Jusczyk, P. W., & Johnson, E. K. (2000). Language discrimination by English learning 5-month-olds: Effects of rhythm and familiarity. *Journal of Memory and Langauge, 43,* 1–19.

Neils, J., & Aram, D. M. (1986). Family history of children with developmental language disorders. *Perceptual and Motor Skills, 63,* 655–658.

Nelson, K. E. (1991). The matter of time: Interdependencies between language and concepts. In S. A. Gelman & J. P. Byrnes (Eds.), *Perspectives on language and thought: Interrelations in development.* New York, NY: Cambridge University Press.

Nelson, K. E., Hampson, J., & Shaw, L. K. (1993). Nouns in early lexicons: Evidence, explanations, and implications. *Journal of Child Language, 20,* 61–84.

Nelson, N. W. (1998). *Childhood language disorders in context: Infancy through adolescence* (2nd ed.). Boston, MA: Allyn & Bacon.

Nelson, N. W. (2000, July). Basing eligibility on discrepancy criteria: A bad idea whose time has passed. *Language Learning and Education, ASHA Division 1 Newsletter,* 8–12.

Nelson, N. W. (2007, June 19). "Be-attitudes" for managing change in school-based practice. *The ASHA Leader,* pp. 20–21.

Netter, F. H. (1953). *The CIBA collection of medical illustrations: Nervous system.* New York, NY: CIBA Pharmaceutical Company.

Neuman, S. B., Copple, C., & Bredekamp, S. (2000). *Learning to read and write: Developmentally appropriate practices for young children*. Washington, DC: National Association for the Education of Young Children.

Neuman, S. B., & Dickinson, D. K. (2001). *Handbook of early literacy research*. New York, NY: Guilford Press.

Newcomer, P. L., & Barenbaum, E. M. (1991). The written composing ability of children with learning disabilities: A review of the literature from 1980 to 1990. *Journal of Learning Disabilities, 24,* 578–593.

Newman, C., Weinstein, B., Jacobson, G., & Hug, G. (1990). The Hearing Handicap Inventory for Adults: Psychometric adequacy and audiometric correlates. *Ear and Hearing, 11,* 430–433.

Nicholas, M., Bath, C., Obler, L. K., Au, R., & Albert, M. J. (1997). Naming in normal aging and dementia of the Alzheimer's type. In H. Goodglass & A. Wingfield (Eds.), *Anomia: Neuroanatomical and cognitive correlates* (pp. 166–188). San Diego, CA: Academic Press.

Nickel, R., & Widerstrom, A. (1997). Developmental disorders in infancy. In A. Widerstrom, B. Mowder, & S. Sandall (Eds.), *Infant development and risk* (2nd ed.). Baltimore, MD: Paul H. Brookes.

Nicosia, M. A., Hind, J. A., Roecker, E. B., Carnes, M., Doyle, J., Dengel, G. A., & Robbins, J. (2000). Age effects on temporal evolution of isometric and swallowing pressure. *Journal of Gerontology, Medical Sciences, 55A,* M634–640.

Nilsson, H., Ekberg, O., Olsson, R., & Hindfelt, B. (1996). Quantitative aspects of swallowing in an elderly non-dysphagia population. *Dysphagia, 11*(3), 180–184.

Nilsson, M., Soil, S. D., & Sullivan, J. A. (1994). Development of the Hearing in Noise Test for the measurement of speech reception thresholds in quiet and in noise. *Journal of the Acoustical Society of America, 95,* 1085–1099.

Ninio, A., & Bruner, J. S. (1978). The achievements and antecedents of labeling. *Journal of Child Language, 5,* 1–16.

Nippold, M. A. (1988a). Figurative language. In M. A. Nippold (Ed.), *Later language development: Ages nine through nineteen*. Boston, MA: College-Hill Press.

Nippold, M. A. (1988b). Verbal reasoning. In M. A. Nippold (Ed.), *Later language development: Ages nine through nineteen*. Boston, MA: College-Hill Press.

Nippold, M. A. (1998). *Later language development* (2nd ed.). Austin, TX: Pro-Ed.

Nippold, M. A. (2007). *Later language development: School-aged children, adolescents, and young adults* (3rd ed.). Austin, TX: ProEd.

Nippold, M. A., Hegel, S. L., Sohlberg, M. M., & Schwarz, I. E. (1999). Defining abstract entities: Development in pre-adolescents, adolescents, and young adults. *Journal of Speech, Language, and Hearing Research, 42,* 473–481.

Nippold, M. A., Hesketh, L. J., Duthie, J. K., & Mansfield, T. C. (2005). Conversational vs. expository discourse: A study of syntactic development in children, adolescents, and adults. *Journal of Speech, Language, and Hearing Research, 48,* 1048–1064.

Nippold, M. A., & Serajul Haq, F. (1996). Proverb comprehension in youth: The role of concreteness and familiarity. *Journal of Speech and Hearing Research, 39,* 166–176.

Nippold, M. A., & Taylor, C. L. (1995). Idiom understanding in youth: Further examination of familiarity and transparency. *Journal of Speech, Language, and Hearing Research, 38,* 426–433.

Nippold, M. A., Taylor, C. L., & Baker, J. M. (1995). Idiom understanding in Australian youth: A cross-cultural comparison. *Journal of Speech, Language, and Hearing Research, 39,* 442–447.

No Child Left Behind Act. (2001). P. L. 107–110.

Norris, J. A., & Damico, J. S. (1990). Whole language in theory and practice: Implications for language intervention. *Language, Speech, and Hearing Services in Schools, 21,* 212–220.

Northern, J. L., & Downs, M. P. (1991). *Hearing in children* (4th ed.). Baltimore, MD: Williams & Wilkins.

Northern, J. L., & Downs, M. P. (2001). *Hearing in children* (5th ed.). Baltimore, MD: Williams & Wilkins.

Notari-Syverson, A., O'Connor, R., & Vadasy, P. F. (1998). *Ladders to literacy: A preschool activity book*. Baltimore, MD: Paul H. Brookes.

O'Donnell, J. P., Armson, J., & Kiefte, M. (2008). The effectiveness of Speech Easy during situations of daily living, *Journal of Fluency Disorders, 33,* 99–119.

O'Neill, D. K., & Topolovec, J. C. (2000). Two-year-old children's sensitivity to the referential (in)efficacy of their own pointing gestures. *Journal of Child Language, 28,* 1–28.

Obler, L. K., & Albert, M. L. (1981). Language and aging: A neurobehavioral analysis. In D. Beasley & G. Davis (Eds.), *Aging: Communication processes and disorders*. New York, NY: Grune & Stratton.

Odom, A. C., & Upthegrove, M. (1997). Moving toward employment using AAC: Case study. *AAC, 13,* 258–262.

Odom, S. L., & McLean, M. E. (1996). *Early intervention/early childhood special education: Recommended practices*. Austin, TX: Pro-Ed.

Oetting, J., & Horohov, J. (1997). Past tense marking by children with and without specific language impairment. *Journal of Speech and Hearing Research, 40,* 62–74.

Oller, D. K., & Delgado, R. (1992). *LIPP: Logical international phonetic programs*. Miami, FL: Intelligent Hearing Systems.

Olsson, C., & Granlund, M. (2003). Presymbolic communication intervention. In R. W. Schlosser (Ed.), *The efficacy of augmentative and alternative communication: Toward evidence-based practice* (pp. 299–322). San Diego, CA: Academic Press.

Olswang, L. B., & Bain, B. (1996). Assessment information for predicting upcoming change in language production. *Journal of Speech and Hearing Research, 39,* 414–423.

Olswang, L. B., Long, S., & Fletcher, P. (1997). Verbs in the emergence of word combinations in young children with specific expressive language impairment. *European Journal of Disorders of Communication, 32,* 15–33.

Olswang, L. B., Rodriguez, B., & Timler, G. (1998). Recommending intervention for toddlers with specific language learning difficulties: We may not have all the answers, but we know a lot. *American Journal of Speech-Language Pathology, 7,* 23–32.

Onslow, M., Packman, A., & Harrison, E. (2003). *The Lidcombe Programme of early childhood stuttering intervention: A clinician's guide.* Austin, TX: Pro-Ed.

Orton, S., & Travis, L. E. (1929). Studies in stuttering: IV. Studies of action currents in stutterers. *Archives of Neurology and Psychiatry, 21,* 61–68.

Ourand, P. R., & Gray, S. (1997). Funding and legal issues in augmentative and alternative communication. In S. L. Glennen & D. C. DeCoste (Eds.), *Handbook of augmentative and alternative communication* (pp. 335–360). San Diego, CA: Singular Publishing Group.

Owens, E., Kessler, D., Roggio, M., & Schubert, E. (1985). Analysis and revision of the minimal auditory capabilities (MAC) battery. *Ear and Hearing, 6,* 280–287.

Owens, R. (1978). *Speech acts in the early language of non-delayed and retarded children: A taxonomy and distributional study* (Unpublished doctoral dissertation). The Ohio State University, Columbus.

Owens, R. (1999). *Language disorders: A functional approach to assessment and intervention* (3rd ed.). Boston, MA: Allyn & Bacon.

Owens, R. (2010). *Language development: An introduction* (7th ed.). Boston, MA: Allyn & Bacon.

Owens, R. E., Jr. (2001). *Language development: An introduction* (5th ed.). Boston, MA: Allyn & Bacon.

Owens, R. E., Jr. (2002). Development of communication, language, and speech. In G. H. Shames & N. B. Anderson (Eds.), *Human communication disorders: An introduction* (6th ed.). Boston, MA: Allyn & Bacon.

Owens, R. E., Jr. (2010). *Language disorders: A functional approach to assessment and intervention* (5th ed.). Boston, MA: Pearson.

Owens, R. E., Jr., & House, L. I. (1984). Decision-making processes in augmentative communication. *Journal of Speech and Hearing Disorders, 49,* 18–25.

Oxford, M., & Spieker, S. (2006). Preschool language development among children of adolescent mother. *Applied Developmental Psychology, 27,* 165–182.

Özçaliskan, S., & Goldin-Meadow, S. (2005). Do parents lead their children by the hand? *Journal of Child Language, 32,* 481–505.

Palmer, J. B. (1989). Electromyography of the muscles of oropharyngeal swallowing: Basic concepts. *Dysphagia, 3,* 192–198.

Pamplona, M. C., Ysuna, A., & Uriostegui, C. (1996). Linguistic interaction: The active role of parents in speech therapy for cleft palate patients. *International Journal of Pediatric Otorhinolaryngology, 37*(1), 17–27.

Pan, B. A., Rowe, M. L., Singer, J. D., & Snow, C. E. (2005). Maternal correlates of growth in toddler vocabulary production in low income families. *Child Development, 76,* 763–782.

Pannebacker, M. (1998). Voice treatment techniques: A review and recommendations for outcome studies. *American Journal of Speech-Language Pathology, 7*(3), 49–64.

Papaeliou, C., Minadakis, G., & Cavouras, D. (2002). Acoustic patterns of infant vocalizations expressing emotions and communicative functions. *Journal of Speech, Language, and Hearing Research, 45,* 311–317.

Papaeliou, C. F., & Trevarthen, C. (2006) Prelinguistic pitch patterns expressing "communication" and "apprehension." *Journal of Child Language, 33,* 163–178.

Paradis, M. (2004). *A neurolinguistic theory of bilingualism.* Amsterdam, The Netherlands: John Benjamins.

Paradise, J. L., Bluestone, C. D., & Felder, H. (1969). The universality of otitis media in 50 infants with cleft palate. *Pediatrics, 44*(1), 35–42.

Paradise, J. L., & McWilliams, B. J. (1974). Simplified feeder for infants with cleft palate. *Pediatrics, 53,* 566–568.

Patterson, J. L. (2002). Relationships of expressive vocabulary to frequency of reading and television experience among bilingual toddlers. *Applied Psycholinguistics, 23,* 493–508.

Paul, D., Frattali, C., Holland, A., Thompson, C., Caperton, C., & Slater, S. (2004). *Quality of communication life scale.* Rockville MD: American Speech-Language-Hearing Association.

Paul, P., & Quigley, S. (1990). *Education and deafness* (pp. 127–150). New York, NY: Longman.

Paul, R. (1991). Profiles of toddlers with slow expressive language development. *Topics in Language Disorders, 11,* 1–13.

Paul, R. (2000). Disorders in communication. In M. Lewis (Ed.), *Child and adolescent psychiatry* (3rd ed.). Baltimore, MD: Williams & Wilkins.

Paul, R. (2007). *Language disorders from infancy through adolescence: Assessment and intervention* (3rd ed.). St. Louis, MO: Mosby.

Paul, R., & Shriberg, L. (1982). Associations among pragmatic functions, linguistic stress, and natural phonological processes in speech-delayed children. *Journal of Speech and Hearing Research, 25,* 536–547.

Paulson, D. M. (1991). *Phonological systems of Spanish-speaking Texas preschoolers* (Thesis). Texas Christian University.

Payne, K. (1997). Considerations for speech and language assessment of multicultural populations following stroke. In *Communication disorders and stroke in African American and other cultural group* (pp. 85–94). Bethesda, MD: National Institutes of Health.

Peets, K. F. (2009). The effects of context on the classroom discourse skills of children with language impairment. *Language, Speech, and Hearing Services in Schools, 40,* 5–16.

Paradis, M. (2004). *A neurolinguistic theory of bilingualism.* Amsterdam, The Netherlands: John Benjamins.

Peña, E. D., & Valles, L. (1995). Language assessment and instructional programming for linguistically different learners: Proactive classroom processes. In H. Kayser (Ed.), *Bilingual speech-language pathology: An Hispanic focus* (pp. 129–152). San Diego, CA: Singular Publishing Group.

Pence, K. L., & Justice, L. M. (2008). *Language development from theory to practice.* Upper Saddle River, NJ: Person.

Pendergast, K., Dickey, S., Selmar, T., & Soder, A. (1969). *The photo articulation test* (2nd ed.). Danville, IL: Interstate Press.

Perkins, W. H., Kent, R. D., & Curlee, R. F. (1991). A theory of neuropsycholinguistic function in stuttering. *Journal of Speech and Hearing Research, 34,* 734–752.

Perkins, W. H., Ruder, J., Johnson, L., & Michael, W. (1976). Stuttering: Discoordination of phonation with articulation and respiration. *Journal of Speech and Hearing Research, 19,* 509–522.

Perlman, A. (1991). The neurology of swallowing. In B. C. Sonies (Ed.), *Seminar in speech and language: Swallowing disorders* (pp. 171–185). New York, NY: Thieme.

Perlman, A. L., Schultz, J. G., & VanDaele, D. J. (1993). Effects of age, gender, bolus volume and bolus viscosity on oropharyngeal pressure during swallowing. *Journal of Applied Physiology, 75,* 33–37.

Persson, C., Elander, A., Lohmander-Agerskov, A., & Soderpalm, E. (2002). Speech outcomes in isolated cleft palate: Impact of cleft extent and additional malformations. *Cleft Palate–Craniofacial Journal, 39(4),* 397–408.

Pigott, R. W. (1969). The nasendoscopic appearance of the normal palatopharyngeal valve. *Plastic Reconstructive Surgery, 43,* 19–24.

Pigott, R. W., & Makepeace, A. P. (1982). Some characteristics of endoscopic and radiological systems used in elaboration of the diagnosis of velopharyngeal incompetence. *British Journal of Plastic Surgery, 35,* 19–32.

Pine, J. M. (1990). *Non-referential children: Slow or different?* Paper presented at the Fifth International Congress for the Study of Child Language, Budapest, Hungary.

Plante, E. (1991). MRI findings in the parents and siblings of specifically language-impaired boys. *Brain and Language, 41,* 67–80.

Plante, E., Swisher, L., & Vance, R. (1989). Anatomical correlates of normal and impaired language in a pair of dizygotic twins. *Brain and Language, 37,* 643–655.

Plante, E., Swisher, L., Vance, R., & Rapcsak, S. (1991). MRI findings in boys with specific language impairments. *Brain and Language, 41,* 52–66.

Plunkett, K. (1993). Lepical segmentation and vocabulary growth in early language acquisition. *Journal of Child Language, 20,* 43–60.

Pokorni, J. L., Worthington, C. K., & Jamison, P. J. (2004). Phonological awareness intervention: Comparison of Fast ForWord, Earobics, and LiPS. *The Journal of Educational Research, 97(3),* 147–157.

Pollack, M., & Shprintzen, R. J. (1981). Velopharyngeal insufficiency in neurofibromatosis. *International Journal of Pediatric Otorhinolaryngology, 3,* 257–262.

Pollard, R., Ellis, J. B., Finan, D., Ramig, P. R. (2009). Effects of the Speech Easy on objective and perceived aspects of stuttering: A six-month, Phase I Clinical trial in naturalistic environments. *Journal of Speech, Language, and Hearing Research, 52,* 516–533.

Porch, B. E. (1967). *Porch Index of Communicative Ability.* Palo Alto, CA: Consulting Psychologists Press.

Postma, A., & Kolk, H. H. J. (1993). The covert repair hypothesis: Prearticulatory repair processes in normal and stuttered disfluencies. *Journal of Speech and Hearing Research, 36,* 472–487.

Powers, G. R. (2000). Communication sciences and disorders: The discipline. In R. B. Gillam, T. P. Marquardt, & F. N. Martin (Eds.), *Communication sciences and disorders: From science to clinical practice, Instructors version.* Clifton Park, NY: Thomson Delmar Learning.

Powers, M. (1971). Clinical educational procedures in functional disorders of articulation. In L. Travis (Ed.), *Handbook of speech pathology and audiology.* Englewood Cliffs, NJ: Prentice-Hall.

Prasada, S., & Ferenz, K. S. (2002). Singular or plural? Children's knowledge of the factors that determine the appropriate form of count nouns. *Journal of Child Language, 29,* 49–70.

Preisler, G. M. (1995). The development of communication in blind and deaf infants—Similarities and differences. *Child Care, Health, and Development, 21(2),* 79–110.

Preminger, J. E. (2003). Should significant others be encouraged to join adult group audiologic rehabilitation classes? *Journal of the American Academy of Audiology, 10,* 545–555.

Prentke Romich Company. (1989). *How to obtain funding for augmentative communication devices.* Wooster, OH: Author.

Prieve, B., & Fitzgerald, T. (2009). Otoacoustic emissions. In J. Katz, L. Medwetsky, R. Burkard, & L. Hood (Eds.), *Handbook of clinical audiology* (pp. 497–528). Baltimore, MD: Lippincott Williams & Wilkins.

Prizant, B. M., & Rydell, P. J. (1993). Assessment and intervention considerations for unconventional verbal behavior. In S. F. Warren & J. Reichle (Series Eds.), J. Reichle & D. Wacker (Vol. Eds.), *Communication and Language Intervention Series: Vol. 3. Communicative alternatives to challenging behavior: Integrating functional assessment and intervention strategies* (pp. 263–297). Baltimore, MD: Paul H. Brookes.

Prizant, B. M., & Wetherby, A. (1987). Communicative intent: A framework for understanding social-communicative behavior in autism. *Journal of the American Academy of Child Psychiatry, 26,* 472–479.

Project SEEL. Accessed from education.byu.edu/literacy/index.html

Pruess, J., Vadasy, P., & Fewell, R. (1987). Language development in children with Down syndrome: An overview of recent research. *Education and Training of the Mentally Retarded, 22,* 44–55.

Pulvermüller, F., Neininger, B., Elbert, T. E., Mohr, B., Rockstroh, B., Koebbel, P., & Taub, E. (2001). Constraint-induced therapy of chronic aphasia following stroke. *Stroke, 32,* 1621–1626.

Queisser-Luft, A., Eggers, I., Stolz, G., Kieninger-Baum, D., & Schlaefer, K. (1996). Serial examination of 20,248 newborn fetuses and infants: Correlations between drug exposure and major malformations. *American Journal of Medical Genetics, 63(1),* 268–76.

Quinn, R. (1995). "Early intervention? Que quiere decir eso?" What does that mean? In H. Kayser (Ed.), *Bilingual speech-language pathology: An Hispanic focus.* San Diego, CA: Singular Publishing Group.

Quist, R. W., & Lloyd, L. L. (1997). Principles and uses of technology. In L. L. Lloyd, D. R. Fuller, & H. H. Arvidson (Eds.), *Augmentative and alternative communication: A handbook of principles and practices.* Boston, MA: llyn & Bacon.

Ramig, L. O., Countryman, S., O'Brien, C., Hoehn, M., & Thompson, L. (1996). Intensive speech treatment for patients with Parkinson disease: Short and long-term comparison of two techniques. *Neurology, 47,* 1496–1504.

Ramig, L.O., Sapir, S., Countryman, S., Pawlas, A. A., O'Brien, C., Hoehn, M., & Thompson, L. L. (2001). Intensive voice treatment (LSVT) for patients with Parkinson's disease: A 2 year follow up. *Journal of Neruology, Neurosurgery, and Psychiatry, 17*(4), 493–498.

Ramig, L. O. Sapir, S., Fox, C., & Countryman, S. (2001). Changes in vocal intensity following intensive voice treatment (LSVT) in individuals with Parkinson disease: A comparison with untreated patients and normal age-matched controls. *Movement Disorders, 16,* 79–83.

Ramig, L. O., & Verdolini, K. (2004). *Treatment efficacy summary: Laryngeal-based voice disorders.* Retrieved July 2004, from www.asha.org/members/slp/healthcare/efficacy.htm

Ramig, P. R. (1993). High reported spontaneous stuttering recovery rates: Fact or fiction? *Language, Speech, and Hearing Services in Schools, 24,* 156–160.

Ramig, P. R. (1994). *To parents of the nonfluent child.* Unpublished manuscript.

Ramig, P. R., & Adams, M. R. (1981). Vocal characteristics of normal speakers and stutterers during choral reading. *Journal of Fluency Disorders, 6,* 15–33.

Ramig, P. R., & Bennett, E. (1995). Working with 7- to 12-year-old children who stutter: Ideas for intervention in the public schools. *Language, Speech, and Hearing Services in Schools, 26,* 138–150.

Ramig, P. R., & Bennett, E. (1997). Clinical management of children: Direct management strategies. In R. Curlee & G. Siegel (Eds.), *Nature and treatment of stuttering: New directions* (2nd ed.). Boston, MD: Allyn & Bacon.

Ramig, P. R., Krieger, S. M., & Adams, M. R. (1982). Vocal changes in stutterers and non-stutterers when speaking to children. *Journal of Fluency Disorders, 7,* 369–384.

Rammage, L., Morrison, M., & Nichol, H. (2001). *Management of the voice and its disorders.* Vancouver, Canada: Singular Thomson Learning.

Read, C. (1971). Preschool children's knowledge of English phonology. *Harvard Educational Review, 41,* 1–34.

Reed, C. M. (1995). Tadoma: An overview of research. In G. Plant & K. E. Spens (Eds.), *Profound deafness and speech communication.* London, England: Whurr.

Reed, V. (1986). An introduction to language. In V. Reed (Ed.), *An introduction to children with language disorders.* New York, NY: Macmillan.

Reichle, J., & Karlan, G. (1985). The selection of an augmentative system in communication intervention: A critique of decision rules. *Journal of the Association for Persons with Severe Handicaps, 10,* 146–156.

Reichle, J., & Wacker, D. P. (1993). *Communicative alternatives to challenging behavior: Integrating functional assessment and intervention strategies.* Baltimore, MD: Paul H. Brookes.

Reichle, J., York, J., & Sigafoos, J. (1991). *Implementing augmentative and alternative communication: Strategies for learners with severe disabilities.* Baltimore, MD: Paul H. Brookes.

Reid, D. K. (2000). The development of discourse: Conversations, stories, and explanations. In K. Fahey & D. K. Reid (Eds.), *Language development, differences and disorders.* Austin, TX: Pro-Ed.

Reinhartsen, D. B., Edmondson, R., & Crais, E. R. (1997). Developing assistive technology strategies for infants and toddlers with communication difficulties. *Seminars in Speech and Hearing, 18,* 283–301.

Remen, R. N. (1996, Spring). In the service of life. *Noetic Sciences Review, 37,* 24–25. Retrieved November 3, 2003, from www.theinterpretersfriend.com/Terpsnet/11.html

Remen, R. N. (2001, January). Recapturing the soul of medicine. *Western Journal of Medicine, 174,* 4–5. Retrieved June 24, 2004, from www.rachelremen.com/recapturing.html

Ren, Y. F., Isberg, A., & Henningsson, G. (1995). Velopharyngeal incompetence and persistent hypernasality after adenoidectomy in children without palatal defect. *Cleft Palate–Craniofacial Journal, 32*(6), 476–482.

Rescorla, L. (2005). Age 13 language and reading outcomes in late-talking children. *Journal of Speech, Language, and Hearing Research, 48,* 459–472.

Rescorla, L. (2009). Age 17 language and reading outcomes in late-talking toddlers: Support for a dimensional perspective on language delay. *Journal of Speech, Language, and Hearing Research, 52,* 16–30.

Reyes, B. (1995). Consideration in the assessment and treatment of neurogenic disorders in bilingual adults. In H. Kayser (Ed.), *Bilingual speech-language pathology: An Hispanic focus.* San Diego, CA: Singular Publishing Group.

Rice, M. (1984). Cognitive aspects of communicative development. In R. Schiefelbusch & J. Pickar (Eds.), *The acquisition of communicative competence.* Baltimore, MD: University Park Press.

Rice, M., Taylor, C., & Zubrick, S. (2008). Language outcomes comes of 7-year-old children with or without a history of late language emergence at 24 months. *Journal of Speech, Language, and Hearing Research, 51,* 394–407.

Rice, M. L., Alexander, A., & Hadley, P. (1993). Social biases toward children with speech and language impairments: A correlative causal model of language limitation. *Applied Psycholinguistics, 14,* 473–488.

Rice, M. L., & Hadley, P. A. (1995). Language outcomes of the language-focused curriculum. In M. L. Rice & K. A. Wilcox (Eds.), *Building a language-focused curriculum for the preschool classroom: A foundation for lifelong communication* (pp. 155–170). Baltimore, MD: Paul H. Brookes.

Rice, M. L., Wexler, K., & Hershberger, S. (1998). Tense over time: The longitudinal course of tense acquisition in children with specific language impairment. *Journal of Speech, Language, and Hearing Research, 41,* 1412–1431.

Rispoli, M. (2005). When children reach beyond their grasp: Why some children make pronoun case errors and others don't. *Journal of Child Language, 32,* 93–116.

Robb, M. P., Bauer, H. R., & Tyler, A. A. (1994). A quantitative analysis of the single-word stage. *First Language, 14,* 37–48.

Robbins, J, Gangnon, R., Theis, S., Kayst, S., Hewitt, A., & Hind, J. (2005). The effects of lingual exercise on swallowing in older adults. *Journal of the American Geriatrics Society, 53,* 1483–1489.

Robbins, J., Gensler, G., Hind, J., Logemann, J., Lindblad, D., Baum, H., . . . Gardner, P. (2008). Comparison of 2 interventions for liquid aspiration on pneumonia incidence. *Annals of Internal Medicine, 148,* 509–518.

Robbins, J. A., Hamilton, J. W., Lof, G. L., & Kempster, G. B. (1992). Oropharyngeal swallowing in normal adults of different ages. *Gastroenterology, 103,* 823–829.

Robbins, J. A., & Levine, R. L. (1988). Swallowing after unilateral stroke of the cerebral cortex: Preliminary experience. *Dysphagia, 3,* 11–17.

Robbins, J. A., Levine, R. L., Maser, A., Rosenbek, J. C., & Kempster, G. L. (1993). Swallowing after unilateral cerebral stroke. *Archives of Physical and Medical Rehabilitation, 74,* 1295–1300.

Robbins, J. A., Levine, R. L., Wood, J., Roecker, E. B., & Luschei, E. (1995). Age effects on lingual pressure generation as a risk factor for dysphagia. *Journal of Gerontology, 50,* M257–M262.

Robbins, J. A., Logemann, J. A., & Kirshner, H. S. (1986). Swallowing and speech production in Parkinson's disease. *Annals of Neurology, 19,* 283-287.

Roberts, J., Rescorla, L., Giroux, J., & Stevens, L. (1998). Phonological skills of children with specific expressive language impairment (SLI-E): Outcome at age 3. *Journal of Speech, Language, and Hearing Research, 41,* 374–384.

Roberts, J. E., Mirrett, P., Anderson, K., Burchinal, M., & Neebe, E. (2002). Early communication, symbolic behavior and social profiles of young males with fragile X syndrome. *American Journal of Speech-Language Pathology, 11,* 295–304.

Roberts, J. E., Mirrett, P., & Burchinal, M. (2001). Receptive and expressive communication development of young males with fragile X syndrome. *American Journal on Mental Retardation, 106,* 216–230.

Roberts, K., & Horowitz, F. (1986). Basic level categorization in seven- and nine-month-old infants. *Journal of Child Language, 13,* 191–208.

Roberts, P. M. (2001). Aphasia assessment and treatment for bilingual and culturally diverse clients. In R. Chapey, *Language intervention strategies in aphasia and related neurogenic communication disorders* (4th ed.) pp. 208–234). New York, NY: Lippincott, Williams & Wilkins.

Robey, R. (1998). A meta-analysis of clinical outcomes in the treatment of aphasia. *Journal of Speech and Hearing Research, 40,* 172–187.

Robinson, T. L., & Crowe, T. A. (2000). Multicultural issues and speech fluency. In T. J. Coleman (Ed.), *Clinical management of communication disorders in culturally diverse children* (pp. 251–269). Boston, MA: Allyn & Bacon.

Rollins, P. R. (2003). Caregivers' contingent comments to 9-month-old infants: Relationships with later language. *Applied Psycholinguistics, 24,* 221–234.

Rollnick, B. R., & Pruzansky, S. (1981). Genetic services at a center for craniofacial anomalies. *Cleft Palate Journal, 18*(4), 304–313.

Rome-Flanders, T., & Cronk, C. (1995). A longitudinal study of infant vocalizations during mother-infant games. *Journal of Child Language, 22,* 259–274.

Rondal, J., Ghiotto, M., Bredart, S., & Bachelet, J. (1987). Age-relation, reliability and grammatical validity of measures of utterance length. *Journal of Child Language, 14,* 433–446.

Rönnberg, J., & Brog, E. (2001). A review and evaluation of research on the deaf-blind from perceptual, communicative, social and rehabilitive perspectives. *Scandinavian Audiology 30,* 67–77.

Roseberry-McKibbin, C. (2002). *Multicultural students with special needs: Practical strategies for assessment and intervention.* Oceanside, CA: Academic Communication Associates.

Roseberry-Mckibbin, C. (2007). *Language disorders in children: A multicultural and case perspective.* Boston, MA: Pearson.

Rosenbek, J. C., Robbins, J. A., Roecker, E. B., Coyle, J. C., & Wood, J. L. (1996). A penetration-aspiration scale. *Dysphagia, 11,* 93–96.

Rosenbek, J. C., Roecker, E., Wood, J., & Robbins, J. (1996). Thermal application reduces the duration of stage transition in dysphagia after stroke. *Dysphagia, 11,* 225–233.

Rosetti, L. M. (1996). *Communication intervention: Birth to three.* San Diego, CA: Singular Publishing Group.

Ross, M., & Lerman, J. (1970). A picture identification test for hearing impaired children. *Journal of Speech and Hearing Research, 13,* 44–53.

Roth, F. P. (2000). Narrative writing: Development and teaching with children with writing difficulties. *Topics in Language Disorders, 20,* 15–28.

Roth, F. P. (2009). Early oral stories and expository narratives. In P. Rhymer (Ed.), *Emergent and early literacy acquisition: Making the connection.* New York, NY: Guilford Press.

Roth, F. P., & Baden, B. (2001). Investing in emergent literacy intervention: A key role for speech-language pathologists. *Seminars in Speech and Language, 22,* 163–174.

Roth, F. P., Speece, D. L., & Cooper, D. H. (2002). A longitudinal analysis of the connection between oral language and early reading. *Journal of Educational Research, 95,* 259–272.

Roth, F. P., Speece, D. L., Cooper, D. H., & De La Paz, S. (1996). Unresolved mysteries: How do metalinguistic and narrative skills connect with early reading? *Journal of Special Education, 30,* 257–277.

Roth, F. P., & Spekman, N. J. (1986). Narrative discourse: Spontaneously generated stories of learning disabled and normally achieving students. *Journal of Speech and Hearing Disorders, 51,* 8–23.

Roth, F. P., Spekman, N. J., & Fye, E. C. (1992, November). *Patterns of oral and written stories of learning disabled students.* Paper presented to the American Speech-Language-Hearing Association, San Antonio, TX.

Roth, F. P., & Troia, G. A. (2009). Applications of responsiveness to intervention and the speech-language pathologist in elementary school settings. *Seminars in Speech and Language, 30,* 75–89.

Roth, F. P., Troia, G. A., Worthington, C. K., & Dow, K. A. (2002). Promoting awareness of sounds of speech: An initial report of an early intervention program for children with speech and language impairments. *Applied Psycholinguistics, 23,* 535–565.

Roth, F. P., Troia, G. A. Worthington, C. K., & Handy, D. (2006). Promoting awareness of sound in speech: A follow-up report of an early intervention program for children with speech and language impairments. *Learning Disability Quarterly, 29,* 67–88.

Rowland, C. F., Pine, J. M., Lieven, E. V. M., & Theakston, A. L. (2005). The incidence of error in young children's wh-questions. *Journal of Speech, Language, and Hearing Research, 48,* 384–404.

Roy, N., Ford, C. N., & Bless, D. M. (1996). Muscle tension dysphonia and spasmodic dysphonia: The role of manual laryngeal tension reduction in diagnosis and management, *Annals of Otology, Rhinology, and Laryngology, 105(11),* 851–856.

Roy, N., Gray, S. D., Simon, M., Dove, H., Corbin-Lewis, K., & Stemple, J. C. (2001). An evaluation of the effects of two treatment approaches for teachers with voice disorders: A prospective randomized clinical trial. *Journal of Speech, Language, and Hearing Research, 44(2),* 286–296.

Roy, N., Mauszycki, S. C., Merrill, R. M., Gouse, M., & Smith, M. E. (2007). Toward improved differential diagnosis of adductor spasmodic dysphonia and muscle tension dysphonia. *Folia Phoniatrica et Logopaedia, 59(2),* 83–90.

RTI Action Network. (2009). Retrieved April 7, 2009, from rtinetwork.org

Ryalls, B., & Pisoni, D. (1997). The effect of talker variability on word recognition in preschool children. *Development Psychology, 33,* 441–452.

Sander, E. (1972). When are speech sounds learned? *Journal of Speech and Hearing Disorders, 37,* 55–63.

Sanders, L. D., & Neville, H. J. (2000). Lexical, syntactic, and stress-pattern cues for speech segmentation. *Journal of Speech, Language, and Hearing Research, 43,* 1301–1321.

Sanford, A. J., & Garrod, S. M. (1998). The role of scenario mapping in text comprehension. *Discourse Processes, 26,* 159–190.

Saunders, N. C., Hartley, B. E., Sell, D., & Sommerlad, B. (2004). Velopharyngeal insufficiency following adenoidectomy. *Clinical Otolaryngology and Allied Sciences, 29(6),* 686–688.

Scanlon, D. M., Vellutino, F. R., Small, S. G., Fanuele, D. P., & Sweeney, J. M. (2005). Severe reading difficulties—Can they be prevented? A comparison of prevention and intervention approaches. *Exceptionality, 13,* 209–227.

Scarborough, H. S. (1998). Early identification of children at risk for reading disabilities. In B. K. Shapiro, P. J. Accardo, & A. J. Capute (Eds.), *Specific reading disability: A view of the spectrum* (pp. 75–119). Timonium, MD: York Press.

Scarborough, H. S. (2001). Connecting early language and literacy to later reading (dis)abilities: Evidence, theory, and practice. In S. B. Neuman & D. K. Dickinson (Eds.), *Handbook of early literacy research* (pp. 97–110). New York, NY: Guilford Press.

Scarborough, H. S. (2005). Developmental relationship between language and reading: Reconciling a beautiful hypothesis with some ugly facts. In H. W. Catts & A. G. Kamhi (Eds.), *The connections between language and reading disabilities* (pp. 3–240) Mahwah, NJ: Laurence Erlbaum.

Scarborough, H. S., & Dobrich, W. (1990). Development of children with early language delay. *Journal of Speech and Hearing Research, 33,* 70–83.

Schafer, G. (2005). Infants can learn decontextualized words before their first birthday. *Child Development, 76,* 87–96.

Scherer, N. J. (2003). *Early speech intervention: Effects of a parent implemented treatment.* Paper presented at the conference of the American Cleft Palate Association, Asheville, NC.

Schlesinger, I. (1971). Production of utterances and language acquisition. In D. Slobin (Ed.), *The ontogenesis of grammar.* New York, NY: Academic Press.

Schlosser, R. W. (1997). Communication-based approaches to problem behavior. In L. L. Lloyd, D. R. Fuller, & H. H. Arvidson (Eds.), *Augmentative and alternative communication: A handbook of principles and practices* (pp. 445–473). Boston, MA: Allyn & Bacon.

Schlosser, R. W. (2003a). Effects of AAC on natural speech development. In R. W. Schlosser (Ed.), *The efficacy of augmentative and alternative communication: Toward evidence-based practice* (pp. 404–425). San Diego, CA: Academic Press.

Schlosser, R. W. (2003b). *The efficacy of augmentative and alternative communication: Toward evidence-based practice.* San Diego, CA: Academic Press.

Schlosser, R. W. (2003c). Outcomes measurement in AAC. In J. C. Light, D. R. Beukelman, & J. Reichle (Eds.), *Communicative competence for individuals who use AAC: From research to practice* (pp. 479–513). Baltimore, MD: Paul H. Brookes.

Schlosser, R. W. (2003d). Speech output: Taking stock and moving forward [Special issue]. *Augmentative and Alternative Communication, 19(1)2.*

Schlosser, R. W., & Blischak, D. (2001). Is there a role for speech output in interventions for persons with autism? A review. *Focus on Autism and Other Developmental Disabilities, 16,* 170–178.

Schlosser, R. W., & Goetze, H. (1992). Effectiveness and treatment validity of interventions addressing self-injurious behavior: From narrative reviews to meta-analyses. In T. E. Scruggs, & M. A. Mastropieri (Eds.), *Advances in learning and behavioral disabilities* (Vol. 7, pp. 135–175). Greenwich, CT: JAI Press.

Schlosser, R. W., & Raghavendra, P. (2003). Toward evidence-based practice in AAC. In R. W. Schlosser (Ed.), *The efficacy* of augmentative and alternative communication: Toward evidence-based practice (pp. 260–297). San Diego, CA: Academic Press.

Schober-Peterson, D., & Johnson, C. (1989). Conversational topics of 4-year-olds. Journal of Speech and Hearing Research, 32, 857–870.

Schory, M. (1990). Whole language and the speech-language pathologist. Language, Speech, and Hearing Services in Schools, 21, 206–211.

Schow, R. L., & Nerbonne, M. A. (2002). Introduction to audiologic rehabilitation. Boston, MA: Allyn & Bacon.

Schuler, A. L., & Prizant, B. M. (1985). Echolalia. In E. Schopler & G. Mesibov (Eds.), Communication problems in autism (pp. 163–184). New York, NY: Plenum.

Schulze-Delrieu, K. S., & Miller, R. (1997). Clinical assessment of dysphagia. In A. L. Perlmann & K. Shultze-Delrieu (Eds.), Deglutition and its disorders: Anatomy, physiology, clinical diagnosis and management (pp. 125–152). San Diego, CA: Singular Publishing Group.

Schwartz, R. (1992). Clinical applications of recent advances in phonological theory. Language, Speech, and Hearing Services in Schools, 23, 269–276.

Schwartz, R. G., Mody, M., & Petinou, K. (1998). Phonological acquisition in children with OME: Speech perception and speech production. In J. Roberts & I. Wallace (Eds.), Otitis media, language, and learning in young children. Baltimore, MD: Paul H. Brookes.

Schwartz, R., Messick, C., & Pollock, K. (1983). Some non-phonological aspects of assessment. In J. Locke (Ed.), Assessment of phonological disorders: Seminars in speech, language and hearing. New York, NY: Thieme-Stratton.

Sciortino, K. F., Liss, J. M., Case, J. L., Gerritsen, K. G. M., & Katz, R. C. (2003). Effects of mechanical, cold, gustatory, and combined stimulation to the human anterior faucial pillars. Dysphagia, 18, 16–26.

Scollon, R., & Scollon, S. (1981). Narrative, literacy, and face in interethnic communication. Norwood, NJ: Ablex.

Scott, C. (1988). Producing complex sentences. Topics in Language Disorders, 8(2), 44–62.

Scott, C. (1994). A discourse continuum for school-age students. In G. Wallach & K. Butler (Eds.), Language learning disabilities in school-age children and adolescents. New York, NY: Macmillan.

Scott, C. (2004). Syntactic ability in children and adolescents with language and learning disabilities. In R. Berman (Ed.), Language development across childhood and adolescence. Philadelphia, PA: John Benjamins.

Scott, C., & Windsor, J. (2000). General language performance measures in spoken and written narrative and expository discourse of school-age children with language learning disabilities. Journal of Speech, Language, and Hearing Research, 43, 324–339.

Scott, C. M. (2005). Learning to write. In H. W. Catts & A. G. Kamhi (Eds.), Language and reading disabilities (2nd ed., pp. 224–258). Boston, MA: Allyn & Bacon.

Scott, J., Flower, E. A., & Bums, J. (1987, November). A quantitative study of histalogical changes in the human parotid gland occurring with adult age. Journal of Oral Pathology, 16(10), 505–510.

Scott, J. A., & Ehri, L. C. (1990). Sight word reading in prereaders: Use of logographic vs. alphabetic access routes. Journal of Reading Behavior, 22, 149–166.

Seewald, R. C. (2004). Treatment efficacy summary: Hearing aids for infants and children. Retrieved July 2004, from www.asha.org/members/slp/healthcare/efficacy.htm

Semel, E. M., Wiig, E. H., & Secord, W. A. (1995). Clinical evaluation of language fundamentals–3. San Antonio, TX: Psychological Corp.

Senechal, M., LeFevre, L., Hudson, E., & Lawson, E. P. (1996). Knowledge of storybooks as a predictor of young children's vocabulary. Journal of Educational Psychology, 88, 520–538.

Seymour, H. N. (1986). Clinical intervention for language disorders among nonstandard speakers of English. In O. L. Taylor (Ed.), Treatment of communication disorders in culturally and linguistically diverse populations (pp. 135–152). San Diego, CA: College-Hill Press.

Seymour, H. N., Roper, T. W., & de Villiers, J. (2003). Diagnostic evaluation of language variation: Examiner's manual. San Antonio, TX: Psychological Corp.

Shaker, R., Easterling, C., Kern, M., Nitschke, T., Massey, B., Daniels, S., … Dikeman, K. (2002). Rehabilitation of swallowing by exercise in tube-fed patients with pharyngeal dysphagia secondary to abnormal UES opening. Gastroenterology, 122, 1314–1321.

Shaker, R., Ren, J., Podvrsan, B., Dodds, W. J., Hogan, W. J., Kern, M., … Hintz, J. (1993). Effect of aging and bolus variables on pharyngeal and upper esophageal sphincter motor function. American Journal of Physiology, 264, G427–G432.

Shames, G. H. (1979). Relapse in stuttering. Paper presented at Banff International Conference on Maintenance of Fluency, Banff, Canada.

Shames, G. H. (1989). Stuttering: An RFP for a cultural perspective. Journal of Fluency Disorders, 14, 67–77.

Shames, G. H. (2000). Counseling the communicatively disabled and their families. Boston, MA: Allyn & Bacon.

Shane, H. C., & Bashir, A. S. (1980). Election criteria for the adoption of an augmentative communication system: Preliminary considerations. Journal of Speech and Hearing Disorders, 45, 408–414.

Shapiro, D. (1999). Stuttering intervention. Austin: Pro-Ed.

Shaw, D. W., Cook, I. J., Gabb, M., Holloway, R. H., Simula, M. E., Panagopoulous, V., & Dent, J. (1995). Influence of normal aging on oral-pharyngeal and upper esophageal sphincter function during swallowing. American Journal of Physiology, 268(31), G389–G396.

Sheahan, P., Miller, I., Earley, M. J., Sheahan, J. N., & Blayney, A. W. (2004). Middle ear disease in children with congenital velopharyngeal insufficiency. Cleft Palate–Craniofacial Journal, 41(4), 364–367.

Sheehan, J. G. (1953). Theory and treatment of stuttering as an approach–avoidance conflict. *Journal of Psychology, 36,* 27–49.

Sheng, L., McGregor, K. K., & Mariam, V. (2006). Lexical-semantic organization in bilingual children: Evidence from a repeated work task. *Journal of Speech, Language, and Hearing Research, 49,* 572–587.

Sherzer, J. (1983). *Kuna ways of speaking: An ethnographic perspective.* Austin, TX: University of Texas Press.

Shine, R. (1980). *Systematic fluency training for young children.* Tigard, OR: C. C. Publications.

Shipley, K. G., & McAfee, J. G. (1998). *Assessment in speech-language pathology: A resource manual* (2nd ed.). San Diego, CA: Singular Publishing group.

Shonkoff, J. P., Phillips, D. A., & Keilty, B. (Eds.). (2000). *Early childhood intervention: Views from the field.* Washington, DC: National Academy Press.

Shprintzen, R. J. (1979). Hypernasal speech in the absence of overt or submucous cleft palate: The mystery solved. In R. Ellis & R. Flack (Eds.), *Diagnosis and treatment of palatoglossal malfunction* (pp. 37–54). London, England: College of Speech Therapists.

Shprintzen, R. J. (1982). Palatal and pharyngeal anomalies in craniofacial syndromes. *Birth Defects, 18*(1), 53–78.

Shprintzen, R. J. (1989). Nasopharyngoscopy. In K. R. Bzoch (Ed.), *Communicative disorders related to cleft lip and palate* (3rd ed.). Boston, MA: College-Hill Press.

Shprintzen, R. J. (1997). *Genetics, syndromes, and communication disorders.* San Diego, CA: Singular Publishing Group.

Shprintzen, R. J. (2000a). *Syndrome identification for speech-language pathology: Illustrated pocketguide.* San Diego, CA: Singular Publishing group.

Shprintzen, R. J. (2000b). Velocardiofacial syndrome. *Otolaryngology Clinics of North America, 33,* 1217–1240.

Shprintzen, R. J. (2001). Velo-cardio-facial syndrome. In S. B. Cassidy & J. Allanson (Eds.), *Management of genetic syndromes* (pp. 495–517). Hoboken, NJ: Wiley.

Shprintzen, R. J. (2003). The origin of speech ease: Evolution of the human upper airway and its functional implications for obstructive sleep apnea. *Sleep Medicine, 4,* 171–173.

Shprintzen, R. J., Croft, C. B., Berkman, M. D., & Rakoff, S. J. (1980). Velopharyngeal insufficiency in the facio-auriculo-vertebral malformation complex. *Cleft Palate Journal, 17*(2), 132–137.

Shprintzen, R. J., Goldberg, R. B., Lewin M. L., Sidoti, E. J., Berkman, M. D., Argamaso, R. V., & Young, D. (1978). A new syndrome involving cleft palate, cardiac anomalies, typical facies, and learning disabilities: Velo-cardio-facial syndrome. *Cleft Palate Journal, 15*(1), 56–62.

Shprintzen, R. J., Lewin, M. L., Croft, C. B., Daniller, A. I., Argamaso, R. V., Ship, A. G., & Strauch, B. (1979). A comprehensive study of pharyngeal flap surgery: Tailor-made flaps. *Cleft Palate Journal, 16*(1), 46–55.

Shprintzen, R. J., Schwartz, R. H., Daniller, A., & Hoch, L. (1985). Morphological significance of bifid uvula. *Pediatrics 75,* 553–561.

Shprintzen, R. J., Sher, A. E., & Croft, C. B. (1987). Hypernasal speech caused by hypertrophic tonsils. *International Journal of Pediatric Otorhinolaryngology, 14,* 45–56.

Shprintzen, R. J., Siegel-Sadewitz, V. L., Amato, J., & Goldberg, R. B. (1985). Retrospective diagnoses of previously missed syndromic disorders amongst 1,000 patients with cleft lip, cleft palate, or both. *Birth Defects, 21*(2), 85–92.

Shriberg, L. D. (1975). A response evocation program for /ʒ/. *Journal of Speech and Hearing Disorders, 40*(1), 92–105.

Shriberg, L. D. (1986). *PEPPER: Programs to examine phonetic and phonologic evaluation records.* Madison, WI: Software Development and Distribution Center, University of Wisconsin.

Shriberg, L. D. (1991). Directions for research in developmental phonological disorders. In J. Miller (Ed.), *Research on child language disorders* (pp. 267–276). Austin, TX: Pro-Ed.

Shriberg, L. D., Aram, D., & Kwiatkowski, J. (1997a). Developmental apraxia of speech: I. Descriptive and theoretical perspectives. *Journal of Speech, Language, and Hearing Research, 40,* 273–285.

Shriberg, L. D., Aram, D. M., & Kwiatkowski, J. (1997b). Developmental apraxia of speech: II. Toward a diagnostic marker. *Journal of Speech, Language, and Hearing Research, 40,* 286–312.

Shriberg, L. D., Aram, D. M., & Kwiatkowski, J. (1997c). Developmental apraxia of speech: III. A subtype marked by inappropriate stress. *Journal of Speech, Language, and Hearing Research, 40,* 313–337.

Shriberg, L. D., & Austin, D. (1998). Comorbidity of speech-language disorder: Implications for a phenotype marker for speech delay. In R. Paul (Ed.), *The speech-language connection* (pp. 73–117). Baltimore, MD: Paul H. Brookes.

Shriberg, L. D., Friel-Patti, S., Flipsen, P., Jr., & Brown, R. L. (2000). Otitis media, fluctuant hearing loss, and speech-language outcomes: A preliminary structural equation model. *Journal of Speech, Language, and Hearing Research, 43,* 100–120.

Shriberg, L. D., & Kwiatkowski, J. (1980). *Natural Process Analysis: A procedure for phonological analysis of continuous speech samples.* New York, NY: Macmillan.

Shriberg, L. D., Kwiatkowski, J., Best, S., Hengst, J., & Terselic-Weber, B. (1986). Characteristics of children with phonologic disorders of unknown origin. *Journal of Speech and Hearing Disorders, 51,* 140–161.

Shriberg, L. D., Paul, R., McSweeny, J. L., Klin, A., & Cohen, D. J. (2001). Speech and prosody characteristics of adolescents and adults with high-functioning autism and asperger syndrome. *Journal of Speech, Language, and Hearing Research, 44,* 1097–1115.

Shriberg, L. D., Tomblin, J. B., & McSweeney, J. L. (1999). Prevalence of speech delay in 6-year-old children and comorbidity with language impairment. *Journal of Speech, Language, and Hearing Research, 42,* 1461–1481.

Shriberg, L., & Widder, C. (1990). Speech and prosody characteristics of adults with mental retardation. *Journal of Speech, Language, and Hearing Research, 35,* 627–653.

Siedlecki, T., & Bonvillian, J. D. (1998). Homonymy in the lexicons of young children acquiring American Sign Language. *Journal of Psycholinguistic Research, 27,* 47–65.

Siegel-Sadewitz, V. L., & Shprintzen, R. J. (1982). Nasopharyngoscopy of the normal velopharyngeal sphincter: An experiment of biofeedback. *Cleft Palate Journal, 19,* 194–201.

Siegel-Sadewitz, V. L., & Shprintzen, R. J. (1986). Changes in velopharyngeal valving with age. *International Journal of Pediatric Otorhinolaryngology, 11,* 171–182.

Sigafoos, J. (1999). Creating opportunities for augmentative and alternative communication: Strategies for involving people with development disabilities. *AAC, 15,* 183–190.

Sigafoos, J., Drasgow, E., & Schlosser, R. W. (2003). Strategies for beginning communicators. In R. W. Schlosser (Ed.), *The efficacy of augmentative and alternative communication: Toward evidence-based practice* (pp. 324–346). San Diego, CA: Academic Press.

Silliman, E. R. (1989). Narratives: A window on the oral substrate of written language disabilities. *Annals of Dyslexia, 39,* 125–139.

Silliman, E. R., & Wilkinson, L. C. (1991). *Communicating for learning: Classroom observation and collaboration.* Gaithersburg, MD: Aspen.

Silliman, E. R., & Wilkinson, L. C. (1994). Discourse scaffolds for classroom intervention. In G. P. Wallach & K. G. Butler (Eds.), *Language learning disabilities in school-age children and adolescents* (pp. 27–52). Boston, MA: Allyn & Bacon.

Silverman, F. L. (2004). Stuttering and other fluency disorders. Long Grove, IL: Waveland Press.

Simon, C. S. (1998). When big kids don't learn: Contextual modifications and intervention strategies for age 8–18 at-risk students. *Clinical Linguistics and Phonetics, 12,* 249–280.

Simon, C. S., & Myrold-Gunyuz, P. (1990). *Into the classroom: The speech-language pathologist in the collaborative role.* Tucson, AZ: Communication Skill Builders.

Singer, B., & Bashir, A. S. (1999, July). What are executive functions and self-regulation and what do they have to do with language-learning disorders? *Language, Speech, and Hearing Services in Schools, 30,* 265–373.

Singer, M. I., & Blom, E. D. (1980). An endoscopic technique for restoration of voice after laryngectomy. *Annals of Otology, Rhinology and Laryngology, 89*(6), 529–533.

Singh, R., Cohen, S. N., & Krupp, R. (1996). Racial differences in cerebrovascular disease. *Neurology, 46* (Suppl. 2), A440–A441.

Sininger, Y. S. (2002). Otoacoustic emissions in the diagnosis of hearing disorder in infants. *The Hearing Journal, 55*(11), 22–26.

Skelly, M. (1979). *Amer-Ind gestural code based on universal American Indian hand talk.* New York, NY: Elsevier.

SKI-HI Institute. (n.d.). *SKI-HI Institute.* Retrieved February 22, 2004, from www.skihi.org

Skolnick, M. L. (1969). Video velopharyngography in patients with nasal speech, with emphasis on lateral pharyngeal motion in velopharyngeal closure. *Radiology, 93,* 747–755.

Skolnick, M. L. (1970). Videofluoroscopic examination of the velopharyngeal portal during phonation in lateral and base projections—A new technique for studying the mechanics. *Cleft Palate Journal, 7,* 803–816.

Skolnick, M. L., & Cohn, E. R. (1989). *Videofluoroscopic studies of speech in patients with cleft palate.* New York, NY: Springer-Verlag.

Skolnick, M. L., McCall, G. N., & Barnes, M. (1973). The sphincteric mechanism of velopharyngeal closure. *Cleft Palate Journal, 10,* 286–305.

Smit, A. B. (1986). Ages of speech sound acquisition: Comparisons and critiques of several normative studies. *Language, Speech, and Hearing Services in Schools, 17,* 175–186.

Smit, A. B., Hand, L., Freilinger, J., & Bernthal, J. (1990). The Iowa Articulation Norms Project and its Nebraska replication. *Journal of Speech, Language, and Hearing Research, 55,* 779–798.

Smith, L., & von Tetzchener, S. (1986). Communicative, sensorimotor and language skills of young children with Down syndrome. *American Journal of Mental Deficiency, 91,* 57–66.

Smith, M. M. (1992). Reading abilities of non-speaking students: Two case studies. *Augmentative and Alternative Communication, 8,* 57–66.

Smith, M. M., & Blischak, D. M. (1997). Literacy. In L. L. Lloyd, D. R. Fuller, & H. H. Arvidson (Eds.), *Augmentative and alternative communication: A handbook of principles and practices.* Boston, MA: Allyn & Bacon.

Smith, V., Mirenda, P., & Zaidman-Zait, A. (2007). Predictors of expressive vocabulary growth in children with autism. *Journal of Speech, Language, and Hearing Research, 50,* 149–160.

Smitheran, J., & Hixon, T. J. (1981). A clinical method for estimating laryngeal airway resistance during vowel production. *Journal of Speech and Hearing Disorders, 46,* 138–146.

Smitherman, G., & Van Dijk, T. (1988). *Discourse and discrimination.* Detroit, MI: Wayne State University Press.

Smyth, R., Jacobs, G., & Rogers, H. (2003). Male voices and perceived sexual orientation: An experimental and theoretical approach. *Language in Society, 32,* 329–350.

Snidecor, J. C. (1962). *Speech rehabilitation of the laryngectomized.* Springfield, IL: Charles C. Thomas.

Snidecor, J. C. (1971). Speech without a larynx. In L. E. Travis (Ed.), *Handbook of speech pathology and audiology.* East Norwalk, CT: Appleton-Century-Crofts.

Snow, C. (1986). Conversations with children. In P. Fletcher & M. Garman (Eds.), *Language acquisition* (2nd ed.). New York, NY: Cambridge University Press.

Snow, C., Burns, S., & Griffin, P. (Eds.). (1998). *Preventing reading difficulties in young children.* Washington, DC: National Academy Press.

Snow, C. E. (1991). The theoretical basis for the relationships between language and literacy in development. *Journal of Research in Child Education, 6,* 5–10.

Snow, K. (1961). Articulation proficiency in relation to certain dental abnormalities. *Journal of Speech and Hearing Disorders, 26,* 209–212.

Snowling, M., Bishop, D. V. M., & Stothard, S. E. (2000). Is preschool language impairment a risk factor for dyslexia in adolescence? *Journal of Child Psychiatry and Psychology, 41,* 5, 587-600.

Sonies, B. C. (1991a). Instrumental procedures for dysphagia and diagnosis. In B. C. Sonies (Ed.), *Seminars in speech and language: Swallowing disorders* (pp. 185–199). New York, NY: Thieme.

Sonies, B. C. (1991b). The aging oropharyngeal system. In D. N. Ripich (Ed.), *Handbook of geriatric communication disorders* (pp. 187–203). Austin, TX: Pro-Ed.

Sonies, B. C. (1992a). Oropharyngeal dysphagia in the elderly. In B. J. Baum (Ed.), *Clinics in geriatric medicine* (pp. 569–579). Philadelphia, PA: W. B. Saunders.

Sonies, B. C. (1992b). Swallowing and speech disturbances. In I. Litvan & Y. Agid (Eds.), *Progressive supranuclear palsy: Clinical and research approaches* (pp. 240–253). New York, NY: Oxford University Press.

Sonies, B. C. (1994). Dysphagia: A model for differential diagnosis for adults and children. In L. R. Cherney (Ed.), *Clinical management of dysphagia in adults and children* (pp. 133–152). Gaithersburg, MD: Aspen.

Sonies, B. C. (1995). Long-term effects of post-polio on oral-motor and swallowing function. In L. S. Halstead & G. Grimby (Eds.), *Post-polio syndrome* (pp. 125–140). Philadelphia, PA: Hanley & Belfus.

Sonies, B. C. (1997). *Dysphagia: A continuum of care.* Gaithersburg, MD: Aspen.

Sonies, B. C., & Dalakas, M. C. (1991). Dysphagia in patients with the post-polio syndrome. *New England Journal of Medicine, 324,* 1162–1167.

Sonies, B. C., & Dalakas, M. C. (1995). Progression of oral-motor and swallowing symptoms in the post-polio syndrome. *Annals of the New York Academy of Sciences, 753,* 87–95.

Sonies, B. C., Fishman, G. C., & Miller, J. L. (2003). Ultrasound imaging and swallowing. In B. Jones (Ed.), *Normal and abnormal swallowing* (pp. 83–90). New York, NY: Springer-Verlag.

Sonies, B. C., Parent, L. J., Morrish, K., & Baum, B. J. (1988). Durational aspects of the oral-pharyngeal phase of swallow in normal adults. *Dysphagia, 3,* 1–10.

Sonies, B. C., Stone, M., & Shawker, T. (1984). Speech and swallowing in the elderly. *Gerontology, 3*(2), 115–124.

Soto, B., Huer, M. B., & Taylor, O. (1997). Multicultural issues in augmentative and alternative communication. In L. L. Lloyd, D. R. Fuller, & H. H. Arvidson (Eds.), *Augmentative and alternative communication: A handbook of principles and practices.* Boston, MA: Allyn & Bacon.

Sparks, R., Helm, N., & Albert, M. (1974). Aphasia rehabilitation resulting from melodic intonation therapy. *Cortex, 10,* 303–310.

Spector, C. C. (1996). Children's comprehension of idioms in the context of humor. *Language, Speech, and Hearing Services in Schools, 27,* 307–315.

Spracher, M. (2000). Learning about literacy: SLPs play key role in reading, writing. *The American Speech-Language-Hearing Association Leader, 8,* 1–18.

Stanovich, K. (1986). Matthew effects in reading: Some consequences of individual differences in the acquisition of literacy. *Reading Research Quarterly, 21,* 360–406.

Stein, C. M., Schick, J. H., Taylor, H. G., Shriberg, L. D., Millard, C., Kundtz-Kluge, A., … Iyengar, S. K. (2004). Pleiotropic effects of a chromosome 3 locus on speech-sound disorder and reading. *American Journal of Human Genetics, 74*(2), 283–297.

Stein, N. L., & Glenn, C. G. (1979). An analysis of story comprehension in elementary school children. In R. O. Freedle (Ed.), *New directions in discourse processing* (pp. 53–120). Norwood, NJ: Ablex.

Stemberger, J. (1988). Between word processes in child phonology. *Journal of Child Language, 15,* 39–61.

Stemple, J. C. (1984). *Clinical voice pathology.* New York, NY: Merrill/Macmillan.

Stemple, J. C., Lee, L., D'Amico, B., & Pickup, B. (1994). Efficacy of vocal function exercise as a method of improving voice production. *Journal of Voice, 8*(3), 271–278.

Stevens, C., Sanders, L., & Neville, H. (2006). Neurophysiological evidence for selective auditory attention deficits in children with specific language impairment. *Brain Research, 1111,* 143–152.

Stevens, J. C., & Cain, W. S. (1986). Smelling via the mouth: Effect of aging. *Perception and Psychophysics, 40*(3), 142–146.

Stewart, J. E. (1983). Communication disorders in American Indian populations. In D. R. Omark & J. G. Erickson (Eds.), *The bilingual exceptional child.* San Diego, CA: College-Hill Press.

Stoel-Gammon, C. (1989). Prespeech development of two late talkers. *First Language, 9,* 207–224.

Stoel-Gammon, C. (2001). Down syndrome phonology: Developmental patterns and intervention strategies. *Down Syndrome Research to Practice, 7,* 93–100.

Stoel-Gammon, C., & Dunn, C. (1985). *Normal and disordered phonology in children.* Baltimore, MD: University Park Press.

Storey, K., Ezell, H., & Lengyel, L. (1995). Communication strategies for increasing the integration of persons in supported employment: A review. *American Journal of Speech-Language Pathology, 4,* 45–54.

Storkel, H. L. (2001). Learning new words: Phonetactic probability in language development. *Journal of Speech, Language, and Hearing Research, 44,* 1321–1337.

Storkel, H. L. (2002). Restructuring of similarity neighbourhoods in the developing mental lexicon. *Journal of Child Language, 29,* 251–274.

Storkel, H. L., & Morrisette, M. L. (2002). The lexicon and phonology: Interactions in language acquisition. *Language, Speech, and Hearing Services in Schools, 33,* 24–37.

Strain, P., McGee, G., & Kohler, F. (2001). Inclusion of children with autism in early intervention environments. In M. Guralnick (Ed.), *Early childhood inclusion: Focus on change* (pp. 337–363). Baltimore, MD: Paul H. Brookes.

Strand, E. A., Miller, R. M., Yorkston, K. M., & Hillel, A. D. (1996). Management of oral pharyngeal dysphagia symptoms in amyotrophic lateral sclerosis. *Dysphgaia, 11*(2), 129–139.

Strauss, R. P. (1995). Evolving across disciplines. *Cleft Palate–Craniofacial Journal, 32,* 268.

Streissguth, A. (1997). *Fetal alcohol syndrome: A guide for families and communities.* Baltimore, MD: Paul H. Brookes.

Striano, T., Rochat, P., & Legerstee, M. (2003). The role of modeling and request type on symbolic comprehension of objects and gestures in young children. *Journal of Child Language, 30,* 27–45.

Strunk, T. L., & Fullwood, H. L. (2000). The impact of early intervention on children with Down syndrome, birth to three years of age. *Catalyst for Change, 30,* 14–16.

Stuchell, R. N., & Mandel, I. D. (1988). Salivary gland dysfunction and swallowing disorders. *Otolaryngologic Clinics of North America, 21*(4), 649–661.

Sturm, J. M., & Clendon, S. A. (2004). Augmentative and alternative communication, language, and literacy: Fostering the relationship. *Topics in Language Disorders, 24,* 76–91.

Sulzby, E., & Teale, W. (1991). Emergent literacy. In R. Barr, M. Kamil, P. B. Mosenthal, & P. D. Pearson (Eds.), *Handbook of reading research* (pp. 727–757). New York, NY: Longman.

Sutherland-Cornett, B. S., & Chabon, S. S. (1988). *The clinical practice of speech-language pathology.* Columbus, OH: Merrill.

Sutton-Smith, B. (1986). The development of fictional narrative performances. *Topics in Language Disorders, 7*(1), 1–10.

Suzuki, M., Asada, Y., Ito, J., Hayashi, K., Inoue, H., & Kitano, H. (2003). Actviation of cerebellum and basal ganglia on volitional swallowing detected by functional magnetic resonance imaging. *Dysphagia, 18,* 71–77.

Sweetow, R. (1999). *Counseling for hearing aid fittings.* San Diego, CA: Singular Publishing Group.

Talbot, R. E. (2002). Listening to the ear "talk": The message of OAEs. *The Hearing Journal, 55*(3), 10–19.

Talkington, L. W., Hall, S., & Altman, R. (1971). Communication deficits and aggression in the mentally retarded. *American Journal of Mental Deficiency, 76,* 235–237.

Tallal, P., Hirsch, L. S., Realpe-Bonilla, T., Miller, S., Brzustowicz, L. M., Bartlett, C., & Flax, J. F. (2001). Familial aggregation in specific language impairment. *Journal of Speech, Language, and Hearing Research, 44,* 1172–1182.

Tannen, D. (1981). Implications of the oral/literate continuum for cross-cultural communication. In J. Alatis (Ed.), *Current issues in bilingualism: Georgetown University roundtable on languages and linguistics, 1980.* Washington, DC: Georgetown University Press.

Tannen, D. (1982). Oral and literate strategies in spoken and written narratives. *Language, 58,* 1–21.

Tannock, R., & Girolametto, L. (1992). Reassessing parent-focused language intervention programs. In S. R. Warren & J. Reichle (Eds.), *Communication and Language Intervention Series: Vol. 1. Causes and effects in communication and language intervention* (pp. 49–80). Baltimore, MD: Paul H. Brookes.

Taylor, O. L. (1986a). *Treatment of communication disorders in culturally and linguistically diverse populations.* San Diego, CA: College-Hill Press.

Taylor, O. L. (Ed.). (1986b). *Nature of communication disorders in culturally and linguistically diverse populations.* San Diego, CA: College-Hill Press.

Taylor, O. L., & Leonard, L. B. (1999). *Language acquisition across North America: Cross-cultural and cross-linguistic perspectives.* San Diego, CA: Singular Publishing Group.

Teasell, R., Foley, N., Fisher, J., & Finestone, H. (2002). The incidence management and complications of patients with medullary strokes admitted to a rehabilitation unit. *Dysphagia, 17,* 115–120.

Templin, M. (1957). *Certain language skills in children.* Minneapolis, MN: University of Minnesota.

Templin, M. C., & Darley, F. L. (1969). *The Templin-Darley tests of articulation* (2nd ed.). Iowa City, IA: University of Iowa, Bureau of Educational Research and Service, Division of Extension and University Services.

Thal, D. J., & Flores, M. (2001). Development of sentence interpretation strategies by typically developing and late-talking toddlers. *Journal of Child Language, 28,* 173–193.

Thal, D., & Katich, J. (1996). Predicaments in early identification of specific language impairment: Does the early bird always catch the worm? In K. Cole, P. Dale, & D. Thal (Eds.), *Assessment of communication and language* (pp. 1–28). Baltimore, MD: Paul H. Brookes.

Thal, D., & Tobias, S. (1992). Communicative gestures in children with delayed onset of oral expressive vocabulary. *Journal of Speech and Hearing Research, 37,* 157–170.

Thompson, C., Shapiro, L., Kiran, S., & Sobecks, J. (2003). The role of syntactic complexity in treatment of sentence deficits in agrammatic aphasia: The complexity account of treatment efficacy (CATE). *Journal of Speech, Language, and Hearing Research, 46,* 591–607.

Thompson-Ward, E. C., & Murdoch, B. E. (1998). Instrumental assessment of the speed mechanism. In B. E. Murdoch (Ed.), *Dysarthria: A physiological approaches to assessment and treatment.* Cheltenham, England: Stanley-Thornes.

Thornton, J. (2008). Working with transgender voice: The role of the speech and language therapist. *Sexologies, 17*(4), 271–276.

Thresher, A. R., & Popovic, M. R. (2004, June). Electrical stimulation and neuroprosthesis for restoring swallowing function. *Perspectives on Swallowing and Swallowing Disorders, ASHA Division 13,* Newsletter, *13*(2), 28–31.

Thurlow, M. L., Elliott, J. L., & Ysseldyke, J. E. (1998). *Testing students with disabilities: Practical strategies for complying with district and state requirements.* Thousand Oaks, CA: Corwin Press.

Tiegerman-Farber, E., & Radziewicz, C. (2008). *Language disorders in children: Real families, real issues, and real interventions.* Upper Saddle River, NJ: Pearson.

Timler, G. (2008a, November 4). Social communication: A framework for assessment and intervention. *The ASLHA Leader*, pp. 10–13.

Timler, G. (2008b). Social knowledge in children with language impairments: Examination of strategies, predicted consequences, and goals in peer conflict situations. *Clinical Linguistics and Phonetics, 22*, 741–763.

Timler, G. R., Olswang, L. B., & Coggins, T. E. (2005). "Do I know what I need to do?" A social communication intervention for children with complex clinical profiles. *Language, Speech, and Hearing Services in Schools, 36*, 73–85.

Tomasello, M., & Slobin, D. I. (Eds.) (2005). *Beyond nature–nurture: Essays in honor of Elizabeth Bates.* Mahwah, NJ: Lawrence Erlbaum.

Tomblin, J. B., Records, N., Buckwalter, P., Zhang, X., Smith, E., & O'Brien, M. (1997). Prevalence of specific language impairment in kindergarten children. *Journal of Speech, Language, and Hearing Research, 40*, 1245–1260.

Tompkins, C. A. (1994). *Right hemisphere communication disorders.* San Diego, CA: Singular Publishing Group.

Torgesen, J. K., & Davis, C. (1996). Individual difference variables that predict response to training in phonological awareness. *Journal of Experimental Child Psychology, 63*, 1–21.

Torgesen, J. K., Wagner, R. K., & Rashotte, C. A. (1994). Longitudinal studies of phonological processing and reading. *Journal of Learning Disabilities, 27*, 276–286.

Tough, J. (1977). *The development of meaning.* New York, NY: Halsted Press.

Towbin, K. E., Mauk, J. E., & Batshaw, M. L. (2002). Pervasive developmental disorders. In M. L. Batshaw (Ed.), *Children with disabilities* (5th ed., pp. 365–387), Baltimore, MD: Paul H. Brookes.

Travis, L. E. (1957). The unspeakable feeling of people with special reference to stuttering. In L. E. Travis (Ed.), *Handbook of speech pathology.* East Norwalk, CT: Appleton-Century-Crofts.

Turkstra, L., Ciccia, A., & Seaton, C. (2003). Interactive behaviors in adolescent conversation dyads. *Language, Speech, and Hearing Services in Schools, 34*, 117–127.

Tye-Murray, N. (1998). *Foundations of aural rehabilitation: Children, adults and their family members.* San Diego, CA: Singular Publishing Group.

Tyler, A., Edwards, M. L., & Saxman, J. (1987). Clinical application of two phonologically based treatment procedures. *Journal of Speech and Hearing Disorders, 52*, 393–409.

Ukrainetz, T. A. (2006a). Assessment and intervention within a contextualized skill framework. In T. A. Ukrainetz (Ed.), *Contextualized language intervention: Scaffolding preK–12 literacy achievement.* Eau Claire, WI: Thinking Publications.

Ukrainetz, T. A. (Ed.), (2006b). *Contextualized language intervention: Scaffolding preK–12 literacy achievement.* Eau Claire, WI: Thinking Publications.

U. S. Department of Energy (DOE). (2003). *Genomics and its impact on science and society: The Human Genome Project and beyond, 1-12.* www.ornl.gov/hgmis/publicat/primer

U. S. Department of Education, National Assessment of Educational Progress, (2002). *The nation's report card: Fourth grade reading.* Accessed from www.nces.ed.gov/nationsreportcard

U. S. Department of Education, National Center for Education Statistics, (2002). *National assessment of educational progress.* Accessed from www.nces.ed.gov

U. S. Department of Education, National Center for Education Statistics. (2003). *The nation's report card: Reading 2002* (NCES 2003-521). Retrieved from nces.ed.gov

U. S. Department of Education, National Center for Education Statistics. (2008). The condition of education 2008 in brief. Accessed from nces.ed.gov/pubsearch/pubsinfo.asp?pubid=2008032

Uziel, A., Mondain, M., Hagen, P., Dejean, F., & Doucet, G. (2003). Rehabilitation for high-frequency sensorineural hearing impairment in adults with the symphonix vibrant soundbridge: A comparative study. *Otology and Neurology, 24*, 775–783.

Vaiman, M., Eviatar, E., & Segal, S. (2004). Evaluation of normal deglutition with the help of rectified surface electromyography records. *Dysphagia, 19*, 125–132.

Valdez, F. M., & Montgomery, J. K. (1997). Outcomes from two treatment approaches for children with communication disorders in Head Start. *Journal of Children's Communication Development, 18*, 65–71.

Valente, M., & Mispagel, K. M. (2008). Unaided and aided performance with a directional open-fit hearing aid. *International Journal of Audiology, 47*, 329–336.

Valian, V., & Aubry, S. (2005). When opportunity knocks twice: Two-year-olds' repetition of sentence subjects. *Journal of Child Language, 32*, 617–641.

Van Bergeijk, W. A., Pierce, J. R., & David, E. E. (1960). *Waves and the ear.* New York, NY: Doubleday.

van der Wal, K. G., & van der Meulen, B. D. (2001). Eruption of canines through alveolar bone grafts in cleft lip and palate. *Nederlands Tijdschrift voor Tandheelkunde, 108*(10), 401–403.

van Kleeck, A. (1994a). Metalinguistic development. In G. Wallach & K. Butler (Eds.), *Language learning disabilities in school-age children and adolescents.* New York, NY: Macmillan.

van Kleeck, A. (1994b). Potential cultural bias in training parents as conversational partners with their children who have delays in language development. *American Journal of Speech-Language Pathology, 3*, 67–78.

van Kleeck, A., & Bryant, D. (1983, October). *A diary study of very early emerging metalinguistic skills.* Paper presented at the Eighth Annual Boston University Conference on Language Development, Boston, MA.

van Kleeck, A., & Schuele, C. M. (1987). Precursors to literacy: Normal development. *Topics in Language Disorders, 7*(2), 13–31.

van Kleeck, A., & VanderWoude, J. (2003). Book sharing with preschool children with language delays. In A. van Kleeck, S. A. Stahl, & E. B. Bauer (Eds.), *On reading books to children: Parents and teachers.* Mahwah, NJ: Lawrence Erlbaum.

Van Meter, A. M., & Nelson, N. (1998). *Language learning possibilities in narrative and expository discourse.* American Speech-Language-Hearing Association Convention, San Antonio, TX.

Van Riper, C. (1973). *The treatment of stuttering.* Englewood Cliffs, NJ: Prentice-Hall.

Van Riper, C. (1978). *Speech correction: Principles and methods* (6th ed.). Englewood Cliffs, NJ: Prentice-Hall.

Van Riper, C. (1982). *The nature of stuttering.* Englewood Cliffs, NJ: Prentice-Hall.

Van Riper, C. (1990). Final thoughts about stuttering. *Journal of Fluency Disorders, 15,* 317–318.

Van Riper, C., & Emerick, L. (1984). *Speech correction: An introduction to speech pathology and audiology.* Englewood Cliffs, NJ: Prentice-Hall.

Vanderheiden, G. C., & Lloyd, L. L. (1986). Nonspeech modes and systems. In S. W. Blackstone (Ed.), *Augmentative communication* (pp. 49–161). Rockville, MD: American Speech-Language-Hearing Association.

Vaughn, B., & Horner, R. H. (1995). Effects of concrete versus verbal choice systems on problem behavior. *AAC, 11,* 89–100.

Vellutino, F. R., & Scanlon, D. M. (1987). Phonological coding, phonological awareness and reading ability: Evidence from longitudinal and experimental studies. *Merrill-Palmer Quarterly, 33,* 99–133.

Vento, A. R., La Brie, R. A., & Mulliken, J. B. (1991). The O. M. E. N. S. classification of hemifacial microsomia. *Cleft Palate–Craniofacial Journal, 28,* 68.

Ventry, I., & Weinstein, B. (1982). The hearing handicap inventory for the elderly: A new tool. *Ear and Hearing, 3,* 128–134.

Verdolini Abbott, K. (2000). Case study: Resonant voice therapy. In J. Stemple (Ed.), *Voice therapy: Clinical studies* (*2nd ed.*, pp. 46–62). San Diego, CA: Singular Publishing Group.

Vitevitch, M. S. (2002). The influence of phonological similarity neighborhoods on speech production. *Learning, Memory, and Cognition, 28,* 735–747.

Vitevitch, M. S., & Luce, P. A. (1999). Probabilistic phonotactics and neighborhood activism in spoken word recognition. *Journal of Memory and Language, 40,* 374–408.

Vitevitch, M. S., Luce, P. A., & Pisoni, D. B. (1999). Phonotactics, neighborhood activation and lexical access for spoken words. *Brain and Language, 68,* 306–311.

Vygotsky, L. S. (1986). *Thought and language.* Cambridge, MA: MIT Press.

Wagner, R. K., & Torgesen, J. K. (1987). The nature of phonological processing and its causal role in the acquisition of reading skills. *Psychological Bulletin, 101,* 192–212.

Wagner, R. K., Torgesen, J. K., & Rashotte, C. A. (1994). Development of reading-related phonological processing abilities: New evidence of bi-directional causality from a latent variable longitudinal study. *Developmental Psychology, 30,* 73–87.

Wakefield, J., & Wilcox, M. (1995). Brain maturation and language acquisition: A theoretical model and preliminary investigation. In D. McLaughlin & S. McEwen (Eds.), *Proceeding of the 19th annual Boston University Conference on Language Development* (Vol. 2, pp. 643–654). Somerville, MA: Cascadilla Press.

Walden, B., Demorest, M., & Hepler, E. (1984). Self-report approach to assessing benefit from amplification. *Journal of Speech and Hearing Research, 27,* 49–56.

Walker, D., Greenwood, C., Hart, B., & Carta, J. (1994). Prediction of school outcomes based in early production and socioeconomic factors. *Child Development, 65,* 606–621.

Wall, B., & Barnett, S. (1998). Toward a sociolinguistic perspective on augmentative and alternative communication. *AAC, 14,* 200–211.

Wallach, G. P., & Butler, K. G. (Eds.). (1994). *Language learning disabilities in school-age children and adolescents.* Boston, MA: Allyn & Bacon.

Wallach, G. P., & Ehren, B. (1997, November). *Moving the literacy agenda in schools.* Short course presented at the Annual Convention of American Speech-Language-Hearing Association, Boston, MA.

Wallach, G. P., & Miller, L. (1988). *Language intervention and academic success.* Boston, MA: College-Hill Press.

Walley, A. (1993). The role of vocabulary development in children's spoken word recognition and segmentation ability. *Developmental Review, 13,* 286–350.

Wang, W. L., Bernas, R., & Eberhard, P. (2001). Effects of teachers' verbal and non-verbal scaffolding on everyday classroom performances of students with Down syndrome. *International Journal of Early Years Education, 9,* 71–80.

Wasson, C. A., Arvidson, H. H., & Lloyd, L. L. (1997). Augmentative and alternative communication assessment process. In L. L. Lloyd, D. R. Fuller, & H. H. Arvidson (Eds.), *Augmentative and alternative communication: A handbook of principles and practices.* Boston, MA: Allyn & Bacon.

Watkins, R., Rice, M., & Moltz, C. (1993). Verb use by language impaired and normally developing children. *First Language, 13,* 133–143.

Watson, A. C., Nixon, C. L., Wilson, A., & Capage, L. (1999). Social interaction skills and theory of mind in young children. *Developmental Psychology, 35,* 386–391.

Waxman, S., & Booth, A. (2003). The origins and evolution of links between word learning and conceptual organization: New evidence from 11-month-olds. *Developmental Science, 6,* 128–135.

Webb, M. W., & Irving, R. W. (1964). Psychologic and anamnestic patterns characteristic of laryngectomies: Relation to speech rehabilitation. *Journal of American Geriatric Society, 12,* 303–322.

Webster, E., & Larkins, P. (1979). *Counseling aphasic families* [Videotape lecture].

Wehren, A., De Lisi, R., & Arnold, M. (1981). The development of noun definition. *Journal of Child Language, 8,* 165–175.

Weiffenbach, J. M. (1984). Taste and smell perception in aging. *Gerodontology, 3*(2), 137–146.

Weiner, F. F. (1981). Treatment of phonological disability using the method of meaningful minimal contrast. *Journal of Speech and Hearing Disorders, 46,* 97–103.

Weiner, F. F., & Bankson, N. (1978). Teaching features. *Language, Speech and Hearing Services in Schools, 9,* 29–34.

Weinstein, B. E. (1996). Treatment efficacy: Hearing aids in the management of hearing loss in adults. *Journal of Speech and Hearing Research, 39,* S37–S45.

Weinstein, B. E. (2004). *Treatment efficacy summary: Hearing loss and hearing aids in adults.* Retrieved July 2004, from www.asha.org/members/slp/healthcare/efficacy.htm

Wells, G. (1985). *Language development in the preschool years.* New York, NY: Cambridge University Press.

Wells, G., Barnes, S., Gutfreund, M., & Sutterly, D. (1983). Characteristics of adult speech which predict children's language development. *Journal of Child Language, 10,* 65–84.

West, R. (1958). An agnostic's speculations about stuttering. In J. Eisenson (Ed.), *Stuttering: A symposium.* New York, NY: Harper & Row.

Westby, C. E. (1986). Cultural differences affecting communication development. In L. Cole & V. Deal (Eds.), *Communication disorders in multicultural populations.* Washington, DC: American Speech-Language-Hearing Association.

Westby, C. E. (1991). Learning to talk—Talking to learn: Oral-literate language differences. In C. Simon (Ed.), *Communication skills and classroom success: Therapy methodologies for language learning disabled students* (pp. 181–218). San Diego, CA: College-Hill Press.

Westby, C. E. (1994). The effects of culture on genre, structure, and type of oral and written texts. In G. P. Wallach & K. G. Butler (Eds.), *Language learning disabilities in school-age children and adolescents* (pp. 180–218). Boston, MA: Allyn & Bacon.

Westby, C. E. (1998, May). Language in critical literacy: Issues in LLD, ADJD, and dyslexia. *Language Learning and Education, ASHA Division 1 Newsletter,* 22–24.

Weston, A., & Irwin, J. (1971). Use of paired-stimuli in modification of articulation. *Perceptual and Motor Skills, 32,* 947–957.

Wetherby, A. (2002). Communication disorders in infants, toddlers, and preschool children. In G. Shames & N. Anderson (Eds.), *Human communication disorders: An introduction* (6th ed., pp. 186–217). Boston, MA: Allyn & Bacon.

Wetherby, A., Prizant, B., & Schuler, A. (2000). Understanding the nature of the communication and language impairments. In A. Wetherby & B. Prizant (Eds.), *Autism spectrum disorders: A transactional developmental perspective* (pp. 109–141). Baltimore, MD: Paul H. Brookes.

Wetherby, A., Reichle, J., & Pierce, P. L. (1998). The transition to symbolic communication. In S. F. Warren & J. Reichle (Series Eds.), A. Wetherby, S. Warren, & J. Reichle (Vol. Eds.), *Communication and Language Intervention Series: Vol. 7. Transitions in prelinguistic communication* (pp. 197–230). Baltimore, MD: Paul H. Brookes.

Wetherby, A., Yonclas, D., & Bryan, A. (1989). Communicative profiles of handicapped preschool children: Implications for early identification. *Journal of Speech and Hearing Disorders, 54,* 148–158.

Whitehurst, G. J. (1996). Language processes in context: Language learning in children reared in poverty. In L. B. Adamson & M. A. Romski (Eds.), *Research on communication and language disorders: Contributions to theories of language development.* Baltimore, MD: Paul H. Brookes.

Whitehurst, G. J., Epstein, J. N., Angell, A. L., Payne, A. C., Crone, D. A., & Fischel, J. E. (1994). Outcomes of an emergent literacy intervention in Head Start. *Journal of Educational Psychology, 86,* 542–555.

Whitehurst, G. J., & Lonigan, C. J. (1998). Child development and emergent literacy. *Child Development, 69,* 848–872.

Whitehurst, G. J., & Lonigan, C. J. (2001). Emergent readers: Development from prereaders to readers. In S. B. Neuman & D. K. Dickinson (Eds.), *Handbook of early literacy research* (pp.11–29). New York, NY: Guilford, Press.

Widerstrom, A. H., & Nickel, R. E. (1997). Determinants of risk in infancy. In A. Widerstrom, B. Mowder, & S. Sandall (Eds.), *Infant development and risk: An introduction* (2nd ed.) Baltimore, MD: Paul H. Brookes.

Wiig, E. (1990). *Wiig criterion referenced inventory of language.* San Antonio, TX: Psychological Corp.

Wiig, E., & Secord, W. (1992). *Measurement and assessment: Making sense of test results.* Buffalo, NY: Educom Associates.

Wiig, E., & Secord, W. (1998). Language disabilities in school-age children. In G. Shames, E. Wiig, & W. Secord (Eds.), *Human communication disorders* (5th ed., pp. 185–226). Boston, MA: Allyn & Bacon.

Wilcox, M., Kouri, T., & Caswell, S. (1991). Early language intervention: A comparison of classroom and individual treatment. *American Journal of Speech-Language Pathology, 1,* 49–62.

Wilcox, M. J., & Shannon, M. S. (1996). Integrated early intervention practices in speech-language pathology. In R. A. McWilliam (Ed.), *Rethinking pull-out services in early intervention: A professional resource* (pp. 217–242). Baltimore, MD: Paul H. Brookes.

Wilcox, M. J., & Shannon, M. S. (1998). Facilitating the transition from prelinguistic to linguistic communication. In S. F. Warren & J. Reichle (Series Eds.), A. Wetherby, S. Warren, & J. Reichle (Vol. Eds.), *Communication and Language Intervention Series: Vol. 7. Transitions in prelinguistic communication* (pp. 385–416). Baltimore, MD: Paul H. Brookes.

Williams, C. A., Zori, R. T., Stone, J. W., Gray, B. A., Cantu, E. S., & Ostrer, H. (1990). Maternal origin of 15q11-13 deletions in Angelman syndrome suggests a role for genomic imprinting. *American Journal of Medical Genetics, 35,* 350–353.

Williams, D. F. (2006). *Stuttering recovery: Personal and empirical perspectives.* Mahwah, NJ: Waveland Press.

Williams, J. P., Lauer, K. D., Hall, K. M., Lord, K. M., Gugga, S. S., Bak, S., ... decani, J. S. (2002) Teaching elementary school students to identify story themes. *Journal of Educational Psychology, 94,* 235–248.

Williams, R., & Wolfram, W. (1977). *Social dialects: Differences vs. disorders.* Washington, DC: American Speech and Hearing Association.

Wilson, S. (2003). Lexically specific constructions in the acquisition of inflection in English. *Journal of Child Language, 30,* 75–115.

Wilson, W. F., Wilson, J. R., & Coleman, T. J. (2000). Culturally appropriate assessment: Issues and strategies. In T. J. Coleman (Ed.), *Clinical management of communication disorders in culturally diverse children* (pp. 101–127). Boston, MA: Allyn & Bacon.

Wingate, M. (1959). Calling attention to stuttering. *Journal of Speech and Hearing Research, 2,* 326–335.

Wingate, M. E. (1964). A standard definition of stuttering. *Journal of Speech and Hearing Disorders, 29,* 484–489.

Wingate, M. (1969). Stuttering as phonetic transition defect. *Journal of Speech and Hearing Disorders, 34,* 107–108.

Winitz, H. (1961). Repetitions in the vocalizations and speech of children in the first two years of life. *Journal of Speech and Hearing Disorders* (Monograph Suppl. 7), 55–62.

Winitz, H. (1969). *Articulation acquisition and disorders.* New York, NY: Appleton-Century-Crofts.

Winitz, H. (1989). Auditory considerations in treatment. In N. Creaghead, P. Newman, & W. Secord (Eds.), *Assessment and remediation of articulatory and phonological disorders* (2nd ed.). Columbus, OH: Merrill.

Wisconsin Department of Public Instruction. (2003). *Linguistically and culturally diverse populations: African American and Hmong.* Madison, WI: Author.

Witt, P. D., O'Daniel, T. G., Marsh, J. L., Grames, L. M., Muntz, H. R., & Pilgram, T. K. (1997). Surgical management of velopharyngeal dysfunction: Outcome analysis of autogenous posterior pharyngeal wall augmentation. *Plastic and Reconstructive Surgery, 99*(5), 1287–1296; discussion 1297–3000.

Wolfram, W., & Fasold, R. W. (1974). *The study of social dialects in American English.* Englewood Cliffs, NJ: Prentice-Hall.

Wood, C., Storr, J., & Reich, P. A. (Eds.). (1992). *Blissymbol reference guide.* Toronto, Canada: Blissymbolics Communication International.

Woods, J. (2008, March 25). Providing early intervention in natural environments. *The ASHA Leader,* pp. 14–17, 23.

Woods, J., & Wetherby, A. (2003). Early identification of and intervention for infants and toddlers who are at risk for autism spectrum disorder. *Language, Speech, and Hearing Services in Schools, 34,* 180–193.

Wyatt, T. (1998). Assessment issues with multicultural populations. In D. E. Battle (Ed.), *Communication disorders in multicultural populations* (pp. 379–426). Boston, MA: Butterworth-Heinemann.

Wynder, E. L., Covey, L. S., Mabuchi, K., & Mushinski, M. (1976). Environmental factors in cancer of the larynx: A second look. *Cancer, 38,* 1591–1601.

Wyszynski, D. F., Beaty, T. H., & Maestri, N. E. (1996). Genetics of nonsyndromic oral clefts revisited. *Cleft Palate–Craniofacial Journal, 33*(5), 407–417.

Yairi, E. (1983). The onset of stuttering in two- and three-year-old children: A preliminary report. *Journal of Speech and Hearing Disorders, 48,* 171–177.

Yairi, E. P. Ambrose, (2005). *Early childhood stuttering.* Austin, TX: ProEd.

Yamashita, R. P., & Trindade, I. E. (2008). Long-term effects of pharyngeal flaps on the upper airways of subjects with velopharyngeal insufficiency. *Cleft Palate–Craniofacial Journal, 45*(4), 364–370.

Yeargin-Allsopp, M., Rice, C., Karapurkar, T., Doernberg, N., Boyle, C., & Murphy, C. (2003). Prevalence of autism in a U.S. metropolitan area. *Journal of the American Medical Association, 289,* 49–55.

Ylvisaker, M., & Feeney, T. (1998). *Collaborative brain injury intervention: Positive everyday routines.* San Diego, CA: Singular Publishing Group.

Yorkston, K. M. (2004). *Treatment efficacy summary: Dysarthria (Neurological motor speech impairment).* Retrieved July 2004, from www.asha.org/members/slp/healthcare/efficacy.htm

Yoshinago-Itano, C. (2003). Early intervention after universal neonatal hearing screening: Impact on outcomes. *Mental Retardation and Developmental Disabilities Research Reviews, 9,* 252–266.

Zajac, D. J., Warren, D. W., & Hinton, V. A. (2009). Aerodynamic assessment of motor speech disorders. In M. R. McNeil (Ed.), *Clinical management of sensorimotor speech disorders* (2nd ed.). New York, NY: Thieme.

Zangari, C., & Kangas, K. A. (1997). Intervention principles and procedures. In L. L. Lloyd, D. R. Fuller, & H. H. Arvidson (Eds.), *Augmentative and alternative communication: A handbook of principles and practices.* Boston, MA: Allyn & Bacon.

Zangari, C., & Wasson, C. A. (1997). Service delivery and funding. In L. L. Lloyd, D. R. Fuller, & H. H. Arvidson (Eds.), *Augmentative and alternative communication: A handbook of principles and practices* (pp. 389–405). Boston, MA: Allyn & Bacon.

Zanzi, M., Cherpillod, J., & Hohlfeld, J. (2002). Phonetic and otological results after early palate closure in 18 consecutive children presenting with cleft lip and palate. *International Journal of Pediatric Otorhinolaryngology, 66*(2), 131–137.

Author Index

Subject Index